Injury Rehabilitation and Sports Medicine

Injury Rehabilitation and Sports Medicine

Editor: Gael Martin

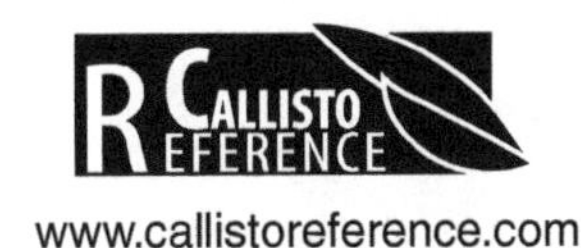

www.callistoreference.com

Callisto Reference,
118-35 Queens Blvd., Suite 400,
Forest Hills, NY 11375, USA

Visit us on the World Wide Web at:
www.callistoreference.com

© Callisto Reference, 2017

This book contains information obtained from authentic and highly regarded sources. Copyright for all individual chapters remain with the respective authors as indicated. All chapters are published with permission under the Creative Commons Attribution License or equivalent. A wide variety of references are listed. Permission and sources are indicated; for detailed attributions, please refer to the permissions page and list of contributors. Reasonable efforts have been made to publish reliable data and information, but the authors, editors and publisher cannot assume any responsibility for the validity of all materials or the consequences of their use.

ISBN: 978-1-63239-879-6 (Hardback)

The publisher's policy is to use permanent paper from mills that operate a sustainable forestry policy. Furthermore, the publisher ensures that the text paper and cover boards used have met acceptable environmental accreditation standards.

Trademark Notice: Registered trademark of products or corporate names are used only for explanation and identification without intent to infringe.

Printed in the United States of America.

Cataloging-in-Publication Data

Injury rehabilitation and sports medicine / edited by Gael Martin.
p. cm.
Includes bibliographical references and index.
ISBN 978-1-63239-879-6
1. Sports medicine. 2. Sports injuries. 3. Medical rehabilitation. 4. Sports--Physiological aspects.
5. Physical fitness. 6. Physical education and training. I. Martin, Gael.

RC1210 .I65 2017
617.102 7--dc23

Table of Contents

Preface .... **IX**

Chapter 1 **Changes in breaststroke swimming performances in national and international athletes competing between 1994 and 2011 -a comparison with freestyle swimming performances** **1**
Mathias Wolfrum, Christoph Alexander Rüst, Thomas Rosemann, Romuald Lepers and Beat Knechtle

Chapter 2 **Cognitive-motor integration deficits in young adult athletes following concussion** **15**
Jeffrey A. Brown, Marc Dalecki, Cindy Hughes, Alison K. Macpherson and Lauren E. Sergio

Chapter 3 **Ultrasonic assessment of exercise-induced change in skeletal muscle glycogen content** **27**
David C Nieman, R Andrew Shanely, Kevin A Zwetsloot, Mary Pat Meaney and Gerald E Farris

Chapter 4 **Transport choice when travelling to a sports facility: the role of perceived route features** **34**

Ellen L de Hollander, Eline Scheepers, Harm J van Wijnen, Pieter JV van Wesemael, Albertine J Schuit, Wanda Wendel-Vos and Elise EMM van Kempen

Chapter 5 **The effect of the stay active advice on physical activity and on the course of acute severe low back pain** **45**
Patricia Olaya-Contreras, Jorma Styf, Daniel Arvidsson, Karin Frennered and Tommy Hansson

Chapter 6 **Can supplementation with vitamin C and E alter physiological adaptations to strength training?** **54**
Gøran Paulsen, Kristoffer T Cumming, Håvard Hamarsland, Elisabet Børsheim, Sveinung Berntsen and Truls Raastad

Chapter 7 **A pilot study on biomarkers for tendinopathy: lower levels of serum TNF-α and other cytokines in females but not males with Achilles tendinopathy** **66**
James E. Gaida , Håkan Alfredson, Sture Forsgren and Jill L. Cook

Chapter 8 **Is a threshold-based model a superior method to the relative percent concept for establishing individual exercise intensity?** **76**
Ali E. Wolpern, Dara J. Burgos, Jeffrey M. Janot and Lance C. Dalleck

Chapter 9 **Comparison of three activity monitors for estimating sedentary time among children** 85
Jarle Stålesen, Frøydis Nordgård Vik, Bjørge Herman Hansen and Sveinung Berntsen

Chapter 10 **Associations between poor oral health and reinjuries in male elite soccer players** 91
Henny Solleveld, Arnold Goedhart and Luc Vanden Bossche

Chapter 11 **The child and adolescent athlete: a review of three potentially serious injuries** 99
Dennis Caine, Laura Purcell and Nicola Maffulli

Chapter 12 **Reliability of the Q Force; a mobile instrument for measuring isometric quadriceps muscle strength** 109
K. W. Douma, G. R. H. Regterschot, W.P. Krijnen, G. E. C. Slager, C. P. van der Schans and W. Zijlstra

Chapter 13 **Biomechanical symmetry in elite rugby union players during dynamic tasks: an investigation using discrete and continuous data analysis techniques** 121
Brendan Marshall, Andrew Franklyn-Miller, Kieran Moran, Enda King, Chris Richter, Shane Gore, Siobhán Strike and Éanna Falvey

Chapter 14 **Metastability in plyometric training on unstable surfaces** 134
Armin Kibele, Claudia Classen, Thomas Muehlbauer, Urs Granacher and David G Behm

Chapter 15 **Reliability and validity of ten consumer activity trackers** 145
Thea J. M. Kooiman, Manon L. Dontje, Siska R. Sprenger, Wim P. Krijnen, Cees P. van der Schans and Martijn de Groot

Chapter 16 **The effect of external ankle support on the kinematics and kinetics of the lower limb during a side step cutting task in netballers** 156
Andrew John Greene, Max Christian Stuelcken, Richard Murray Smith and Benedicte Vanwanseele

Chapter 17 **Age profiles of sport participants** 166
Rochelle M. Eime, Jack T. Harvey, Melanie J. Charity, Meghan M. Casey, Hans Westerbeek and Warren R. Payne

Chapter 18 **Pre-pubertal males practising Taekwondo exhibit favourable postural and neuromuscular performance** 176
Mohamed Chedly Jlid, Nicola Maffulli, Nisar Souissi, Mohamed Souheil Chelly and Thierry Paillard

Chapter 19 **Joint torque variability and repeatability during cyclic flexion-extension of the elbow** 183
Laurent Ballaz, Maxime Raison, Christine Detrembleur, Guillaume Gaudet and Martin Lemay

Chapter 20 **Cancer patients participating in a lifestyle intervention during chemotherapy greatly over-report their physical activity level** 191
Karianne Vassbakk-Brovold, Christian Kersten, Liv Fegran, Odd Mjåland, Svein Mjåland, Stephen Seiler and Sveinung Berntsen

Chapter 21 **Effect of fatigue caused by a simulated handball game on ball throwing velocity, shoulder muscle strength and balance ratio** 200
Marília Santos Andrade, Fabiana de Carvalho Koffes, Ana Amélia Benedito-Silva, Antonio Carlos da Silva and Claudio Andre Barbosa de Lira

Chapter 22 **Maximal strength training as physical rehabilitation for patients with substance use disorder** 207
Runar Unhjem, Grete Flemmen, Jan Hoff and Eivind Wang

Chapter 23 **A systematic review of financial incentives given in the healthcare setting; do they effectively improve physical activity levels?** 217
Claudia C. M. Molema, G. C. Wanda Wendel-Vos, Lisanne Puijk, Jørgen Dejgaard Jensen, A. Jantine Schuit and G. Ardine de Wit

Permissions

List of Contributors

Index

Preface

The purpose of the book is to provide a glimpse into the dynamics and to present opinions and studies of some of the scientists engaged in the development of new ideas in the field from very different standpoints. This book will prove useful to students and researchers owing to its high content quality.

Sports injury rehabilitation is the practice of treating pain and discomfort effectively with the purpose to return to normal function. This book on injury rehabilitation and sports medicine discusses topics related to the early detection and treatment of sports injuries and the technology and treatments that are involved with the same. Research in this field deals with minor and major injuries ranging from strains and sprains to tendon and ligament tears and traumatic head injuries. Chapters in this book strive to provide knowledge for the prevention, evaluation and treatment of sports injuries. It is a vital tool for all researching and studying this field. This book attempts to assist those with a goal of delving into the field of sports medicine and injury rehabilitation.

At the end, I would like to appreciate all the efforts made by the authors in completing their chapters professionally. I express my deepest gratitude to all of them for contributing to this book by sharing their valuable works. A special thanks to my family and friends for their constant support in this journey.

Editor

1

Changes in breaststroke swimming performances in national and international athletes competing between 1994 and 2011 –a comparison with freestyle swimming performances

Mathias Wolfrum[1,2], Christoph Alexander Rüst[1], Thomas Rosemann[1], Romuald Lepers[3] and Beat Knechtle[1,4*]

Abstract

Background: The purpose of the present study was to analyse potential changes in performance of elite breaststroke swimmers competing at national and international level and to compare to elite freestyle swimming performance.

Methods: Temporal trends in performance of elite breaststroke swimmers were analysed from records of the Swiss Swimming Federation and the FINA (Fédération Internationale de Natation) World Swimming Championships during the 1994–2011 period. Swimming speeds of elite female and male breaststroke swimmers competing in 50 m, 100 m, and 200 m were examined using linear regression, non-linear regression and analysis of variance. Results of breaststroke swimmers were compared to results of freestyle swimmers.

Results: Swimming speed in both strokes improved significantly ($p < 0.0001$-0.025) over time for both sexes, with the exception of 50 m breaststroke for FINA men. Sex differences in swimming speed increased significantly over time for Swiss freestyle swimmers ($p < 0.0001$), but not for FINA swimmers for freestyle, while the sex difference remained stable for Swiss and FINA breaststroke swimmers. The sex differences in swimming speed decreased significantly ($p < 0.0001$) with increasing race distance.

Conclusions: The present study showed that elite male and female swimmers competing during the 1994–2011 period at national and international level improved their swimming speed in both breaststroke and freestyle. The sex difference in freestyle swimming speed consistently increased in athletes competing at national level, whereas it remained unchanged in athletes competing at international level. Future studies should investigate temporal trends for recent time in other strokes, to determine whether this improvement is a generalized phenomenon.

Keywords: Swimming speed, Sex-related difference, Gender difference, Men, Women

Background

Improved understanding of performance by top athletes, including long-term changes and sex-related differences, can help athletes and coaches to estimate performance limits, to choose appropriate training protocols, and to set realistic goals. During the past 30 years, several studies investigated human limits in various sports such as running [1-3], track and field [4], tennis [4], and swimming [3]. However, the results were inconsistent. For example, Whipp and Ward [5] predicted that there would be no limits to human performance in running, and women would eventually run faster than men, while Cheuvront *et al.* [2] concluded that running performances by both men and women had already reached a plateau. Similarly, Nevill *et al.* [3] suggested that freestyle swimming performance had reached the limits of human capability. World record speeds improved significantly during the 1960s and 1970s, but levelled off early in the 21st century [3]. This conclusion was further supported by Seiler *et al.* [6] and

* Correspondence: beat.knechtle@hispeed.ch
[1]Institute of General Practice and for Health Services Research, University of Zurich, Zurich, Switzerland
[4]Gesundheitszentrum St. Gallen, Vadianstrasse 26, 9001 St. Gallen, Switzerland
Full list of author information is available at the end of the article

Johnson *et al.* [7]. However, temporal trends have not been examined in other strokes, and in fact, new world records in breaststroke and freestyle swimming were set by both men and women during the 2012 Olympic Games [8], suggesting that swimming performance has not reached its limit.

For swimmers, changes in performance over time have mainly been investigated in freestyle swimming [3,9-11]. Nevill *et al.* reported that the 10% faster performance in men compared to women in various freestyle swimming events remained unchanged during the last 60 years [3]. However, it is not known whether or not this is also true for breaststroke swimming. Differences between freestyle and breaststroke do exist in terms of technique, energy cost and stroke length [12]. It has been shown that freestyle is the most economic stroke, followed by backstroke, butterfly and breaststroke [13].

The changes in swimming performance have been investigated for freestyle swimmers competing at international top level [3,9,10]. Little data is known for changes in freestyle swimming performance across years for swimmers competing at national level [11] and no data exist for changes in swimming performance over time for other strokes such as breaststroke [14]. Differences in performance between athletes competing at international and national level are related to differences in the energetic and biomechanical profiles of these athletes [15-18]. Considering breaststroke, Seifert *et al.* [19] reported differences in the elbow-knee continuous relative phase in breaststroke swimmers of different performance levels. Furthermore, recent studies reported greater sex-related differences in swimming speed for freestyle than for breaststroke for swimmers at national level, but not for swimmers competing at international level [14]. This finding might be attributed to the biomechanics of the two swimming styles [20,21]. However, there is now comprehensive data about the temporal trend over recent years for the sex differences in breaststroke and freestyle swimming.

The purpose of the present study was to investigate the changes in breaststroke swimming performance in athletes competing at both national and international level and to compare breaststroke swimming performance to freestyle swimming performance. We therefore analyzed changes in freestyle and breaststroke performance of the annual top ten Swiss swimmers (*i.e.* national level) and the eight finalists in the Fédération Internationale de Natation (FINA) World Championships (*i.e.* international level) during the 1994–2011 period for 50 m, 100 m, and 200 m. The aims of the present study were to investigate (*i*) potential changes in breaststroke swimming performance across years in national and international athletes and to compare to potential changes in freestyle swimming performance, (*ii*) differences in swimming performance between national and international athletes and (*iii*) differences in swimming performance between women and men. We hypothesized that (*i*) performance in breaststroke swimmers would improve over time, (*ii*) national athletes would compete slower that international athletes and (*iii*) men would be faster than women for all distances with a constant sex difference in swimming performance.

Methods

Ethics

All procedures used in the study were approved by the Institutional Review Board of Kanton St. Gallen, Switzerland with a waiver of the requirement for informed consent of the participants given the fact that the study involved the analysis of publicly available data.

Subjects and design

Race times on long courses for the annual top ten men and women in breaststroke and freestyle swimming recorded in the Swiss high score list between 1994 and 2011 were obtained per civil year from the website of the Swiss Swimming Federation [22]. The Swiss Swimming Federation records only the annual best swimming performance for each athlete, so no Swiss athlete was included more than once in the same year. Race times for the eight female and male finalists competing on international level in breaststroke and freestyle in the FINA (Fédération Internationale de Natation) World Swimming Championships between 1994 and 2011 were obtained from the website of the FINA [23]. Race times for athletes competing on national level were available annually for swimmers for both breaststroke and freestyle and all distances (*i.e.* 50 m, 100 m, and 200 m). For FINA finalists, race times were available from the World Championships in Rome (1994), Perth (1998) Fukuoka (2001), Barcelona (2003), Montreal (2005), Melbourne (2007), Rome (2009) and Shanghai (2011). The 50 m breaststroke was held for the first time in the 2001 World Championships.

Methodology

Since races in breaststroke swimming were held for 50 m, 100 m and 200 m but freestyle races for 50 m, 100 m, 200 m, 400 m, 800 m and 1,500 m, we analysed freestyle swimming races only for 50 m, 100 m, and 200 m to compare with breaststroke swimming results. To allow a comparison of swimming performance for different styles and distances, race times were transformed to swimming speed by dividing race distance by time. To determine temporal trends, we compared the average annual swimming speed for each stroke and race distance, by the top ten Swiss men and top ten Swiss women, and by the eight men and eight women competing in the FINA finals. To analyse the maximum overall swimming performance, we averaged the fastest ten swimming speeds in each stroke for four groups: Swiss women, Swiss men, FINA women, and FINA men. Sex-related differences were calculated using the equation [(women swimming speed) – (men swimming speed)]/(men swimming speed) × 100. The calculation was performed for pairs of equally placed athletes during each year, *e.g.*, the fastest women and men, the second fastest women and men, etc. The absolute value of the sex-related difference for each pair was used to calculate the annual mean and standard deviation.

Statistical analyses

Prior to statistical analyses, each data set was tested for normal distribution and homogeneity of variances. Normal distribution was tested using a D'Agostino and Pearson omnibus normality test. Homogeneity of variances was tested using a Levene's test, in cases with two groups, and with a Bartlett's test, in cases with more than two groups. A potential change in swimming speed across years was investigated using regression analyses. Since the change in sex difference in endurance is assumed to be non-linear [24], we additionally calculated the non-linear regression model that fits the data best. For swimmers at national level, polynomial regressions from 2nd to 17th degree were calculated; for swimmers at international level, polynomial regressions from 2nd to 7th degree were calculated. Additionally, LOWESS (*i.e.* locally weighted scatterplot smoothing) and 64 further standard models were used. We compared the best-fit non-linear models to the linear models using Akaike's Information Criteria (AIC) and F-test in order to show which model (*i.e.* linear versus non-linear) would be the most appropriate to explain the trend of the data. One-way analysis of variance (ANOVA) with subsequent Tukey-Kramer post-hoc tests were used to compare data for multiple groups. A two-way ANOVA with a Bonferroni post-hoc test was used to determine the significance of interactive effects of swimming style and sex on performance. Significance of all statistical tests was accepted at $p < 0.05$. Statistical analyses were performed using IBM SPSS Statistics (Version 19 and 20, IBM SPSS, Chicago, IL, USA) and GraphPad Prism (Version 5 and 6.01, GraphPad Software, La Jolla, CA, USA). Data are reported in the text and figures as mean ± standard deviation (SD).

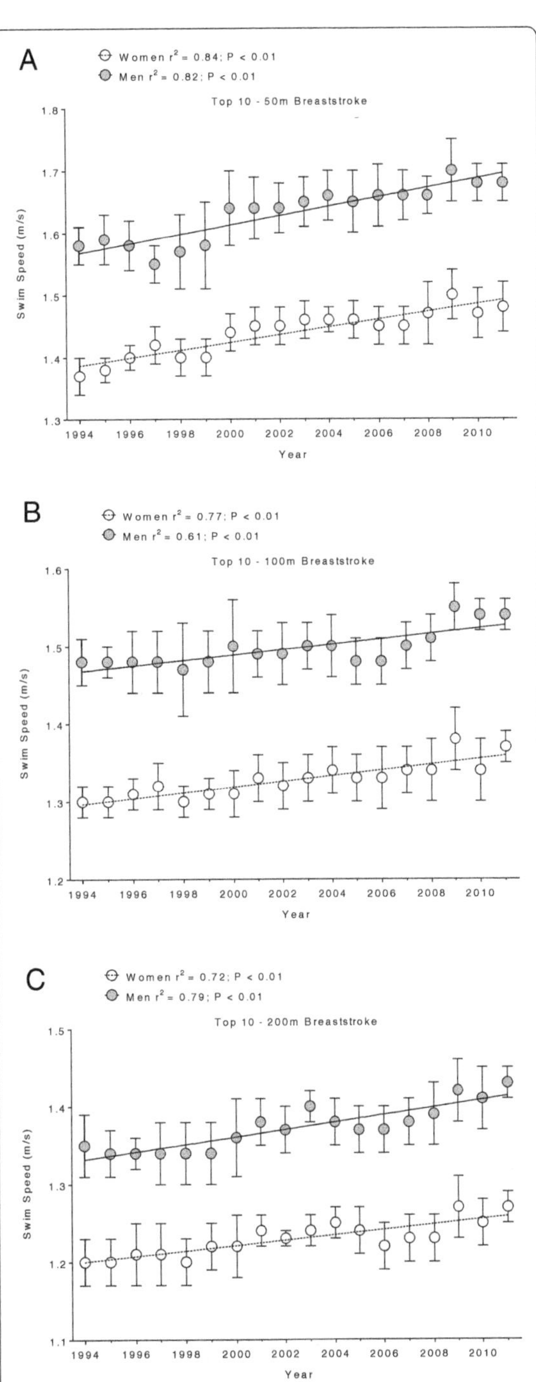

Figure 1 Swimming speeds of Swiss top ten breaststroke swimmers for 50 m (Panel A), 100 m (Panel B) and 200 m (Panel C). Results are presented as mean ± SD.

Results

Changes in breaststroke and freestyle swimming speed across the years

Figure 1,2,3 and 4 present the changes in swimming speeds for breaststroke (Figure 1) and freestyle (Figure 2) in Swiss swimmers and for breaststroke (Figure 3) and freestyle (Figure 4) in FINA swimmers for 50 m (Panels A), 100 m (Panels B) and 200 m (Panels C). Swimming speed

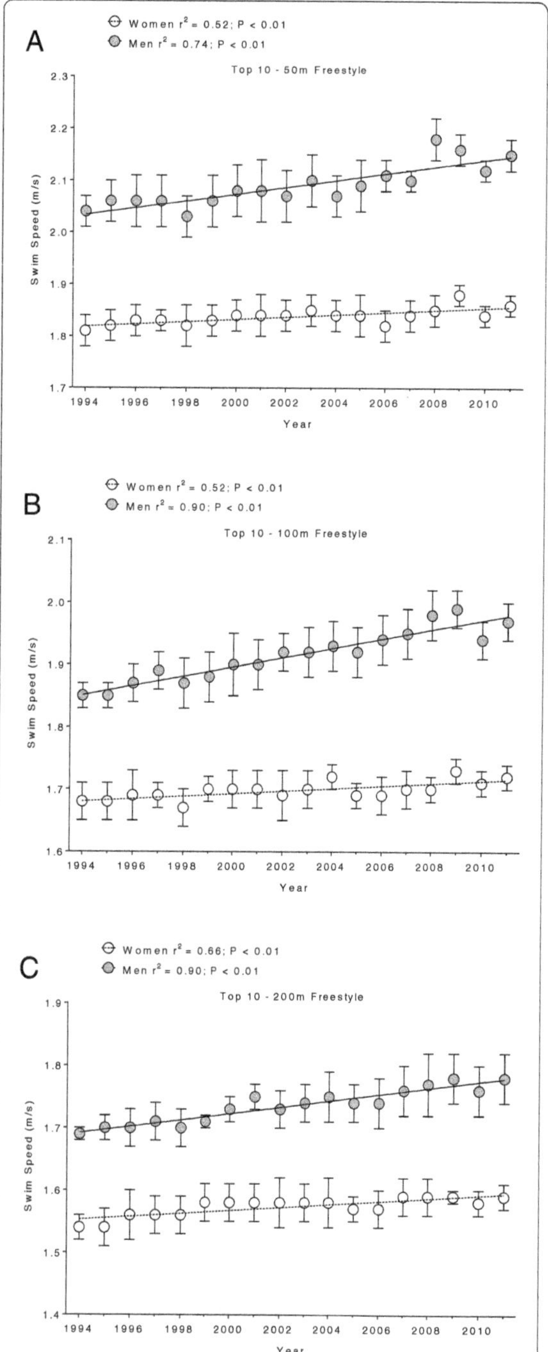

Figure 2 Swimming speeds of Swiss top ten freestyle swimmers for 50 m (Panel A), 100 m (Panel B) and 200 m (Panel C). Results are presented as mean ± SD.

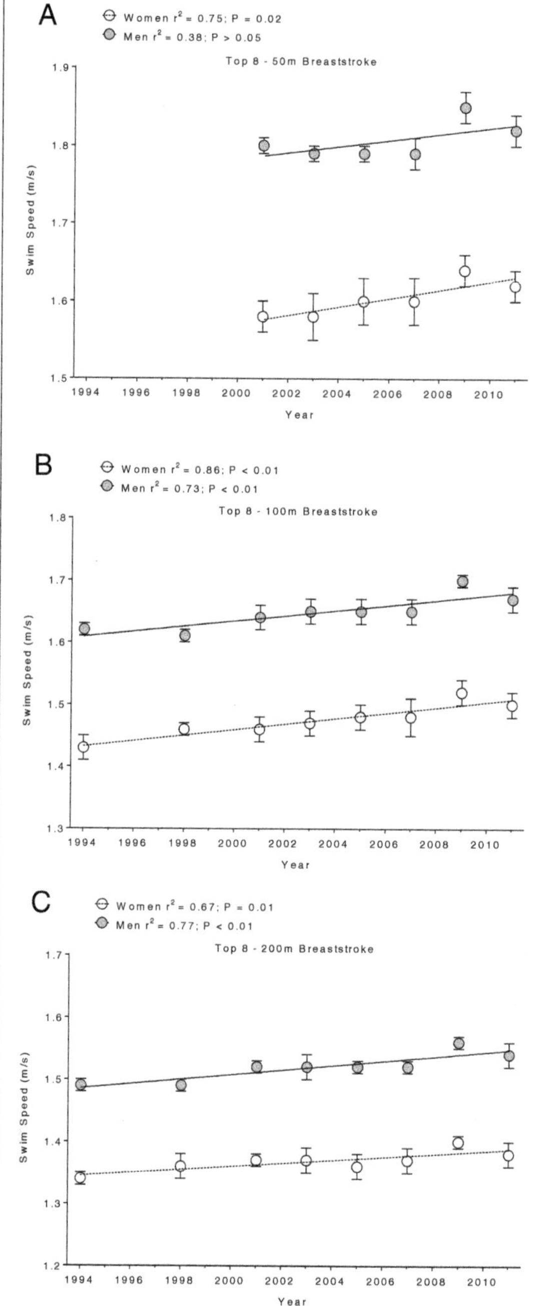

Figure 3 Swimming speeds of breaststroke FINA finalists for 50 m (Panel A), 100 m (Panel B) and 200 m (Panel C). Results are presented as mean ± SD.

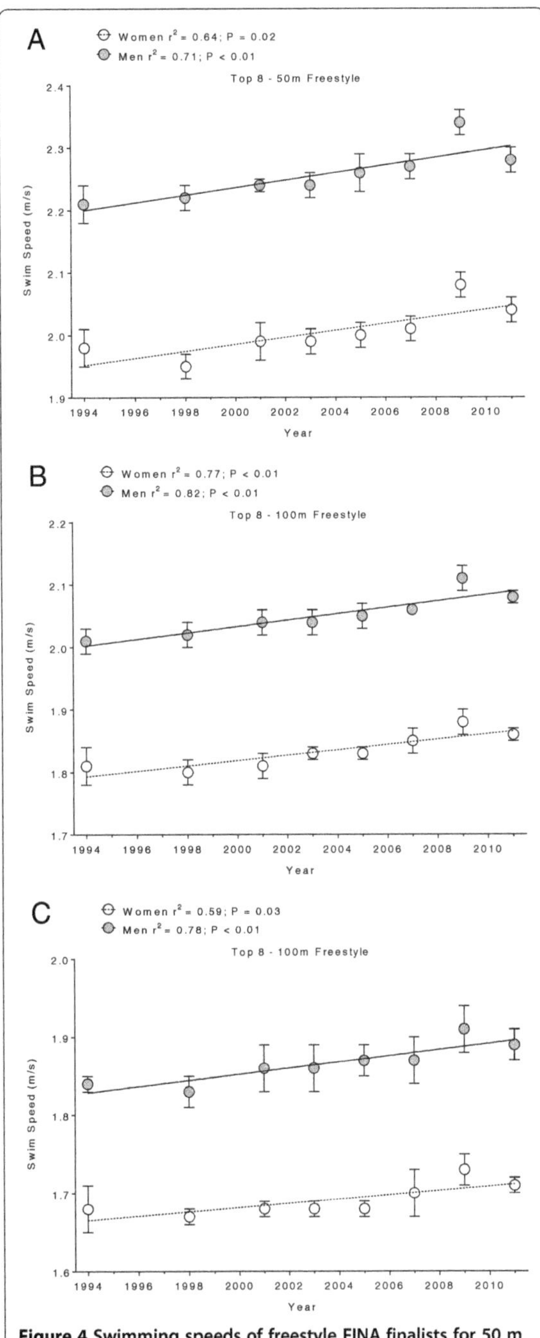

Figure 4 Swimming speeds of freestyle FINA finalists for 50 m (Panel A), 100 m (Panel B) and 200 m (Panel C). Results are presented as mean ± SD.

increased linearly for Swiss swimmers in breaststroke (Table 1) and freestyle (Table 2). In FINA finalists, swimming speed increased also linearly in breaststroke (Table 3) and freestyle (Table 4), with the exception of male FINA swimmers in the 50 m breaststroke (Figure 3A).

In breaststroke, male Swiss swimmers increased their swimming speed by 0.008 $m \cdot s^{-1}$, 0.004 $m \cdot s^{-1}$, and 0.005 $m \cdot s^{-1}$ *per annum* in 50 m, 100 m, and 200 m, respectively, and female swimmers by 0.006 $m \cdot s^{-1}$, 0.004 $m \cdot s^{-1}$, 0.004 $m \cdot s^{-1}$ *per annum*, respectively. Male FINA swimmers increased swimming speed by 0.004 $m \cdot s^{-1}$ *per annum* over 100 m and 200 m, respectively, and female swimmers by 0.005 $m \cdot s^{-1}$, 0.004 $m \cdot s^{-1}$, 0.003 $m \cdot s^{-1}$ *per annum* in 50 m, 100 m, and 200 m, respectively. In freestyle, male Swiss swimmers increased swimming speed by 0.007 $m \cdot s^{-1}$, 0.008 $m \cdot s^{-1}$, and 0.005 $m \cdot s^{-1}$ *per annum* in 50 m, 100 m, and 200 m, respectively, and female swimmers by 0.002 $m \cdot s^{-1}$ *per annum* for all distances. Male FINA swimmers increased swimming speed by 0.006 $m \cdot s^{-1}$, 0.005 $m \cdot s^{-1}$, and 0.004 $m \cdot s^{-1}$ *per annum* in 50 m, 100 m, and 200 m, respectively, and female swimmers by 0.006 $m \cdot s^{-1}$, 0.004 $m \cdot s^{-1}$, and 0.003 $m \cdot s^{-1}$ *per annum*, respectively.

Sex differences in breaststroke and freestyle swimming speed

Men swam consistently faster than women for both strokes and all distances. In Swiss swimmers, swimming speed in breaststroke showed no changes across years (Figure 5 and Table 5). In freestyle, however, the sex difference in swimming speed increased linearly (Table 6) for all distances (Figure 6). In FINA finalists, the sex differences in swimming speed showed no significant trends over time (Table 6) for breaststroke (Figure 7) and for freestyle (Figure 8). Sex differences in both breaststroke and freestyle performance decreased significantly ($p < 0.0001$) with increasing race distance for both Swiss (Figure 9) and FINA swimmers (Figure 10) (*i.e.* for breaststroke at national level 50 m 11.8%, 100 m 11.4% and 200 m 10.5%; international level 50 m 11.2%, 100 m 10.6% and 200 m 9.9%; for freestyle at national level 50 m 12.0%, 100 m 11.3% and 200 m 9.3%, international level 50 m 11.3%, 100 m 10.6%, 200 m 9.4%, respectively).

Interaction between style and sex

Based on the fastest breaststroke and freestyle swimmers, swimming style and sex had a significant interactive effect on swimming speed for both Swiss (F = 15.13, Dfn = 1, DFd = 2156, $p = 0.0001$) and FINA athletes (F = 6.77, Dfn = 1, DFd = 732, $p = 0.0094$) (Table 7). In Swiss swimmers, style accounted for 61.9% of the total variance of race time (F = 5753.7, Dfn = 1, DFd = 732, $p < 0.0001$) and sex for 14.7% of total variance (F = 1365.6, Dfn = 1, DFd = 2156, $p < 0.0001$), while the interaction accounted for 0.16% (F = 15.1, Dfn = 1, DFd = 2156, $p = 0.0001$). In the FINA swimmers, style accounted for 59.5% of the total variance of race time (F = 1691.3, Dfn = 1, DFd = 732, $p < 0.0001$), sex accounted for 14.5% (F = 412.2,

Table 1 Comparison of linear and non-linear regression analysis of changes in swimming speed for female and male breast stroke swimmers at national level across years to determine which model is the best

	Kind of regression	Sum of Squares	DOF	AICC	Best regression AIC-Test	Best regression F-Test	Delta	Probability	Likelihood
50 m breaststroke	polynomial	0.0035	12	−138.34	linear	linear	2.80	0.19	80.3%
male Swiss swimmers	linear	0.0062	16	−141.15					
100 m breaststroke	polynomial	0.0009	0	−144.16	linear	undetermined	5.72	0.054	94.6%
male Swiss swimmers	linear	0.0038	16	−149.88					
200 m breaststroke	polynomial	0.0011	0	−139.69	linear	undetermined	13.48	0.0011	99.88%
male Swiss swimmers	linear	0.0032	16	−153.17					
50 m breaststroke	polynomial	0.0011	0	−140.12	linear	undetermined	6.62	0.035	96.5%
female Swiss swimmers	linear	0.0045	16	−146.74					
100 m breaststroke	polynomial	0.0018	0	−131.76	linear	undetermined	29.91	3.19 e^{-07}	100%
female Swiss swimmers	linear	0.0019	16	−161.67					
200 m breaststroke	polynomial	0.0014	0	−135.81	linear	undetermined	22.41	1.35 e^{-05}	99.99%
female Swiss swimmers	linear	0.0024	16	−158.22					

For all distances, the changes in swimming speed were linear.

Dfn = 1, DFd = 732, $p < 0.0001$), and the interaction accounted for 0.24% (F = 6.8, Dfn = 1, DFd = 732, $p = 0.009$).

Discussion

The present study examined temporal changes in breaststroke swimming speed for top Swiss and FINA finalists and compared to freestyle swimming speed. The results showed that (*i*) swimming speed increased for both national and international swimmers during the 1994–2011 period for both women and men with the exception for male FINA swimmers in 50 m breaststroke, (*ii*) the sex difference in swimming speed did not change significantly over time except for Swiss freestyle swimmers and (*iii*) the sex-related difference in swimming speed consistently decreased with increasing race distance from 50 m to 200 m for both freestyle and breaststroke.

Temporal changes in breaststroke and freestyle swimming speed

The increased swimming speed of women and men in freestyle and breaststroke swimming during the 1994–2011 period as well as the new world records during the 2012 Olympic Games [8] are partly attributable to technological advances. Deeper deck-level pools, more effective anti-wave lane ropes, and improved swimming suits reducing drag, improving buoyancy, and enhancing body compression, contributed to the enhanced swimming performance [3,25]. Full-body, polyurethane, technical swimsuits were

Table 2 Comparison of linear and non-linear regression analysis of changes in swimming speed for female and male freestyle swimmers at national level across years to determine which model is the best

	Kind of regression	Sum of Squares	DOF	AICC	Best regression AIC-Test	Best regression F-Test	Delta	Probability	Likelihood
50 m freestyle	polynomial	0.0067	0	−108.11	linear	undetermined	29.06	4.87 e^{-07}	100%
male Swiss swimmers	linear	0.0077	16	−137.18					
100 m freestyle	polynomial	0.0002	2	−45.86	linear	linear	21.05	2.67 e^{-05}	99.99%
male Swiss swimmers	linear	0.0013	6	−66.92					
200 m freestyle	polynomial	0.0015	0	−134.90	linear	linear	32.22	1.005 e^{-07}	100%
male Swiss swimmers	linear	0.0014	16	−167.13					
50 m freestyle	polynomial	0.0016	0	−132.88	linear	undetermined	27.20	1.23 e^{-06}	99.99%
female Swiss swimmers	linear	0.0021	16	−160.08					
100 m freestyle	polynomial	0.0027	0	−124.34	linear	undetermined	28.91	5.26 e^{-07}	99.99%
female Swiss swimmers	linear	0.0031	16	−153.25					
200 m freestyle	polynomial	0.0006	0	−152.27	linear	undetermined	14.68	0.00064	99.93%
female Swiss swimmers	linear	0.0014	16	−166.95					

For all distances, the changes were linear.

Table 3 Comparison of linear and non-linear regression analysis of changes in swimming speed for female and male breast stroke swimmers at international level across years to determine which model is the best

	Kind of regression	Sum of Squares	DOF	AICC	Best regression AIC-Test	Best regression F-Test	Delta	Probability	Likelihood
50 m breaststroke	polynomial	0.00042	1	−9.35	linear	linear	35.83	1.65 e^{-08}	100%
male FINA finalists	linear	0.00190	4	−45.19					
100 m breaststroke	polynomial	0.00035	2	−40.28	linear	linear	23.83	6.66 e^{-06}	99.99%
male FINA finalists	linear	0.00180	6	−64.12					
200 m breaststroke	polynomial	0.00014	2	−47.16	linear	linear	23.19	9.18 e^{-06}	99.99%
male FINA finalists	linear	0.00086	6	−70.35					
50 m breaststroke	polynomial	0.00027	0	−49.89	linear	undetermined	1.51	0.31	68.04%
female FINA finalists	linear	0.00069	4	−51.41					
100 m breaststroke	polynomial	0.00034	2	−40.31	linear	linear	30.66	2.19 e^{-07}	100%
female FINA finalists	linear	0.00080	6	−70.97					
200 m breaststroke	polynomial	8.76 e^{-05}	2	−51.37	linear	linear	18.04	0.00012	99.98%
female FINA finalists	linear	0.00097	6	−69.41					

For all distances, the changes were linear.

most probably an important contributor to the unprecedented run of broken records from 1990 to 2009 [26]. A full-body suit improves performance by 3.2 ± 2.4% and reduces drag by 6.2 ± 7.9% for distances from 25 m to 800 m leading to a reduction of energy costs [27]. Indeed, FINA's release of new rules in 2010 limiting the types of technical swimsuits that could be worn by athletes was followed by a downward trend in performance [26]. However, since 2010, there were still world records in 50 m pools achieved. Especially, world records in breaststroke swimming were improved. For women, Katie Ledecky improved the world records in 800 m and 1,500 m freestyle in 2013, Missy Frankling in 2012 for 200 m backstroke, Ruta Meilutyte in 2013 for 50 m and 100 m breaststroke and Rikke Møller Pederson for 200 m breaststroke. For butterfly, Dana Vollmer improved the world record for 100 m in 2012. For men, Sun Yang improved the 1,500 m freestyle world record in 2012, Cameron van der Burgh in 2012 the world record in 100 m breaststroke, Akihiro Yamaguchi also in 2012 for 200 m breaststroke and Ryan Lochte in 2011 for 200 m individual medley [8].

In addition to technological advances, swimming speed during the 1994–2011 period could have been affected by changes in anthropometric and physiological characteristics [28], improvements in training [29], competition psychology [30,31], and sports nutrition [32], as well as increased access to the sport by a larger number of athletes [4]. A study of 6–17 year-old children during

Table 4 Comparison of linear and non-linear regression analysis of changes in swimming speed for female and male freestyle swimmers at international level across years to determine which model is the best

	Kind of regression	Sum of Squares	DOF	AICC	Best regression AIC-Test	Best regression F-Test	Delta	Probability	Likelihood
50 m freestyle	polynomial	0.00061	2	−35.82	linear	linear	23.53	7.76 e^{-06}	99.99%
male FINA finalists	linear	0.00340	6	−59.35					
100 m freestyle	polynomial	0.00017	2	−45.86	linear	linear	32.22	1.005 e^{-07}	100%
male FINA finalists	linear	0.00130	6	−66.92					
200 m freestyle	polynomial	0.00020	2	−44.73	linear	linear	23.55	7.69 e^{-06}	99.99%
male FINA finalists	linear	0.00110	6	−68.28					
50 m freestyle	polynomial	0.00039	2	−39.26	linear	linear	18.46	9.76 e^{-05}	99.99%
female FINA finalists	linear	0.00420	6	−57.73					
100 m freestyle	polynomial	0.00019	2	−44.78	linear	linear	22.05	1.62 e^{-05}	99.99%
female FINA finalists	linear	0.00130	6	−66.84					
200 m freestyle	polynomial	1.58 e^{-05}	2	−65.03	linear	polynomial	1.24	0.34	65.08%
female FINA finalists	linear	0.00140	6	−66.27					

The changes were linear for all distances.

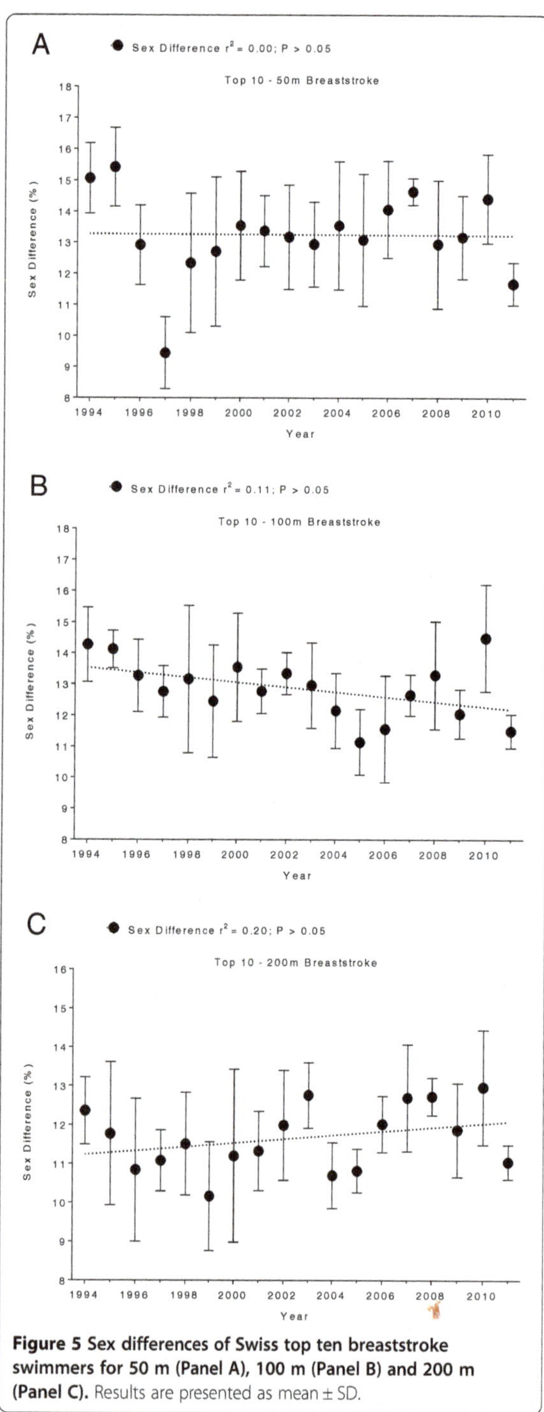

Figure 5 Sex differences of Swiss top ten breaststroke swimmers for 50 m (Panel A), 100 m (Panel B) and 200 m (Panel C). Results are presented as mean ± SD.

20th century found an increase of 1–2 cm in body height and 0.5-1.5 kg in body weight per decade [33], a trend which could have led to the improved performances observed in our study. Charles and Bejan [34] observed that the mean body height of champion swimmers in 100 m freestyle increased by 11.4 cm since 1912, and predicted that the fastest athletes would become heavier and taller in future. If available, anthropometric data for Swiss and FINA competitors during the 1994–2011 period could be used to test these assumptions. Due to the linear increase in swimming speed for both national and international swimmers for both breaststroke and freestyle, we may assume that the limits of performance have not reached yet a limit with the exception of the 50 m breaststroke in FINA finalists where the limit of performance may be been reached. However, the period of 1994–2011 might be too short to define whether the change was really linear. Nevill *et al.* [3] investigated the changes in swimming speeds in 100 m, 200 m, and 400 m freestyle world records from 1957 to 2006 and found that a flattened 'S-shaped curve' logistic curve best described the changes.

Sex differences in breaststroke and freestyle swimming

Results of previous studies reporting that the difference between men and women's world freestyle records remained stable during the past 60 years [3,4,26], were confirmed by results of the present study showing that sex-related differences in breaststroke - and in freestyle swimming by FINA athletes - remained relatively constant over time. The temporal increase in the sex-related difference in freestyle performance by Swiss swimmers is difficult to explain. Different levels of freestyle swimming performance by the variations of velocity, stroke rate, and especially stroke length were found in 100 m freestyle for male swimmers of differing skills (*i.e.* national versus international level) [35]. Additionally, international swimmers are able to maintain a higher energetic and biomechanical capacity than national swimmers [15] and high-speed swimmers have a higher and more stable stroke length and index of coordination than low-speed swimmers [36].

Sex-related differences in performance are largely explained by sex-specific differences in body dimensions, swimming speed, buoyancy, stroke mechanics, stroke length, starts and turn time, basic and specific endurance, anaerobic power and capacity, muscle power, and flexibility [3,37-39]. Young male swimmers have a higher speed fluctuation, active drag, power needed to overcome and technique drag index than young female swimmers [40]. Male freestyle swimmers have also a greater stroke length than female swimmers [36]. Male athletes exhibit greater left ventricular end-diastolic volume than female athletes, resulting in higher stroke volume at rest and during exercise, and higher cardiac output in absolute and relative terms [41]. Men also have 5-10% higher haemoglobin content, which increases oxygen carrying capacity at sub-maximal oxygen uptake levels. These factors lead to greater peak aerobic

Table 5 Comparison of linear and non-linear regression analysis of changes in sex difference for freestyle and breaststroke swimmers at national level across years to determine which model is the best

	Kind of regression	Sum of Squares	DOF	AICC	Best regression AIC-Test	Best regression F-Test	Delta	Probability	Likelihood
50 m breaststroke	polynomial	10.02	0	23.45	linear	undetermined	21.71	1.92 e^{-5}	99.99%
Swiss swimmers	linear	17.49	16	1.73					
100 m breaststroke	polynomial	2.78	0	0.40	linear	linear	13.75	0.0010	99.89%
Swiss swimmers	linear	7.56	16	−13.35					
200 m breaststroke	polynomial	3.80	0	6.03	linear	undetermined	22.42	1.34 e^{-5}	99.99%
Swiss swimmers	linear	6.38	18	−16.39					
50 m freestyle	polynomial	7.20	0	17.51	linear	undetermined	24.94	3.83 e^{-6}	99.99%
Swiss swimmers	linear	10.51	16	−7.42					
100 m freestyle	polynomial	3.93	13	−16.30	linear	linear	1.30	0.34	65.7%
Swiss swimmers	linear	5.97	16	−17.61					
200 m freestyle	polynomial	1.90	0	−6.42	linear	undetermined	18.32	0.00010	99.98%
Swiss swimmers	linear	4.01	16	−24.74					

The changes were linear for all distances.

power, accounting for sex-related differences in the contribution of aerobic energy to exercise [42,43], a factor that is particularly relevant to longer race distances (*i.e.* 100 m-200 m). It has also been reported that pacing strategy differed between women and men [44]. Men applied a positive pacing strategy whereas women applied a negative pacing strategy in 200 m and 400 m medley between 2000 and 2011 for international races [44]. However, it is unlikely that these factors changed significantly during 1994–2011, especially as the change would have had to be greater in Swiss men than in Swiss women to explain the observed results. The gains in swimming speed during the early 21st century following the introduction of new technological swim suits were greater for men than for women in freestyle swimming, while the gains in breaststroke was similar for the two sexes [45]. Although these technological effects might explain the increase in the sex-related difference in Swiss freestyle swimmers, the explanation is countered by the lack of a concomitant increase in FINA swimmers. Differential access to competitive swimming and/or improved training concepts might partly explain the increasing sex-related difference in Swiss freestyle swimming. However, participation in Swiss swimming competition showed a steady annual increase of 3% by both sexes, during 1994–2011 [46].

The stable sex difference at international level is in agreement with previous investigations [4,6,26]. In this

Table 6 Comparison of linear and non-linear regression analysis of changes in sex difference for freestyle and breaststroke swimmers at international level across years to determine which model is the best

	Kind of regression	Sum of Squares	DOF	AICC	Best regression AIC-Test	Best regression F-Test	Delta	Probability	Likelihood
50 m breaststroke	polynomial	0.037	1	17.53	linear	linear	23.80	6.75 e^{-6}	99.99%
FINA finalists	linear	1.27	4	−6.26					
100 m breaststroke	polynomial	0.17	2	9.28	linear	linear	15.80	0.00036	99.96%
FINA finalists	linear	2.53	6	−6.51					
200 m breaststroke	polynomial	0.21	3	−7.73	linear	linear	3.24	0.16	83.5%
FINA finalists	linear	1.45	6	−10.98					
50 m freestyle	polynomial	0.16	2	9.13	linear	linear	20.57	3.41 e^{-5}	99.99%
FINA finalists	linear	1.37	6	−11.44					
100 m freestyle	polynomial	0.56	0	−7.19	linear	undetermined	3.61	0.14	85.9%
FINA finalists	linear	1.48	6	−10.81					
200 m freestyle	polynomial	0.60	0	−6.60	linear	undetermined	6.38	0.039	96.1%
FINA finalists	linear	1.13	6	−12.98					

The changes were all linear.

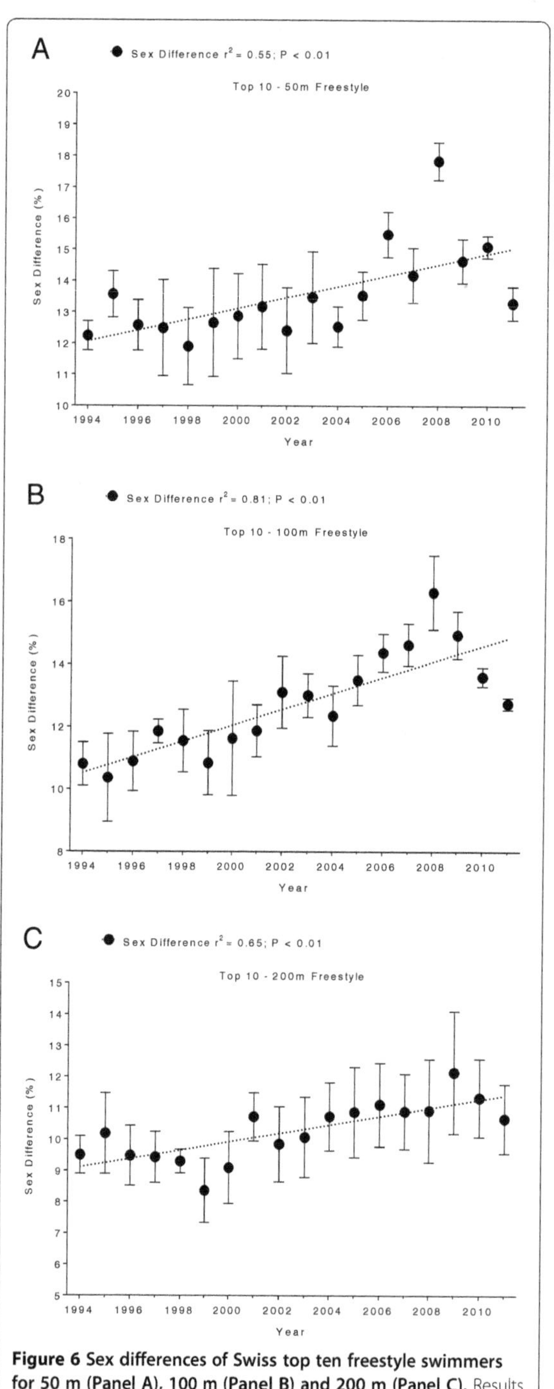

Figure 6 Sex differences of Swiss top ten freestyle swimmers for 50 m (Panel A), 100 m (Panel B) and 200 m (Panel C). Results are presented as mean ± SD.

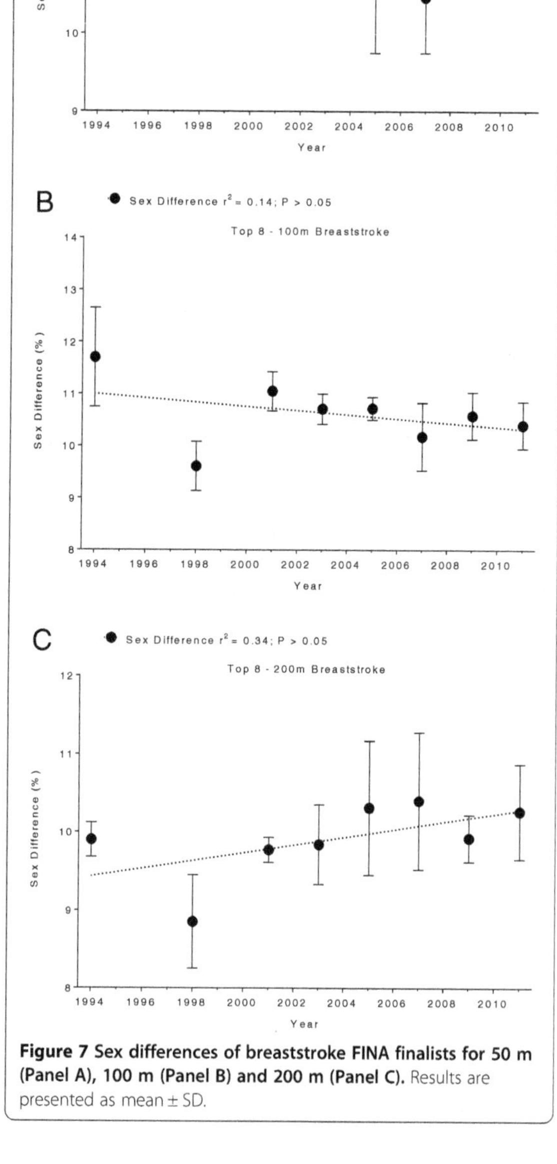

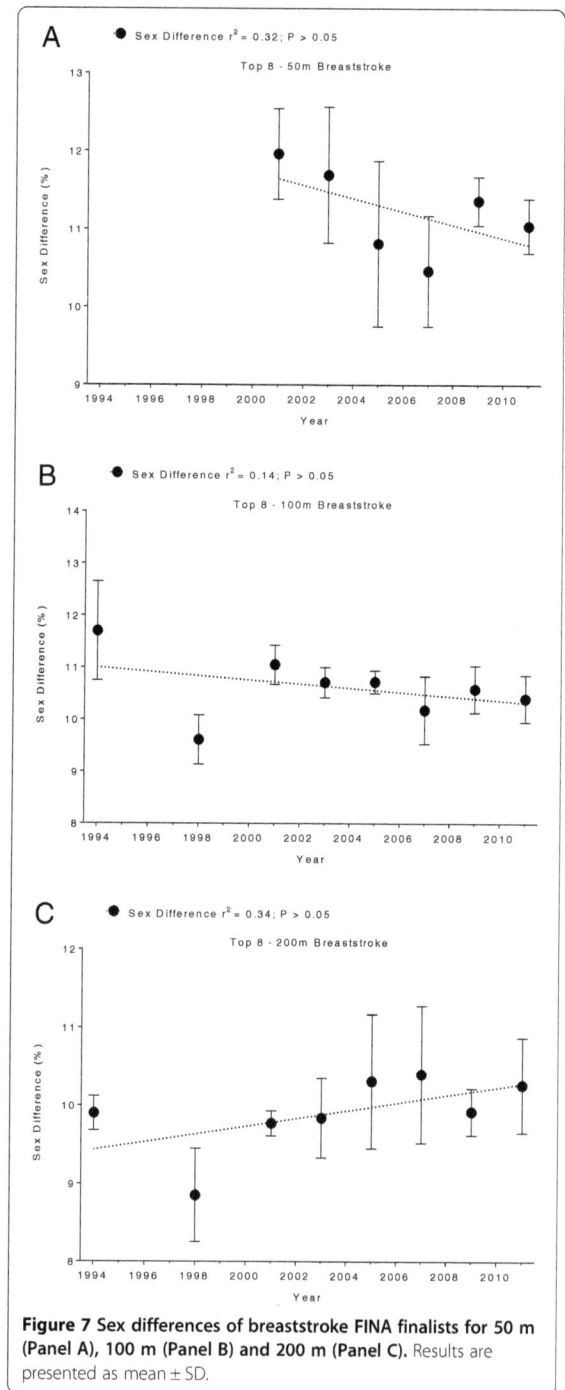

Figure 7 Sex differences of breaststroke FINA finalists for 50 m (Panel A), 100 m (Panel B) and 200 m (Panel C). Results are presented as mean ± SD.

highly competitive and demanding environment both men and women have the same access to state-of-the-art training and equipment. It remains to be explored, why at national level men showed a higher increase in swim speed compared to women. Although the sex difference in sport is closing, it remains due to biological differences affecting performance. However, the sex difference is also influenced by reduced opportunity and

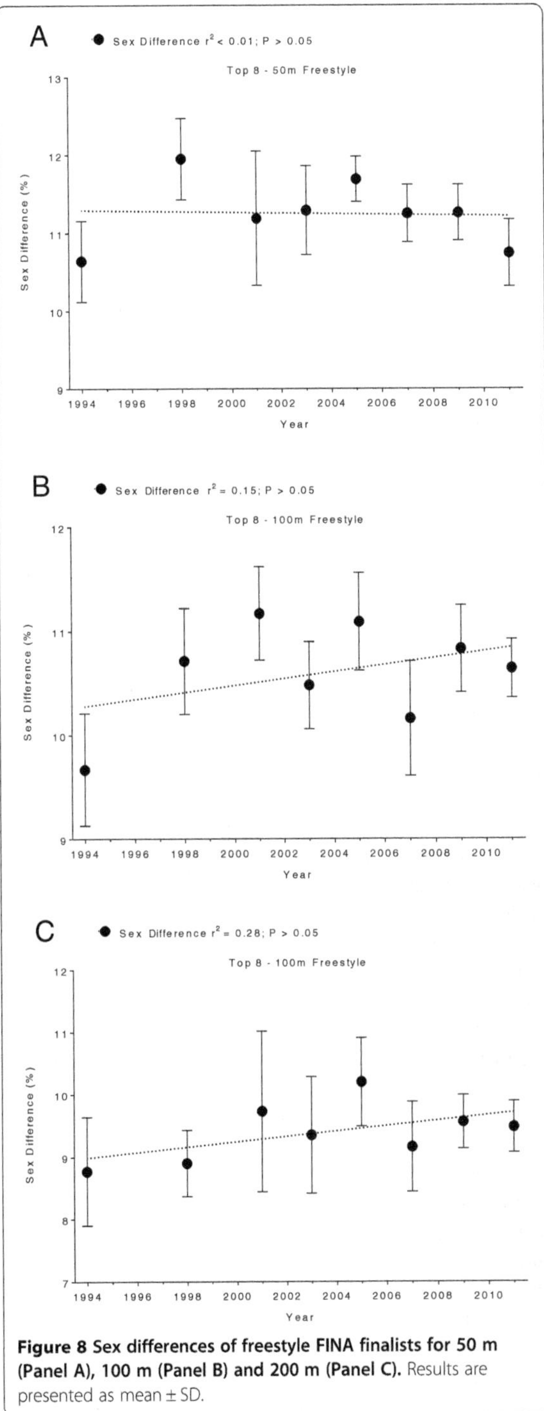

Figure 8 Sex differences of freestyle FINA finalists for 50 m (Panel A), 100 m (Panel B) and 200 m (Panel C). Results are presented as mean ± SD.

socio-political factors that influence full female participation across a range of sports around the world [47].

There is also indirect evidence that the sex-related difference might be different in breaststroke compared to

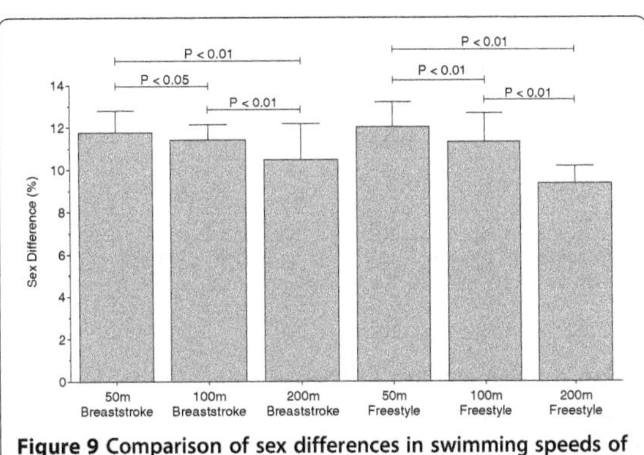

Figure 9 Comparison of sex differences in swimming speeds of the top ten Swiss breaststroke and freestyle swimmers for 50 m, 100 m and 200 m. Results are presented as mean ± SD.

freestyle swimming. Active drag coefficient (C_d) as a measure of technique and performance was lower for faster swimmers [48]. Havriluk found that C_d was similar for men and women in freestyle swimming, but that women had a significantly lower C_d than men in breaststroke [49]. Therefore, the greater power of men, which allows them to outperform women in freestyle swimming, might not provide such a great advantage in breaststroke.

Sex difference in swimming performance decreased with increasing distance

The results of the present study showed a decrease in sex-related difference with increasing distance for both breaststroke and freestyle swimming. These results confirm the conclusions of Tanaka and Seals [38] reporting a decrease in the sex-related difference in freestyle performance with increasing race distance from 50 m to 1,500 m. The decrease was attributed to the fact that women were swimming more efficiently than men, and so show relative improvement in performance as distance increases. The more efficient swimming of women

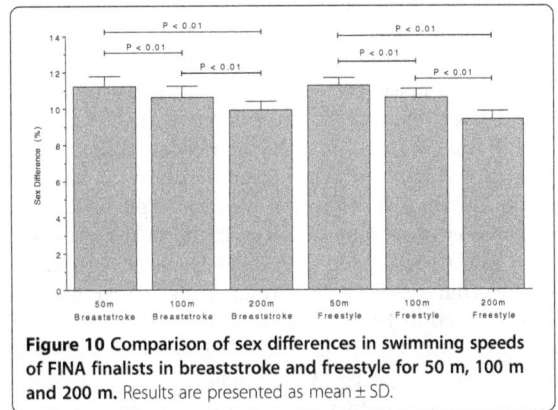

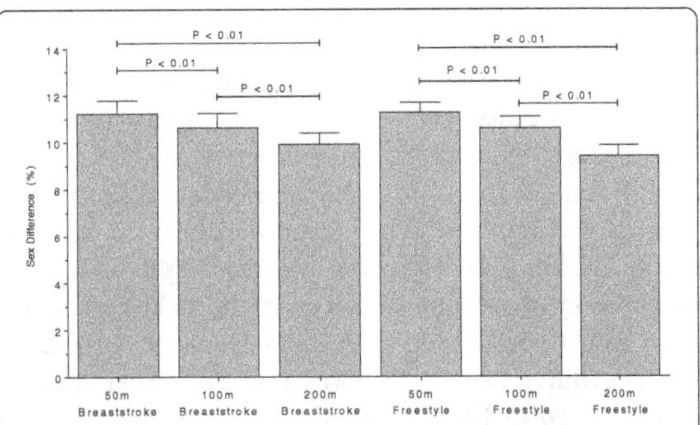

Figure 10 Comparison of sex differences in swimming speeds of FINA finalists in breaststroke and freestyle for 50 m, 100 m and 200 m. Results are presented as mean ± SD.

Table 7 Mean speed ± SD (m/s) of the top breaststroke and freestyle swimmers over 50 m-200 m distances, at FINA and Swiss competitions during the 1994–2011 period

	Speed of Swiss swimmers (m/s)*		Speed of FINA swimmers (m/s) **	
	Breaststroke	Freestyle	Breaststroke	Freestyle
Men	1.50 ± 0.12	1.91 ± 0.15	1.64 ± 0.10	2.06 ± 0.16
Women	1.33 ± 0.09	1.70 ± 0.11	1.47 ± 0.10	1.84 ± 0.13

All main effects of stroke and sex on swimming speed were highly significant (2-way ANOVA, $p < 0.0001$). A significant interactive effect of swim style x sex is indicated by *($p = 0.0001$) and **($p = 0.009$).

is due to their greater fat percentage, shorter legs, and smaller body density, resulting in a more horizontal and streamlined position and smaller body size, which reduces body drag [50,51].

Differences in upper body power might also play a role in the decreasing sex-related difference with increasing race distance [52]. It has been shown that swimming performance was associated with dry land strength of the upper body such as mean power of lat pull down back in elite male freestyle swimmers [53]. Freestyle swimming performance was positively correlated with upper body power in races from 50 m to 400 m [52], but the correlation weakened with increasing race distance [52]. Thus, the greater muscle power of men might become less important with increasing swim distance [54].

It has been assumed that women would be able to outrun men in ultra-marathon running and it was suggested that the sex difference in running would disappear with increasing running distance particularly in distances longer than the marathon [55]. However, a very recent study investigating the sex differences in ultra-marathon running from 50 km to 1,000 km showed that the sex differences in running speeds decreased non-linearly in 50 km and 100 km but remained unchanged in 200 km and 1,000 km [56]. Furthermore, the sex differences in running speeds showed no change with increasing length of the race distance [56]. The findings suggested that it would very unlikely that women will ever outrun men in ultra-marathons held from 50 km to 100 km [56]. For ultra-swimming, however, very recent studies showed that elite female open-water ultra-distance swimmers improved in 10 km but impaired in 25 km leading to a linear decrease in sex difference in 10 km and a linear increase in sex difference in 25 km [57]. The linear changes in sex differences suggest that women will improve in the near future in 10 km, but not in 25 km [57]. However, women might be able to beat men in longer ultra-distances. In the 36 km 'Maratona del Golfo Capri-Napoli' race held from 1954 to 2013, the sex difference in performance decreased linearly from ~38.2% in 1963 to ~6.0% in 2013 [58]. The linear change in both race times and sex differences suggested that women might be able to achieve men's performance or even to outperform men in the near future in open-water ultra-distance swimming. Indeed, in the 46 km 'Manhattan Island Marathon Swim' held in water temperatures <20°C held between 1983 and 2013, the best women were ~12-14% faster than the best men [59]. Most probably the low water temperatures and the higher body fat enable women to beat men in ultra-distance swimming in cold water.

Limitations and implications for future research

This study has three major limitations. First, we investigated the ten fastest swimmers competing at national level and the eight finalists in the World Championships. The mean of eight swimmers might give a different result compared to the mean of ten swimmers. The 10th fastest woman is not comparable, in terms of level and performance, to the 10th fastest man; this might have influenced the sex difference. Future studies might also normalize the performance (*i.e.* percent of the best performance of each year) which could actually show a better improvement in women's performance. Second, we used swimming speed as variable to express swimming performance. However, in swimmers, performance could also be compared using FINA points [23]. The 'FINA Points Table' allows comparisons of results among different events. The FINA Points Table assigns point values to swimming performances, more points for world class performances typically 1000 or more and fewer points for slower performances [23]. For future studies, performance could be better compared using the 'FINA Points Table'. Future studies should investigate temporal trends in other swimming styles to determine whether temporal improvement is a generalized phenomenon. Potentially influential factors such as anthropometric characteristics, training, motivation, and nutrition should be included to elucidate the mechanisms underlying temporal changes in athletic performance [16]. Third, we used a time frame of 18 years (1994 to 2011) and investigated the changes across years using linear and non-linear regression analyses. Interestingly, we found only linear changes for both swimming speed and sex difference. In contrast, Nevill *et al.* [3] and Stanula *et al.* [9] reported non-linear changes in freestyle swimming speeds. However, Nevill *et al.* [3] investigated a time period of 50 years (1957–2006) and Stanula *et al.* [9] of 113 years (1986–2008). The shorter time frame in our study most probably explains why we found linear trends and the other authors [3,9] in contrast non-linear trends. The investigation of longer time frames for breaststroke swimmers might show a non-linear trend in both swimming speed and sex difference in swimming speed.

Conclusion

The results of the present study showed that swimming performance in athletes competing at national and international level improved in freestyle and breaststroke during the 1994–2011 period. The improvement might be related to technological advances, changes in anthropometric and physiological characteristics, improved training methods and competition psychology, improved sports nutrition, and/or increased access to the sport by a larger number of athletes. The sex-related difference in swimming performance did not change significantly over time in breaststroke, or in freestyle swimming by FINA competitors, but increased significantly in Swiss freestyle swimmers. Finally, the sex-related difference in performance declined with increasing race distance in both swim styles.

Competing interests

The authors declare that they have no competing interests.

Authors' contributions

All authors have been involved in collecting data, writing, drafting and revising the manuscript. MW interpreted the data, drafted and revised the manuscript. CAR carried out the data collection, statistical analysis and interpretation. TR participated in its design and revised the manuscript critically for important intellectual content. RL participated in designing and coordinating the study and revised the manuscript critically. BK conceived, designed, coordinated the study and revised the manuscript. All authors read and approved the final manuscript.

Author details

[1]Institute of General Practice and for Health Services Research, University of Zurich, Zurich, Switzerland. [2]Cardiovascular Center Cardiology, University Hospital Zürich, Zürich, Switzerland. [3]INSERM U1093, Faculty of Sport Sciences, University of Burgundy, Dijon, France. [4]Gesundheitszentrum St. Gallen, Vadianstrasse 26, 9001 St. Gallen, Switzerland.

References

1. Chatterjee S, Chatterjee S: **New Lamps for Old: An Exploratory Analysis of Running Times in Olympic Games.** *Appl Statist* 1982, **31**:14–22.
2. Cheuvront SN, Carter R, Deruisseau KC, Moffatt RJ: **Running performance differences between men and women: an update.** *Sports Med* 2005, **35**:1017–1024.
3. Nevill AM, Whyte GP, Holder RL, Peyrebrune M: **Are there limits to swimming world records?** *Int J Sports Med* 2007, **28**:1012–1017.
4. Schulz R, Curnow C: **Peak performance and age among superathletes: track and field, swimming, baseball, tennis, and golf.** *J Gerontol* 1988, **43**:P113–120.
5. Whipp BJ, Ward SA: **Will women soon outrun men?** *Nature* 1992, **355**:25.
6. Seiler S, De Koning JJ, Foster C: **The fall and rise of the gender difference in elite anaerobic performance 1952–2006.** *Med Sci Sports Exerc* 2007, **39**:534–540.
7. Johnson B, Edmonds W, Jain S, Cavazos J: **Analyses of elite swimming performances and their respective between-gender differences over time.** *J Quant Anal Sports* 2009, **5**:1–18.
8. *FINA, website.* http://www.fina.org/H2O/docs/WR_Oct82013.pdf.
9. Stanula A, Maszczyk A, Roczniok R, Pietraszewski P, Ostrowski A, Zając A, Strzała M: **The development and prediction of athletic performance in freestyle swimming.** *J Hum Kinet* 2012, **32**:97–107.
10. Mytton G, Archer D, Thompson K, Gibson AS: **Reliability of retrospective performance data in elite 400-m swimming and 1500-m running.** *Br J Sports Med* 2013, **47**(17):e4.
11. Rüst CA, Knechtle B, Rosemann T, Lepers R: **The changes in age of peak swim speed for elite male and female Swiss freestyle swimmers between 1994 and 2012.** *J Sports Sci* 2014, **32**:248–258.
12. Barbosa TM, Fernandes RJ, Keskinen KL, Vilas-Boas JP: **The influence of stroke mechanics into energy cost of elite swimmers.** *Eur J Appl Physiol* 2008, **103**:139–149.
13. Barbosa TM, Fernandes R, Keskinen KL, Colaço P, Cardoso C, Silva J, Vilas-Boas JP: **Evaluation of the energy expenditure in competitive swimming strokes.** *Int J Sports Med* 2006, **27**:894–899.
14. Wolfrum M, Knechtle B, Rüst CA, Rosemann T, Lepers R: **Sex-related differences and age of peak performance in breaststroke versus freestyle swimming.** *BMC Sports Sci Med Rehabil* 2013, **5**:29.
15. Costa MJ, Bragada JA, Mejias JE, Louro H, Marinho DA, Silva AJ, Barbosa TM: **Tracking the performance, energetics and biomechanics of international versus national level swimmers during a competitive season.** *Eur J Appl Physiol* 2012, **112**:811–820.
16. Costa MJ, Bragada JA, Marinho DA, Silva AJ, Barbosa TM: **Longitudinal interventions in elite swimming: a systematic review based on energetics, biomechanics, and performance.** *J Strength Cond Res* 2012, **26**:2006–2016.
17. Pozo J, Bastien G, Dierick F: **Execution time, kinetics, and kinematics of the mae-geri kick: comparison of national and international standard karate athletes.** *J Sports Sci* 2011, **29**:1553–1561.
18. Jennings DH, Cormack SJ, Coutts AJ, Aughey RJ: **International field hockey players perform more high-speed running than national-level counterparts.** *J Strength Cond Res* 2012, **26**:947–952.
19. Seifert L, Leblanc H, Herault R, Komar J, Button C, Chollet D: **Inter-individual variability in the upper-lower limb breaststroke coordination.** *Hum Mov Sci* 2011, **30**:550–565.
20. Lätt E, Jürimäe T, Mäestu J, Purge P, Rämson R, Haljaste K, Keskinen KL, Rodriguez FA, Jürimäe T: **Physiological, biomechanical and anthropometrical predictors of sprint swimming performance in adolescent swimmers.** *J Sports Sci Med* 2010, **9**:398–404.
21. Psycharakis SG, Cooke CB, Paradisis GP, O'Hara J, Phillips G: **Analysis of selected kinematic and physiological performance determinants during incremental testing in elite swimmers.** *J Strength Cond Res* 2008, **22**:951–957.
22. *Swiss Swimming Federation.* website http://rankings.fsn.ch/.
23. *Fédération Internationale de Natation.* website http://www.fina.org/.
24. Reinboud W: **Linear models can't keep up with sport gender gap.** *Nature* 2004, **432**(7014):147.
25. FINA: *Report from the FINA Dubai, UAE: Swimwear Approval Commission.* 2010:1–12. http://www.fina.org/H2O/docs/misc/Dubai-FINA-Bureau-SAC_1210_v13d_s-2%20in1.pdf.
26. O'Connor LM, Vozenilek JA: **Is it the athlete or the equipment? An analysis of the top swim performances from 1990 to 2010.** *J Strength Cond Res* 2011, **25**:3239–3241.
27. Chatard JC, Wilson B: **Effect of fastskin suits on performance, drag, and energy cost of swimming.** *Med Sci Sports Exerc* 2008, **40**:1149–1154.
28. Caspersen C, Berthelsen PA, Eik M, Pâkozdi C, Kjendlie PL: **Added mass in human swimmers: age and gender differences.** *J Biomech* s, **43**(12):2369–2373.
29. Issurin VB: **New horizons for the methodology and physiology of training periodization.** *Sports Med* 2010, **40**:189–206.
30. Psychountaki M, Psychountaki: **Competitive worries, sport confidence, and performance ratings for young swimmers.** *Percept Mot Skills* 2000, **91**:87.
31. Sheard M, Golby J: **Effect of a psychological skills training program on swimming performance and positive psychological development.** *Int Rev Sport Exerc Psychol* 2006, **4**:149–169.
32. Stellingwerff T, Maughan RJ, Burke LM: **Nutrition for power sports: Middle-distance running, track cycling, rowing, canoeing/kayaking, and swimming.** *J Sports Sci* 2011, **29**:S79–S89.
33. Kagawa M: **Secular changes in growth among Japanese children over 100 years (1900–2000).** *Asia Pac J Clin Nutr* 2011, **20**:180–189.

34. Charles JD, Bejan A: **The evolution of speed, size and shape in modern athletics.** *J Exp Biol* 2009, **212:**2419–2425.
35. Chollet D, Pelayo P, Delaplace C, Tourny C, Sidney M: **Stroking characteristic variations in the 100-M freestyle for male swimmers of differing skill.** *Percept Mot Skills* 1997, **85:**167–177.
36. Seifert L, Chollet D, Chatard JC: **Kinematic changes during a 100-m front crawl: effects of performance level and gender.** *Med Sci Sports Exerc* 2007, **39:**1784–1793.
37. Smith DJ, Norris SR, Hogg JM: **Performance evaluation of swimmers: scientific tools.** *Sports Med* 2002, **32:**539–554.
38. Tanaka H, Seals DR: **Age and gender interactions in physiological functional capacity: insight from swimming performance.** *J Appl Physiol* 1997, **82:**846–851.
39. Zampagni ML, Casino D, Benelli P, Visani A, Marcacci M, De Vito G: **Anthropometric and strength variables to predict freestyle performance times in elite master swimmers.** *J Strength Cond Res* 2008, **22:**1298–1307.
40. Barbosa TM, Costa MJ, Morais JE, Morouço P, Moreira M, Garrido ND, Marinho DA, Silva AJ: **Characterization of speed fluctuation and drag force in young swimmers: A gender comparison.** *Hum Mov Sci* 2013, **32:**1214–1225.
41. Whyte GP, George K, Sharma S, Firoozi S, Stephens N, Senior R, McKenna WJ: **The upper limit of physiological cardiac hypertrophy in elite male and female athletes: the British experience.** *Eur J Appl Physiol* 2004, **92:**592–597.
42. Gastin PB: **Energy system interaction and relative contribution during maximal exercise.** *Sports Med* 2001, **31:**725–741.
43. Maglischo E: *Swimming Fastest.* Champaign: Human Kinetics; 2003.
44. Saavedra JM, Escalante Y, Garcia-Hermoso A, Arellano R, Navarro F: **A 12-year analysis of pacing strategies in 200- and 400-m individual medley in international swimming competitions.** *J Strength Cond Res* 2012, **26:**3289–3296.
45. Berthelot G, Len S, Hellard P: **Technology & swimming: 3 steps beyond physiology.** *Mater Today* 2010, **13:**46–51.
46. SwissSwimming: *Jahresbericht 2011.* Schweizer Schwimmverband; 2011. http://www.swiss-swimming.ch/desktopdefault.aspx/tabid-612/720_read-7404/.
47. Capranica L, Piacentini MF, Halson S, Myburgh KH, Ogasawara E, Millard-Stafford M: **The gender gap in sport performance: equity influences equality.** *Int J Sports Physiol Perform* 2013, **8:**99–103.
48. Havriluk R: *Performance level differences in swimming drag coefficient.* Athens: Paper presented at the VIIth IOC Olympic World Congress on Sport Sciences; 2003.
49. Havriluk R: *Performance level differences in swimming: relative contributions of strength and technique.* Oslo: XIth International Symposium for Biomechanics and Medicine in Swimming; 2010.
50. Lavoie JM, Montpetit RR: **Applied physiology of swimming.** *Sports Med* 1986, **3**(3)**:**165–189.
51. Pendergast DR, Di Prampero PE, Craig AB Jr, Wilson DR, Rennie DW: **Quantitative analysis of the front crawl in men and women.** *J Appl Physiol* 1977, **43:**475–479.
52. Hawley JA, Williams MM: **Relationship between upper body anaerobic power and freestyle swimming performance.** *Int J Sports Med* 1991, **12:**1–5.
53. Morouço P, Neiva H, González-Badillo JJ, Garrido N, Marinho DA, Marques MC: **Associations between dry land strength and power measurements with swimming performance in elite athletes: a pilot study.** *J Hum Kinet* 2011, **29A:**105–112.
54. Gursoy R, Gursoy: **Sex differences in relations of muscle power lung function, and reaction time in athletes.** *Percept Mot Skills* 2010, **110:**714–720.
55. Bam J, Noakes TD, Juritz J, Dennis SC: **Could women outrun men in ultramarathon races?** *Med Sci Sports Exerc* 1997, **29:**244–247.
56. Zingg MA, Karner-Rezek K, Rosemann T, Knechtle B, Lepers R, Rüst CA: **Will women outrun men in ultra-marathon road races from 50 km to 1,000 km?** *Springerplus* 2014, **3:**97.
57. Zingg MA, Rüst CA, Rosemann T, Lepers R, Knechtle B: **Analysis of sex differences in open-water ultra-distance swimming performances in the FINA World Cup races in 5 km, 10 km and 25 km from 2000 to 2012.** *BMC Sports Sci Med Rehabil* 2014, **6:**7.
58. Rüst CA, Lepers R, Rosemann T, Knechtle B: **Will women soon outperform men in open-water ultra-distance swimming in the 'Maratona del Golfo Capri-Napoli'?** *Springerplus* 2014, **3:**86.
59. Knechtle B, Rosemann T, Lepers R, Rüst CA: **Women outperform men in ultra-distance swimming - The 'Manhattan Island Marathon Swim' from 1983 to 2013.** *Int J Sports Physiol Perform* 2014. Epub ahead of print.

2

Cognitive-motor integration deficits in young adult athletes following concussion

Jeffrey A. Brown[1], Marc Dalecki[1,2], Cindy Hughes[1,3], Alison K. Macpherson[1,3] and Lauren E. Sergio[1,2,3,4*]

Abstract

Background: The ability to perform visually-guided motor tasks requires the transformation of visual information into programmed motor outputs. When the guiding visual information does not align spatially with the motor output, the brain processes rules to integrate the information for an appropriate motor response. Here, we look at how performance on such tasks is affected in young adult athletes with concussion history.

Methods: Participants displaced a cursor from a central to peripheral targets on a vertical display by sliding their finger along a touch sensitive screen in one of two spatial planes. The addition of a memory component, along with variations in cursor feedback increased task complexity across conditions.

Results: Significant main effects between participants with concussion history and healthy controls without concussion history were observed in timing and accuracy measures. Importantly, the deficits were distinctly more pronounced for participants with concussion history compared to healthy controls, especially when the brain had to control movements having two levels of decoupling between vision and action. A discriminant analysis correctly classified athletes with a history of concussion based on task performance with an accuracy of 94 %, despite the majority of these athletes being rated asymptomatic by current standards.

Conclusions: These findings correspond to our previous work with adults at risk of developing dementia, and support the use of cognitive motor integration as an enhanced assessment tool for those who may have mild brain dysfunction. Such a task may provide a more sensitive metric of performance relevant to daily function than what is currently in use, to assist in return to play/work/learn decisions.

Keywords: Mild traumatic brain injury, Prediction model, Movement control, Return to play protocol, Eye-hand coordination

Background

Concussion can be defined as a rapid onset brain injury leading to short-lived impairment of neurological function that resolves spontaneously [1]. With concussion, function may be interrupted but there is no obvious structural damage to the brain using current structural neuroimaging techniques [2], although recent imaging and behavioral studies have found alterations in both function and anatomy in particular brain regions following concussion [3–5]. Moreover, concerns over the short and long term effects of the concussion suffered by professional athletes have been highly influential in bringing concerns about concussion in sport to the global scale. Recent media attention has focused on the short-term memory loss, headache, and migraine suffered 10–20 years following concussion in sports such as football and hockey [6]. Recent behavioral studies have found up to a five-fold increase in mild cognitive impairment (MCI) and earlier onset of Alzheimer's disease (AD) among retired football athletes [7]. It is also recognized that concussions are cumulative; once one has had a concussion, it is easier to get another one, with symptoms often lasting longer. For example, football players with three concussions were three times as likely to suffer another one relative to a player with no concussion [8, 9]. The neurological reasons underlying this increased vulnerability are poorly understood.

While at present the Return to Play or Return to Work protocols are fairly well-established, there remains a lack

* Correspondence: lsergio@yorku.ca
[1]School of Kinesiology and Health Science, York University, 357 Bethune College, 4700 Keele Street, Toronto M3J 1P3ON, Canada
[2]Centre for Vision Research, York University, Toronto, Canada
Full list of author information is available at the end of the article

of robust metrics for use by clinicians to thoroughly assess function following a mild brain injury prior to safe resumption of pre-injury activities [1]. Current neurocognitive testing reports (balance, vestibular, oculomotor, symptoms, neuropsychological tests) measure cognitive and motor abilities separately. However, in daily life, and particularly during many sport activities, there occur several situations where the brain needs to integrate both cognition and movement control concurrently. This rule-based motor performance can occur for example when the brain has to decouple vision from action (e.g., gaze and hand motion are in different directions and spatial locations) [10]. One might argue that if the brain is 'pushed' to think and act concurrently following a concussion, there may occur functionally relevant performance deficits, ones which currently used metrics testing cognitive and motor abilities separately do not find. If so, more sensitive performance metrics testing cognitive and motor abilities concurrently could, arguably, reduce the potential for re-injury.

Previously, our group has indeed examined rule-based motor performance ("cognitive-motor integration") in adults affected by age-related mild brain dysfunction [11–14]. Such integration is often required when performing non-standard visuomotor tasks, where a rule is used to align the required motor output to the guiding visual information [15]. A standard task refers to one which involves direct interaction with an object, such as reaching for a coffee cup in front of you; the eye and hand end at the same spatial location. A non-standard task results in different final spatial locations for the eye and hand, such as making a horizontal movement with a computer mouse in order to vertically displace the cursor viewed on the monitor. In our research to date we have observed that reaching and gross motor movements made under congruent, standard conditions are *not* impaired in early Alzheimer's disease (eAD) and mild cognitive impairment (MCI) relative to healthy aging. Significantly, however, we have found that as soon as an element of dissociation is introduced into a reaching task (the guiding visual information is spatially decoupled from the required motor act, such as using a computer mouse or parking a car using a rear-view mirror), eAD performance declines precipitously relative to healthy adults, whose performance also declines but much less so [11, 16]. Our more recent results suggest that adults with MCI, and even healthy adults with a familial dementia risk, also show a decline in performance, albeit less dramatically [12–14]. Thus there appears to be an impaired ability to integrate rules into coordinated motor tasks with the presence of mild brain dysfunction.

To date, there has been little research examining the utility of assessing mild brain dysfunction brought on by concussion using cognitive-motor integration [17]. Concussion's longer term effects on cognitive ability and cognitive-motor integration are poorly understood and not fully characterized. Indeed, there is a limited amount of information on functional problems associated with having a history of concussion. A more sensitive quantification of function post-concussion would in turn assist in return-to-play/work/learn decisions. In the present study, we address this gap in knowledge by studying the performance of university varsity athletes both with a history of concussion and healthy age matched controls without concussion history on a movement coordination task requiring rule integration. Based on our previous work, we hypothesize that cognitive-motor integration is affected in athletes with a history concussion when compared to healthy age-matched controls without concussion history. Specifically we predict that, like older adults at risk for developing dementia, these athletes with concussion history will show degraded movement planning and movement execution performance when there are two or more levels of decoupling between vision and action. To find out, we used in the present study the same cognitive-motor integration task as in our previous work, which has proven to produce valid and reliable data and to be effective at quantifying subtle cognitive-motor integration changes in those at risk of, or in the early stages of dementia [11–13, 16]. Therefore, it was an additional aim of our study to assess the effectiveness of our computer-based task and to find out if we are able to distinguish between participants with concussion history and with no-history of concussion. Here we report that in support of our prediction, athletes with a concussion history - most of whom were asymptomatic by current measures-nevertheless displayed significant performance impairment when required to think and move at the same time.

Methods

Participants

We recruited 18 athletes with a history of concussion (Age: 21.44 ± 4.29 years; 2 female, 16 male) and 17 healthy control participants (Age: 20.44 ± 2.43 years; 9 female, 8 male) for this study. All participants of both groups were recruited from the York Lions varsity sport teams (including football, hockey, rugby, basketball, volleyball, track and field and field hockey) at York University Toronto, ON, Canada. Potential participants were approached during their routine pre-season baseline medical testing, and their concussion history was unknown to the experimenter at the time of testing. The participants were free of neurological conditions excluding concussion history. All participants' concussions were being managed by the York University Sport Medicine team. Within the concussion history participant group, 13 were asymptomatic and were already progressing through the return to play protocols at the time of testing, and five participants were still symptomatic at the time of testing and had not begun the Return to Play protocols. Details for the participants with a history of concussion are summarized in Table 1. All participants signed a consent form to participate in the experiment, approved by the York University review board.

Procedure

While performing the experiment, participants were seated at a desk so that they could comfortably reach a laptop computer with two touch-sensitive screens, one in the vertical and one in the horizontal plane (ACER brand computer, Model: Iconia 6120). For all conditions in the experimental task, participants were instructed to slide their index finger along one of the touch screens in order to displace a cursor as quickly and accurately as possible from a central circle to one of four peripheral targets (all 20 mm diameter) that were presented on the vertical screen. The targets were located 75 mm directly to the left, right, above, or below the home target. A yellow home target was presented in the center of the vertical tablet and participants touched the home target (either directly or with the cursor using the horizontal tablet depending on the condition), which then changed to green. After holding the home target for 4000 ms a red peripheral target was presented and the home target disappeared, serving as a 'go-signal' for participants to look towards the visual target and slide their finger along the touchscreen in order to direct the cursor to the target. Once the cursor reached the peripheral target and remained for 500 ms, it disappeared and the trial ended. The next trial began with the presentation of the home target after an inter trial interval of 2000 ms. To ensure smooth movement of the finger during the experiment task, participants wore a capacitive-touch glove on their preferred hand.

Different experimental conditions with different levels of decoupling of vision and action were used. The decoupling was achieved by either changing the plane on which the finger moved (vertical V, or horizontal H), changing the direction of cursor visual feedback (veridical or 180° rotated R, i.e. to move cursor right, slide finger left.), or inserting a memory delay (M) between target presentation and go signal (cf. Fig. 1a). These conditions were performed in a randomized block design. All combinations of the spatial correspondence, visual feedback, and memory conditions were tested to make seven conditions: V (vertical), VR (vertical rotated), VM (vertical memory delay), VRM (vertical rotated memory delay), H (horizontal), HR (horizontal rotated), and HM (horizontal memory delay). There were a total of 140 trials for each participant (4 directions × 5 trials × 7 conditions). Note that within the seven conditions only V represents

Table 1 Characteristics and concussion incidence for participants with concussion history

Part.	Age	# of Conc.	Time since last Conc. (months)	Symp./Asymp.	Symptoms	Sport
1	21	1	2	Asymp.	-	B
2	19	1	7	Asymp.	-	H
3	34	8	5	Symp.	Headache, light-sensitivity, fatigue	H
4	20	3	0.5	Asymp.	-	H
5	22	6	15	Asymp.	-	F
6	19	2	0.5	Asymp.	-	H
7	18	1	84	Asymp.	-	F
8	20	1	0.75	Symp.	Headache, dizziness	V
9	27	1	0.25	Symp.	Headache, light-sensitivity, dizziness	NV
10	22	1	6	Asymp.	-	F
11	18	2	9	Asymp.	-	F
12	23	3	48	Asymp.	-	F
13	20	2	48	Asymp.	-	F
14	18	1	108	Asymp.	-	F
15	21	1	0.25	Asymp.	-	FH
16	18	1	0.5	Symp.	Headache	R
17	28	1	0.1	Symp.	Headache	NV
18	18	4	1	Asymp.	-	F
Mean ± SD	21.4 ± 4.3	2.2 ± 1.9	18.66 ± 32.07			

Part. participant, *#* number, *Conc.* concussion, *Symp.* symptomatic, *Asympt* asymptomatic, *B* basketball, *H* hockey, *F* football, *V* volleyball, *NV* non-varsity, *FH* field hockey, *R* rugby

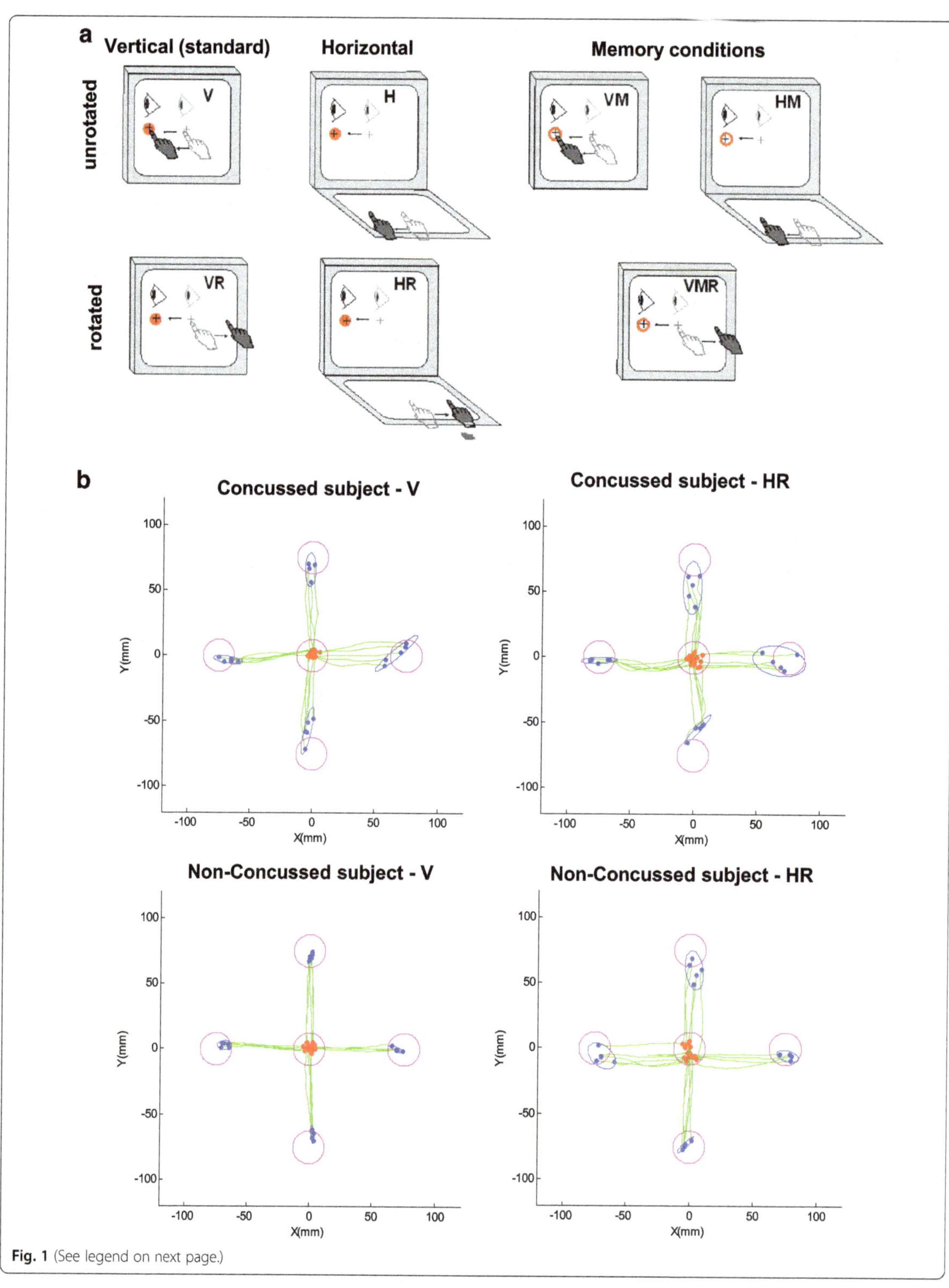

Fig. 1 (See legend on next page.)

(See figure on previous page.)
Fig. 1 Drawing of experimental conditions and example of typical hand path data. **a** Schematic drawing of the experimental conditions. Visual stimuli were presented on the vertical monitor for all conditions. Light grey cursor, eye, and hand symbols denote the starting position for each trial (home target). Dark grey eye and hand symbols denote the instructed eye and hand movements for each task. Red circles denote the peripheral (reach) target, presented randomly in one of four locations (left, up, right, down). The dark crosshair denotes the cursor feedback provided during each condition. The open circles denote the cued position before the movement (seen in memory conditions). **b** Typical hand path data of one participant with concussion history and one participant with no-history of concussion performing the V and HR condition. Note the poorer performance in condition HR compared to V, particularly in the concussed participant

a standard visuomotor mapping, where eye and hand movements were congruent in direction and plane. All other conditions required cognitive-motor integration in order to successfully perform a movement where the effector was decoupled from the guiding visual information. In the memory conditions, the target center appeared, and once the participants positioned the cursor in the central target, the peripheral target stayed for 2000 ms, followed by the removal of the peripheral target. The participants had to hold the cursor within the target for an additional 2000 ms and then it disappeared, serving as a go signal to move to the remembered target location.

Prior to each experimental condition, participants were allowed two practice trials in each direction (i.e., eight practice trials for each condition). Due to the possibility of cervical soft-tissue injury following concussion and the need for portability, eye-tracking was not feasible. Participant's eye movements were monitored by the experimenter and if incorrect movements were made in the non-standard conditions, participants were reminded to always look towards the target and not at their hand; these trials were excluded from further data analyzing.

Data processing and analysis

Movement trajectories and timing

The custom-written (C++) acquisition software used the touch-screen computer's internal CPU clock to align the finger's X-Y screen position to exact sampling times. The sampling rate was approximately 55 Hz. Individual movements paths derived from the cursor location were first low-pass Butterworth filtered at 10Hz (filfilt function, Matlab, Mathworks Inc.). Custom software was then used to generate a computerized velocity profile of each trial's movement, with movement onset and end being recorded at 10 % peak velocity. These profiles were then verified by visual inspection and corrections were performed when necessary. Reaction time (RT) was calculated as the time interval (milliseconds; ms) between the central target disappearance and the point at which the finger velocity reached 10 % peak velocity. Movement time (MT) was the time (milliseconds; ms) between onset and offset, thereby representing the 'ballistic' initial movement without corrective adjustments. Pathlength (PL) was recorded for each trial, and was quantified as the distance (millimeter; mm) between start and the first correction of the initial cursor movement. The constant error (CE, i.e., movement accuracy) was determined as the distance (millimeter; mm) between the average movement endpoint for each target location (Σ x/n, Σ y/n) and the actual target central location. Variable error (VE, i.e., movement precision), was determined as the distance (millimeter; mm) between the endpoints of the individual movements (σ2) from their mean movement endpoint.

Direction reversals and task completion error counts

Direction reversals errors (DR) were calculated when there was a deviation of more than ±45° from the line between center of central and peripheral target during the first half of each movement. Failed trials were counted for each condition. Failures were: failure to start trial within 10,000 ms of onset, failure to remain in the central target for 2000 ms (4000 ms M conditions), leaving start < 150 ms after the go signal, leaving the start > 5,000 ms after the go signal, or exceeding the maximum movement time to a target (>10,000 ms).

Statistical analyses

For all dependent variables, main effects of Group (Non-history, Concussion history) and Condition (V, VR, VM, VRM, H, HR, HM) were analyzed using repeated-measures mixed ANOVA. Additionally, initial separate analyses using sex or symptomatic/asymptomatic as a main effect were run. Trials whose value was >2 standard deviations (SDs) away from the mean for a given condition in a given group were considered outliers and removed before statistical analysis. All remaining data were checked for normal distribution (Shapiro-Wilk's test) and sphericity (Mauchly's test), and were Greenhouse-Geisser corrected where necessary. Statistical significance levels were set to 0.05, and all analyses were performed using SPSS software (IBM corp.).

Level of dissociation

We grouped the conditions by 'level of eye-hand dissociation' in order to test our hypothesis that performance declines would be significant for only the most decoupled situations. For this analysis, we compared participants' performance as a function of their change from the most direct condition (no decoupling, standard mapping), similar to our previous studies. Specifically, we subtracted out the result on the V condition from the other six conditions for a given dependent measure. We grouped these six 'delta' conditions into 1 level (VM, H, VR) and 2 levels (HM, VRM, HR) of dissociation and performed a repeated-measures mixed ANOVA with the within factor Level (1 level, 2 levels) and the between factor Group (No-history, Concussion history).

Discriminant analysis

In order to test if our task was sensitive enough to predict a presence of concussion history based on performance, we performed separate stepwise discriminant analyses testing different combinations of dependent measures between the no-history of concussion and the concussion history group.

Results

The two analyses using sex or symptomatic/asymptomatic status as a main effect yielded no significant differences for any dependent variable (all $p > 0.05$), supporting the decision to merge data across sexes and status. Examples of typical movement trajectories of one subject with concussion history and one subject with no-history of concussion performing the V and HR conditions are presented in Fig. 1b-e. Statistical outcomes of the repeated mixed measures ANOVA for Group (No-history, Concussion history) and Condition (V, VR, VM, VRM, H, HR, HM) and significant pair-wise comparisons are summarized in Table 2, and the according descriptive statistics in Table 3.

Table 2 Statistical outcome repeated-measures mixed ANOVA of Group (Concussion history, No-history) and Condition (V, VR, VM, VRM, H, HR, HM) for all dependent variables (RT, MT, PL, CE, VE, DR)

Parameter	Group	Condition	Group × Condition
RT	$F(1,33) = 9.28^{**}$	$F(6, 198) = 20.77^{***}$	$F(6, 198) = 1.56^{n.s.}$
MT	$F(1,33) = 15.25^{***}$	$F(6, 198) = 11.79^{***}$	$F(6, 198) = 3.59^{**}$
PL	$F(1,33) = 3.75^{n.s.}$	$F(6, 198) = 2.94^{**}$	$F(6, 198) = 0.53^{n.s.}$
CE	$F(1,33) = 1.55^{n.s.}$	$F(6, 198) = 10.30^{***}$	$F(6, 198) = 0.84^{n.s.}$
VE	$F(1,33) = 1.15^{n.s.}$	$F(6, 198) = 12.30^{***}$	$F(6, 198) = 3.30^{**}$
DR	$F(1,33) = 1.80^{n.s.}$	$F(6, 198) = 1.13^{n.s.}$	$F(6, 198) = 0.64^{n.s.}$
Parameter	**Condition**	**Group**	
RT	VR	$F(1,33) = 5.48^{*}$	
	VM	$F(1,33) = 6.70^{*}$	
	VRM	$F(1,33) = 7.51^{*}$	
	HM	$F(1,33) = 13.50^{**}$	
MT	V	$F(1,33) = 7.38^{*}$	
	VRM	$F(1,33) = 19.47^{***}$	
	H	$F(1,33) = 7.32^{*}$	
	HM	$F(1,33) = 9.62^{**}$	
VE	V	$F(1,33) = 10.53^{**}$	
	VR	$F(1,33) = 8.94^{**}$	
	H	$F(1,33) = 17.63^{***}$	
	HR	$F(1,33) = 4.52^{*}$	

Significant outcomes of pair-wise comparisons for Group (Concussion history, No-history) of all variables and conditions
RT reaction time, *MT* movement time, *CE* endpoint accuracy, *VE* endpoint precision, *DR* direction reversal errors, *PL* pathlength, *V* vertical, *VR* vertical rotated, *VM* vertical memory, *VRM* vertical rotated memory, *H* horizontal, *HR* horizontal rotated, *HM* horizontal memory, *n.s.* non significant. Asterisks represent * < 0.05, ** < 0.01, *** < 0.001

Performance timing

Repeated-measures mixed ANOVA revealed significant effects for RT for both Group ($p < 0.01$) and Condition ($p < 0.001$), but not for Group × Condition ($p > 0.05$). ANOVA yielded a main effect of Group ($p < 0.001$) and Condition ($p < 0.001$) for MT and a Group × Condition interaction ($p < 0.01$). Pair-wise comparisons of Group showed significant differences between no-history and concussion history for RT in condition VR ($p < 0.05$), VM ($p < 0.05$), VRM ($p < 0.05$) and HM ($p < 0.01$), and for MT in condition V ($p < 0.05$), VRM ($p < 0.001$), H ($p < 0.05$) and HM ($p < 0.01$). Both performance timing measures, RT and MT increased with increasing task difficulty, and were, across conditions, longer for concussion history participants compared to healthy controls with no-history of concussion (cf. Fig. 2a, b).

Performance execution

Repeated-measures mixed ANOVA revealed significant effects of PL for Condition ($p < 0.01$), both not for Group and Group × Condition (both $p > 0.05$). Repeated-measures mixed ANOVA for CE (i.e. movement accuracy) revealed a main effect of Condition ($p < 0.001$), but no effects of Group and Group × Condition (both $p > 0.05$). Repeated-measures mixed ANOVA for VE (i.e. movement precision) revealed a main effect of Condition ($p < 0.001$), and an interaction between Group × Condition ($p < 0.01$), but no significant effect of Group ($p > 0.05$). Pair-wise comparisons showed no significant Group differences of PL for all variables (all $p < 0.05$), but significant differences between no-history and concussion history group for VE in condition V ($p < 0.01$), VR ($p < 0.01$), H ($p < 0.001$) and HR ($p < 0.05$). Increasing the task complexity lengthened the pathlength, and had a detrimental effect on endpoint accuracy and precision. Endpoint accuracy (CE) and endpoint precision (VE) decreased both with task difficulty for no-history and concussion history participants, however endpoint precision (VE) was lower for the participants with concussion history (cf. Fig. 2c).

Table 3 Descriptive statistics of main repeated-mixed ANOVA for all conditions vand groups (Concussion history, No-history) of all dependent variables (RT, MT, PL, CE, VE, DR)

Parameter	Condition	No-history	Concussion history
		[ms]	[ms]
RT	V	392.04 ± 90.98	426.82 ± 65.90
	VR	470.86 ± 69.63	548.87 ± 119.50
	VM	376.45 ± 105.34	466.05 ± 99.49
	VRM	369.49 ± 88.06	451.99 ± 89.04
	H	403.92 ± 87.56	443.80 ± 92.98
	HR	497.75 ± 98.40	536.55 ± 62.10
	HM	336.76 ± 74.29	440.56 ± 91.41
MT	V	336.53 ± 91.07	436.03 ± 122.31
	VR	475.99 ± 178.49	554.01 ± 160.76
	VM	466.45 ± 247.88	550.76 ± 174.42
	VRM	450.10 ± 163.19	775.07 ± 225.34
	H	402.15 ± 189.70	573.52 ± 184.97
	HR	526.44 ± 278.17	710.44 ± 270.83
	HM	427.62 ± 192.04	680.46 ± 279.42
		[mm]	[mm]
PL	V	88.88 ± 4.58	89.21 ± 2.91
	VR	88.57 ± 6.00	89.51 ± 6.27
	VM	89.88 ± 5.61	92.03 ± 5.03
	VRM	88.95 ± 8.98	90.18 ± 4.66
	H	84.40 ± 7.66	88.27 ± 6.82
	HR	87.60 ± 5.44	90.70 ± 5.53
	HM	86.89 ± 4.96	88.34 ± 5.05
CE	V	10.67 ± 2.93	9.51 ± 2.90
	VR	14.05 ± 3.14	14.88 ± 4.84
	VM	10.87 ± 3.17	10.73 ± 3.86
	VRM	12.70 ± 3.16	15.13 ± 5.27
	H	13.04 ± 4.53	15.51 ± 4.44
	HR	14.02 ± 3.55	15.58 ± 4.63
	HM	12.84 ± 4.09	13.67 ± 4.46
VE	V	6.90 ± 1.17	9.71 ± 3.38
	VR	6.53 ± 1.51	8.35 ± 2.04
	VM	9.41 ± 1.78	9.95 ± 2.93
	VRM	10.27 ± 1.91	10.07 ± 3.10
	H	6.77 ± 1.12	10.45 ± 3.44
	HR	8.01 ± 2.79	9.88 ± 2.40
	HM	8.18 ± 1.81	8.16 ± 2.30
		[count]	[count]
DR	V	0.00 ± 0.00	0.17 ± 0.38
	VR	0.18 ± 0.53	0.44 ± 1.25
	VM	0.12 ± 0.33	0.06 ± 0.24
	VRM	0.00 ± 0.00	0.28 ± 0.75
	H	0.06 ± 0.24	0.00 ± 0.00
	HR	0.12 ± 0.33	0.28 ± 0.96
	HM	0.06 ± 0.24	0.17 ± 0.51

RT reaction time (ms), *MT* movement time (ms), *CE* endpoint accuracy (% target distance), *VE* endpoint precision (% target distance), *DR* direction reversal errors (count), *PL* pathlength (mm), *V* vertical, *VR* vertical rotated, *VM* vertical memory, *VRM* vertical rotated memory, *H* horizontal, *HR* horizontal rotated, *HM* horizontal memory

Direction reversals, and Task Completion Error Counts

Repeated-measures mixed ANOVA for direction reversals revealed no significant effects of Condition, Group or Group × Condition (all p > 0.05). We also did not find any significant group differences in the number of remaining error types (all p > 0.05).

Performance as a Function of Level of Dissociation

Statistical outcomes of the repeated mixed measures ANOVA for the level of dissociation are summarized in Table 4, and descriptive statistics for all dependent variables of Group and Level are summarized in Table 5. We observed a main effect of Group (No-history, Concussion history) for RT ($p < 0.05$) and CE ($p < 0.05$), a main effect of Level (1 level, 2 levels) for MT ($p < 0.001$), and notably a significant Group × Level interaction for MT ($p < 0.001$) and VE ($p < 0.05$). Pair-wise comparisons of Group showed significant differences between no-history and concussion history participants of MT for 2 levels ($p < 0.01$), of CE for 1 level and 2 levels (both $p < 0.05$), and of VE for 1 level ($p < 0.05$).

Most importantly, the change between non-standard-mapping and standard mapping condition for MT increased dramatically in the concussion history group in going from 1 level of dissociation to 2 levels of dissociation, while there was no significant MT increase in no-history control participants' MT (cf. Fig. 3 and Table. 5). Across groups, the change between non-standard-mapping and standard mapping condition for MT was significant longer in the 2 level (203.743 ± 25.05 ms) than in the 1 level (117.54 ± 18.17 ms) condition. Across levels, the change between non-standard-mapping and standard mapping condition for RT was significantly longer in the concussion history (54.42 ± 12.17 ms) compared to no-history of concussion group (17.17 ± 12.52 ms), and movement accuracy (CE) was significantly less in the concussion history group (4.75 ± 0.68 mm) compared to no-history controls (2.25 ± 0.70 mm). Interestingly, movement precision (VE) showed the opposite effect, increasing from a very small amount (precise) for no-history control participants in the 1 level condition to a much greater amount (imprecise) in the 2 level condition ($p < 0.05$), an increase not seen for concussion

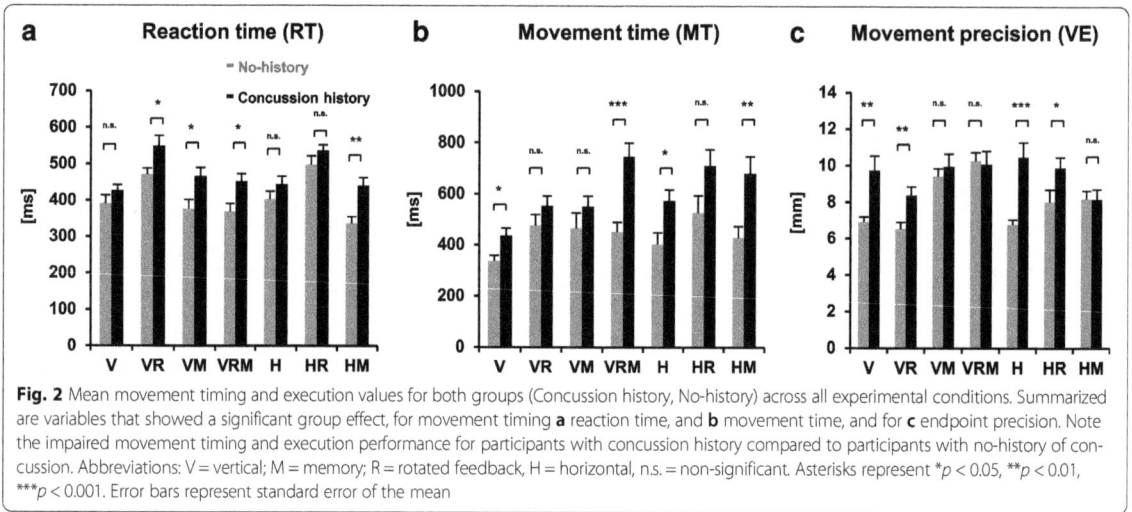

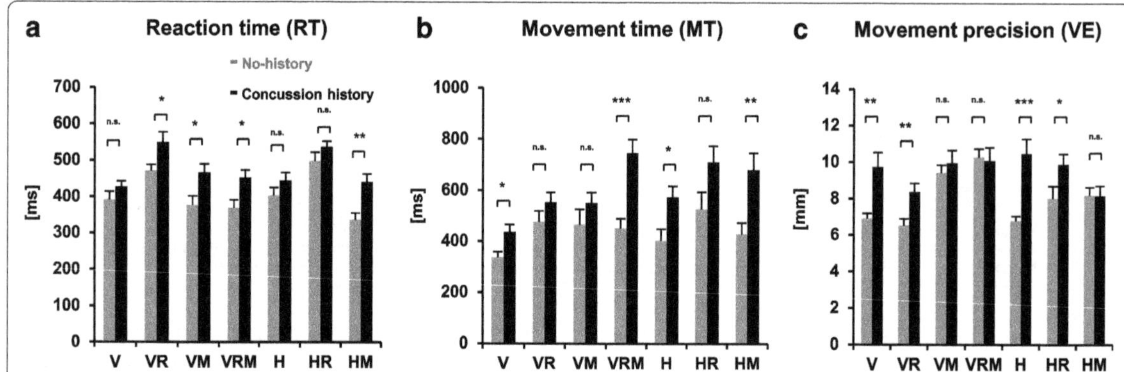

Fig. 2 Mean movement timing and execution values for both groups (Concussion history, No-history) across all experimental conditions. Summarized are variables that showed a significant group effect, for movement timing **a** reaction time, and **b** movement time, and for **c** endpoint precision. Note the impaired movement timing and execution performance for participants with concussion history compared to participants with no-history of concussion. Abbreviations: V = vertical; M = memory; R = rotated feedback, H = horizontal, n.s. = non-significant. Asterisks represent $*p < 0.05$, $**p < 0.01$, $***p < 0.001$. Error bars represent standard error of the mean

history participants, whose values were in the middle range relative to no-history control performance (cf. Tab. 5).

Discriminant analysis

The discriminant analysis performed for the concussion history group demonstrated good separation from the no-history control group. Based on the outcome of the dependent variable analyses, the predictors supplied to the discriminant function classifying concussion history *versus* no-history control participants were VE and MT in the H condition, and MT in the VRM condition. Using these variables, the outcome of the discriminant analyses showed that our assessment tool was able to discriminate athletes with a history of concussion from athletes with no-history of concussion with an accuracy of 94 % (for details please see Table. 6 and Fig. 4).

Table 4 Statistical outcome of repeated-measures mixed ANOVA for Level (1 level, 2 levels) and Group (Concussion history, No-history)

Parameter	Group	Level	Group × Level
RT	F (1,33) = 4.55*	F (1,33) = 2.05$^{n.s.}$	F (1,33) = 0.10$^{n.s.}$
MT	F (1,33) = 3.77$^{n.s.}$	F (1,33) = 25.05***	F (1,33) = 14.84***
PL	F (1,33) = 1.32$^{n.s.}$	F (1,33) = 0.00$^{n.s.}$	F (1,33) = 0.09$^{n.s.}$
CE	F (1,33) = 6.509*	F (1,33) = 3.38$^{n.s.}$	F (1,33) = 0.40$^{n.s.}$
VE	F (1,33) = 2.76$^{n.s.}$	F (1,33) = 2.85$^{n.s.}$	F (1,33) = 5.75*
DR	F (1,33) = 0.23$^{n.s.}$	F (1,33) = 0.00$^{n.s.}$	F (1,33) = 0.49$^{n.s.}$
Parameter	Level	Condition effect	
MT	2 levels	F (1,33) = 8.31**	
CE	1 level	F (1,33) = 5.54*	
CE	2 levels	F (1,33) = 5.45*	
VE	2 levels	F (1,33) = 6.53*	

Level represent dependent variable values averaged across one (VM, H, HM) and two levels (VR, VRM, HR) of dissociation between vision and action, distracted from V

Significant outcomes of pair-wise comparisons for Group (Concussion history, No-history) of all variables and both levels (1 level, 2 levels)

RT reaction time, *MT* movement time, *CE* endpoint accuracy, *VE* endpoint precision, *DR* direction reversal errors, *PL* pathlength, *V* vertical, *VR* vertical rotated, *VM* vertical memory, *VRM* vertical rotated memory, *H* horizontal, *HR* horizontal rotated, *HM* horizontal memory, *n.s.* non significant. Asterisks represent * < 0.05, ** < 0.01, *** < 0.001

Table 5 Descriptive statistics of the ANOVA for 1 level and 2 levels of disassociation for both groups (Concussion history, No-history)

Parameter	Level	Concussed	Non-concussed
		[ms]	[ms]
RT	1 level	59.42 ± 55.12	25.03 ± 50.98
	2 levels	49.43 ± 58.23	9.29 ± 66.83
MT	1 level	123.41 ± 79.55	111.67 ± 130.73
	2 levels	275.96 ± 152.01	131.53 ± 143.85
		[mm]	[mm]
PL	1 level	−1.26 ± 4.91	0.73 ± 3.48
	2 levels	−1.06 ± 6.67	0.54 ± 4.43
CE	1 level	4.20 ± 2.59	1.99 ± 2.97
	2 levels	5.29 ± 3.49	2.52 ± 3.53
VE	1 level	−0.13 ± 4.02	0.67 ± 1.61
	2 levels	−0.34 ± 3.35	1.92 ± 1.47
		[count]	[count]
DR	1 level	0.00 ± 0.30	0.12 ± 0.26
	2 levels	0.07 ± 0.72	0.06 ± 0.13

RT reaction time, *MT* movement time, *CE* endpoint accuracy, *VE* endpoint precision, *DR* direction reversal errors, *PL* pathlength, 1 *level* mean across conditions requiring 1 level of disassociation between vision and action, 2 *levels* mean across conditions requiring 2 levels of disassociation between vision and action

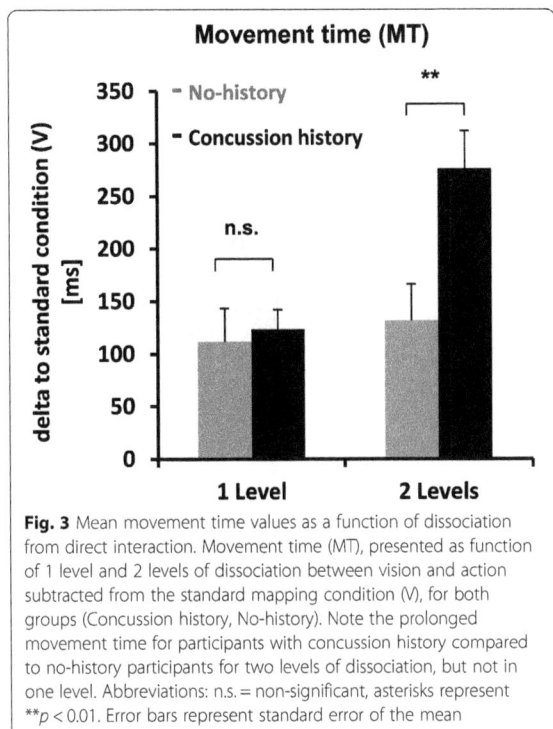

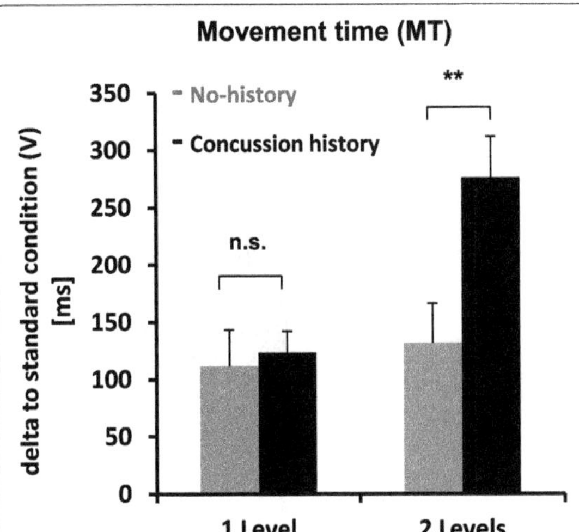

Fig. 3 Mean movement time values as a function of dissociation from direct interaction. Movement time (MT), presented as function of 1 level and 2 levels of dissociation between vision and action subtracted from the standard mapping condition (V), for both groups (Concussion history, No-history). Note the prolonged movement time for participants with concussion history compared to no-history participants for two levels of dissociation, but not in one level. Abbreviations: n.s. = non-significant, asterisks represent $^{**}p < 0.01$. Error bars represent standard error of the mean

DISCUSSION

The main aim of this study was to determine whether participants with a history of concussion had deficits in a cognitive-motor integration task when compared to healthy controls without a history of concussion. A second aim of this study was to assess the effectiveness of our computer-based task to detect cognitive-motor integration deficits in participants with concussion history, which has proven effective at quantifying subtle cognitive-motor integration changes in those at risk of, or in the early stages of dementia [11–13, 16]. We observed differences in performance on complex visuomotor tasks between varsity-level athletes with a history of concussion and healthy age-matched adults with no-history of concussion. Specifically, participants with a concussion history had difficulty executing visually-guided movements when there was a single level of dissociation between the guiding visual information and the required motor action. In support of our hypothesis, participants with a concussion history also displayed both impaired movement planning and execution when the brain had to control a movement with the highest level of dissociation between vision and action. Notably, our assessment tool was able to discriminate between athletes with a history of concussion – most of whom are asymptomatic by current measures–and athletes with no-history of concussion with 94 % accuracy.

Table 6 Classification results [a,c] of stepwise discriminant analyses

		Group	Predicted Group Membership		Total
			Conc.	Control	
Original	Count	Conc.-H.	16	1	17
		No-H.	2	16	18
	%	Conc.-H.	94.1	5.9	100
		No-H.	11.1	88.9	100
Classification[b]	Count	Conc.-H.	15	2	17
		No-H.	2	16	18
	%	Conc.-H.	88.2	11.8	100
		No-H.	11.1	88.9	100

[a]91.4 % of original grouped cases correctly classified
[b]Cross validation is done only for those cases in the analysis. In cross validation, each case is classified by the functions derived from all cases other than that case
[c]88.6 % of cross-validated grouped cases correctly classified
Conc.-H. concussion history, *No-H.* no-history of concussion

Our present findings complement those of our previous studies on adults at-risk (through an MCI diagnosis or family history) for the development of Alzheimer's disease [12, 13]. While similar behavioural deficits between these otherwise very different groups do not mean the mechanism underlying motor impairment is the same, it does suggest that young athletes with a history of concussion are neurologically fragile, even when they are asymptomatic and in the late period of the return to play/work schedule. A task which 'pushes the system' appears to bring out behavioural deficits across a range of mild brain dysfunction. We propose that the present results reflect a problem in the *communication* between brain regions responsible for planning and executing skilled movement when there is an element of cognition involved. This proposal is based on recent work on brain networks for cognitive-motor integration in both human- and non-human primates [14, 18–24]. In particular, our behavioural results may arise from impairments in parietal-frontal networks as well as communication between cortical and subcortical movement control regions due to cellular damages following concussion. Cellular changes are well known following concussion, with an initial reduction in cerebral blood flow and cerebral glucose utilization followed by membrane depolarization and excess excitatory neurotransmitter release [25–28]. Such changes could lead to problems in ATP metabolism [28] and in long-term potentiation (LTP) of the brain [29–31]. While the long-term effects of subtle hypoxia on brain tissue are not fully understood, it is becoming increasingly clear that oxidative stress may trigger neuropathological processes both local and distal to the site of mild brain contusion, effects which may only manifest themselves months to years later [31]. Indeed, recent studies of brain metabolism in adults with concussion history have found

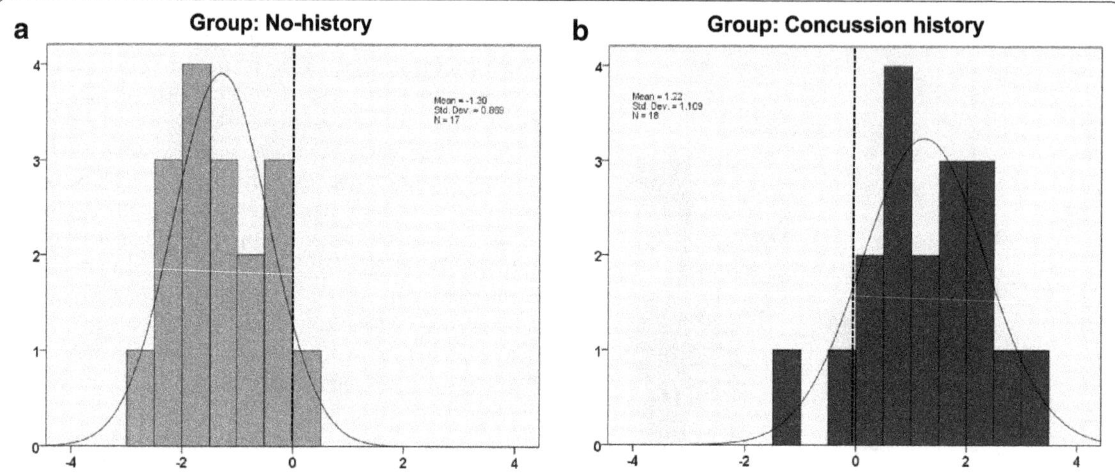

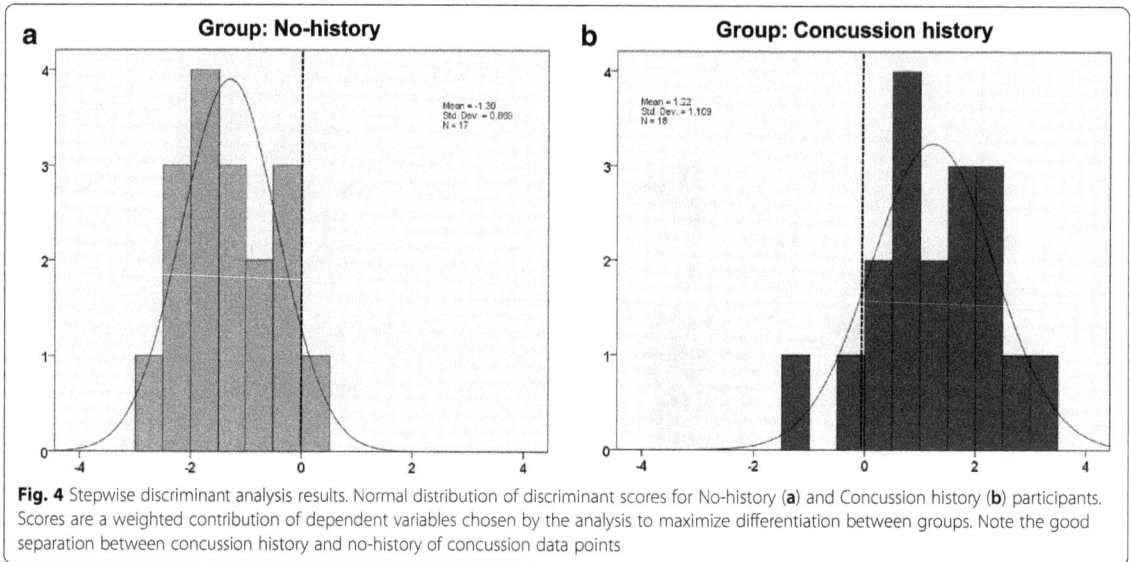

Fig. 4 Stepwise discriminant analysis results. Normal distribution of discriminant scores for No-history (**a**) and Concussion history (**b**) participants. Scores are a weighted contribution of dependent variables chosen by the analysis to maximize differentiation between groups. Note the good separation between concussion history and no-history of concussion data points

concurrent motor skill deficits and primary motor cortex metabolism abnormalities related to deficits in motor learning [32]. Lingering abnormalities in not only individual brain areas but the pathways between them may thus underly problems in more complex behaviour manifested following concussion.

In support of our proposal, imaging and brain function studies have found alterations in both function and anatomy in particular brain regions following concussion. Studies have found increased and more widespread activation of pre-frontal cortex (PFC), dorsolateral prefrontal cortex, and cerebellum for a variety of tasks in concussed *versus* non-concussed populations [3–5]. These authors suggested that the additional and more elaborate network activations may reflect compensatory mechanisms to accommodate functional and/or structural deficits in the brain's default networks as a result of concussion. In terms of networks that may relate specifically to cognitive-motor integration, imaging studies have found increased activation in parietal, frontal, as well as cerebellar regions in concussed individuals compared to pre-injury fMRI data, although no cognitive performance deficits were noted [33]. Further, recent anatomical studies have found altered white matter integrity in concussed adolescents, younger adults with concussion history, and older adults with concussion history that involved those pathways connecting frontal and parietal regions [34–37]. These data complement our group's findings on the crucial role played by such fronto-parietal networks in integrating thought and action [10, 14, 19, 20, 38].

A notable aspect to the group of athletes examined in this study is that the majority of our athletes with a concussion history were classified as "asymptomatic" by current testing standards (computerized cognitive testing alone, balance/coordination testing alone), which suggests that the current testing standards are examining individual brain regions. When one is forced to integrate one's behavior across the traditionally segregated domains of cognition and action, something which athletes and skilled workers are often called upon to do in the course of their actual activities, the integrity of brain connections between regions is likely crucial for successful performance. We suggest that multi-domain tasks such as the one used here are more effective at assessing function prior to a return to activity, in that they allow one to test communication between brain regions needed for the control of complex skilled action. Further studies are needed to better understand the detailed neural mechanisms that are involved in cognitive-motor integration following concussion. These further studies should taking into account number of concussions and aspects of one's medical history, specifics of the concussive event itself, as well as severity and time since last concussion.

Conclusions

The present data suggest that our cognitive-motor integration task is able to sensitively detect concussion-related functional performance changes, important for the safe return to play/work. Additionally, our assessment tool was able to discriminate between athletes with concussion history–most of whom are asymptomatic by current measures–and athletes with no-history of concussion with 94 % accuracy. This type of evaluation in domains crucial for safe performance (e.g. sports, military, industry, rehabilitation settings) represents a clinically efficient approach to concussion recovery assessment. Based on our "level of disassociation" analysis, it is feasible to reduce the experiment conditions used here (i.e., one standard-mapping condition and one non-standard mapping condition requiring two levels of disassociation), to allow a simple, quick assessment tool for the both clinical and field settings.

Competing interests

The authors declare that they have no financial or non-financial competing interests in relation to this manuscript.

Authors' contributions

JB carried out the data collection, initial data analysis, and drafted the manuscript. MD contributed to the data analysis and manuscript preparation. CH assisted in study design, data collection, and study coordination. AM assisted with data analysis and manuscript preparation. LS conceived of the study, and participated in its design, data collection, data analysis, and manuscript preparation. All authors read and approved the final manuscript.

Acknowledgements

The authors gratefully acknowledge Laura Cruz, MD and Tracey Meloche, CATA for their assistance with the athletes, and the York University Lions organization. Funding provided by the Ontario Neurotrauma Foundation (JB), Canadian Institutes of Health Research operating grant #125915 (LS, AM), and the Donald Sanderson Memorial Trust (LS, AM, CH).

Author details

[1]School of Kinesiology and Health Science, York University, 357 Bethune College, 4700 Keele Street, Toronto M3J 1P3ON, Canada. [2]Centre for Vision Research, York University, Toronto, Canada. [3]York University Sport Medicine Team, York University, Toronto, Canada. [4]Southlake Regional Health Centre, Newmarket, ON, Canada.

References

1. McCrory P, Meeuwisse WH, Aubry M, Cantu RC, Dvořák J, Echemendia RJ, et al. Consensus statement on concussion in sport: the 4th International Conference on Concussion in Sport held in Zurich, November 2012. Br J Sports Med. 2013;47(5):250–8.
2. McCrory P, Johnston KM, Mohtadi NG, Meeuwisse W. Evidence-based review of sport-related concussion: basic science. Clin J Sport Med. 2001;11(3):160–5.
3. McAllister TW, Sparling MB, Flashman LA, Guerin SJ, Mamourian AC, Saykin AJ. Differential working memory load effects after mild traumatic brain injury. Neuroimage. 2001;14(5):1004–12.
4. Chen J-K, Johnston KM, Frey S, Petrides M, Worsley K, Ptito A. Functional abnormalities in symptomatic concussed athletes: an fMRI study. Neuroimage. 2004;22(1):68–82.
5. Zhang K, Johnson B, Pennell D, Ray W, Sebastianelli W, Slobounov S. Are functional deficits in concussed individuals consistent with white matter structural alterations: combined FMRI & DTI study. Exp Brain Res. 2010;204(1):57–70.
6. Meehan 3rd WP, Bachur RG. Sport-related concussion. Pediatrics. 2009;123(1):114.
7. Guskiewicz KM, Marshall SW, Bailes J, McCrea M, Cantu RC, Randolph C, et al. Association between recurrent concussion and late-life cognitive impairment in retired professional football players. Neurosurgery. 2005;57(4):719–26.
8. Guskiewicz KM, McCrea M, Marshall SW, Cantu RC, Randolph C, Barr W, et al. Cumulative effects associated with recurrent concussion in collegiate football players: the NCAA Concussion Study. JAMA. 2003;290(19):2549–55.
9. Karlin AM. Concussion in the pediatric and adolescent population: "different population, different concerns.". PM R. 2011;3(10 Suppl 2):S369–79.
10. Gorbet DJ, Sergio LE. The behavioural consequences of dissociating the spatial directions of eye and arm movements. Brain Res. 2009;1284:77–88.
11. Tippett WJ, Krajewski A, Sergio LE. Visuomotor integration is compromised in Alzheimer's disease patients reaching for remembered targets. Eur Neurol. 2007;58(1):1–11.
12. Salek Y, Anderson ND, Sergio L. Mild cognitive impairment is associated with impaired visual-motor planning when visual stimuli and actions are incongruent. Eur Neurol. 2011;66(5):283–93.
13. Hawkins KM, Sergio LE. Visuomotor impairments in older adults at increased Alzheimer's disease risk. J Alzheimers Dis. 2014;42(2):607–21.
14. Hawkins KM, Goyal AI, Sergio LE. Diffusion tensor imaging correlates of cognitive-motor decline in normal aging and increased Alzheimer's disease risk. J Alzheimers Dis. 2015;44(3):867–78.
15. Wise SP, Di Pellegrino G, Boussaoud D. The premotor cortex and nonstandard sensorimotor mapping. Can J Physiol Pharmacol. 1996;74(4):469–82.
16. Tippett WJ, Sergio LE. Visuomotor integration is impaired in early stage Alzheimer's disease. Brain Res. 2006;1102(1):92–102.
17. Locklin J, Bunn L, Roy E, Danckert J. Measuring deficits in visually guided action post-concussion. Sports Med. 2010;40(3):183–7.
18. Hawkins KM, Sayegh P, Yan X, Crawford JD, Sergio LE. Neural activity in superior parietal cortex during rule-based visual-motor transformations. J Cogn Neurosci. 2013;25(3):436–54.
19. Sayegh PF, Hawkins KM, Hoffman KL, Sergio LE. Differences in spectral profiles between rostral and caudal premotor cortex when hand-eye actions are decoupled. J Neurophysiol. 2013;110(4):952–63.
20. Sayegh PF, Hawkins KM, Neagu B, Crawford JD, Hoffman KL, Sergio LE. Decoupling the actions of the eyes from the hand alters beta and gamma synchrony within SPL. J Neurophysiol. 2014;111(11):2210–21.
21. Gail A, Klaes C, Westendorff S. Implementation of spatial transformation rules for goal-directed reaching *via* gain modulation in monkey parietal and premotor cortex. J Neurosci. 2009;29(30):9490–9.
22. Gorbet DJ, Staines WR, Sergio LE. Brain mechanisms for preparing increasingly complex sensory to motor transformations. Neuroimage. 2004;23(3):1100–11.
23. Gorbet DJ, Sergio LE. Preliminary sex differences in human cortical BOLD fMRI activity during the preparation of increasingly complex visually guided movements. Eur J Neurosci. 2007;25(4):1228–39.
24. Werner C, Engelhard K. Pathophysiology of traumatic brain injury. Br J Anaesth. 2007;99(1):4–9.
25. Bartnik BL, Hovda DA, Lee PWN. Glucose metabolism after traumatic brain injury: estimation of pyruvate carboxylase and pyruvate dehydrogenase flux by mass isotopomer analysis. J Neurotrauma. 2007;24(1):181–94.
26. Bergsneider M, Hovda DA, Lee SM, Kelly DF, McArthur DL, Vespa PM, et al. Dissociation of cerebral glucose metabolism and level of consciousness during the period of metabolic depression following human traumatic brain injury. J Neurotrauma. 2000;17(5):389–401.
27. Giza CC, Hovda DA. The Neurometabolic Cascade of Concussion. J Athl Train. 2001;36(3):228–35.
28. Verweij BH, Muizelaar JP, Vinas FC, Peterson PL, Xiong Y, Lee CP. Mitochondrial dysfunction after experimental and human brain injury and its possible reversal with a selective N-type calcium channel antagonist (SNX-111). Clin Neurol Neurosurg. 1997;99:102.
29. D'Ambrosio R, Maris DO, Grady MS, Winn HR, Janigro D. Selective loss of hippocampal long-term potentiation, but not depression, following fluid percussion injury. Brain Res. 1998;786(1):64–79.
30. Sick TJ, Pérez-Pinzón MA, Feng Z-Z. Impaired expression of long-term potentiation in hippocampal slices 4 and 48 h following mild fluid-percussion brain injury *in vivo*. Brain Res. 1998;785(2):287–92.
31. McKee AC, Cantu RC, Nowinski CJ, Hedley-Whyte ET, Gavett BE, Budson AE, et al. Chronic traumatic encephalopathy in athletes: progressive tauopathy after repetitive head injury. J Neuropathol Exp Neurol. 2009;68(7):709–35.
32. De Beaumont L, Tremblay S, Henry LC, Poirier J, Lassonde M, Theoret H. Motor system alterations in retired former athletes: the role of aging and concussion history. BMC Neurol. 2013;13:109.
33. Jantzen KJ, Anderson B, Steinberg FL, Kelso JA. A prospective functional MR imaging study of mild traumatic brain injury in college football players. AJNRAmerican J Neuroradiol. 2004;25(5):738–45.
34. Virji-Babul N, Borich MR, Makan N, Moore T, Frew K, Emery CA, et al. Diffusion tensor imaging of sports-related concussion in adolescents. Pediatr Neurol. 2013;48(1):24–9.
35. Chamard E, Lassonde M, Henry L, Tremblay J, Boulanger Y, De Beaumont L, et al. Neurometabolic and microstructural alterations following a sports-related concussion in female athletes. Brain Inj. 2013;27(9):1038–46.

36. Tremblay S, De Beaumont L, Henry LC, Boulanger Y, Evans AC, Bourgouin P, et al. Sports concussions and aging: a neuroimaging investigation. Cereb Cortex. 2013;23(5):1159–66.
37. Tremblay S, Henry LC, Bedetti C, Larson-Dupuis C, Gagnon JF, Evans AC, et al. Diffuse white matter tract abnormalities in clinically normal ageing retired athletes with a history of sports-related concussions. Brain. 2014;137(11):2997–3011.
38. Granek J, Pisella L, Stemberger J, Vighetto A, Rossetti Y, Sergio LE. Decoupled visually-guided reaching in optic ataxia: Differences in motor control between canonical and non-canonical orientations in space. PLoS One. 2013;8(12):1–18.

3

Ultrasonic assessment of exercise-induced change in skeletal muscle glycogen content

David C Nieman[1*], R Andrew Shanely[2], Kevin A Zwetsloot[2], Mary Pat Meaney[1] and Gerald E Farris[3]

Abstract

Background: Ultrasound imaging is a valuable tool in exercise and sport science research, and has been used to visualize and track real-time movement of muscles and tendons, estimate hydration status in body tissues, and most recently, quantify skeletal muscle glycogen content. In this validation study, direct glycogen quantification from pre- and post-exercise muscle biopsy samples was compared with glycogen content estimates made through a portable, diagnostic high-frequency ultrasound and cloud-based software system (MuscleSound®, Denver, CO).

Methods: Well-trained cyclists (N = 20, age 38.4 ± 6.0 y, 351 ± 57.6 $watts_{max}$) participated in a 75-km cycling time trial on their own bicycles using CompuTrainer Pro Model 8001 trainers (RacerMate, Seattle, WA). Muscle biopsy samples and ultrasound measurements were acquired pre- and post-exercise. Specific locations on the vastus lateralis were marked, and a trained technician used a 12 MHz linear transducer and a standard diagnostic high resolution GE LOGIQ-e ultrasound machine (GE Healthcare, Milwaukee, WI) to make three ultrasound measurements. Ultrasound images were pre-processed to isolate the muscle area under analysis, with the mean pixel intensity averaged from the three scans and scaled (0 to 100 scale) to create the glycogen score. Pre- and post-exercise muscle biopsy samples were acquired at the vastus lateralis location (2 cm apart) using the suction-modified percutaneous needle biopsy procedure, and analyzed for glycogen content.

Results: The 20 cyclists completed the 75-km cycling time trial in 168 ± 26.0 minutes at a power output of 193 ± 57.8 watts (54.2 ± 9.6% $watts_{max}$). Muscle glycogen decreased 77.2 ± 17.4%, with an absolute change of 71.4 ± 23.1 mmol glycogen per kilogram of muscle. The MuscleSound® change score at the vastus lateralis site correlated highly with change in measured muscle glycogen content ($R = 0.92$, $P < 0.001$).

Conclusions: MuscleSound® change scores acquired from an average of three ultrasound scans at the vastus lateralis site correlated significantly with change in vastus lateralis muscle glycogen content. These data support the use of the MuscleSound® system for accurately and non-invasively estimating exercise-induced decreases in vastus lateralis skeletal muscle glycogen content.

Keywords: Cycling, Muscle biopsy, Vastus lateralis, Skeletal muscle, Sonography

Background

Muscle glycogen content is important for high-intensity exercise, and low levels are related to fatigue [1]. Muscle glycogen content is typically analyzed in research settings using muscle samples obtained with percutaneous biopsy needles, imposing significant participant burden in terms of discomfort and time, especially when repeated measurements are made [2,3]. Magnetic resonance spectroscopy (MRS) is used to non-invasively measure tissue glycogen using: 1) ^{13}C natural abundance levels, or ^{13}C atoms incorporated into glycogen by ^{13}C substrate received through ingestion or intravenous administration; and 2) the water signal with chemical exchange saturation transfer imaging (glycoCEST) [4-6]. These MRS techniques involve significant investments in terms of equipment expenditure and technician training, and are not available in portable form for use in athletic settings.

Ultrasound or sonography is widely used in medicine, and has several advantages compared to other prominent methods of imaging including portability, low cost, the absence of harmful ionizing radiation, the provision

* Correspondence: niemandc@appstate.edu
[1]Appalachian State University, Human Performance Lab, North Carolina Research Campus, 600 Laureate Way, Kannapolis, NC 28081, USA
Full list of author information is available at the end of the article

of images in real-time, no discomfort or long-term side effects to the participant, and widely available equipment. In exercise and sport science research, ultrasound imaging is used for a wide variety of applications including evaluation of the cardiovascular status of athletes, musculoskeletal pathology diagnosis and therapeutic interventions, and to visualize and track real-time movement of muscles and tendons [7,8]. The ultrasonographic image of muscles is distinct and can easily be discriminated from surrounding tissues such as bone, nerves, blood vessels, and subcutaneous fat [9]. Ultrasound velocity can be used to assess hydration status in body tissues including muscle that contains 70-80% water [10,11], and detect structural muscle changes caused by neuromuscular disease [12].

MuscleSound® utilizes portable, diagnostic high-frequency ultrasound technology and cloud-based software to non-invasively measure change in muscle glycogen content. This methodology is based upon measurement of the water content associated with glycogen in muscle. When muscle glycogen content is high, the ultrasound image is hypoechoic (dark), and with glycogen depletion and water loss, the image is hyperchoic (brighter). The MuscleSound® software quantifies change in muscle glycogen content using image processing and analysis through segmentation of the region of interest and measurement of the mean signal intensities. One previous study using muscle biopsy samples taken from the rectus femoris in 22 cyclists before and after 90 minutes of steady-state cycling showed a correlation of 0.81 between the modest change in muscle glycogen content and the glycogen change score calculated with MuscleSound® technology [13]. Muscle biopsy samples are typically taken from the vastus lateralis, and the present study extended these results by comparing estimation of change in muscle glycogen content from the MuscleSound® device with direct glycogen content quantification from pre- and post-exercise muscle biopsies taken from the vastus lateralis muscles of cyclists participating in a 75-km cycling time trial.

Methods

Subjects and baseline testing

Subjects included 20 male cyclists (ages 18 to 55 y) who regularly competed in road races and had experience with long distance cycling time trials. Subjects voluntarily provided informed consent and all study procedures were approved by the Institutional Review Board at Appalachian State University. One week prior to the 75-km time trial, each athlete completed orientation/baseline testing in the North Carolina Research Campus Human Performance Laboratory operated by Appalachian State University in Kannapolis, NC. Demographic and training histories were acquired with questionnaires. During baseline testing, maximal power, oxygen consumption, ventilation, and heart rate were measured during a graded exercise test (25 Watts increase every two minutes, starting at 150 Watts) with the Cosmed Quark CPET metabolic cart (Rome, Italy) and the Lode cycle ergometer (Lode Excaliber Sport, Lode B.V., Groningen, Netherlands). Body composition was measured with the Bod Pod body composition analyzer (Life Measurement, Concord, CA).

75-km cycling time trial

One week following baseline testing, subjects participated in a 75-km cycling time trial on their own bicycles on CompuTrainer Pro Model 8001 trainers (RacerMate, Seattle, WA). A mountainous 75-km course with moderate difficulty was chosen and programmed into the software system. Heart rate and rating of perceived exertion (RPE) were recorded at 15 minutes, and every 60 minutes thereafter, and workload in watts was continuously monitored using the CompuTrainer MultiRider software system (version 3.0). Oxygen consumption and ventilation were measured using the Cosmed Quark CPET metabolic cart (Rome, Italy) after 16 km and 55 km cycling. Subjects were allowed to ingest water ad libitum during the 75-km cycling time trial.

Blood sample analysis

Blood samples were collected pre- and post-exercise and analyzed for plasma glucose, plasma lactate, serum cortisol, and serum myoglobin. Plasma glucose and lactate were analyzed using the YSI 2300 STAT Plus Glucose and Lactate analyzer (Yellow Springs, OH). Serum myoglobin was measured using an LX-20 clinical analyzer (Beckman Coulter Electronics, Brea, CA), and cortisol with an electrochemiluminescence immunoassay (ECLIA) through a commercial lab (LabCorp, Burlington, NC).

Skeletal muscle ultrasound procedures

Ultrasound measurements and muscle biopsy samples were taken pre-exercise and within 20 to 30 minutes post-exercise. Specific locations on the vastus lateralis and rectus femoris were marked with indelible ink, followed by three ultrasound measurements at each site by a trained technician using a 12 MHz linear transducer and a standard diagnostic high resolution GE LOGIQ-e ultrasound machine (GE Healthcare, Milwaukee, WI). After calculating statistics on the colorbar to determine the general brightness settings of the machine, images were pre-processed and segmented to isolate the muscle area under analysis using a center crop within the muscle section 25 mm from the top muscle sheath (Figure 1). As shown in Figure 2, pre-exercise muscle with high glycogen stores display darker pixel

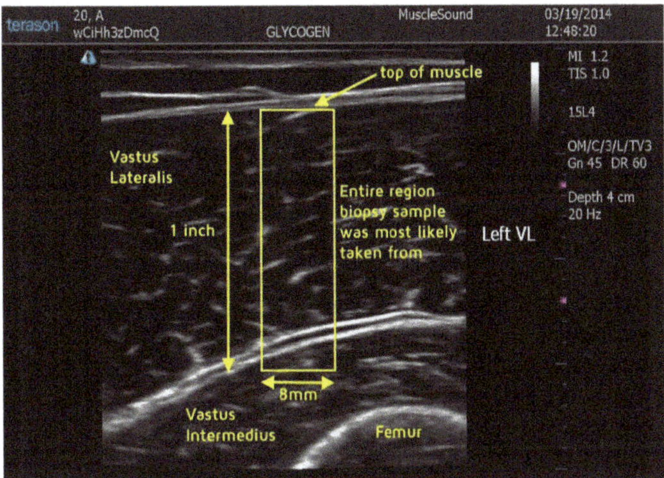

Figure 1 Ultrasonic scan from a subject with the rectangle area representing where images were segmented to isolate the muscle area under analysis using a center crop within the muscle section 25 mm from the top of the muscle sheath.

intensities. Figure 3 shows that post-exercise muscle with lower glycogen stores display brighter pixel intensities. The pixel intensity of the muscle fibers was measured to quantify the amount of glycogen stores within the region of interest (Figure 4). The mean pixel intensity was averaged from the three cropped and segmented scans, and scaled (0 to 100 scale) to create the glycogen score with MuscleSound® software.

Muscle biopsy procedures

Following the ultrasound scans, pre- and post-exercise muscle biopsy samples were acquired on the same leg at the same vastus lateralis locations (2 cm apart). Local anesthesia (1% xylocaine, Hospira, Inc., Lake Forest, IL) was injected subcutaneously. After a small incision, a muscle biopsy sample was obtained using the suction-modified percutaneous needle biopsy procedure [14].

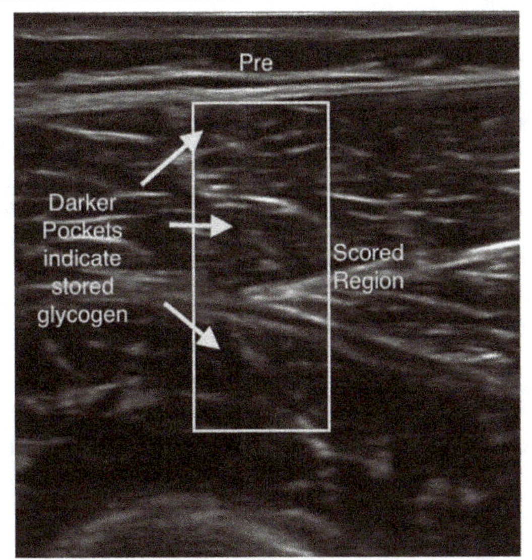

Figure 2 Pre-exercise muscle with high glycogen stores display darker pixel intensities.

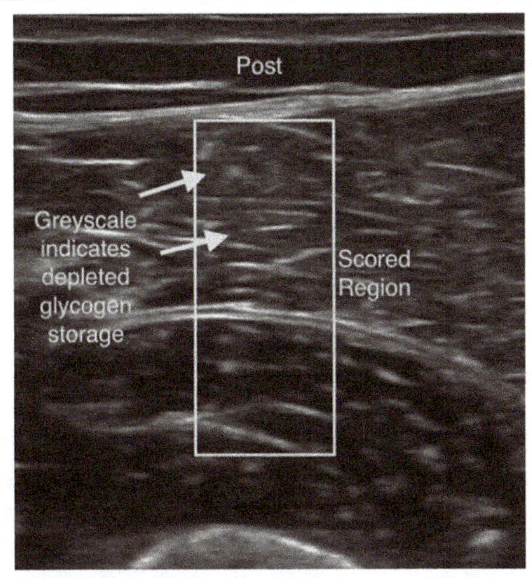

Figure 3 Post-exercise muscle with lower glycogen stores display brighter pixel intensities.

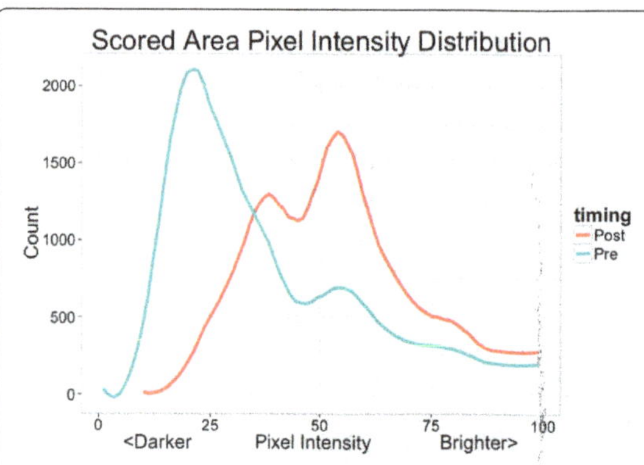

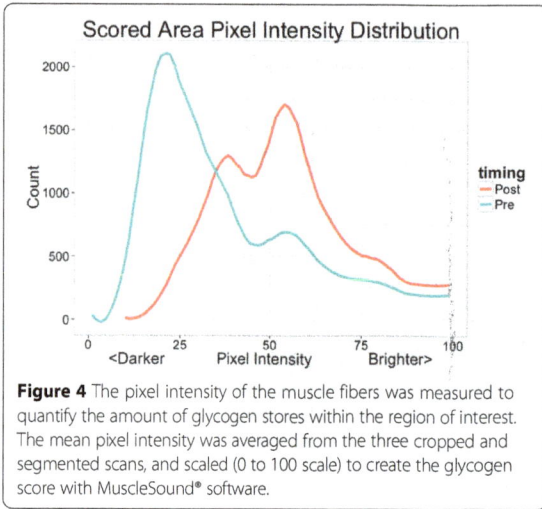

Figure 4 The pixel intensity of the muscle fibers was measured to quantify the amount of glycogen stores within the region of interest. The mean pixel intensity was averaged from the three cropped and segmented scans, and scaled (0 to 100 scale) to create the glycogen score with MuscleSound® software.

Muscle was trimmed of connective tissue and fat and immediately frozen in liquid nitrogen. Samples were stored at −80°C until subsequent analysis. A glycogen assay kit (Catalog #MAK016, Sigma-Aldrich, St. Louis, MO) was used to determine the concentration of glycogen in vastus lateralis muscle homogenates. In this coupled enzyme assay, glucoamylase hydrolyzed glycogen to glucose, and then the glucose was oxidized to yield a product that reacted with a probe to generate a color detectable with a microplate reader (Synergy H1 Hybrid Reader, BioTek Instruments, Inc., Winooski, VT) at 570 nm.

Statistical analysis

Data are expressed as mean ± SD. Pre- and post-exercise data were tested for change using paired t-tests, with Pearson correlations used to test relationships between MuscleSound® glycogen scores and muscle glycogen content measured through biochemical techniques.

Table 1 Subject characteristics (N = 20)

Variable	Mean±SD
Age	38.4 ± 6.0
Height (m)	1.82 ± 0.7
Weight (kg)	83.3 ± 7.2
Body fat (%)	20.3 ± 5.9
VO_{2max} (ml·kg^{-1} min^{-1})	47.9 ± 7.8
Maximal heart rate (beats/min)	179 ± 8.6
$Watts_{max}$	351 ± 57.6
Maximal ventilation (L/min)	128 ± 17.1
Maximal respiratory rate (breaths/min)	46.7 ± 7.4
Training (km/wk)	154 ± 93.5

Table 2 Performance variables averaged for entire 75 km cycling time trial

Variable	Mean±SD
VO_2 (ml·kg^{-1} min^{-1})	33.2 ± 6.4
VO_2 (%VO_{2max})	69.6 ± 10.3
Watts	193 ± 57.8
% $Watts_{max}$	54.2 ± 9.6
HR (beats/min)	160 ± 11.5
%HR_{max}	89.4 ± 5.9
Ventilation (L/min)	74.0 ± 16.7
Rating Perceived Exertion	14.7 ± 1.6

Results

Table 1 summarizes subject characteristics, Table 2 performance outcomes, and Table 3 data from the blood samples. The 20 cyclists completed the 75-km cycling time trial in 168 ± 26.0 minutes. Table 2 indicates that oxygen consumption (taken at 16 and 55 km) averaged 69.6 ± 10.3% VO_{2max}, with a heart rate of 160 ± 11.5 bpm (89.4 ± 5.9% maximal heart rate). Power output was measured continuously, and averaged 193 ± 57.8 watts, representing 54.2 ± 9.6% $watts_{max}$ on the mountainous course. Subjects reported an RPE of 12.4 ± 1.5 at 15 minutes, 13.1 ± 1.5 at 60 minutes, 14.6 ± 1.8 at 120 minutes, and 17.6 ± 0.7 ("very hard") at the end of the 75-km cycling trial. Serum cortisol increased 165%, serum myoglobin 654%, and plasma lactate 108% (Table 3), providing further support that the subjects engaged in an intensive and prolonged exercise bout.

Muscle glycogen decreased 77.2 ± 17.4% (Figure 5), with an absolute change of 71.4 ± 23.1 mmol glycogen per kilogram wet weight of muscle ($P < 0.001$). The absolute change in muscle glycogen varied substantially between subjects (32 to 110 mmol/kg).

The MuscleSound® change score at the vastus lateralis site correlated highly with change in vastus lateralis muscle glycogen content ($r = 0.92$, $P < 0.001$) (Figure 6). The MuscleSound® change score at the rectus femoris site also correlated highly with change in vastus lateralis muscle glycogen content ($r = 0.87$, $P < 0.001$) (data not shown). Figures 7 and 8 indicates that strong, positive

Table 3 Cortisol, myoglobin, lactate, and glucose data from blood samples (mean ± SD)

Variable	Pre-75 km cycling	Post-75-km cycling	P-value
Serum cortisol (μg/dl)	10.7 ± 4.3	28.4 ± 10.5	<0.001
Serum myoglobin (ng/mL)	32.1 ± 14.7	242 ± 216	<0.001
Plasma lactate (mmol/L)	0.97 ± 0.3	2.02 ± 1.0	<0.001
Plasma glucose (mmol/L)	3.88 ± 0.78	4.25 ± 0.75	0.185

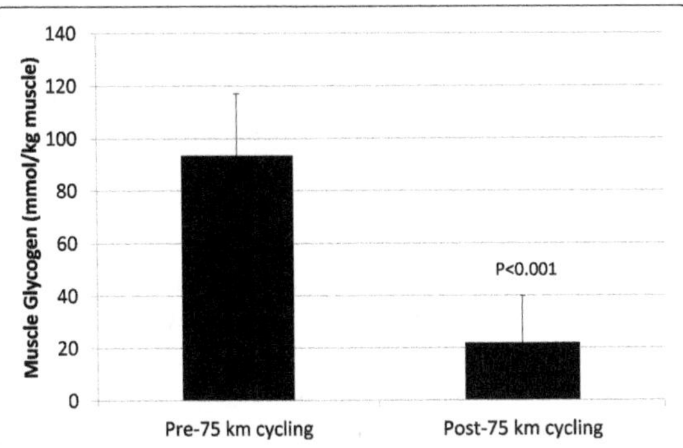

Figure 5 Vastus lateralis muscle glycogen content data pre- and post-exercise, indicating a 77.2 ± 17.4% decrease and an absolute change of 71.4 ± 23.1 mmol glycogen per kilogram of muscle (P < 0.001), as measured by biochemical assay.

correlations were measured for vastus lateralis MuscleSound® scores and muscle glycogen content for pre-exercise and post-exercise time points (r = 0.92, r = 0.90, respectively, P < 0.001).

Discussion

The 20 cyclists completed the mountainous 75-km cycling time trial in an average of 2.8 hours at a power output of 54% $watts_{max}$ Serum cortisol and plasma lactate increased 165% and 108% in response to this intensive and prolonged exercise bout, and the cyclists experienced an average decrease of approximately three-fourths of glycogen content in the vastus lateralis, as determined directly with pre- and post-exercise skeletal muscle biopsies. The absolute decrease in muscle glycogen content varied widely between subjects. MuscleSound® glycogen change scores acquired non-invasively from an average of three ultrasound scans at the vastus lateralis and rectus femoris sites correlated significantly with change in vastus lateralis muscle glycogen content. Additionally, pre- and post-exercise MuscleSound® glycogen scores were highly correlated with direct muscle glycogen measurements.

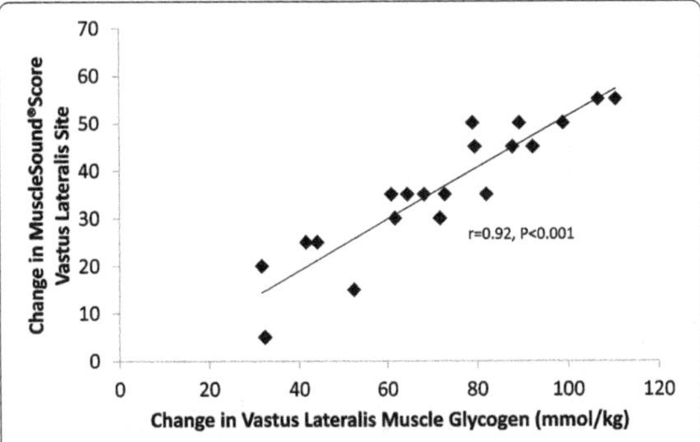

Figure 6 Correlation of the change in vastus lateralis MuscleSound® glycogen score with change in vastus lateralis muscle glycogen content (r = 0.92, P < 0.001).

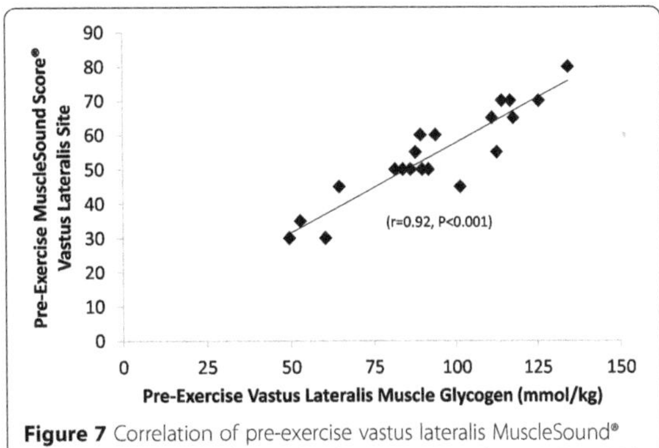

Figure 7 Correlation of pre-exercise vastus lateralis MuscleSound® scores and vastus lateralis muscle glycogen content (r = 0.92, P < 0.001).

These data support the use of the MuscleSound® system for accurately estimating quadriceps muscle glycogen content and exercise-induced decreases in muscle glycogen content despite the wide variation in glycogen depletion following the rigorous 75-km cycling time trial. Hill et al. [13] reported a correlation of 0.81 between change in muscle glycogen content obtained from rectus femoris biopsy samples and the MuscleSound® glycogen change score in 22 cyclists following 90 minutes of steady-state exercise. Glycogen change in the Hill et al. [13] study was modest, and an ultrasound-guided muscle biopsy technique was used to access the rectus femoris without compromising major vascular structures. Muscle biopsy samples are more easily acquired from the vastus lateralis [14], and our data support that ultrasound scans taken at both the vastus lateralis and rectus femoris correlate strongly with change in muscle glycogen content within the vastus lateralis. Few studies have compared exercise-induced glycogen depletion simultaneously in the vastus lateralis and rectus femoris. Kim et al. [15] showed that

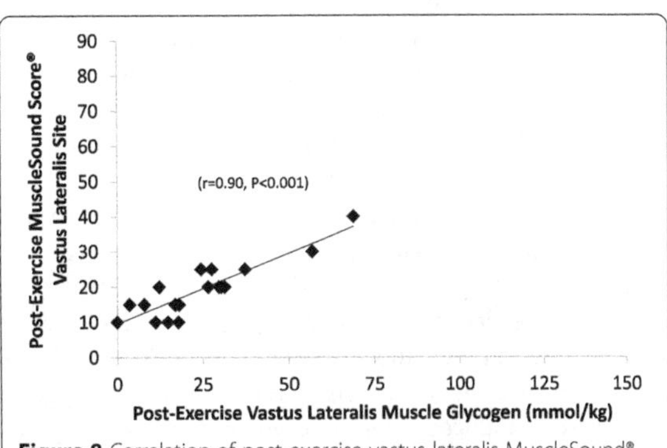

Figure 8 Correlation of post-exercise vastus lateralis MuscleSound® scores and vastus lateralis muscle glycogen content (r = 0.90, P < 0.001).

functional electrical stimulation (FES) but not voluntary dynamic unilateral knee-extensor exercise for 60 minutes decreased muscle glycogen in both the vastus lateralis and rectus femoris to a similar extent. We did not obtain muscle biopsies from the gastrocnemius muscle, a site often used in studies evaluating skeletal muscle glycogen change in runners [16]. Additional research with runners is needed to determine if our muscle glycogen and MuscleSound® data from the vastus lateralis in cyclists can be extrapolated to the gastrocnemius muscle in long distance runners.

Muscle glycogen is the primary source of fuel during prolonged and intensive exercise, and the relationship between muscle glycogen and fatigue resistance is supported through several lines of experimental evidence including alterations in pre-exercise muscle glycogen content by dietary and exercise interventions [1-3,16,17], and the development of profound fatigue during exercise in individuals with McArdle disease which restricts glycogen metabolism [18]. As demonstrated in the current study, glycogen depletion rates during exercise vary widely between athletes, even when duration and intensity are controlled, and this could be due to multiple factors including variance in pre-exercise muscle glycogen levels and ability to beta-oxidize fatty acids [2,3,13]. Use of the suction-modified Bergström percutaneous needle biopsy technique to obtain skeletal muscle tissue samples from the vastus lateralis of human subjects imposes significant subject burden, typically requires physician involvement and oversight, and is costly in terms of supplies and personnel [14]. These barriers are largely removed through utilization of high frequency musculoskeletal ultrasound for non-invasive muscle glycogen assessment with the MuscleSound® system.

MuscleSound® methodology is based upon measurement of the water content associated with glycogen in the muscle. This study and that of Hill et al. [13] support a strong correlation between ultrasound- and biochemical-based measurements of skeletal muscle glycogen. Additional research is needed to determine how exercise-induced changes in muscle water content influence this relationship. Skeletal muscle water content can vary depending on the hydration status of the athlete, and the influence of acute exercise and disease states [10,11]. Ultrasound velocity in the soleus muscle has been shown to correspond to changes in urine osmolarity and specific gravity during acute dehydration and rehydration in collegiate wrestlers [19]. The strong positive correlations demonstrated in our study between MuscleSound® glycogen scores and vastus lateralis glycogen content suggests that exercise-induced alterations in muscle tissue hydration has little effect on the pixel intensity used to calculate the glycogen score.

Conclusions

In this validation study, MuscleSound® change scores acquired from an average of three ultrasound scans at the vastus lateralis site correlated significantly with change in vastus lateralis muscle glycogen content assessed through a biochemical assay. These data extend the findings of Hill et al. [13] and support the use of the MuscleSound® system to accurately and non-invasively estimate exercise-induced decreases in vastus lateralis skeletal muscle glycogen content. Further research is needed with additional muscle groups and a wide variety of athletes under varying environmental conditions to confirm the within-subject and between-subject value of using ultrasound scans for muscle glycogen determination.

Abbreviations

ECLIA: Electrochemiluminescence immunoassay; EDTA: Ethylenediaminetetraacetic acid; glycoCEST: Use of the water signal by magnetic resonance spectroscopy for glycogen analysis; MRS: Magnetic resonance spectroscopy; RPE: Rating of perceived exertion.

Competing interests

None of the authors had any personal or financial conflicts of interest. Funding for the study was provided by MuscleSound® (Denver, CO). The funders provided a technician to conduct the ultrasound scans but had no other role in the study's design, conduct, analysis, interpretation of the data, or reporting beyond approval of the scientific protocol.

Authors' contributions

DCN was the primary investigator, conceived and designed the study, conducted the statistical analysis, and wrote the paper. RAS, KAZ, and MPM helped conceive the study, participated in data collection, and assisted GF in acquiring muscle biopsies. RAS, KAZ, MPM, and GF assisted in interpreting the data and reviewing and edited the manuscript. RAS, KAZ, and MPM coordinated analysis of the glycogen content of the muscle biopsies. All authors read and approved the final manuscript.

Acknowledgements

We acknowledge the assistance of Dustin Dew, Pierre Sarnow, Zach Snyder, Beth Swiatek, and Mitch Tanaka during the data collection phase of this study. This study was funded by a grant from MuscleSound (Denver, CO). One technician from MuscleSound (Zach Snyder) acquired the ultrasound images from the subjects, and a second MuscleSound technician (Pierre Sarnow) calculated the glycogen scores from the ultrasound images. All other aspects of the study, manuscript preparation, and the decision to submit the manuscript for publication were coordinated by the primary investigator, Dr. David Nieman.

Author details

[1]Appalachian State University, Human Performance Lab, North Carolina Research Campus, 600 Laureate Way, Kannapolis, NC 28081, USA. [2]Department of Health and Exercise Science, Appalachian State University, Boone, NC, USA. [3]Department of Emergency Medicine, Carolinas Medical Center NorthEast, Concord, NC, USA.

References

1. Conlee RK. Muscle glycogen and exercise endurance: a twenty-year perspective. Exerc Sport Sci Rev. 1987;15:1–28.
2. Nieman DC, Davis JM, Henson DA, Gross SJ, Dumke CL, Utter AC, et al. Muscle cytokine mRNA changes after 2.5 h of cycling: influence of carbohydrate. Med Sci Sports Exerc. 2005;37:1283–90.
3. Nieman DC, Davis JM, Henson DA, Walberg-Rankin J, Shute M, Dumke CL, et al. Carbohydrate ingestion influences skeletal muscle cytokine mRNA and plasma cytokine levels after a 3-h run. J Appl Physiol. 2003;94:1917–25.

4. Avison MJ, Rothman DL, Nadel E, Shulman RG. Detection of human muscle glycogen by natural abundance ^{13}C NMR. Proc Natl Acad Sci U S A. 1988;85:1634–6.
5. Van Zijl PC, Jones CK, Ren J, Malloy CR, Sherry AD. MRI detection of glycogen in vivo by using chemical exchange saturation transfer imaging (glycoCEST). Proc Natl Acad Sci U S A. 2007;104:4359–64.
6. Kogan F, Hariharan H, Reddy R. Chemical Exchange Saturation Transfer (CEST) Imaging: Description of technique and potential clinical applications. Curr Radiol Rep. 2013;1:102–14.
7. Sikdar S, Wei Q, Cortes N. Dynamic ultrasound imaging applications to quantify musculoskeletal function. Exerc Sport Sci Rev. 2014;42:126–35.
8. Yim ES, Corrado G. Ultrasound in sports medicine: relevance of emerging techniques to clinical care of athletes. Sports Med. 2012;42:665–80.
9. Lopata RG, van Dijk JP, Pillen S, Nillesen MM, Maas H, Thijssen JM, et al. Dynamic imaging of skeletal muscle contraction in three orthogonal directions. J Appl Physiol. 2010;109:906–15.
10. Sarvazyan A, Tatarinov A, Sarvazyan N. Ultrasonic assessment of tissue hydration status. Ultrasonics. 2005;43:661–71.
11. Topchyan A, Tatarinov A, Sarvazyan N, Sarvazyan A. Ultrasound velocity in human muscle in vivo: perspective for edema studies. Ultrasonics. 2006;44:259–64.
12. Arts IM, Pillen S, Schelhaas HJ, Overeem S, Zwarts MJ. Normal values for quantitative muscle ultrasonography in adults. Muscle Nerve. 2010;41:32–41.
13. Hill JC, Millán IS. Validation of musculoskeletal ultrasound to assess and quantify muscle glycogen content. A novel approach Phys Sportsmed. 2014;42(3):45–52.
14. Shanely RA, Zwetsloot KA, Triplett NT, Meaney MP, Farris GE, Nieman DC. Human skeletal muscle biopsy procedures using the modified Bergström technique. J Vis Exp. 2014: (91). doi: 10.3791/51812
15. Kim CK, Bangsbo J, Strange S, Karpakka J, Saltin B. Metabolic response and muscle glycogen depletion pattern during prolonged electrically induced dynamic exercise in man. Scand J Rehabil Med. 1995;27:51–8.
16. Sherman WM, Doyle JA, Lamb DR, Strauss RH. Dietary carbohydrate, muscle glycogen, and exercise performance during 7 d of training. Am J Clin Nutr. 1993;57:27–31.
17. Duhamel TA, Green HJ, Stewart RD, Foley KP, Smith IC, Ouyang J. Muscle metabolic, SR Ca(2+) -cycling responses to prolonged cycling, with and without glucose supplementation. J Appl Physiol. 2007;103:1986–98.
18. Lewis SF, Haller RG. The pathophysiology of McArdle's disease: clues to regulation in exercise and fatigue. J Appl Physiol. 1986;61:391–401.
19. Utter AC, McAnulty SR, Sarvazyan A, Query MC, Landram MJ. Evaluation of ultrasound velocity to assess the hydration status of wrestlers. J Strength Cond Res. 2010;24:1451–7.

4

Transport choice when travelling to a sports facility: the role of perceived route features - Results from a cross-sectional study in the Netherlands

Ellen L de Hollander[1*], Eline Scheepers[1,2], Harm J van Wijnen[3], Pieter JV van Wesemael[4], Albertine J Schuit[1,2], Wanda Wendel-Vos[2] and Elise EMM van Kempen[3]

Abstract

Background: Physical activity and sedentary behaviour are independently associated with health outcomes, where physical activity (PA) is associated with health benefits and sedentary behaviour is associated with health risks. One possible strategy to counteract sedentary behaviour is to stimulate active transport use. As monitoring studies in the Netherlands have shown that among sedentary people the proportion of adults who engage in sports (hereafter: sports practitioners) is 62.3%, sports practitioners seem a feasible target group for this strategy. Previous studies have generally reported associations between neighbourhood characteristics and active transport use. However, the neighbourhood covers only part of the route to a certain destination. Therefore, we examined the association between perceived route features and transport choice when travelling up to 7.5 kilometres to a sports facility among sports practitioners.

Methods: For 1118 Dutch sports practitioners – who indicated that they practice a sport and travel to a sports facility – age 18 and older, data on transport choice and perceived features of the route to a sports facility were gathered. Participants were classified into one of three transport groups based on their transport choice: car users, cyclists and walkers. Participants were asked whether perceived route features influenced their transport choice. Logistic regression was used to model the odds of cycling versus car use and walking versus car use in the association with perceived route features, adjusted for potential confounders.

Results: Perceived traffic safety was associated with lower odds of cycling (OR: 0.36, 95% CI: 0.15-0.86). Perceived route duration was associated with lower odds of both cycling (OR: 0.54, 95%CI: 0.39-0.75) and walking (OR: 0.60, 95%CI: 0.36-1.00). Perceived distance to a sports facility and having to make a detour when using other transport modes than the chosen transport mode were associated with higher odds of both cycling and walking (OR_{range}: 1.82-5.21). What and who people encountered during their trip (i.e. visual aspects) was associated with higher odds of both cycling and walking (OR_{range}: 2.40-3.69).

Conclusions: Perceived traffic safety, duration, distance, detour, and visual aspects, when travelling to a sports facility were associated with transport choice. Therefore, the perception of route features should be considered when stimulating active transport use among sports practitioners.

Keywords: Car use, Walking, Cycling, Active transportation, Physical activity, Sports, Transport choice, Route features

* Correspondence: ellen.de.hollander@rivm.nl
[1]National Institute for Public Health and the Environment, Centre for Nutrition, Prevention and Health Services, PO Box 1, 3720 BA Bilthoven, Netherlands
Full list of author information is available at the end of the article

Background

Physical activity (PA) is associated with health benefits, such as the prevention of chronic diseases and an improved quality of life. Moreover, increasing the amount of PA can result in additional health benefits [1]. Sedentary behaviour is associated with health risks, such as an increased risk of type 2 diabetes, all-cause and CVD mortality [2]. These two behaviours, i.e. physical activity (PA) and sedentary behaviour, are independently associated with health outcomes [3–5]. Therefore, it is important to stimulate PA in both physically active persons, who can increase their PA levels, as well as in sedentary persons.

In the Netherlands, monitoring studies have shown that among sedentary people the proportion of adults who engage in sports (hereafter referred to as: sports practitioners) is 62.3% [6]. This indicates that a substantial proportion of sedentary people, who gain the most by increasing their PA levels, are sports practitioners. Therefore, sports practitioners may constitute a specific target population to increase their physical activity levels and decrease their sedentary behaviour despite the fact that they are actively involved in sports.

One way to increase PA levels is to stimulate active transport use. Stimulating active transport use has become a popular policy strategy and can be carried out by replacing short-distance car trips with cycling or walking [7]. A distance up to 7.5 kilometres may be considered feasible; it represents a maximum of 30 minutes of cycling at an average speed [8]. However, one set of barriers that may hamper active transport use lies in the physical environment. Previous studies have reported an association between neighbourhood characteristics, such as accessibility of facilities, availability of cycling and walking paths, safety (traffic and crime), and the aesthetic quality of the built environment and active transport use for different trip purposes [9–11]. However, the neighbourhood covers only part of the route to a certain destination (also referred to as 'trip purpose' in travel surveys). Moreover, factors influencing active transport use differ by trip purpose [12]. Therefore, insight into route features and the association with active transport use for specific trip purposes is needed.

In this study, we focus specifically on the associations between perceived route features when travelling to a sports facility and transport choice among sports practitioners. Findings from our study may be important for public health, as it can give guidance for policy programmes such as the Dutch national policy programme 'Sports and Physical Activity in the Neighbourhood' that stimulates physical activity by making the healthy choice, the easy choice (e.g. providing sports fields in the neighbourhood and improving the infrastructure to enhance physical activity) [13, 14].

Methods

Study design

This study was part of the Dutch 'impActs of actiVE traNsport in Urban Environments' (AVENUE) project. The aim of the AVENUE project is to provide in-depth information on characteristics of short car and active (cycling and walking) transport trips and the feasibility of replacing short car trips with short trips by active transport by using a multidisciplinary approach, including a combination of qualitative (focus groups, policy analysis) and quantitative methods (systematic literature review, questionnaire and (secondary) data analysis). In this study, we used the data obtained from the questionnaire that was designed by the AVENUE project group. The questionnaire was distributed by IPSOS-Nederland [15] among a random sample from their internet panel (Scheepers CE, Wendel-Vos GCW, van Kempen EEMM, de Hollander EL, van Wijnen HJ, Maas J, den Hertog FRJ, Staatsen BAM, Stipdonk HL, Int Panis LLR, van Wesemael PJV, Schuit AJ: Perceived Accessibility is An Important Factor in Transport Choice — Results from the AVENUE Project, Submitted). IPSOS-Nederland applies the Personal Data Protection Act [15] and gathered the informed consent from the participants in this study. As an Institutional Review Board (IRB) approval is only needed when the daily life of participants is influenced or participants are required to perform specific actions, an IRB approval was not warranted and therefore not obtained. The data were anonymised prior to the moment that the AVENUE project group received the dataset from IPSOS-Nederland. The authors did not have access to any identifying information.

For 3,663 adults age 18 and older, data were collected using an online questionnaire administered during one calendar year that started in July 2012. Data included information about individual characteristics, environmental characteristics, trip purposes, transport mode, factors influencing transport choice separately for car, bicycle and walking, health, and lifestyle.

In this study, we focussed on route features when travelling to a sports facility. Thus, participants who answered that they travelled a distance up to 7.5 kilometres to a sports facility directly from home and who filled in a sport they practiced at least on a weekly basis were selected and defined as 'sports practitioners' (N = 1190; Fig. 1).

Transport mode

Participants were classified into one of three transport groups based on their transport choice: car users (passive transport), cyclists and walkers (active transport). Their choice was inferred from their self-reported frequency of using the car, cycling, or walking when travelling to a sports facility. When participants used two or more transport modes equally frequent, they were categorised as a car user if one of the transport modes was a car, and as a cyclist in all other cases.

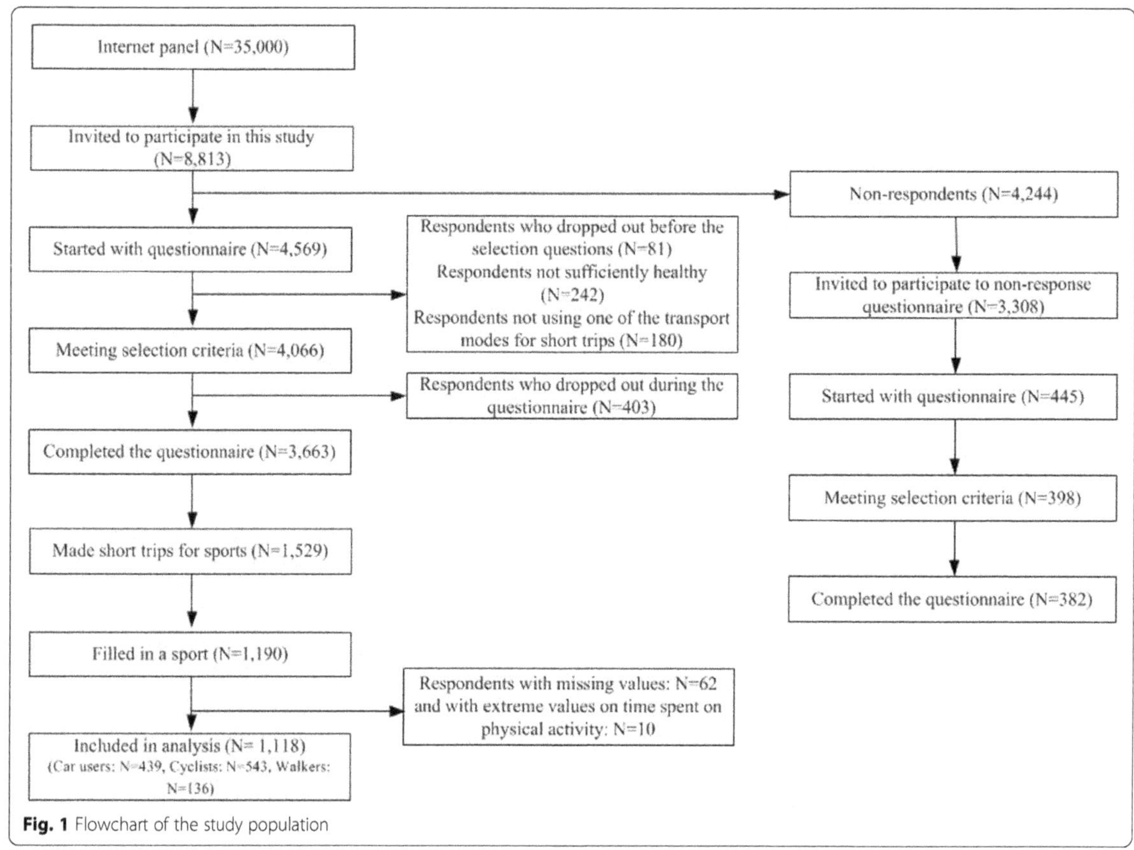

Fig. 1 Flowchart of the study population

Perceived route features

In the questionnaire, 13 items were included inquiring about the influence of route features on transport choice (see Table 1). These items included subjects with regard to safety, bother by noise, odour and vibrations, route convenience, and visual aspects. Answers were rated on a four-point category scale ('(almost) never', 'sometimes', 'often','always').

If participants indicated that they used multiple transport modes when travelling to a sports facility, they initially answered the 13 questions for each transport mode, because the questions were formulated from the perspective of one transport mode. For example, if someone was categorised as a car user, the following question was asked: 'If you travel to the sports facility within a radius of 7.5 kilometres, do you choose *to use the car* because you think traffic safety is inadequate when travelling *by bicycle or foot*?' When someone was categorised as a cyclist or walker, 'to use the car' in the question was replaced by 'to cycle' or 'to walk'. The part 'by bicycle or on foot' in the previous question was then replaced by 'by car or on foot', or by 'by car or bicycle', respectively. For the statistical analysis, we only used the answers to the questions that belonged to the transport mode categorisation of a participant. The answers for every item were dichotomised into 0 ('(almost) never' and 'sometimes') and 1 ('often' and 'always').

Covariates

Individual characteristics

Gender, age, educational level, household composition, and physical activity level were obtained from the questionnaire. Educational level was categorised into: low (primary school and lower general secondary education), medium (intermediate vocational education, higher general secondary education, and pre-university education), and high (higher vocational education and university, reference). Household composition was categorised into: living alone, with a partner, with children under 18, with other adults (parents, children age 18 and older, or other adults; reference). Physical activity was assessed with the validated 'Short QUestionnaire to ASsess Health-enhancing physical activity' (SQUASH), which contains questions about multiple activities including commuting, household, leisure time and sport activities referring to a normal week in the past months [16, 17]. Results from the SQUASH were converted to time spent (hours per week) on total physical activity [16–18].

Table 1 Characteristics of the population by transport choice when travelling to a sports facility

	Car use (n = 439)	Bicycling (n = 543)	Walking (n = 136)	$P_{car\ vs\ cycling}$	$P_{car\ vs\ walking}$
Individual characteristics					
Men, %	53.3	49.0	55.2	0.18	0.71
Age (yrs), mean (SD)	48.4 (13.4)	45.7 (14.7)	46.6 (14.1)	<0.01	0.17
Educational level, %				0.22	0.98
High	35.5	40.7	34.6		
Medium	43.3	41.1	44.1		
Low	21.2	18.2	21.3		
Household composition, %				<0.01	0.03
living alone	17.3	21.6	26.5		
with a partner	39.0	37.0	36.0		
with children under 18	31.9	20.8	.22.1		
with other adults	11.9	20.6	15.4		
Physical activity (h/wk), mean (SD)	20.4 (15.2)	24.3 (18.2)	24.0 (19.7)	<0.01	0.03
Characteristics of the direct living environment					
Neighbourhood typology, %				0.32	0.02
rural	7.3	6.3	4.4		
village-centre	33.0	30.4	25.0		
urban-green	15.0	12.3	10.3		
urban-outside centre	37.8	42.0	47.5		
urban-centre	6.8	9.0	12.5		
Age of the neighbourhood, %				0.18	0.23
<1910	8.0	7.7	8.8		
1910-1939	29.4	29.3	22.8		
1940-1969	41.5	35.7	39.0		
1970-1984	18.7	24.9	27.2		
≥1985	2.5	2.4	2.2		
Availability cycling paths (km/km²), mean (SD)	1.5 (0.8)	1.6 (1.0)	1.9 (1.1)	0.01	<0.01
Availability walking paths (km/km²), mean (SD)	1.1 (0.8)	1.3 (1.0)	1.6 (1.1)	<0.01	<0.01
Availability of sports facilities (#/km²), mean (SD)	0.6 (0.3)	0.6 (0.4)	0.7 (0.4)	0.03	<0.01
Availability of public natural spaces (km²/km²), mean (SD)	0.1 (0.1)	0.1 (0.1)	0.2 (0.1)	0.55	0.07
Distance to a sports facility (km), mean (SD)	1.7 (1.5)	1.4 (1.5)	0.9 (1.2)	<0.01	<0.01
Motivational and situational factors (% that answered often or always)					
Do the following factors influence whether you choose *this transport mode*[a] when travelling these distances?'					
The weather	51.0	36.1	21.3	<0.01	<0.01
I am used to travelling by this transport mode	66.7	85.6	71.3	<0.01	0.32
It depends on whether I feel like using this transport mode	21.4	28.6	27.9	0.01	0.11
My health/health in general	15.5	62.8	57.4	<0.01	<0.01
Whether there is a cycle parking at my destination	7.1	13.8	8.1	<0.01	0.69
Season				0.96	0.08
Winter	28.7	27.8	18.4		
Spring	21.6	20.8	26.5		
Summer	24.8	26.0	24.3		
Autumn	24.8	25.4	30.9		

Table 1 Characteristics of the population by transport choice when travelling to a sports facility *(Continued)*

Perceived route features (% that answered often or always)					
If you travel to the sports facility within a radius of 7.5 km, do you choose *this transport mode*[a] because you…					
Safety					
Consider the road traffic situation unsafe when using the other 2 transport modes[b]	5.2	2.4	4.4	0.02	0.70
Feel unsafe when travelling by the other 2 transport modes[b] because of criminality	3.4	2.4	2.9	0.34	0.79
Bother by noise, odour and vibrations					
Are bothered by noise when travelling by the other 2 transport modes[b]	1.1	2.0	2.2	0.28	0.35
Are bothered by odour when travelling by the other 2 transport modes[b]	1.4	1.8	2.2	0.56	0.49
Are bothered by vibrations when travelling by the other 2 transport modes[b]	1.1	1.5	1.5	0.65	0.76
Do the following factors influence your choice of using this transport mode when you travel these distances?					
Route convenience					
Whether the distance to my destination is shorter	15.7	38.1	44.1	<0.01	<0.01
Whether it takes less time to reach my destination	54.0	44.8	39.7	<0.01	<0.01
Whether my destination is easy to reach	44.2	52.1	51.5	0.01	0.14
Whether I encounter a lot of traffic lights	8.4	11.8	10.3	0.09	0.50
Whether I encounter obstacles aimed at speed reduction (such as bumps in the road or road narrowings)	6.4	9.0	8.1	0.13	0.49
Whether I am forced to make a detour to reach my destination would I use either of the other 2 transport modes[b]	6.8	15.3	13.2	<0.01	0.02
Visual aspects					
What I see/encounter during the trip	4.3	14.0	13.2	<0.01	<0.01
Who I see/encounter during the trip	3.4	12.0	9.6	<0.01	<0.01

yrs = years; SD = standard deviation; h/wk = hour per week; wk = week; km = kilometre; # = number

[a]In this question, the interpretation of 'this transport mode' depends on the categorisation of the respondent into a transport mode (i.e. car user, cyclist, walker). If someone was a car user, this transport mode was replaced by 'to use the car'; if someone was a cyclist, it was replaced by 'to cycle'; and if someone was a walker, it was replaced by 'to walk'

[b]If someone was categorised as a car user, the 2 other transport modes are cycling and walking; if someone was a cyclists, the other 2 transport modes are using the car and walking, if someone was a walker the other transport mode are using the car and cycling

Motivational and situational factors

Motivational and situational factors that could influence transport choice were also measured with the questionnaire (see Table 1 for the 10 questions). As was the case for the questions regarding route features, we only used the answers to the questions that belonged to the transport mode categorisation of a participant. For example, if someone was categorised as a car user, the following question was asked: 'Do the following factors influence whether you choose *to use the car* when travelling these distances?' If someone was categorised as a cyclist or walker, *'to use the car'* in the question was replaced by *'to cycle'* or *'to walk'*. Answers were rated on a four-point category scale ('(almost) never', 'sometimes', 'often', 'always'). The answers for every item were dichotomised into 0 ('(almost) never' and 'sometimes') and 1 ('often' and 'always'). Because of possible autocorrelation, we checked how these 10 items were correlated with each other (Additional file 1: Table S1). Because of a lack of power, we set the threshold of the Spearman's Rho at ≥0.5 instead of ≥0.8 to exclude correlated items. Additional file 1: Table S1 shows that multiple items were correlated. As a consequence, some items were excluded, which is described in Additional file 1. The remaining items were 'the weather', 'I am used to travelling by this transport mode', 'I feel like using this transport mode', 'my health/health in general', and 'cycle parking at destination'. The answers for these items were dichotomised into 0 ('(almost) never' and 'sometimes') and 1 ('often' and 'always').

Finally, the season was derived from the date the questionnaire was filled in. Seasons were categorised into: winter, spring, summer, and autumn (reference).

Characteristics of the living environment

In the Netherlands, postal codes consist of a six-digit postal code starting with four numbers (four-digit postal code), followed by two letters (six-digit-postal code). The six-digit postal code reflects a smaller area within the four-digit postal code, and is thereby more specific than the four-digit postal code. The surface of the four-digit and six-digit areas differs across the Netherlands as will be illustrated next. There are 4000 four-digit postal codes, representing on average 1,772 households each. In urban areas, this four-digit postal code represents only one neighbourhood, whereas in rural areas this postal code can represent a whole village. Each six-digit postal code represents on average 15 to 20 households. In our study, the six-digit postal code of each respondent's home was available.

To determine neighbourhood typology, we merged our dataset with a dataset from ABF Research (2009) using the four-digit postal code. The data source (ABF Research) provided five different typologies based on density, accessibility/connectivity, land use mix and quality of buildings: 1) Urban – centre, 2) Urban – outside centre, 3) Urban – green, 4) Village-centre, and 5) Rural [19].

For the following characteristics of the living environment, we used the six-digit postal codes of the home address in ArcGIS 10.1.

Another proxy to characterise the neighbourhood was determined: age of the respondents' neighbourhood. In the Netherlands, the layout of a neighbourhood depends highly on the period in which a neighbourhood was built. Therefore, we categorised the six-digit postal code areas into the following historical periods of urban planning: <1910, 1910–1939, 1940–1969, 1970–1984, ≥1985. We obtained the age of all buildings from the Dutch Registration of Addresses and Buildings (in Dutch: "Basisregistratie Adressen en Gebouwen (BAG)") [20]. First, we categorised the buildings into the historical periods. Then, the historical period in which most buildings were built was assigned to that area. If the number of buildings between historical periods were equal, the oldest historical period was assigned.

Availability of cycling and walking paths were calculated by summing up the total length of the paths within a circle with a 7.5-km radius originating from the midpoint of the six-digit postal codes of the home addresses (hereafter: living environment). OpenStreetMap [21] was used, which gives detailed information about separate walking and cycle paths. For 10 % of the participants, a proportion of the surface of the living environment was located outside the borders of the Netherlands. As we had no information available about environmental characteristics outside the borders, the length of cycling and walking paths was divided by the surface that was located within the Netherlands.

The availability of sports facilities was assessed by counting the number of sports facilities within the living environment by using the Sports Accommodation Monitor (in Dutch: "Accommodatie Monitor Sport) (Additional file 2: Table S2.1, Table S2.2). Because practicing sports like Nordic walking or mountain biking can take place in public natural spaces, the availability of public natural spaces was assessed by calculating the squared kilometres of public natural spaces within the living environment. The surface of the public natural spaces was obtained from a map of TOP10NL [22], and the function from a map of Statistics Netherlands [23]. The availability of sports facilities and natural public spaces was then corrected for the surface that was located within the Netherlands as described above (calculation density walking/cycling paths).

The distance to the nearest sports facility was assessed by calculating the straight-line distance using the midpoints of the six-digit postal codes of the home address and the sports facility. Sports accommodations and the types of sports that were available per accommodation were registered in the Sports Accommodation Monitor (Additional file 2: Table S2.1, Table S2.2). The sport that the respondent was practicing was obtained from the questionnaire. The facility that offered the sport they were practicing and was closest to the home address was then linked to the information of the respondent in 1187 of 1190 cases. This also included public natural spaces for sports such as running and cycling (see Additional file 2: Table S2.1, Table S2.2 for classification and an explanation of the sports and the accompanying facilities).

Statistical analysis

Six participants had missing values on individual characteristics and 56 participants had missing values on the distance to a specific sports facility (including the three participants who could not be linked to a sports facility). Finally, 10 participants with extreme values on time spent on physical activity (>112 hrs/wk) were excluded, leaving 1118 participants for the analysis (Fig. 1). Descriptive statistics were carried out for study characteristics. The differences of study characteristics between transport modes were examined with an ANOVA for continuous variables and a χ^2 test for categorical variables ($P < 0.05$).

To examine the association between perceived route features and transport choice, we used logistics regression analysis resulting in odds ratios (OR) and their confidence intervals (95 % CI) of cycling versus car use and walking versus car use. The ORs can be interpreted as the likelihood of an average person in our dataset choosing active transport use over car use for trips up to 7.5 kilometres. The ORs were adjusted for individual characteristics, motivational and situational factors and characteristics of the living environment, as previous literature reported that these can influence transport use [9–12]. The 13 perceived route features were entered separately in the model. The statistical analyses were carried out in SAS statistical software, version 9.3.

Results

Study characteristics

Table 1 presents characteristics of the participants and the direct living environment and it presents the motivational and situational factors and perceived route features that could influence transport choice when travelling to a sports facility.

Cyclists (mean: 46 yrs) were younger than car users (mean: 48 yrs, $p = 0.01$). Walkers ($p = 0.03$) and cyclists ($p < 0.01$) had a different household composition as compared to car users, i.e. walkers lived alone more often (26.5 % vs. 17.3 %) and cyclists lived more often with other adults (20.6 % vs. 11.9 %), whereas car users more often had children (31.9 $\%_{car}$ vs 20.8 $\%_{cyclists}$, 22.1 $\%_{walkers}$). Both cyclists (24.3 h/wk, $p < 0.01$) and walkers (24.0 h/wk, $p = 0.03$) were more physically active than car users (20.4 h/wk).

Walkers lived more often in urban- (outside-) centre areas than car users (47.5% vs. 37.8 %), and had a higher availability of cycling paths (1.9 km/km^2 vs 1.5 km/km^2) and walking paths (1.6 km/km^2 vs 1.1 km/km^2), sports facilities (0.7 $\#/km^2$ vs 0.6 $\#/km^2$) and public natural spaces (0.2 km^2/km^2 vs 0.1 km^2/km^2) ($p \leq 0.02$), and they lived closer to a sports facility (0.9 km vs 1.7 km, $p \leq 0.07$). Cyclists also had a higher availability of cycling paths (1.6 km/km^2 vs 1.5 km/km^2) and walking paths (1.3 km/km^2 vs 1.1 km/km^2), sports facilities (0.6 $\#/km^2$ vs 0.6 $\#/km^2$) and public natural spaces (0.1 km^2/km^2 vs 0.1 km^2/km^2), and they also lived closer to sports facilities than car users did (1.4 km vs 1.7 km) ($p \leq 0.03$).

All situational and motivational factors were rated differently between cyclists (13.8-85.6 %) and car users (7.1-66.7 %) ($p \leq 0.01$) except for the season ($p = 0.96$). Walkers rated only the situational and motivational factors such as 'the weather' (21.3 %), and 'my health' (57.4 %) differently from car users (51.0 % and 15.5 %, respectively, $p < 0.01$).

Seven out of thirteen perceived route features were rated differently between cyclists and car users, whereas five out of these seven perceived route features were rated differently between walkers and car users. Car users (5.2 %) more often answered that considering the traffic situation unsafe influenced their transport choice than cyclists did (2.4 %, $p = 0.02$). Most features of perceived route convenience (i.e. distance, time, easy to reach, and detour) were rated differently by car users (15.7 %, 54.0 %, 44.2 %, 6.8 % respectively) than by cyclists (38.1 %, 44.8 %, 52.1%, 15.3 %, respectively, $p \leq 0.01$). Walkers only rated distance (44.1 %), time (39.7 %), and detour (13.2 %, $p \leq 0.01$) differently from car users. The proportion of car users answering that the two perceived visual aspects of the route influenced their transport choice (3.4 %, 4.3 %) was lower than that of active transport users (9.6-14.0 %, $p < 0.01$).

The association between perceived route features and transport choice

In Table 2, the associations between perceived route features and the odds of cycling and walking as compared to using the car are presented.

Perceiving the road traffic situation as being unsafe was associated with lower odds of cycling (OR: 0.36, 95 % CI: 0.15-0.86), but not with the odds of walking (1.45, 95 % CI: 0.44-4.80).

Three aspects of perceived route convenience were associated with transport choice. 'The trip taking less time' was associated with lower odds of cycling (OR: 0.54, 95 % CI: 0.39-0.75) and walking (OR: 0.60, 95 % CI: 0.36-1.00). 'The distance to their destination being shorter' was associated with higher odds of both cycling (2.91, 95 % CI: 1.97-4.30) and walking (5.21, 95 % CI: 2.85-9.52). 'Being forced to make a detour when using the other two transport modes than the chosen transport mode' was associated with higher odds of cycling (1.82, 95 % CI: 1.06-3.15) and near statistically significant with walking (2.36, 95 %: 0.91-5.08).

Perceived visual aspects, i.e. what and who the participants see/encounter during the trip, were associated with higher odds of both cycling (2.40, 95 % CI: 1.27-4.53; 2.77, 95 % CI: 1.34-5.27) and walking (3.34, 95 % CI: 1.27-8.76; 3.69, 95 % CI: 1.29-10.52).

Perceived route features in terms of safety from criminality, bother by noise, odour, and vibrations, and route convenience aspects such as easy to reach their destination, traffic lights and obstacles, were not associated with cycling or walking.

Discussion

In this study, perceived route features in terms of traffic safety, some aspects of route convenience, and visual aspects were associated with transport choice when travelling to a sports facility. When traffic safety was perceived as unsafe or taking the car took less time, participants were more likely to choose the car than active transport modes. When the distance by using active transport was perceived shorter, or a detour had to be made when using the car, participants were more likely to choose active transport modes over the car. When participants considered what and who they may see/encounter during the trip to be important when making a transport choice, they were more likely to choose active transport modes over the car.

Strengths and limitations

In our study, we used a questionnaire that was specially designed to examine transport choice for specific trip purposes (i.e. sports). In addition, we were able to study the association between perceived route features and transport choice independent of individual, motivational and situational factors as well as physical characteristics of the built environment, which have been shown to be associated with active transport [9, 11, 24, 25]. Data were collected for all days during a full year, which enabled correction for seasonal influences. Moreover, data were

Table 2 Association* between perceived route features and active transport

	OR (95 % CI) $_{cycling\ vs\ car}$	OR (95 % CI) $_{cycling\ vs\ car}$
If you travel to the sports facility within a radius of 7.5 km, do you choose this transport mode[a] because you...		
Safety		
Consider the road traffic situation unsafe when using the other 2 transport modes[b]	0.36 (0.15-0.86)	1.45 (0.44-4.80)
Feel unsafe when travelling by the other 2 transport modes[b] because of criminality	0.71 (0.27-1.87)	1.41 (0.30-6.59)
Bother by noise, odour and vibrations		
Are bothered by noise when travelling by the other 2 transport modes[b]	0.86 (0.24-3.12)	1.33 (0.16-11.11)
Are bothered by odour when travelling by the other 2 transport modes[b]	0.75 (0.21-2.68)	1.29 (0.16-10.51)
Are bothered by vibrations when travelling by the other 2 transport modes[b]	0.65 (0.17-2.51)	0.39 (0.04-3.92)
Do the following factors influence your choice of using this transport mode[a] when you travel these distances?		
Route convenience		
Whether the distance to my destination is shorter	2.91 (1.97-4.30)	5.21 (2.85-9.52)
Whether it takes less time to reach my destination	0.54 (0.39-0.75)	0.60 (0.36-1.00)
Whether my destination is easy to reach	1.06 (0.77-1.48)	1.39 (0.82-2.36)
Whether I encounter a lot of traffic lights	0.92 (0.54-1.59)	0.56 (0.22-1.42)
Whether I encounter obstacles aimed at speed reduction (such as bumps in the road or road narrowings)	1.02 (0.57-1.85)	0.50 (0.18-1.40)
Whether I am forced to make a detour to reach my destination should I use either of the other 2 transport modes[b]	1.82 (1.06-3.15)	2.15 (0.91-5.08)
Visual aspects		
What I see/encounter during the trip	2.40 (1.27-4.53)	3.34 (1.27-8.76)
Who I see/encounter during the trip	2.77 (1.34-5.72)	3.69 (1.29-10.52)

OR = Odds Ratio indicating the odds to choose active transport modes compared to the car; 95%CI = 95% confidence interval; significance was tested at $\alpha = 0.05$
*Adjusted for: sex, age, education level, household composition, physical activity, neighbourhood typology, age of the neighbourhood, and length (km) cycling lane (for cyclists), length (km) walking paths (for walkers), number of sport facilities, and square km of public natural spaces per km^2, and the distance to a sports facility, and factors that influence the transport choice (i.e. the weather, I am used to travelling by this ,transport mode, It depends on whether I feel like using this transport mode, My health/health in general, Whether there is a cycle parking at my destination)
[a]In this question, the interpretation of 'this transport mode' depends on the categorisation of the respondent into a transport mode (i.e. car user, cyclist, walker). If someone was a car user, this transport mode was replaced by 'to use the car'; if someone was a cyclist, it was replaced by 'to cycle'; and if someone was a walker, it was replaced by 'to walk'
[b]If someone was categorised as a car user, the 2 other transport modes are by 'bicycle or on foot'; if someone was a cyclists, the other 2 transport modes are using the car and walking, if someone was a walker the other transport mode are using the car and cycling

collected from adults across the Netherlands, which provides a good representation of the Dutch adult population living in different environments.

Due to missing values, 27% (N = 401) of the participants who indicated that they made a short trip to a sports facility (N = 1529, Fig. 1) were not included in the analysis. The largest proportion (85%, N = 339) of the 401 participants with missing values had missing values on the sport they practiced. A possible explanation is that they did not practice any sport but, for example, made trips to a sports facility to watch a game or bring their children. Of the remaining 62 persons with missing values, six persons had missing data on individual characteristics and 56 persons had missing values on the distance to the sports facility. This latter might be due to a lack of information on the exact destination of our respondents. We assumed that they would go to the nearest sports facility linked to the sport they were participating in by means of the Sports Accommodation Monitor. It might be that their destination, i.e. sports facility, was not in the Sports Accommodation Monitor or that the sports facility was just outside the range of a 7.5-km radius. Moreover, we used straight-line distances instead of route distances, because of a lack of information of the route taken to their destination. In future, studies should consider gathering information about route distances and destinations (for example by using GPS tracking).

Putting results into context of the literature

To our knowledge, only a few studies have examined the association between features of the route and active transport use [26–28]. When comparing these studies with our study, it should be kept in mind that the study design in terms of definitions of active transport use, measures of (perceived) route features, setting (city, or a defined radius from the home address), and country (e.g., the Netherlands is densely populated and known for its unique cycling environment [29]), which can be a part of the explanation of differences in findings.

Traffic safety

When we compare the studies with regard to traffic safety, in the study by Panter and colleagues, less traffic was associated with lower odds of walking to work, which may be explained by the fact that walking to work is probably more prevalent in built-up areas where traffic levels are higher [26]. In the study by Titze and colleagues, students who cycled regularly to the university rated the traffic safety lower as compared to non-cyclists. This may seem odd, but it might be explained by the non-awareness of dangers by non-cyclists who may not have cycled the route to the university, whereas regular cyclists probably are aware of the dangers [27]. In our study, traffic safety was inversely associated with cycling as compared to using the car indicating that those who travel by car to a sports facility more often perceive the traffic situation as unsafe as compared to those who travel by bicycle. This suggests that the experience of safety may be different between trip purposes, as in our study where people travel for recreational purposes (i.e. sports), thinking the traffic situation being unsafe was associated with passive transport use, whereas in the other two studies high traffic volume or unsafe traffic situations did not stop the participants from walking or cycling to work or the university.

Route convenience

With regard to perceived route convenience, Panter and colleagues found higher odds for both '1-149 min/wk' cycling and ' ≥150 min/wk' cycling if participants indicated that 'there are convenient routes for cycling' [26]. In the Norfolk study, both men and women who lived a relatively short distance from work were more likely to actively commute, whereas having a main or secondary road on the route to work was associated with a decreased likelihood of active commuting [28]. The latter may be explained by safety concerns as the presence of these roads could reflect unpleasant traffic interaction (busy, noise, high speeds) when actively commuting [28], or by the fact that access to their destination is simply easier by car because of these roads. In our study, we also found aspects of route convenience (i.e. distance, time and detour) to be associated with active transport use. However, other aspects of perceived route convenience such as easy to reach, traffic lights, and obstacles to reduce speeding were not associated with active transport use. Similarly, Titze and colleagues found no association between perceived traffic flow (continuous cycling, presence of traffic lights) and connectivity (shortcuts, quickness compared to driving a car) and active commuting [27]. From a previous review with objectively measured neighbourhood characteristics, it was shown that residents from communities with higher density, greater connectivity and more land use mix more often used active transport than low-density, poorly connected, and single land use neighbourhoods [25], raising the expectations that perceived route convenience, such as connectivity and easy to reach could be of importance in using active transport. This mismatch between perceived and objective accessibility measures has previously been shown [30, 31]. In addition, a recent study within the AVENUE project has shown that perceived accessibility, irrespective of objective accessibility, was strongly associated with transport choice for trips with the purpose of shopping, sports or public natural spaces (Scheepers CE, Wendel-Vos GCW, van Kempen EEMM, de Hollander EL, van Wijnen HJ, Maas J, den Hertog FRJ, Staatsen BAM, Stipdonk HL , Int Panis LLR, van Wesemael PJV, Schuit AJ: Perceived Accessibility is An Important Factor in Transport Choice — Results from the AVENUE Project, Submitted). This indicates that perceived environmental characteristics cannot be translated to objectively measured environmental characteristics. This can be illustrated by case studies [32, 33]. One study found that cycling commuters were more likely to take a route that was bumpy, but quiet and green, instead of taking the separate cycling lane designed by urban planners [33]. Another case study including different neighbourhoods in Amsterdam, the Netherlands, showed that individuals perceived the distance to be shorter if many people and less traffic were observed along the route [32]. Taking all of these aspects into account, this indicates that determining the contribution of perceived features and the contribution of objective features in stimulating active transport use is difficult as subjective and objective features interact with each other. Future research should incorporate these aspects in order to guide policy makers and urban planners in the development of measures to stimulate active transport use.

Visual aspects

With regard to perceived visual aspects, attractiveness was positively associated with irregular cycling but not with regular cycling compared to non-cycling in the study by Titze et al. [27]. In a previous study, it was shown that physical activity in general is positively associated with attractiveness [34]. Since cycling to work is different from cycling during leisure time (recreation), it seems reasonable that attractiveness is more important for irregular cyclists than for regular cyclists [27]. In our study, visual aspects of the route were positively associated with both cycling and walking as compared to using the car when travelling to a sports facility. This might be explained by visual aspects being more important when travelling for recreational purposes (i.e. to a sports facility) than for school purposes. To illustrate further the importance of the trip purpose in the association between perceived environmental factors and active transport use, previous studies have shown that different perceived environmental factors were associated with different types of walking [24], and the strength of the association of perceived accessibility differed per trip purpose (i.e. shopping, work, public natural spaces and sports facility) (Scheepers CE, Wendel-Vos GCW, van Kempen EEMM, de Hollander EL, van Wijnen HJ, Maas J, den Hertog FRJ, Staatsen BAM, Stipdonk HL, Int Panis LLR, van Wesemael PJV, Schuit AJ: Perceived Accessibility is An Important Factor in Transport Choice — Results from the AVENUE Project, Submitted). Moreover, from exploratory analysis in the AVENUE study, we found that persons who indicated that they travelled for sports and working purposes, the transport choice differed in 33% of the cases. For sports and shopping purposes, the difference was 41% and for sports and public natural spaces purposes 48%. Thus, it is very well possible that not only the experience and importance of route features differ per trip purpose, but that people also choose different transport modes to travel to different destinations. Therefore, future research should take trip purpose into account when examining the associations between route features and active transport use. Consequently, when developing policy measures to stimulate active transport, the target group (workers, students or sports practitioners) should be taken into account.

Conclusions

For Dutch adult sports practitioners, perceived route features in terms of traffic safety, convenience, and visual aspects were associated with transport choice when travelling to a sports facility. This suggests that the perception of different route aspects should be considered when developing measures for stimulating active transport use among sports practitioners.

Additional files

Additional file 1: Table S1. 1Correlations between factors that could influence the choice of transport.

Additional file 2: Table S2. 1Calculating the distance to a sports facility according to different types of sport.

Abbreviations

AVENUE: impActs of actiVE traNsport in Urban Environments; BAG: Dutch Registration of Addresses and Buildings (in Dutch: "Basisregistratie Adressen en Gebouwen); CI: Confidence interval; OR: Odds ratio; PA: Physical activity; SQUASH: Short QUestionnaire to ASsess Health-enhancing physical activity.

Competing interests

The authors declare that they have no competing interests.

Authors' contributions

ELdH wrote the draft version of the manuscript and conducted the statistical analysis. ELdH, ES, WWV, EEMMvK contributed to the statistical analysis and the study concept. All authors contributed to the interpretation of the results and revision of the manuscript, approved the final manuscript and are accountable for all aspects of the work in ensuring that questions related to the accuracy or integrity of any part of the work are appropriately investigated and resolved.

Acknowledgements

The authors thank K. Wezenberg-Hoenderkamp from the Mulier Institute for deriving data on sports facilities from the Sports Accommodation Monitor.

Funding

The authors have no support or funding to report.

Author details

[1]National Institute for Public Health and the Environment, Centre for Nutrition, Prevention and Health Services, PO Box 1, 3720 BA Bilthoven, Netherlands. [2]Department of Health Sciences and EMGO institute for Health and Care Research, VU University Amsterdam, De Boelelaan 1085, 1081 HV Amsterdam, Netherlands. [3]National Institute for Public Health and the Environment, Centre for Sustainability, Environment and Health, PO Box 1, 3720 BA Bilthoven, Netherlands. [4]Department of the Built Environment, Technical University Eindhoven, PO Box 513, 5600 MB Eindhoven, Netherlands.

References

1. Global Recommendations on Physical Activity for Health. Geneva, Switzerland: World Health Organisation; 2010.
2. Proper KI, Singh AS, van Mechelen W, Chinapaw MJ. Sedentary behaviors and health outcomes among adults: a systematic review of prospective studies. Am J Prev Med. 2011;40(2):174–82.
3. Wagner A, Dallongeville J, Haas B, Ruidavets JB, Amouyel P, Ferrieres J, et al. Sedentary behaviour, physical activity and dietary patterns are independently associated with the metabolic syndrome. Diabetes & metabolism. 2012;38(5):428–35.
4. Chau J, van der Ploeg H, Merom D, Chey T, Bauman A. Cross-sectional associations between occupational and leisure-time sitting, physical activity and obesity in working adults. Prev Med. 2012;54:195–200.
5. van der Ploeg H, Chey T, Korda R, Banks E, Bauman A. Sitting Time and All-Cause Mortality Risk in 222 497 Australian Adults. Arch Intern Med. 2012;172(6):494–500.
6. Hendriksen IJ, Bernaards CM, Hildebrandt VH. Lichamelijke inactiviteit en sedentair gedrag in de Nederlandse bevolking. In: De B, editor. Trendrapport Bewegen en Gezondheid 2008/2009. Leiden: TNO Kwaliteit van Leven; 2010.
7. de Nazelle A, Nieuwenhuijsen MJ, Anto JM, Brauer M, Briggs D, Braun-Fahrlander C, et al. Improving health through policies that promote active travel: a review of evidence to support integrated health impact assessment. Environ Int. 2011;37(4):766–77.

8. Scheepers E, Slinger M, Wendel-Vos W, Schuit J. How combined trip purposes are associated with transport choice for short distance trips. Results from a cross-sectional study in the Netherlands. PLoS One. 2014;9(12):e114797.
9. Wendel-Vos W, Droomers M, Kremers S, Brug J, van Lenthe F. Potential environmental determinants of physical activity in adults: a systematic review. Obes Rev. 2007;8(5):425–40.
10. Deforche B, Van Dyck D, Verloigne M, De Bourdeaudhuij I. Perceived social and physical environmental correlates of physical activity in older adolescents and the moderating effect of self-efficacy. Prev Med. 2010;50 Suppl 1:S24–9.
11. Saelens BE, Handy SL. Built environment correlates of walking: a review. Med Sci Sports Exerc. 2008;40(7 Suppl):S550–66.
12. Scheepers E, Wendel-Vos W, van Kempen E, Panis LI, Maas J, Stipdonk H, et al. Personal and environmental characteristics associated with choice of active transport modes versus car use for different trip purposes of trips up to 7.5 kilometers in The Netherlands. PLoS One. 2013;8(9):e73105.
13. Projectbureau Sport en Bewegen in de Buurt: Sport en Bewegen in de buurt. http://www.sportindebuurt.nl/ (2013). Accessed 23 Dec 2015.
14. Schippers E. Kamerbrief over voortgang programma Sport en Bewegen in de Buurt. Den Haag, the Netherlands: Ministerie van Volksgezondheid, Welzijn en Sport; 2014.
15. Ipsos: Over Ipsos. http://www.ipsos-nederland.nl/over-ipsos (2015). Accessed 09 Apr 2015.
16. de Hollander EL, Zwart L, de Vries SI, Wendel-Vos W. The SQUASH was a more valid tool than the OBiN for categorizing adults according to the Dutch physical activity and the combined guideline. J Clin Epidemiol. 2012;65(1):73–81.
17. Wendel-Vos GC, Schuit AJ, Saris WH, Kromhout D. Reproducibility and relative validity of the short questionnaire to assess health-enhancing physical activity. J Clin Epidemiol. 2003;56(12):1163–9.
18. Kemper H, Ooijendijk W, Stiggelbout M. Consensus about the Dutch Physical Activity Guideline. TSG. 2000;78:180–3.
19. ABF Research: ABF Woonmilieutypologie. http://www.abfresearch.nl/media/644840/woonmilieutypologie.pdf (2009). Accessed 23 December 2013.
20. Kadaster: Basisregistratie Adressen en Gebouwen (BAG). http://www.kadaster.nl/bag (2014). Accessed 16 Jan 2014.
21. OpenStreetMap contributors: OpenStreetMap. www.openstreetmap.org (2013). Accessed 01 Oct 2013.
22. Publieke Dienstverlening Op de Kaart: TOP10NL (2008). https://www.pdok.nl/nl/producten/pdok-downloads/basis-registratie-topografie/topnl/topnl-actueel/top10nl. Accessed 01 Nov 2013.
23. Statistics Netherlands: CBS Geoviewer. Bodemgebruik Nederland (2008). http://download.cbs.nl/geoviewer/index.html?config=config-bodemgebruik-2008.xml. Accessed 01 Nov 2013.
24. Owen N, Humpel N, Leslie E, Bauman A, Sallis JF. Understanding environmental influences on walking; Review and research agenda. Am J Prev Med. 2004;27(1):67–76.
25. Saelens BE, Sallis JF, Frank LD. Environmental correlates of walking and cycling: findings from the transportation, urban design, and planning literatures. Ann Behav Med. 2003;25(2):80–91.
26. Panter J, Griffin S, Jones A, Mackett R, Ogilvie D. Correlates of time spent walking and cycling to and from work: baseline results from the commuting and health in Cambridge study. Int J Behav Nutr Phys Act. 2011;8:124.
27. Titze S, Stronegger WJ, Janschitz S, Oja P. Environmental, social, and personal correlates of cycling for transportation in a student population. J Phys Act Health. 2007;4(1):66–79.
28. Panter JR, Jones AP, van Sluijs EM, Griffin SJ, Wareham NJ. Environmental and psychological correlates of older adult's active commuting. Med Sci Sports Exerc. 2011;43(7):1235–43.
29. Pucher J, Buehler R. Making cycling irresistible: lessons form the Netherlands. Denmark and Germany Transport Rev. 2008;28(4):495–528.
30. McCormack GR, Cerin E, Leslie E, Du Toit L, Owen N. Objective versus perceived walking distances to destinations. Correspondence and predictive validity Environment and Behavior. 2008;40(3):294–8.
31. Ball K, Jeffery RW, Crawford DA, Roberts RJ, Salmon J, Timperio AF. Mismatch between perceived and objective measures of physical activity environments. Prev Med. 2008;47(3):294–8.
32. den Hertog F, Bronkhorst M, Moerman M, van Wilgenburg R. De Gezonde Wijk. Een onderzoek naar de relatie tussen fysieke wijkkenmerken en lichamelijke activiteit. Amsterdam, the Netherlands: EMGO Instituut; 2006.
33. van Duppen J, Spierings B. Retracing trajectories: The embodied experience of cycling, urban sensescapes and the commute between 'neighbourhood' and the 'city' in Utrecht. NL Journal of Transport Geography. 2013;30:234–43.
34. Humpel N, Owen N, Iverson D, Leslie E, Bauman A. Perceived environment attributes, residential location, and walking for particular purposes. Am J Prev Med. 2004;26(2):119–25.

5

The effect of the stay active advice on physical activity and on the course of acute severe low back pain

Patricia Olaya-Contreras[1,2,3*], Jorma Styf[1], Daniel Arvidsson[4,5], Karin Frennered[1] and Tommy Hansson[1]

Abstract

Background: Disability due to acute low back pain (ALBP) runs parallel with distress and physical inactivity. If low back pain persists, this may lead to long-term sick leave and chronic back pain. This prospective randomized study evaluated the effect on physical activity and on the course of ALBP of two different treatment advices provided in routine care.

Methods: Ninety-nine patients with acute severe LBP examined within 48 h after pain onset were randomized to the treatment advices "Stay active in spite of pain" (stay active group) or "Adjust activity to the pain" (adjust activity group). Pedometer step count and pain intensity (Numeric Rating Scale, NRS, 0–10) were followed daily during seven days. Linear mixed modeling were employed for statistical analyses.

Results: The step count change trajectory showed a curvilinear shape with a steep initial increase reaching a plateau after day 3 in both groups, followed by an additional increase to day 7 in the stay active group only. At day 1, the step count was 4560 in the stay active group compared to 4317 in adjust activity group ($p = 0.76$). Although there were no statistical differences between the two groups in the parameters describing the change trajectory for step count, the increase in step count was larger in the stay active group. At day 7 the step count was 9865 in the stay active group compared to 6609 in the adjust activity group ($p = 0.008$). The pain intensity (NRS) trajectory was similar in the two groups. Between day 1 and day 7 it decreased linearly from 5.0 to 2.8 in the stay active group ($p < 0.001$), and from 4.8 to 2.3 in the adjust activity group ($p < 0.001$).

Conclusions: Patients with acute severe LBP advised to stay active in spite of the pain exhibited a considerable more active behavior compared to patients adjusting their activity to pain. This result confirms compliance to the treatment advice as well as the utility of the stay active advice to promote additional physical activity for more health benefits in patients with ALBP. There was minimal effect of the treatment advice on the course of ALBP.

Trial registration: ClinicalTrials.gov (NCT02517762).

Background

The prevalence of low back pain (LBP) is around 10 % and it causes more disability than any other condition [1]. The highest prevalence can be found in Western Europe, with almost 16 % of the males and 15 % of the females affected [1]. Acute low back pain (ALBP) defined as an episode of LBP persisting for less than six weeks [2], is commonly encountered in primary care practice. Nevertheless, often the specific cause cannot be identified in spite of a variety of diagnostic methods in general practice. A specific diagnosis can only be reached in around 10–20 % of all patients with LBP. Even though ALBP has good prognosis with normalization of its symptoms usually within few days, as many as 30 % of people with episode of nonspecific LBP do not recover within 1 year [3, 4]. Additionally, the risk for recurrence and development into chronic LBP is between 2 % and 56 % [5–7]. About half of the adult population will suffer

* Correspondence: patricia.olayac@udea.edu.co
[1]Department of Orthopedics, Institute of Clinical Sciences at the Sahlgrenska Academy, University of Gothenburg, Gothenburg, Sweden
[2]Department of Postgraduate Studies, Faculty of Nursing, University of Antioquia, Calle 70 No 52-21, Apartado Aereo, 1226 Medellín, Antioquia, Colombia
Full list of author information is available at the end of the article

from LBP during a 12-month period [8]. In Sweden, the high prevalence of spine problems is a major source of disability and treatment for this necessitates high levels of health care expenditure [9]. Therefore, regimens that accelerate recovery of ALBP would be of profound importance for optimizing clinical practice, which could prevent chronicity of pain and reduce a big amount of disability due to LBP.

There is substantial evidence that physical activity has beneficial effects on most musculoskeletal conditions, including LBP [10]. For that reason, advising the patient to stay active is a crucial part of the recommended treatment of ALBP [2, 11]. However, current evidence in favor for the stay active advise in patients with ALBP is limited, with small or no benefits in pain relief, functional improvement or sick leave compared to rest in bed [12]. Effects in favor for rest in bed has also been reported [12]. In an observational study, lower risk of ALBP and lower rate of recurrence were found among patients advised to stay active compared to patients advised to rest [13]. In these studies, the stay active advice was implemented several days after onset ALBP, and an important part of its effect may therefore have been lost. In addition, as the symptoms of ALBP have a course of days up to a week, late assessment would probably lead to lost treatment opportunities to support patients to stay active and to prevent negative pain behaviors/pain avoidance. Previous studies investigated the effect of the stay active advice after several months [12]. However, to best of our knowledge, no study has actually investigated neither the early implementation of the stay active advice after a severe ALBP, nor followed up its effect on pain or compliance to treatment advice using an objective measure of physical activity, prospectively.

Compliance to the stay active advice could be an important factor influencing the magnitude of the effect on ALBP, but little has been reported. Malmivaara et al. found less hours of bed rest and more hours doing back exercises as measures of compliance in patients with ALBP receiving a stay active advice compared to patients advised to rest in bed. In the referred study, compliance was assessed by means of a questionnaire [14], thus, these questions were not direct measures of whether the patients stayed active and maintained their normal activity levels. Further, questionnaires are prone to recall bias and may exaggerate any intervention effect [15, 16]. It is likely that bed rest is a rather obsolete advice for patients with ALBP today. Currently, stay active or adjust your activity according to the pain are probably the most common clinical advices. However, the definition and implementation of the stay active advice may vary between clinics and investigators. A more cautious attitude among general practitioners may influence the beliefs of the patient and compliance to intentioned treatment [17–20].

Moreover, fear avoidance beliefs have been shown to influence the prognosis of ALBP [21–23]. According to previous research, pain avoidance belief in general practitioners is associated with prescribing sick leave during painful periods of ALBP [24, 25]. Further, management of first time ALBP varies, reflecting uncertainty about the optimal approach [25, 26]. Therefore, there is a need for implementation of early treatments strategies relying on evidence-based knowledge to treat acute problems and lower the risk for recurrence and chronicity of LBP.

The stay active advice may not only be a treatment to improve recovery from ALBP, but also an opportunity to promote physical activity for other health benefits, such as improved cardio-metabolic function, blood pressure, and reduced body fatness [27, 28]. An individual that accumulates at least 10000 steps daily could be defined as being at a health-enhancing level of physical activity [29]. However, a low proportion of the general population actually meets the recommended level of physical activity. Among person with low level of physical activity it has been observed increased risk for LBP, recurrence and disability due to LBP [30].

In the present study, the two treatment advices "Stay as active as possible in spite of the back pain" or "Adjust activity to pain" were implemented early after onset of acute severe LBP. The aims were to evaluate their effect on objectively measured physical activity and on the course of ALBP.

Methods

Design

A prospective randomized study was conducted at the Department of Orthopaedics, Sahlgrenska University Hospital Gothenburg, Sweden, to evaluate the effect on physical activity and on the course of acute severe LBP of two different treatment advices provided in routine care. All patients were followed for seven days from maximum 48 h after the onset of the ALBP. The Regional Ethical Review Board at the University of Gothenburg approved the study protocol. Trial registration: ClinicalTrials.gov (NCT02517762).

Patients and procedures

Participants in the study were recruited consecutively among employees from a large local manufacturing company representing several different factories. All employees had been informed to immediately contact the company physiotherapist or the nurse coordinating the study in case of acute severe pain in the lower back. Eligible participants were subjects between 18 and 65 years of age, with acute severe LPB, with duration from onset less than or equal to 48 h, with or without radiating leg pain, with or without neurological signs, and the pain had to exceed 50 mm on the Visual Analog Scale (VAS).

Patients were requested to fill out and return a seven-day diary and those who did so were included. Excluded were those who had been on sick leave because of LBP in the last month or because of pain in the spine. Employees determined eligible were enrolled in the study after giving informed consent, and were immediately referred to an academic orthopedic department for further examinations. Enrolment took place from March 2005 until December 2008.

At the hospital the patients underwent an X-ray examination of the lumbar spine (frontal and lateral projections and a spot view of the lumbosacral spine) followed by a magnetic resonance imaging (MRI) examination including T1 and T2 weighted and short time inversion recovery (STIR) sequences. They also underwent an extensive physical examination performed in a standardized way by one of three orthopedic spine specialists. The physician explained for the patient the imaging findings as well as the results of the physical examination. The patients were also asked to complete a battery of questionnaires [31] covering history of ALBP, lifestyle characteristics, work place factors, and initial intensity of pain on Visual Analog Scale (VAS), and location of pain on pain drawing. Additional psychosocial factors and psychological variables were asked.

Thereafter, each patient was randomly allocated to one of the two treatment advices, using a random table. A sealed envelope with the treatment assignment was distributed to the physician, who instructed the patient about the content and practical aspects of the actual treatment advice according to protocol (see Treatments below). To obtain as similar information as possible the three physicians coordinated the content of the two treatment advices prior to the study. This coordination was repeated at several occasions during the study period to keep the instruction as constant as possible. The coordinating nurse gave the patient instructions regarding the 7-day diary (see 7-day diary below). The patient was instructed to return the completed diary as soon as possible after the follow-up period. One month after entering the study, each patient had a follow-up appointment with a physiotherapist at the company health center to check the patient's status. Throughout the entire study, the coordinating nurse acted as a study monitor, guiding each patient through the study and providing standardized information. We enrolled and allocated 109 employees to treatment (Fig. 1).

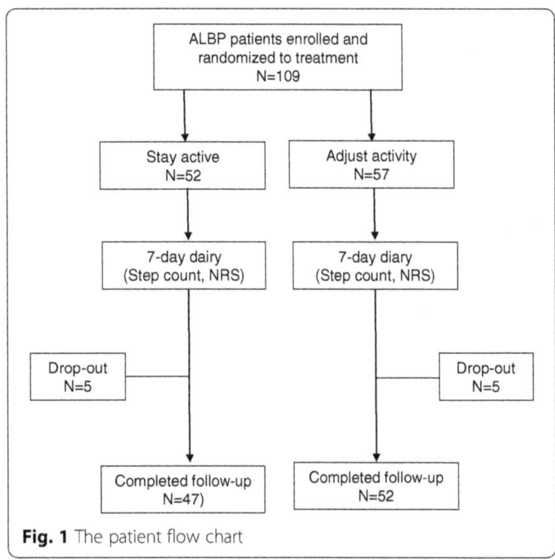

Fig. 1 The patient flow chart

Treatment advices

The patients were advised either to stay as physically active as possible in spite of the LBP (stay active, SA), or to adjust the activity according to the pain (adjust activity, AA). Patients with the AA advice were instructed to avoid activities, movements, or positions that caused or worsened the pain. Of the 109 randomized patients, 52 patients (47.5 %) were allocated the SA advice and 57 patients (52.5 %) to the AA advice.

Medication

All the patients who wanted help with pain relief were prescribed either paracetamol and/or NSAID. The number of prescriptions in the two groups was similar but the use of the drugs was not checked.

7-day diary

After the clinical examinations and the allocation to the treatment, each patient received a diary to record daily step count (pedometer), pain intensity (NRS), pain location and pain-related disability (DRI) during the following 7 days. In addition, they described in the diary all kind of physical activities performed under the 7-day follow-up period.

Physical activity

Step count was used both as a measure of daily physical activity, and as an indicator of compliance to treatment advice over the 7-day follow-up. Each patient received a digital pedometer (LS 2000, Kalmar, Sweden) and was instructed to wear it during all waken hours and to record the daily step count in the diary. This type of pedometer has been validated in previous studies for estimating the total daily number of steps [32, 33]. The daily step count was used to categorize patients according to step count cut-offs for activity levels defined from healthy adults: sedentary <5000, low active 5000–7499, somewhat active 7500–9999, and active ≥10000 [34]. The last category has also been used as the recommended level of step count to promote health. The patients were also asked to report in the diary any other kind of special physical activities that they participated in at work or during leisure (e.g. sporting events, etc.), during the follow up.

Pain intensity

The Numerical Graphic Rating Scale (NRS, 0–10) is a box scale consisting of 11 numbers from 0 (no pain) to 10 (pain as bad as it could be). The patients were asked to place an "X" at the number that represented their pain. The NRS is easy to administer and there is good evidence for its construct validity [35]. The VAS was used to self-assess the patient's pain intensity at the initial clinical examination, and was rated on a 100 mm scale, ranging from 0 (no pain) to 100 (worst possible pain) [35]. In addition, using a full-body drawing in the dorsal and ventral views, the patient marked the location(s) of the pain [35].

Absenteeism

Information regarding work absenteeism and sick leave due to the current back problems was collected from the company records up to one month after the onset of the ALBP episode.

Statistical analyses

Due to the lack of previous information on step count from patients with ALBP, a power calculation was performed as follows. Based on an estimated mean difference in daily step count between the 2 groups of 1000 steps (SD = 2000/day) reported by healthy subjects [36], to achieve a statistical power of 0.80 with a significance level of 0.05, it was estimated that 120 patients would be required for this study [37]. Allowing for a dropout rate of up to 10 %, the target recruitment number was 66 patients in each group.

Group comparisons at baseline were performed using the Chi-squared test (gender, occupation, and type of activity before the LBP), the Mann–Whitney test (NRS, VAS), and the *t*-test (age and days of absenteeism). Linear mixed models (LMM) were used to estimate the shape of the step count and pain intensity (NRS) change trajectories over seven repeated measures (Day, 1–7), as they provide greater flexibility to repeated measures designs and their specific variance structures [38]. A third-order polynomial function provided the best fit to data for the change in step count over time, while a first-order polynomial function provided the best fit to data for pain intensity according to the Bayesian information criterion (BIC) for goodness-of-fit. Models developed included both fixed and random effects for intercepts, and fixed effects for all slope components (linear, quadratic and cubic terms). As we are limited in the number of random effects by the number of repeated measures, a random effect was included only for the linear slope component to describe inter-individual difference in change trajectory [38]. A second step was to include the fixed effect of treatment advice on intercepts and slope components. Maximum likelihood (ML) was used for the estimation of fixed and random effects. For the models developed, day 1 was used as intercept. By also defining the intercept at each of the other days (day 2–7), difference in step count or pain intensity could be statistically tested for each day over the entire follow-up. Statistical significance was set at $p < 0.05$. All statistical analyses were performed using SPSS 22 (IBM Coperation, NY, USA).

Results

Patients and clinical findings

One hundred-and-nine participants with acute (≤48 h) severe LBP (VAS > 50 mm) were enrolled in the study. The mean age for all the participants was 42.1 years (range 20–63). Seventy-two percent were men and 57 % percent were white-collar. Thirty-five percent of the patients claimed that their ALBP arose while working and 32 % reported that their back problems arose without any obvious external exertion. The diagnoses (ICD10 coding) were acute lumbago in 88 % (M545), acute lumbago with sciatica in 10 % (M544), and lumbar spinal stenosis in 2 % (M480). The majority of the patients (76 %) returned directly to work after the clinical examination, whereas 17 % were absent from work less than 5 days, and 7 % were absent from work between 6 to 8 days. The return to work rate was the same in the two treatment groups. There were no differences between the two groups for age, gender or sick leave due to the ALBP ($p > 0.05$). In addition, there were no differences between the groups regarding the reported cause of ALBP, occupation or initial pain intensity (VAS).

Non-response analyses

Ninety-nine patients (91 %) completed and returned the diary with the information regarding step count, pain intensity (NRS) and pain-related disability (DRI). The average age was 37.3 years (range 27–53) for those not returning the diary, and 42.5 years (range 20–63) for those returning the completed diary ($p > 0.05$). There were no statistically significant differences between the responders and non-responders regarding gender or ethnicity ($p > 0.05$). Differences in the initial scores on DRI were found between the groups, where the responders scored higher ($p < 0.05$). For the responders included in the statistical analyses, 47 patients were assigned to the stay active group (SA) and 52 to the adjust activity group (AA) (Fig. 1). Of the 10 non-responders, 5 had been randomized to the SA group and 5 to the AA group.

Physical activity change trajectory

Figure 2 displays the modeled change trajectory of step count over time and is complemented by the results in Table 1. There was a steep initial linear increase (Table 1, Model 1, linear term, $p < 0.001$) that leveled off and reached a plateau after day 3 (quadratic term, $p < 0.001$). From day 6 there was an additional increase in step count (cubic term, $p < 0.001$). However, the change trajectory in step count was not similar in the two treatment groups. At the first follow-up day there was only a small difference of 243 steps between the groups (Model 2, intercept $p = 0.76$). Although there was no statistically significant effect of treatment advice on any of the three change trajectory terms (Model 2, linear $p = 0.30$, quadratic $p = 0.42$, cubic $p = 0.34$), the increase in step count was larger in the SA group compared to the AA group. At the plateau at day 3 the difference between the groups was 1133 steps ($p = 0.09$). Thereafter, the step count increased only in the SA group with statistically significant difference between groups reached at day 6 ($p = 0.02$, Fig. 2). At the last day of the follow-up period the estimated step count in the SA group was 9865 steps which approached the step count cut-off defined as being active, compared to 6609 steps in the AA group remaining in the low active step count category ($p = 0.008$). At the first day of the follow-up, 2 % in the SA group and 8 % in the AA group reached the recommended 10000 steps. At the last day, the corresponding proportions were 39 % in the SA group compared to 8 % in the AA group.

Pain intensity change trajectory

Figure 3 and Table 2 display the modeled change trajectory of pain intensity (NRS) over time. The pain intensity decreased linearly over the follow-up period for all the patients in both groups (Table 2, Model 1, linear term $p < 0.001$). The SA group showed somewhat higher pain intensity and a somewhat slower decrease in pain intensity compared to the AA group, however, there was no statistically significant effect of treatment advice on the pain intensity change trajectory (Model 2, intercept $p = 0.67$, linear term $p = 0.52$). The estimated pain intensity decreased between day 1 and day 7 from 5.0 to 2.8 ($p < 0.001$) in the SA group, and from 4.8 to 2.3 ($p < 0.001$) in the AA group.

Discussion

The present study contributed with the follow-up of the effect of two treatment advices on objectively measured physical activity and on the course of ALBP from early after its onset. The patients advised to stay active (SA) in spite of LBP increased their activity more than the patients advised to adjust activity (AA) to the pain, which confirmed compliance with the advices. Due to this compliance and the early inclusion after the pain onset, it can be stated that the SA advice did not alter the course of ALBP. However, the SA advice promoted a pronounced increase in daily activity among these patients who reached the recommended level of 10000 steps for additional health benefits [34, 36, 39], which has important clinical and public health implications.

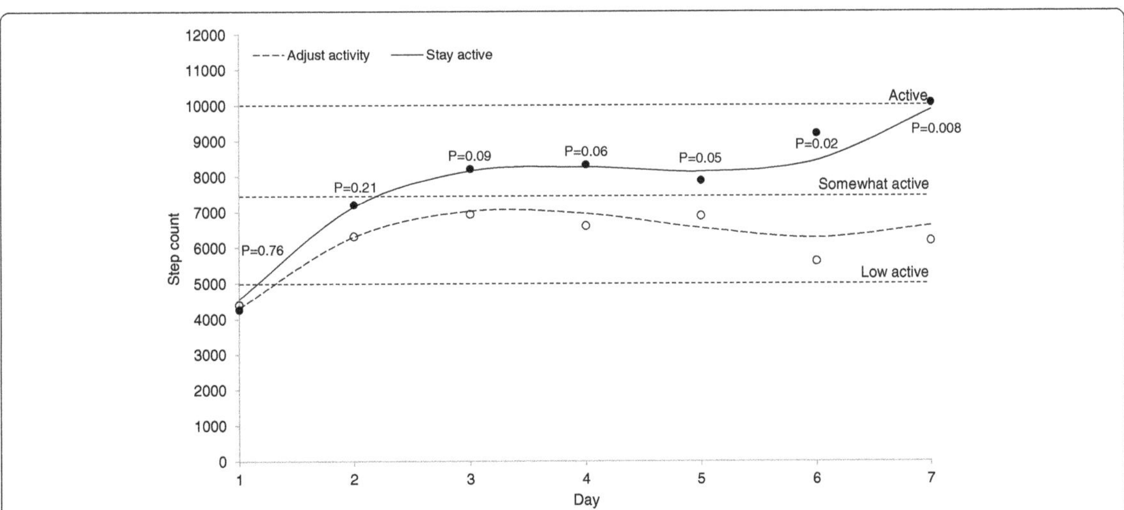

Fig. 2 Modeled daily step count over the 7 days follow-up in patients with ALBP. Solid line represents patients advised to stay active (SA) and dashed line patients advised to adjust activity (AA) to the pain; horizontal lines are cut-offs for daily step count levels; p-values indicate statistical difference between groups of modeled values; circles indicate mean of observed step count (SA = filled, AA = open)

Table 1 Linear mixed models to estimate change in step count over seven days follow-up and the effect of treatment advice (SA = Stay active versus AA = Adjust activity) on this change

$N = 99$	Model 1: Change trajectory		Model 2: Effect of treatment advice	
Fixed effects in model	Estimate (SE)	*p*-value	Estimate (SE)	*p*-value
Day 1 (intercept)	4434 (405)	<0.001	4317 (558)	<0.001
+Stay active advice	-	-	243 (812)	0.76
Day (β, linear term)	3160 (398)	<0.001	2773 (545)	<0.001
+Stay active advice	-	-	824 (796)	0.30
Day^2 (β, quadratic term)	−987 (161)	<0.001	−865 (220)	<0.001
+Stay active advice	-	-	−257 (321)	0.42
Day^3 (β, cubic term)	94 (18)	<0.001	75 (24)	0.002
+Stay active advice	-	-	34 (36)	0.34

Fixed effects in models are presented with step count as outcome
Model 1 is the estimated change trajectory without the effect of treatment advice. Model 2 includes the effect of treatment advice, where the effect of the Adjust activity is presented first followed by the added effect of the Stay active advice
A third-order polynomial function was used with a linear term (Day) describing the initial increase (positive value), a quadratic term (Day^2) describing the level-off of the initial increase (negative value) and a cubic term (Day^3) for the additional final increase in step count over time

In a supportive clinical environment where general practitioners have a positive attitude to active rehabilitation in combination with early assessment and treatment, the fear of motion or avoidance of pain among patients advised to be physically active might be less pronounced [17–20]. Among patients receiving the SA advice, the large increase in step count with a large proportion of patients reaching the recommended level of step count should indicate that they overcame their fear of movement/activity related to pain, in line with previous research [21–23].

Previous research often involved ALBP patients from primary care settings recruited after three or more days of LBP duration [2, 14, 40, 41]. In the present study, the severe pain symptoms were alleviated within hours after presentation and the pain intensity decreased linearly over the follow-up period with the patients being cured or having at most a mild degree of pain at day 7. If the patients would have been examined later than within 48 h after the pain onset, many of them would not have been included in the study. Furthermore, the effect of the SA advice might be underestimated if started at a later stage of the course of ALBP. Our results shown that the SA advice and pedometer, as accessible methods, promoted a considerable larger increase in physical activity among patients in the SA group, even though they exhibited similar experience of pain as did the patients in the AA group. These findings have important clinical implications

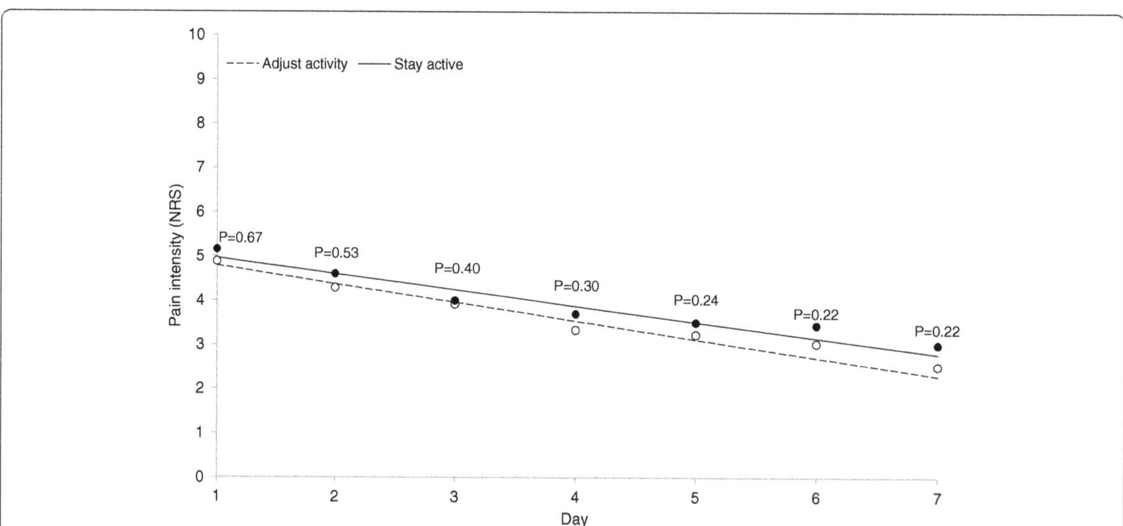

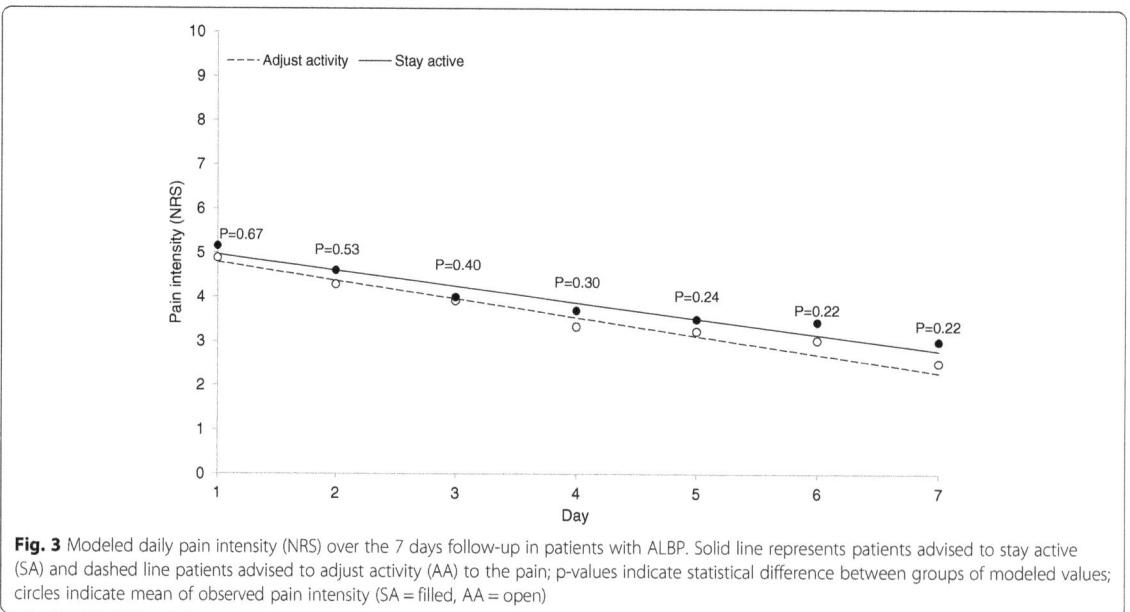

Fig. 3 Modeled daily pain intensity (NRS) over the 7 days follow-up in patients with ALBP. Solid line represents patients advised to stay active (SA) and dashed line patients advised to adjust activity (AA) to the pain; p-values indicate statistical difference between groups of modeled values; circles indicate mean of observed pain intensity (SA = filled, AA = open)

Table 2 Linear mixed models to estimate change in pain intensity (NRS) over seven days follow-up and the effect of treatment advice (SA = Stay active versus AA = Adjust activity) on this change

N = 99	Model 1: Change trajectory		Model 2: Effect of treatment advice	
Fixed effects in model	Estimate (SE)	*p*-value	Estimate (SE)	*p*-value
Day 1 (intercept)	4.9 (0.2)	<0.001	4.8 (0.3)	<0.001
+Stay active advice	-	-	0.2 (0.4)	0.67
Day (β, linear term)	−0.4 (0.04)	<0.001	−0.4 (0.06)	<0.001
+Stay active advice	-	-	0.05 (0.08)	0.52

Fixed effects in models are presented with pain intensity (NRS) as outcome
Model 1 is the estimated change trajectory without the effect of treatment advice. Model 2 includes the effect of treatment advice, where the effect of the Adjust activity is presented first followed by the added effect of the Stay active advice
A first-order polynomial function was used including the linear term (Day) describing a decrease in pain intensity over time (negative values)

and thus, general practitioners should stimulate early activity and return to work among patients with acute lumbago.

One could argue that a patient whose back problem decays within a week is a minor clinical problem. However, even with the very short duration in the majority of patients with ALBP, there is a considerable risk for future recurrence and/or development into chronic LBP, as previously stated [5–7]. The combination of the SA advice and monitoring of step counts is an inexpensive treatment to maintain or even improve daily activity, instead of embracing a pain avoidance attitude, which commonly has been observed among general practitioners [17–20]. The evidence supports the beneficial effects of physical activity on most musculoskeletal conditions, including LBP [10]. Previous studies with a follow-up period of up to 12 weeks found favorable effects of advising the patient to stay active on pain intensity, functional status and sick leave compared to bed rest, although the effects were not consistent across studies [12]. The present study focused on the early, natural course of ALBP. A continuation would be to demonstrate effects of staying active on future recurrences of back pain, functional status, and sick leave among patients with acute severe LBP.

Strengths and limitations

One strength in the herein study is the use of objective measure of physical activity, which has not been used in prior research to confirm compliance with the stay active advice in patients with acute severe LBP. Subjective methods tend to exaggerate intervention effects related to physical activity [16]. The use of pedometer for self-monitoring of behavior is an effective technique in itself to promote physical activity [36, 39], and as all the patients in the present study wore pedometers, the group differences found were likely attributed to the treatment advices. However, we cannot rule out the possibility of synergy between the SA advice and self-monitoring contributing to a larger increase in step count in the SA group. In the present study, the early, careful, and comprehensive examinations by experienced orthopedic spine specialists at a university clinic, which represent an optimal treatment condition for ALBP, could have influenced the compliance with the treatment advices. However, this bias was similar in both groups. Another strength is the inclusion of patients with ALBP from the very earliest hours after onset pain, i.e. referring severe pain, and comparing the treatment advices effect on pain and physical activity, which has not been performed previously. The AA advice might better reflect the advice provided in health care today, rather than the advice to stay in bed that has been used in previous research. The inclusion of patients in the study occurred over an extended period in order to try to reach the numbers determined in the power analysis (See Methods). In spite of the prolonged recruiting time, the study was forced to close before the optimal number of patients was obtained, due to economic and logistic reasons. Still, the effect of the SA advice versus the AA advice largely exceeded the 1000 steps difference considered prior in the power-calculations. The study is limited to the course of ALBP, not allowing conclusions either of long-term effects on pain, or recurrence/work absence due to chronic LBP.

Conclusions

Treatment advice given in acute severe LBP is complied with. Patients advised to stay active showed a more active behavior compared to patients advised to adjust their activity to the pain. A large proportion in the SA group reached recommended level of 10000 steps per day defined for a population without pain. Thus, the stay active advice is appropriate for the early treatment of acute severe LBP and to promote additional physical activity for more health benefits among workers in risk for suffer from LBP.

Practical applications

The present study demonstrates the opportunity within the health care setting to support return to habitual levels of physical activity and early return to work after onset of acute severe LBP, using inexpensive methods in form of the stay active advice and pedometers. It also demonstrates that even higher levels of physical activity can be promoted with these methods to prevent recurrence/chronicity of pain and for additional health benefits.

Abbreviations

AA: Adjust activity; ALBP: Acute low back pain; LBP: Low back pain; NRS: Numeric Rating Scale; SA: Stay active.

Competing interests

The authors disclose no professional relationships with companies or manufacturers who will benefit from the results of the present study.

Authors' contribution

POC contributed to conception and design of study, acquisition of data, analysis and interpretation of data. JS contributed to acquisition of data. DA contributed to analyses and interpretation of data. KF contributed to acquisition of data. TH contributed to conception and design of study, acquisition and interpretation of data. All authors have been involved in drafting and critically revising of manuscript and have given final approval of the version to be published, as well as are accountable for all aspects of the work.

Acknowledgements

This work was supported by the Swedish Council for Working Life and Social Research 2003–0460; AFA, FA 03:02; and ALF, Gothenburg University.

Author details

[1]Department of Orthopedics, Institute of Clinical Sciences at the Sahlgrenska Academy, University of Gothenburg, Gothenburg, Sweden. [2]Department of Postgraduate Studies, Faculty of Nursing, University of Antioquia, Calle 70 No 52-21, Apartado Aereo, 1226 Medellín, Antioquia, Colombia. [3]Unit for Health Promotion Research, University of Southern Denmark, Esbjerg, Denmark. [4]Unit of Clinical Physiology and Nuclear Medicine, Department of Translational Medicine, Lund University, Malmö, Sweden. [5]RICH/EXE, Institute of Sports Science and Clinical Biomechanics, University of Southern Denmark, Odense, Denmark.

References

1. Hoy D, March L, Brooks P, Blyth F, Woolf A, Bain C, et al. The global burden of low back pain: estimates from the Global Burden of Disease 2010 study. Ann Rheum Dis. 2014;73(6):968–74.
2. van Tulder M, Becker A, Bekkering T, Breen A, del Real MT, Hutchinson A, et al. Chapter 3. European guidelines for the management of acute nonspecific low back pain in primary care. Eur Spine J. 2006;15 Suppl 2:S169–191.
3. Henschke N, Maher CG, Refshauge KM, Herbert RD, Cumming RG, Bleasel J, et al. Prognosis in patients with recent onset low back pain in Australian primary care: inception cohort study. BMJ. 2008;337:a171.
4. van Tulder MW, Koes B, Malmivaara A. Outcome of non-invasive treatment modalities on back pain: an evidence-based review. Eur Spine J. 2006;15 Suppl 1:S64–81.
5. Hestbaek L, Leboeuf-Yde C, Manniche C. Low back pain: what is the long-term course? A review of studies of general patient populations. Eur Spine J. 2003;12(2):149–65.
6. Pengel LH, Herbert RD, Maher CG, Refshauge KM. Acute low back pain: systematic review of its prognosis. BMJ. 2003;327(7410):323.
7. Schiøttz-Christensen B, Nielsen GL, Hansen VK, Schødt T, Sørensen HT, Olesen F. Long-term prognosis of acute low back pain in patients seen in general practice: a 1-year prospective follow-up study. Fam Pract. 1999;16(3):223–32.
8. Dannesskiold-Samsøe B. Idiopathic low back pain: classification and differential diagnosis. JMP. 2004;12:93–9.
9. Hansson EK, Hansson TH. The costs for persons sick-listed more than one month because of low back or neck problems. A two-year prospective study of Swedish patients. Eur Spine J. 2005;14(4):337–45.
10. Hagen KB, Dagfinrud H, Moe RH, Østerås N, Kjeken I, Grotle M, et al. Exercise therapy for bone and muscle health: an overview of systematic reviews. BMC Med. 2012;10:167.
11. Bach SM, Holten KB. Guideline update: what's the best approach to acute low back pain? J Fam Pract. 2009;58(12), E1.
12. Dahm KT, Brurberg KG, Jamtvedt G, Hagen KB. Advice to rest in bed versus advice to stay active for acute low-back pain and sciatica. Cochrane Database Syst Rev. 2010;6, CD007612.
13. Matsudaira K, Hara N, Arisaka M, Isomura T. Comparison of physician's advice for non-specific acute low back pain in Japanese workers: advice to rest versus advice to stay active. Ind Health. 2011;49(2):203–8.
14. Malmivaara A, Häkkinen U, Aro T, Heinrichs ML, Koskenniemi L, Kuosma E, et al. The treatment of acute low back pain–bed rest, exercises, or ordinary activity? N Engl J Med. 1995;332(6):351–5.
15. Ainsworth BE, Caspersen CJ, Matthews CE, Mâsse LC, Baranowski T, Zhu W. Recommendations to improve the accuracy of estimates of physical activity derived from self report. J Phys Act Health. 2012;9 Suppl 1:S76–84.
16. Winkler E, Waters L, Eakin E, Fjeldsoe B, Owen N, Reeves M. Is measurement error altered by participation in a physical activity intervention? Med Sci Sports Exerc. 2013;45(5):1004–11.
17. Bishop A, Foster NE, Thomas E, Hay EM. How does the self-reported clinical management of patients with low back pain relate to the attitudes and beliefs of health care practitioners? A survey of UK general practitioners and physiotherapists. Pain. 2008;135(1–2):187–95.
18. Darlow B, Fullen BM, Dean S, Hurley DA, Baxter GD, Dowell A. The association between health care professional attitudes and beliefs and the attitudes and beliefs, clinical management, and outcomes of patients with low back pain: a systematic review. Eur J Pain. 2012;16(1):3–17.
19. Darlow B, Dean S, Perry M, Mathieson F, Baxter GD, Dowell A. Acute low back pain management in general practice: uncertainty and conflicting certainties. Fam Pract. 2014.
20. Linton SJ, Vlaeyen J, Ostelo R. The back pain beliefs of health care providers: are we fear-avoidant? J Occup Rehabil. 2002;12(4):223–32.
21. Grotle M, Vøllestad NK, Brox JI. Clinical course and impact of fear-avoidance beliefs in low back pain: prospective cohort study of acute and chronic low back pain: II. Spine (Phila Pa 1976). 2006;31(9):1038–46.
22. Söderlund A, Asenlöf P. The mediating role of self-efficacy expectations and fear of movement and (re)injury beliefs in two samples of acute pain. Disabil Rehabil. 2010;32(25):2118–26.
23. Swinkels-Meewisse IE, Roelofs J, Verbeek AL, Oostendorp RA, Vlaeyen JW. Fear-avoidance beliefs, disability, and participation in workers and non-workers with acute low back pain. Clin J Pain. 2006;22(1):45–54.
24. Coudeyre E, Rannou F, Tubach F, Baron G, Coriat F, Brin S, et al. General practitioners' fear-avoidance beliefs influence their management of patients with low back pain. Pain. 2006;124(3):330–7.
25. Bishop A, Thomas E, Foster NE. Health care practitioners' attitudes and beliefs about low back pain: a systematic search and critical review of available measurement tools. Pain. 2007;132(1–2):91–101.
26. Deyo RA, Weinstein JN. Low back pain. N Engl J Med. 2001;344(5):363–70.
27. Garber CE, Blissmer B, Deschenes MR, Franklin BA, Lamonte MJ, Lee IM, et al. Medicine ACoS: American College of Sports Medicine position stand. Quantity and quality of exercise for developing and maintaining cardiorespiratory, musculoskeletal, and neuromotor fitness in apparently healthy adults: guidance for prescribing exercise. Med Sci Sports Exerc. 2011;43(7):1334–59.
28. Haskell WL, Lee IM, Pate RR, Powell KE, Blair SN, Franklin BA, et al. Physical activity and public health: updated recommendation for adults from the American College of Sports Medicine and the American Heart Association. Circulation. 2007;116(9):1081–93.
29. Tudor-Locke C, Hatano Y, Pangrazi RP, Kang M. Revisiting "how many steps are enough?". Med Sci Sports Exerc. 2008;40(7 Suppl):S537–543.
30. Hagströmer M, Oja P, Sjöström M. Physical activity and inactivity in an adult population assessed by accelerometry. Med Sci Sports Exerc. 2007;39(9):1502–8.
31. Teichtahl AJ, Urquhart DM, Wang Y, Wluka AE, O'Sullivan R, Jones G, et al. Physical inactivity is associated with narrower lumbar intervertebral discs, high fat content of paraspinal muscles and low back pain and disability. Arthritis Res Ther. 2015;17(1):114.
32. Hansson TH, Hansson EK. The effects of common medical interventions on pain, back function, and work resumption in patients with chronic low back

pain: A prospective 2-year cohort study in six countries. Spine (Phila Pa 1976). 2000;25(23):3055–64.
33. Raustorp A, Ekroth Y. Eight-year secular trends of pedometer-determined physical activity in young Swedish adolescents. J Phys Act Health. 2010;7(3):369–74.
34. Schneider PL, Crouter S, Bassett DR. Pedometer measures of free-living physical activity: comparison of 13 models. Med Sci Sports Exerc. 2004;36(2):331–5.
35. Jensen M, Karoly P. Measurement of pain: self-report scales and procedures for assessing pain in adults. In: Turk D, Melzack R, editors. Handbook of pain assessment. 2dth ed. New York: Guildford Press; 2001. p. 15–34. 760.
36. Bravata DM, Smith-Spangler C, Sundaram V, Gienger AL, Lin N, Lewis R, et al. Using pedometers to increase physical activity and improve health: a systematic review. JAMA. 2007;298(19):2296–304.
37. Altman D. Practical statistics for medical research. London: Chapman and Hall; 1999.
38. Heck R, Thomas S, Tabata L. Multilevel and longitudinal modelling with SPSS, Second edition edn: Taylor & Francis. 2014.
39. Murtagh EM, Murphy MH, Boone-Heinonen J. Walking: the first steps in cardiovascular disease prevention. Curr Opin Cardiol. 2010;25(5):490–6.
40. Grunnesjö MI, Bogefeldt JP, Svärdsudd KF, Blomberg SI. A randomized controlled clinical trial of stay-active care versus manual therapy in addition to stay-active care: functional variables and pain. J Manipulative Physiol Ther. 2004;27(7):431–41.
41. Grunnesjö MI, Bogefeldt JP, Blomberg SI, Strender LE, Svärdsudd KF. A randomized controlled trial of the effects of muscle stretching, manual therapy and steroid injections in addition to 'stay active' care on health-related quality of life in acute or subacute low back pain. Clin Rehabil. 2011;25(11):999–1010.

6

Can supplementation with vitamin C and E alter physiological adaptations to strength training?

Gøran Paulsen[1,2*], Kristoffer T Cumming[1], Håvard Hamarsland[1], Elisabet Børsheim[3], Sveinung Berntsen[4] and Truls Raastad[1]

Abstract

Background: Antioxidant supplementation has recently been demonstrated to be a double-edged sword, because small to moderate doses of exogenous antioxidants are essential or beneficial, while high doses may have adverse effects. The adverse effects can be manifested in attenuated effects of exercise and training, as the antioxidants may shut down some redox-sensitive signaling in the exercised muscle fibers. However, conditions such as age may potentially modulate the need for antioxidant intake. Therefore, this paper describes experiments for testing the hypothesis that high dosages of vitamin C (1000 mg/day) and E (235 mg/day) have negative effects on adaptation to resistance exercise and training in young volunteers, but positive effects in older men.

Methods/design: We recruited a total of 73 volunteers. The participants were randomly assigned to receiving either vitamin C and E supplementation or a placebo. The study design was double-blinded, and the participants followed an intensive training program for 10–12 weeks. Tests and measurements aimed at assessing changes in physical performance (maximal strength) and physiological characteristics (muscle mass), as well as biochemical and cellular systems and structures (e.g., cell signaling and morphology).

Discussion: Dietary supplements, such as vitamin C and E, are used by many people, especially athletes. The users often believe that high dosages of supplements improve health (resistance to illness and disease) and physical performance. These assumptions are, however, generally not supported in the scientific literature. On the contrary, some studies have indicated that high dosages of antioxidant supplements have negative effects on exercise-induced adaptation processes. Since this issue concerns many people and few randomized controlled trials have been conducted in humans, further studies are highly warranted.

Trial registration: ACTRN12614000065695

Keywords: Protocol paper, Antioxidants, Muscle mass, Muscle strength, 1 repetition maximum

Background

Exercise and training have indisputably demonstrated impressive potential in inducing physiological adaptations in both the cardiovascular and muscular systems [1-4]. Nonetheless, researchers still strive to elucidate the most efficient ways to exercise for certain adaptations, such as increased strength and endurance. A prerequisite for optimal effects of training is adequate nutrition, and indeed, the intake of certain types and amounts of macro- and micro-nutrients may modulate the effects of training [5]. Whey protein and creatine supplementation are two examples [6,7]. Antioxidants constitute a central group of micro-nutrients. Several studies have been conducted to explore their effects on health, physical performance, exercise and training [8-13]. The human body definitely requires a variety of antioxidants, but an unanswered question is whether it is beneficial or not to supplement the diet with isolated, highly concentrated antioxidant products, such as vitamin C and E pills [10,14].

Supplementation with different types of antioxidants has been variably shown to have positive effects, no effect, and even negative effects on training adaptation [10,15-17]. Because intensive exercise generates stress in the working muscles [16], it seems logical that antioxidant

* Correspondence: goran.paulsen@olympiatoppen.no
[1]Department of Physical Performance, Norwegian School of Sport Sciences, Oslo, Norway
[2]Norwegian Olympic Sport Center, Oslo, Norway
Full list of author information is available at the end of the article

supplementation could beneficially reduce this stress. On the other hand, it has become clear that cellular stress, which includes increased production of free radicals and oxidative stress, in fact works as a signal to induce important adaptions in muscle cells, including mitochondrial biogenesis and myofiber hypertrophy [13,18]. Thus, if the cells are exposed to high levels of antioxidants this signaling may be blunted or blocked, which in turn may inhibit physiological adaptations. In line with this, Makanae et al. [19] recently reported that high dosages of vitamin C attenuated hypertrophy of overloaded plantaris muscles in rats. The diminished muscle growth appeared to be related to reduced overload-induced phosphorylation of p70S6K. Similar human studies are currently lacking, but Morales-Alamo et al. [20] have recently reported that an antioxidant mix (vitamin C, E and alpha-lipoic acid) blunted the activation of Ca^{2+}/calmodulin-dependent protein kinase II (CaMKII) and AMP-activated protein kinase after maximal sprint exercise. Such signaling could be important for initiating training adaptation, and could explain the abolished training effects observed in anaerobic training combined with antioxidant supplementation (Q-10; [21]).

Hitherto, most investigations on antioxidant supplementation and training in humans have focused on endurance training (for reviews, see [10,15,22]). Only three human training studies have applied a high-force, resistance mode of exercise; i.e., traditional strength training [23,24] and eccentric exercise [25]. In a study by Theodorou et al. [25], no effects of vitamin C and E supplementation (1000 mg and 400 IU, respectively) were found on either recovery after eccentric exercise or adaptation to 4 weeks of eccentric training. Chuin et al. [24] supplemented elderly women (Vitamin C: 1000 mg/d, vitamin E: 600 IU/d) who concomitantly participated in strength training or control groups. The authors only reported results on bone mineral content (BMC), which allegedly was preserved better with C and E vitamin supplementation, but there was no interaction between training and supplementation. Bobeuf et al. [23] observed that vitamin C (1000 mg/d) and E (400 IU/d) supplementation affected neither body composition nor strength gain in elderly participants. Notably, Bobeuf et al. found no clear muscle gain in the placebo group, which means that the antioxidant effect on muscle growth is uncertain.

The effect of antioxidant supplementation and exercise in elderly individuals is indeed elusive. However, Ryan et al. [26] observed that vitamin C and E supplementation improved concentric work capacity in old rats, but not young rats. This suggests that antioxidant supplementation could exert different effects in young and aged muscles; possibly because of low levels of inflammation and augmented oxidative stress levels in aged muscles [27,28]. Consequently, aged muscles seem more likely to respond positively to antioxidant supplementation [29].

In the present study, we aimed to investigate the effects of antioxidant supplementation, in the form of vitamin C and E supplementation, recruiting both young (20–40 years) and elderly (60–80 years) volunteers. The effects of both a training period (10–12 weeks) and an acute exercise session with recovery were examined. Biochemical analyses of blood and muscle were combined with physiological measurements and performance tests.

Based on the notion that antioxidants blunt exercise-induced redox sensitive signaling in young, healthy muscles, but reduce unfavorable oxidative stress in aging muscles, we hypothesized that vitamin C (1000 mg/day) and E (235 mg/day) supplementation would:

(1) inhibit the adaptation to strength training in young, healthy men and women; and (2) augment the adaptation to strength training in healthy, elderly men (60–80 years). Moreover, we hypothesized that "hypertrophic" cell signaling and protein synthetic rate would be blunted in the hours after a single session of strength training in young persons, and, thus, reflect the long-term effects.

Methods

This study comprises three experiments and involves the potential interference of antioxidant supplementation in exercise-induced responses and adaptations to strength training in young and elderly participants.

Participants

A total of 73 participants were recruited to the study (Figure 1).

The young participants (20–45 years of age), both males and females, were healthy and did not use any form of supplements or medications, except contraceptives for women (menstrual cycle was not controlled for). They were all accustomed to strength training (recreationally trained), exercising 1–4 times per week. We excluded volunteers who did more than four strength training sessions per week to avoid including highly trained individuals, who are expected to show little or no progress over 10 weeks of training [4].

The older participants were males aged between 60–80 years. They were healthy, although some medications to treat mildly elevated cholesterol and blood pressure, migraine, and the use of mild antidepressants were accepted. The older participants were not engaged in strength training when they entered the study.

Interested volunteers who already used some kind of supplements, such as vitamins, were allowed to join the study if they immediately stopped using the supplements and went through a wash-out period of at least two weeks.

The young participants filled out a standard health form (developed at the Norwegian School of Sport

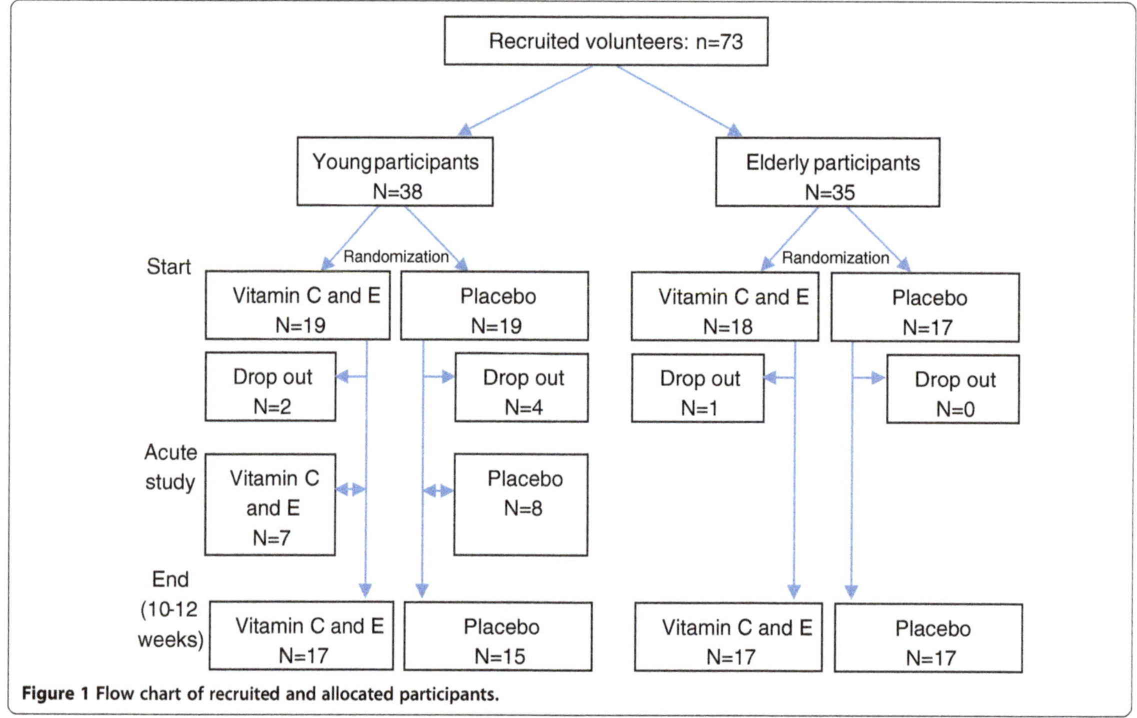

Figure 1 Flow chart of recruited and allocated participants.

Sciences), concerning health status and risk factors (smoking etc.). If a participant had a potential health issue, he or she was examined and cleared for training by a medical doctor before entering the study.

All elderly participants underwent a medical examination before entering the study, including blood pressure assessment, rest and work echocardiogram, as well as vascular ultrasound scans of the carotid arteries and aorta.

All participants signed a written informed consent. The study was approved by the South East Regional Committee for Medical and Health Research Ethics in Norway, and was performed in accordance with the Helsinki Declaration.

Designs

The study defined two training/exercise and antioxidant supplementation interventions:

1. Strength training and vitamin C and E supplementation with young participants
2. Strength training and vitamin C and E supplementation with elderly participants

Tests and assessments were conducted before, during, and after the training periods (10–12 weeks). One to three familiarization sessions were conducted before the strength tests (see description below; Figure 2).

Baseline tests were conducted before group allocation so that the volunteers could be randomly assigned to receive a supplement or placebo, stratified for sex (for the young participants) and muscle strength (1 repetition maximum, 1RM). Research Randomizer (www.randomizer.org/) was applied to perform the randomization procedure. The experiments with young and elderly volunteers were performed separately at two different institutions.

Both experiments (young and elderly volunteers) were carried out in a double blinded fashion. The scientists responsible for the administration of the supplements were not involved in the tests and assessments.

The main outcome of the experiments with both the young and the elderly participants was a change in muscle mass, measured by dual-energy X-ray absorptiometry (DXA; see power calculations under "Statistics"). For assessing local muscle growth, magnetic resonance imaging (MRI) and/or ultrasound were applied. Bio-impedance measurement of body composition was used auxiliary to DXA and to provide midway measurements.

Secondary outcomes were measurements of muscle strength, measured by 1RM and isometric tests (maximal voluntary contraction; MVC), as well as analyses of tissue samples (young participants only). The tissue samples were used for analyses of endogenous antioxidant systems (e.g., glutathione peroxidase).

***Young* participants receiving C and E vitamin or placebo**	Familiarization to tests and exercises	Pre-tests: DXA, Inbody 1RM, MVC, MRI, USI, biopsy and blood samples	Group randomization Start training	Midway tests: and measurements and acute experiment	Post-tests: DXA, Inbody 1RM, MVC, MRI, USI, biopsy and blood samples
	Weeks -2-3	Week -1	Week 1	Week 4-6	Week 10-11

***Elderly* participants receiving C and E vitamin or placebo**	Familiarization to tests and exercises	Pre-tests : DXA, Inbody, 1RM, USI, VO_2, blood sample	Group randomization Start training	Midway tests: Inbody, 1RM, USI	Midway tests: Inbody, 1RM, USI	Post-tests: DXA, Inbody, 1RM, USI, VO_2, blood sample
	Weeks -2-3	Week -1	Week 1	Week 4	Week 8	Week 13-14

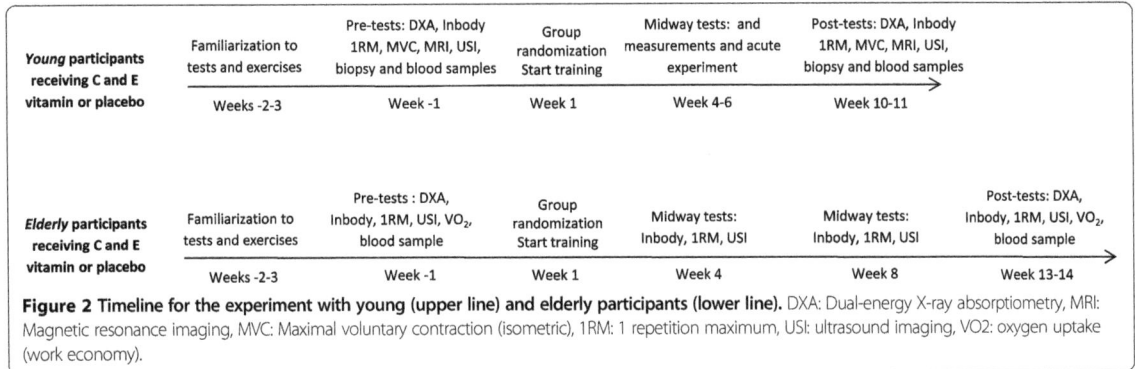

Figure 2 Timeline for the experiment with young (upper line) and elderly participants (lower line). DXA: Dual-energy X-ray absorptiometry, MRI: Magnetic resonance imaging, MVC: Maximal voluntary contraction (isometric), 1RM: 1 repetition maximum, USI: ultrasound imaging, VO2: oxygen uptake (work economy).

Additionally, blood samples were collected from all participants before, midway and after the intervention periods for analyses of endogenous and exogenous (vitamin C and E) antioxidant levels. Work economy during level/uphill walking was measured in the elderly participants only.

Assessments of nutrient intake and level of physical activity were undertaken in order to control for potential confounding factors.

Acute experiment

After 4–6 weeks of training, an "acute" experiment, in the form of a single exercise session, was conducted with a randomly selected subgroup of the young participants (Figure 1).

During the experiment MVC tests were conducted before and in the hours after the exercise session, for assessment of recovery of muscle function. Muscle and blood samples were obtained before and after the exercise session. Supplements were ingested ~3 hours before and immediately after exercise. Figure 3 displays the layout of the experiment.

The rationale for the acute experiment was to elucidate the acute cellular processes (signaling for hypertrophy), and potential correlations with long-term adaptations (increase in muscle mass).

The main outcome in the acute experiment was changes in the fractional synthetic rate of mixed muscle protein (protein synthesis).

Secondary outcomes were recovery of muscle function and assessments of the phosphorylation state of protein kinases (e.g., p70S6K) involved in "hypertrophic" intracellular signaling.

Supplementation

Vitamin C and E supplementation

The vitamin C and E and placebo pills were produced under Good Manufacturing Practice (GMP) requirements at Petefa AB (Västra Frölunda, Sweden). Each vitamin pill contained 250 mg of ascorbic acid and 58.5 mg DL-alpha-tocopherol acetate (all-rac-alpha-tocopheryl acetate); in addition to cellulose, di/tri-calsium phosphate and magnesium stearate. Similar-looking placebo pills contained the same ingredients, except for the vitamins, and were produced by the same manufacturer. The pills were analyzed by a commercial company, Vitas (Oslo, Norway) ~2 years after production, with no sign of degradation of the vitamins (per pill: vitamin C: 255 ± 7 mg, vitamin E: 62 ± 2 mg). The experiments were conducted within this time period. No traces of the vitamins were found in the placebo pills.

The participants ingested two pills (totaling 500 mg of vitamin C and 117.5 mg vitamin E) 1–3 hours before every training session and two pills within the hour after training. On non-training days the participants ingested two pills in the morning and two pills in the evening. The intake of pills was confirmed in a training diary (see below). Thus, the daily dosage was 1000 mg of vitamin C and 235 mg vitamin E.

We divided the intake in two equal dosages to increase the bioavailability of the vitamins [30,31]. Moreover, due

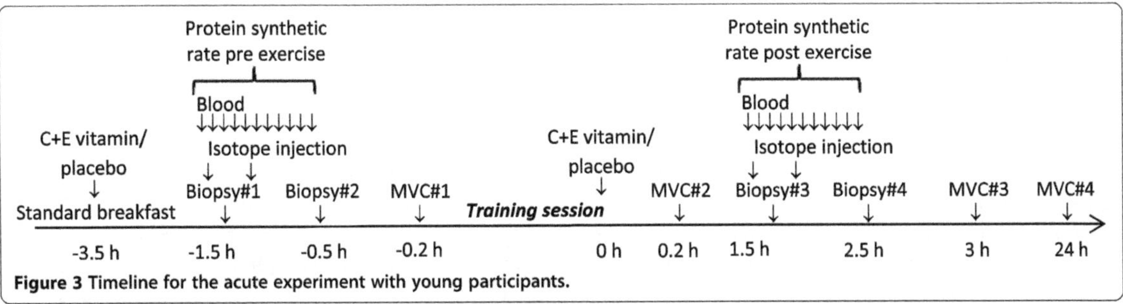

Figure 3 Timeline for the acute experiment with young participants.

to the pharmacokinetics of the water-soluble vitamin C [32], the timing of the intakes was chosen to ensure that the blood levels of the antioxidants were high during exercise and in the first hours of recovery, when oxidative stress is suggested to be at its highest [16].

The participants were given pills for two weeks at a time, and exchanged the empty pill bottle for a new bottle every other week. The investigator who administrated the supplements did not take part in any of the tests or measurements, meaning that all tests were done blinded to group affiliation.

Nutrition

Nutrition restrictions

Participants were asked not to take any form of nutritional supplement apart from those given in the study. They were asked to drink no more than two glasses of juice and four cups of coffee or tea per day. Juices especially rich in antioxidants, such as grape juice, were to be avoided.

Standardized nutrient intake in the acute experiment

In preparation for the acute experiment, the participants ingested the supplements, C and E vitamin or placebo, followed by a standardized breakfast: 3 g oatmeal per kg body weight boiled in water with 10 g sugar, 2 hours before meeting in the laboratory.

Nutrition registration

The young participants completed a four-day weighed food registration dietary assessment [33] at the start and at the end of the training period. The participants used a digital food weighing scale (Vera 67002; Soehnle-Waagen GmbH & Co, Murrhardt, Germany; precision 1 g). The dietary registrations were analyzed using a nutrient analysis program (Mat på data 4.1; LKH, Oslo, Norway). We aimed to keep the participants in energy balance (or in slight positive balance), and to keep the intake of micro- and macro-nutrients, excluding the supplements, within the recommended ranges for Norway (www.helsedirektoratet.no).

Elderly participants registered their food intake using a four-day pre-coded food diary [34]. Diet recordings were performed during the same days as the activity recordings (see below). Daily intake of energy was computed using the food database and software system (KBS, version 4.9.) developed at the Department of Nutrition, University of Oslo, Norway.

A skilled nutritionist educated the participants in the given nutrient restrictions and in the diet registration prior to registration.

Training diary

The participants filled out a training diary. On training days they recorded details about the training (exercises, kg lifted, etc.), as well as their subjective perception of effort during the sessions (Borgs scale [35]), and confirmed intake of pills. On non-training days they confirmed intake of pills and recorded muscle soreness, and if present, any symptoms of injuries/illness/sickness. Soreness and symptoms of injuries/illness/sickness were rated on a scale from 0–10, where 0 is no soreness/symptoms and 10 is extreme soreness and severe symptoms.

The training diary for the young participants was electronically available to the researchers during the training period, while the training diary for elderly participants was registered manually on paper and controlled during each exercise session.

Training regimes

Young participants

The young participants followed a "classical" strength training program with heavy loads (6-11RM) and with short rest periods (1–1.5 min) for four sessions per week (Table 1). Exercises for all major muscle groups were included in a 4-split exercise routine (two upper body and two lower body sessions per week; Table 1). Variation in exercises for the different muscle groups was intended to enhance the exercise stimuli and reduce the risk of injuries. The main goal was to stimulate both increase in maximal strength and muscle growth.

The young volunteers were supervised during the first sessions, and thereafter they had the opportunity to continue supervised training. However, most participants trained unsupervised after the initial supervision. This seemed acceptable, as most of the participants were familiar with strength training and the specific exercises before entering the study. Furthermore, as the recruitment period lasted for about 4 weeks, the volunteers stopped their current training routine and started to follow a simple whole body workout program with 3 sessions per week (8–12 repetitions with approximately 15RM loads), including the main exercises in the intervention program, until pre-testing and group randomization. Thus, this run-in period allowed the participants to become accustomed to the exercises used in the intervention period.

Acute experiment

The exercise sessions consisted of four 10RM sets of leg press and knee-extension, with 1 min rest between sets and 3 min rest between exercises. The participants were verbally encouraged to execute each set to failure. If necessary, manual assistance was given so that the participants were able to complete the final repetition in each set.

Table 1 The training program for young participants

Week	Load (RM)	Sets	Inter-set rest (min)	Sessions per week
1-6	9-11	3	1	4
7-10	6-8	3-4	1.5	4
Upper-body Exercises #1	**Lower-body Exercises #1**	**Upper-body Exercise #2**	**Lower-body Exercises #2**	
Bench press	Squat	Incline chest press	Deadlift	
Dumbbell flyes	Lunge	Pullover	Lunge	
Standing shoulder press	Knee-extension	Lateral rise	Leg press	
Triceps push-down	Straight leg deadlift	Pull-down narrow grip	Knee-flexion	
Seated row	Standing calf raise	Standing bent over row	Standing calf raise	
Pull-down wipe grip	Self-selected abdominal exercise	Biceps curl (scott curl)	Self-selected abdominal exercise	
Self-selected abdominal exercise		Self-selected abdominal exercise		

Elderly participants

The elderly participants followed a daily undulating (non-linear periodized) training program, with three sessions per week (Table 2). The total training volume increased during the first 10 weeks, but was reduced during the two last weeks (tapering). The elderly volunteers were unfamiliar with strength training, and all sessions were supervised by an investigator. As for the young, exercises for all major muscle groups were selected (Table 2), and the main aim was to increase maximal strength and muscle mass.

Table 2 The training program for elderly participants

	Session 1	Session 2	Session 3
Reps.	8-10	13-15	3-5
Rest	1 min	45 sec	2 min
Sets:			
Week 1	1 (warm-up) + 1	1 + 1	
Week 2	1 (warm-up) + 2		1 + 1
Week 3	1 (warm-up) + 2	1 + 2	
Week 4	1 (warm-up) + 2		1 + 2
Week 5	1 (warm-up) + 3	1 + 2	
Week 6	1 (warm-up) + 3		1 + 3
Week 7-8	1 (warm-up) + 3	1 + 3	1 + 3
Week 9	1 (warm-up) + 4	1 + 3	
Week 10	1 (warm-up) + 4		1 + 4
Week 11	1 (warm-up) + 3	1 + 3	
Week 12	1 (warm-up) + 2		1 + 2
Exercises:			
	Bulgarian squat	"Sumo" deadlift w/kettlebells	Knee-extension
	Squat	Lunges	Leg press
	Bench-press	Step up	Chest-press
	Pull-down narrow grip	Flyes	Pull-down wide grip
	Upright row	Seated row machine	Arnold-press
	Calf raise	Lateral raises	Bench press narrow grip
	French press	Triceps pushdown	Scott curl
	Standing biceps curl w/dumbbells	Scott curl	Side-plank (abdominals)
	Quadruped exercise	Plank (abdominals)	

Tests and measurements

Maximal strength testing of young participants

Maximal strength was assessed by 1 repetition maximum (1RM) tests and a maximal isometric voluntary contraction (MVC).

1RM was tested in knee-extension, knee-flexion, biceps curl and elbow extension. Each leg and arm was tested separately (unilateral tests). After a general warm-up (5 min walking or bicycling), a specific warm-up/preparation procedure was performed for each exercise, using loads corresponding to 50%, 70%, 80% and 90% of expected 1RM – conducting 10, 6, 3, and 1 repetitions, respectively. The loads were individually adjusted so the participants did not fatigue their muscles. Optimally, 2–5 attempts were used to establish 1RM. The loads could be adjusted in steps as low as 3%. The left and right leg/arm was tested interchangeably, so that each muscle rested for approximately 2 minutes between attempts. The range of motion was strictly controlled. The coefficient of variation (CV) of these assessments was <5%.

MVC was tested for the knee-extensors. The participants were fixed in a chair with belts over chest and hips, and an angle of 90° in the knee and hip joints. During the unilateral test the participants pressed maximally with their shank against the lever-arm of the apparatus, which was attached to a force-transducer (HBM U2AC2, Darmstadt, Germany). The participants got three 5-seconds attempts to reach MVC; 1 minute rest was given between attempts.

Maximal strength tests in elderly participants

1RM was tested in a similar manner as for the young participants (see above). 1RM was assessed in scott-curl (elbow flexors), leg press and knee-extension.

Assessments of changes in muscle mass

Dual-energy X-ray absorptiometry, DXA

Body composition was measured by DXA (young participants: Hologic Discovery, Waltham, MA, USA; elderly participants: GE-Lunar Prodigy, Madison, WI, USA). Participants were scanned from head to toe in a supine position, providing values for bone mineral content, lean mass, and fat mass. The CV of these assessments was <2%.

Bio-impedance

In addition to the body composition measurements by DXA, a bio-impedance apparatus was used (Inbody 720, Biospace Co., Ltd., Seoul, Korea). The apparatus has been found valid (compared with DXA) for estimating fat mass and lean mass in men and women [36]. Bio-impedance was used on both young and elderly participants.

Magnetic resonance imaging (MRI)

MRI was only conducted on young participants. Transverse section images were captured of the dominant arm and both thighs (GE Signa 1.5 Tesla Echospeed, GE Medical Systems, Madison, Wisconsin, USA), before and after the intervention period. Thigh muscles: Joint gaps were used for reference points and nine images (5 mm) were captured with a 35.5 mm inter-image distance. Upper arm muscles: The os humerus of each participant was sectioned in nine evenly distributed images (5 mm). The images (DICOM) were analyzed using OsiriX 3.9.3 (Pixmeo, Bernex, Switzerland), giving the cross-sectional area of individual muscles. The CV of these assessments was <2%.

Ultrasound imaging

In young participants, the muscle thickness and fascicle angle of m. vastus lateralis was assessed with a 50-mm linear probe (5–12 MHz) connected to a Philips HD11 XE ultrasound apparatus (Royal Philips Electronics, Amsterdam, Netherlands). In elderly participants, the muscle thickness of m. rectus femoris, m. vastus lateralis, and arm flexors (m. brachialis and m. biceps brachii) was assessed using a LogicScan 128 ultrasound apparatus (CEXT-1Z kit, Telemed Ltd., Vilnius, Lithuania) using a 60-mm probe. Fascicle angle was measured only in m. vastus lateralis. Image J software (National Institutes of Health, USA) was utilized to analyze the ultrasound images. The CV of these assessments was <5%.

Work economy measurements of elderly participants

Work economy, determined as body mass adjusted oxygen consumption, was measured while walking on a treadmill (Woodway, Weil am Rhein, Germany), at 5 km/h at three different inclinations: 0%, 4% and 8%; 5 min at each inclination. Finger-stick capillary blood samples were collected and analyzed immediately for lactate concentration using a portable lactate analyzer (Lactate Pro, LT-1710, Arkay KDK, Kyoto, Japan) after finishing each inclination. Heart rate (RS800CX, Polar Electro KY, Kempele, Finland) was recorded continuously. Minute ventilation and respiratory exchange ratio (RER) were recorded continuously during each inclination using an Oxycon Pro (Jaeger BeNeLux, Breda, Netherlands). Equipment calibration was conducted before each test period.

Physical activity level of elderly participants

Habitual physical activity was measured only in the elderly participants, and was measured with a SenseWear™ Pro3 Armband (BodyMedia Inc., Pittsburgh, PA, USA). The recording of physical activity started on a Saturday and included two weekdays and two weekend days. The monitor was worn on the right upper-arm at the midpoint between the acromion and olecranon processes as described previously [37]. Energy expenditure was computed at 1-minute intervals. Cut-off points defining moderate to very vigorous intensity were 3 metabolic equivalents (METs). Data from the monitor was downloaded and analyzed with software developed by the manufacturer (SenseWear Professional Research Software Version 6.1, BodyMedia Inc., Pittsburgh, PA, USA).

Muscle tissue sampling and analyses

In young participants, a biopsy was sampled from the right leg before and after the 10 week training period (Figure 2). The participants who also took part in the acute experiment had four biopsies taken from the left leg (two biopsies before and two after the exercise session; Figure 3). Thus, each participant underwent no more than six biopsies.

Biopsies were taken from the mid-portion of m. vastus lateralis. The insertions for repeated biopsies were always located approximately 3 cm proximal to the previous insertion. The procedure was conducted under local anesthesia (Xylocain adrenalin, 10 mg/ml + 5 μg/ml, AstraZeneca, London, UK). Approximately 200 mg (2–3 × 50–150 mg) of muscle tissue was obtained with a modified Bergström technique. Biopsy samples intended for homogenization were quickly washed in physiological saline and fat, connective tissue, and blood were discarded, before being weighed and quickly frozen in isopentane cooled on dry ice. Muscle biopsies for immunohistochemistry were mounted in a Tissue-Tek compound (Cat#4583, Sakura Finetek, Torrance, CA, USA) and quickly frozen in isopentane cooled on liquid nitrogen. Tissue intended for mRNA analyses were placed in RNAlater (Cat#AM7020, Ambion, Life technologies, Carlsbad, CA, USA). All muscle samples were stored at -80°C for later analyses.

For immunohistochemistry, cross-sections were cut in a cryostat microtome (CM3050, Leica Biosystems GmbH, Wetzlar, Germany), and the samples were stained for dystrophin, SC71 (fiber type II) and CD56/NCAM for analyses of mean fiber area, fiber type distribution and satellite cells; DAPI was used to mark myonuclei (for more details regarding antibodies and procedures, see [38-40]).

Planned analyses by means of western blotting and ELISA, were: Heat shock protein (as previously described [41]), and endogenous antioxidants, such as MnSOD and glutathione peroxidation.

mRNA was analyzed using real time PCR, and generally, the mRNA analyses complemented the protein measurements (e.g., heat shock protein and endogenous antioxidants).

Blood sampling and analyses

Blood was drawn from an antecubital vein into two 4.5 ml EDTA, one 4.5 ml Heparin, one 4.5 ml Stabilyte, and one 9 ml serum vacutainer tube. EDTA blood for hematological analyses was analyzed within 4 h after sampling. To extract plasma and serum the tubes were, after appropriate treatment, centrifuged at 1500 g for 10 min at 4°C. Plasma and serum were then pipetted into Eppendorf tubes and immediately stored at -80°C for later analyses.

Plasma destined for vitamin C analysis was mixed in equal volumes with metaphosphoric acid before storage at -80°C for later analyses. Plasma intended for glutathione analysis was treated in accordance with the procedure described by Sakhi et al. [42]. From the Stabilyte blood, erythrocytes were also collected for glutathione analysis. Other planned plasma/serum analyses included: cholesterol, triglycerides and CRP, plasma uric acid, creatine kinase and total antioxidant capacity (Modell X, MaxMat S.A., Montpellier, France), and various cytokines/chemokines (i.e., IL-6, IL-8, IL-10 and TNF-alpha; Milliplex MAP, Luminex xMAP technology by Millipore, Billerica, MA, USA).

Protein synthesis

The procedure for measuring rate of protein synthesis is described in detail by Zhang et al. [43]. Briefly, a baseline blood sample (2 ml) was taken for background measurement of amino acid enrichment. Thereafter, a bolus injection of $^{13}C_6$-phenylalanine was given at a dose of 50 μmol/kg, followed by a bolus of ^{15}N-phenylalanine (50 μmol/kg) 30 minutes later. All isotopes were from Cambridge Isotope Laboratories (Andover, MA, USA). Biopsies from m. vastus lateralis were collected at 10 and 50 min after the first bolus injection (see description of the biopsy procedure above). Muscle samples were quickly rinsed in cold saline, blotted and immediately frozen in liquid nitrogen and stored at -80°C for later analyses. A total of eleven blood samples (2 ml) were drawn during the procedure. Plasma was separated (as described above) and stored at -80°C for later analysis.

Statistics

The primary outcome was a change in muscle mass (lean mass measured with DXA); with an expected gain of 1.5 kg in lean mass and a standard deviation of 0.7. Sixteen volunteers in each group gave 80% power to detect a difference of approximately 0.7 kg. (alpha: 0.05; two-tailed; StatMate, GraphPad Software, La Jolla, CA, USA).

The secondary outcome was a change in muscle strength (1RM); with an expected standard deviation (SD) of 15, we had 80% power to detect a group difference of 11% with 16 subjects in each group (alpha: 0.05; two-tailed; StatMate, Graphpad software).

The primary and secondary outcome variables were expected to be normally distributed and parametric tests were applied: Student t-tests for relative changes and 2-way ANOVA for comparing pre and post absolute values, as well as repeated measures. Outcome variables that turned out not to be normally distributed were analyzed with appropriate non-parametric tests.

Discussion

In this study we aimed to test the hypothesis that high dosages of antioxidants, in the form of 1000 mg vitamin C and 235 mg of vitamin E (alpha-tocopherol) per day, will inhibit adaptation to strength training in young, healthy volunteers. In contrast, in elderly individuals (60–80 years), where the antioxidant status is expected to be lower, we tested the hypothesis that supplementation with vitamin C and vitamin E would augment the adaptations to strength training.

The supplements

Exercise that challenges the energy systems of muscle cells induces metabolic stress, which includes oxidative stress by the generation of reactive oxygen and nitrogen species (RONS) [16,44]. Several endogenous antioxidants, such as glutathione, superoxide dismutase and catalase, will counteract most of the adverse effects of acute exercise. In addition, cells will take up exogenous antioxidants in the form of vitamins C and E, alpha-lipoic acid, carotenoids, ubiquinones and a range of phytochemicals [45], which will reinforce the cellular antioxidant system. In the present study we selected a vitamin C and E combination. Vitamin C and E are well established supplements and there appear to be no large risks concerning toxic effects, even if the daily dosages are several-fold higher than the recommended amounts [46,47]. Because the water soluble vitamin C and the lipid soluble vitamin E interact with the major endogenous antioxidant glutathione, a combination should be more effective than one single compound given alone. In short, vitamin C regenerates oxidized vitamin E, and oxidized vitamin C is in turn regenerated, although dependent on both the dose and the time elapsed between intake and measurement [32]. In contrast to vitamin E (alpha-tocopherol; [48]), the pharmacokinetics of vitamin C displays a quite rapid increase after oral intake and a gradual reduction during the next hours after intake [32].

Concerning the pharmacokinetics of vitamin C, the timing of intake in regard to exercise sessions should be considered. Some studies have administered supplements in the morning [23,25,49], and 1.5-2 hours before the exercise sessions [50]. Others have chosen two intakes per day [51,52]. In order to maximize the influence of the antioxidant supplementation, it thus seemed reasonable to time the intake so that the plasma concentration was highest just before and during the first hours of recovery after the exercise sessions.

We administered dosages of 1000 mg vitamin C and 235 mg of vitamin E (DL-alpha-tocopherol) per day. These amounts are in line with other recent studies, although our vitamin E dosages could be considered moderate [15].

Participants

In the experiment with young volunteers we included both sexes. This was partly due to there being no obvious reasons to exclude one of the sexes, and partly because it is interesting to look for sex differences, as most studies on antioxidant supplementation and training adaptation have been conducted on males [25,49-54].

In the experiment on the elderly, we chose males only. The main reason for this was that very few studies have investigated interactions between exercise and antioxidant supplementation in elderly participants; however, Bobeuf et al. [23] have conducted studies on elderly males, and we wanted to follow up this study. The second reason was that elderly females appear to have less potential to respond to high intensity resistance exercise with three exercise sessions per week [55,56]. Thus, in order to increase the likelihood of inducing robust muscle growth, we selected elderly males.

We recruited recreationally trained young volunteers, but untrained elderly volunteers. Our motivation for choosing young, trained individuals was that we hypothesized that antioxidant supplementation would affect adaptations in the muscle. Thus, we assumed it was better to test this in trained individuals in whom muscular adaptations are expected to dominant over neural adaptations [57,58]. We chose untrained elderly volunteers, as we expected it would be very difficult to recruit the needed number of trained elderly participants. Furthermore, since we hypothesized that the elderly need more antioxidants to combat an increasing redox state in the aftermath of developing sarcopenia, we included untrained elderly individuals.

High intensity exercise

Based on the theory of hormesis, the advantage of antioxidant supplementation should be largest during high intensity training that induces large oxidative stress; and conversely, low intensity training – that produces low oxidative stress – in combination with antioxidant supplementation should increase the likelihood of blunting or blocking training effects [18]. In our study we wanted to apply training programs that were similar to what dedicated strength-trained individuals use in practice. We therefore designed the training protocols to induce high metabolic and oxidative stress. Accordingly, the strength training program consisted of an energy-demanding, full range of motion exercises and repetition maximum (RM) intensity, as well as short inter-set/-exercise rest periods (see Table 1).

We designed a periodized strength training program, which has been suggested to be superior to non-periodized programs [59,60]. However, there is no consensus concerning what type of periodization is better [59]. For practical reasons, we designed a linear program for the young and an undulating (non-linear) program for the elderly.

Limitations

Supplementation with vitamin C and E is a conservative choice, but the dosages chosen, 1000 mg vitamin C and 235 mg vitamin E (DL-alpha-tocopherol acetate), are in line with previously published studies [24,25,49-51,53,54]. Ideally, a dosage titration would be preferable (i.e., 400 mg, 800 mg and 1600 mg of vitamin C). Moreover, it was of interest to test vitamins C and E both separately and together; and in a stronger study design we would also include groups that received vitamins, but did not follow an exercise intervention. Unfortunately, we did not have the resources to design a study that took all these aspects into account.

We supplemented our participants with DL-alpha-tocopherol acetate, the synthetic form of vitamin E. It has been shown that the biological response to natural (D-alpha-tocopherol/RRR- alpha-tocopherol) may be different [61,62]. Thus, we must be careful when discussing our results alongside studies that have administered the natural form of vitamin E.

Training supervision was optional for the young participants in this study; while the elderly participants were supervised in all sessions. All participants were, however, instructed to keep a training diary in which they logged loads and perceived exertion, and they could request assistance whenever needed. Moreover, the young participants were familiar with strength training before entering the study. Nevertheless, full training supervision is preferable [63], to ensure that all participants follow the training as prescribed and exercise with appropriate lifting techniques and effort.

The training programs for young and elderly participants differed. This means that we cannot easily compare results from young and elderly participants. Such comparisons were not part of our hypotheses, but equal training programs could potentially give more information about the effects of the supplements. However, several practical reasons made us use different training regimes for the two groups of volunteers. Thus, we tried to optimize the training for the two groups independently of each other.

We monitored the influence of antioxidant supplementation over a rather short period of time, and long-term effects cannot be extracted. However, the most significant physiological changes occur typically in the first weeks after embarking on a new training program [58,64,57].

In the acute experiment we tested the response to a single session of strength training. The intention was to investigate the immediate cell signaling (e.g., redox sensitive mitogen activated kinases, MAPKs [65]) and the protein synthetic rate, in order to get a mechanistic insight into the hypothesized effects of the supplements. As the experiment was conducted midway into the intervention period, on the young participants, we realize that we cannot easily differentiate between the potential effects of the supplementation before/after the session and the potential effects of the preceding ~ 4 weeks with supplementation.

Relevance for investigating the effects of vitamin C and E

Vitamin C and E supplements are widely used in the general population and even more so amongst athletes [66-71]. The most common motivation for using antioxidant vitamins such as vitamin C seems to be strengthening the immune system and thereby preventing and treating diseases, especially upper-respiratory infections such as the common cold [72]. Intriguingly, vitamin C supplementation seems at best to have limited clinically relevant effects on "the common man" and on athletes who are otherwise healthy and have a normal diet [72,73]. Some groups, such as the elderly population, are more susceptible to dietary deficiencies of some vitamins and therefore supplementation may be defensible [73,74].

Amongst athletes and people engaged in recreational sport activities, dietary supplements are also used to improve performance and recovery after exercise [9,71]. Equivocal observations have been reported, but vitamin C and E do not seem to have appreciable/consistent ergogenic effects or effects on recovery from exercise [9,14,75,76].

Regardless of the motivation for use, vitamin C and E supplementation is widespread. This fact, combined with recent studies that indicate adverse effects on adaptation to exercise and training [51,53], clearly illuminate and justify further research into the biological effects of vitamin C and E supplementation in humans.

Conclusion

Antioxidant supplementations, such as vitamin C and E, are commonly used by large and divergent groups worldwide (e.g. athletes, elderly, patients etc.). Recently the potential interaction between antioxidant supplementation and training has received increased scientific interest and become a debated topic. Indeed, both animal and human studies have indicated negative effects when vitamin C and/or E are administered in high dosages. The literature is, however, ambiguous and many important questions remain unanswered. Hitherto, human investigations have focused on endurance exercise and training, so the experiments described here should provide novel data and insight into the interactions between antioxidant supplementation and adaptations to strength training.

Competing interests

The authors declare that they have no competing interests.

Authors' contributions

GP contributed to all parts of the study. He currently works with data analysis and writing. KTC took part in the planning and design of the study with young participants. He contributed to the recruitment of volunteers and management of the experiments. KCT currently works with biochemical analyses of blood and muscle, as well as statistical data analysis and writing. KCT's focus is on endogenous antioxidants and heat shock proteins. HH took part in the planning and design of the study with young participants. He contributed to the recruitment of volunteers and management of the experiments. HH currently works with biochemical analyses of muscle, as well as data analysis and writing. HH's focus is on protein signaling after acute resistance exercise sessions. EB took part in the planning and design of the study with young participants. She had a special responsibility for the acute experiment concerning measurements of protein synthesis (stable isotope procedure). EB is currently involved in data analysis and writing. SB took part in the planning and design of the study with elderly participants. SB administered the study with the elderly participants, and is currently involved in data analysis and writing. TR contributed to all parts of the studies, and he was responsible for the biopsy procedure. He currently works with data analysis and writing. All authors read and approved the final manuscript.

Author details

[1]Department of Physical Performance, Norwegian School of Sport Sciences, Oslo, Norway. [2]Norwegian Olympic Sport Center, Oslo, Norway. [3]University of Arkansas for Medical Sciences, Arkansas Children's Nutrition Center, Arkansas Children's Hospital Research Institute, Little Rock, Arkansas, USA. [4]Department of Public Health, Sport and Nutrition, Faculty of Health and Sport Sciences, University of Agder, Kristiansand, Norway.

References

1. Holloszy JO, Coyle EF: **Adaptations of skeletal muscle to endurance exercise and their metabolic consequences.** *J Appl Physiol* 1984, **56:**831–838.
2. Costill DL, Coyle EF, Fink WF, Lesmes GR, Witzmann FA: **Adaptations in skeletal muscle following strength training.** *J Appl Physiol* 1979, **46:**96–99.
3. Pollock ML: **The quantification of endurance training programs.** *Exerc Sport Sci Rev* 1973, **1:**155–188.
4. Deschenes MR, Kraemer WJ: **Performance and physiologic adaptations to resistance training.** *Am J Phys Med Rehabil* 2002, **81:**S3–16.
5. Hawley JA, Tipton KD, Millard-Stafford ML: **Promoting training adaptations through nutritional interventions.** *J Sports Sci* 2006, **24:**709–721.
6. Hulmi JJ, Lockwood CM, Stout JR: **Effect of protein/essential amino acids and resistance training on skeletal muscle hypertrophy: a case for whey protein.** *Nutr Metab (Lond)* 2010, **7:**51.
7. Bemben MG, Lamont HS: **Creatine supplementation and exercise performance: recent findings.** *Sports Med* 2005, **35:**107–125.
8. Rodriguez NR, Di Marco NM, Langley S: **American college of sports medicine position stands nutrition and athletic performance.** *Med Sci Sports Exerc* 2009, **41:**709–731.
9. Clarkson PM, Thompson HS: **Antioxidants: what role do they play in physical activity and health?** *Am J Clin Nutr* 2000, **72:**637S–646S.
10. Peternelj TT, Coombes JS: **Antioxidant supplementation during exercise training: beneficial or detrimental?** *Sports Med* 2011, **41:**1043–1069.
11. Vina J, Gomez-Cabrera MC, Borras C: **Fostering antioxidant defences: up-regulation of antioxidant genes or antioxidant supplementation?** *Br J Nutr* 2007, **98**(Suppl 1):S36–S40.
12. Peake JM, Suzuki K, Coombes JS: **The influence of antioxidant supplementation on markers of inflammation and the relationship to oxidative stress after exercise.** *J Nutr Biochem* 2007, **18:**357–371.
13. Ristow M, Zarse K: **How increased oxidative stress promotes longevity and metabolic health: the concept of mitochondrial hormesis (mitohormesis).** *Exp Gerontol* 2010, **45:**410–418.
14. Braakhuis AJ: **Effect of vitamin C supplements on physical performance.** *Curr Sports Med Rep* 2012, **11:**180–184.
15. Nikolaidis MG, Kerksick CM, Lamprecht M, McAnulty SR: **Does vitamin C and E supplementation impair the favorable adaptations of regular exercise?** *Oxid Med Cell Longev* 2012, **2012:**707941.
16. Fisher-Wellman K, Bloomer RJ: **Acute exercise and oxidative stress: a 30 year history.** *Dyn Med* 2009, **8:**1.
17. Warren JA, Jenkins RR, Packer L, Witt EH, Armstrong RB: **Elevated muscle vitamin E does not attenuate eccentric exercise-induced muscle injury.** *J Appl Physiol* 1992, **72:**2168–2175.
18. Hawley JA, Burke LM, Phillips SM, Spriet LL: **Nutritional modulation of training-induced skeletal muscle adaptations.** *J Appl Physiol* 2011, **110:**834–845.
19. Makanae Y, Kawada S, Sasaki K, Nakazato K, Ishii N: **Vitamin C administration attenuates overload-induced skeletal muscle hypertrophy in rats.** *Acta Physiol (Oxf)* 2013, **208:**57–65.
20. Morales-Alamo D, Ponce-Gonzalez JG, Guadalupe-Grau A, Rodriguez-Garcia L, Santana A, Cusso MR, Guerrero M, Guerra B, Dorado C, Calbet JA: **Increased oxidative stress and anaerobic energy release, but blunted Thr172-AMPKalpha phosphorylation, in response to sprint exercise in severe acute hypoxia in humans.** *J Appl Physiol* 2012, **113:**917–928.
21. Malm C, Svensson M, Ekblom B, Sjodin B: **Effects of ubiquinone-10 supplementation and high intensity training on physical performance in humans.** *Acta Physiol Scand* 1997, **161:**379–384.
22. Braakhuis AJ, Hopkins WG, Lowe TE: **Effects of dietary antioxidants on training and performance in female runners.** *Eur J Sport Sci* 2014, **14:**160–168.
23. Bobeuf F, Labonte M, Dionne IJ, Khalil A: **Combined effect of antioxidant supplementation and resistance training on oxidative stress markers, muscle and body composition in an elderly population.** *J Nutr Health Aging* 2011, **15:**883–889.
24. Chuin A, Labonte M, Tessier D, Khalil A, Bobeuf F, Doyon CY, Rieth N, Dionne IJ: **Effect of antioxidants combined to resistance training on BMD in elderly women: a pilot study.** *Osteoporos Int* 2009, **20:**1253–1258.
25. Theodorou AA, Nikolaidis MG, Paschalis V, Koutsias S, Panayiotou G, Fatouros IG, Koutedakis Y, Jamurtas AZ: **No effect of antioxidant supplementation on muscle performance and blood redox status adaptations to eccentric training.** *Am J Clin Nutr* 2011, **93:**1373–1383.
26. Ryan MJ, Dudash HJ, Docherty M, Geronilla KB, Baker BA, Haff GG, Cutlip RG, Always SE: **Vitamin E and C supplementation reduces oxidative stress, improves antioxidant enzymes and positive muscle work in chronically loaded muscles of aged rats.** *Exp Gerontol* 2010, **45:**882–895.
27. Peake J, Della GP, Cameron-Smith D: **Aging and its effects on inflammation in skeletal muscle at rest and following exercise-induced muscle injury.** *Am J Physiol Regul Integr Comp Physiol* 2010, **298:**R1485–R1495.
28. Gianni P, Jan KJ, Douglas MJ, Stuart PM, Tarnopolsky MA: **Oxidative stress and the mitochondrial theory of aging in human skeletal muscle.** *Exp Gerontol* 2004, **39:**1391–1400.
29. Gomez-Cabrera MC, Ferrando B, Brioche TS-GF, Vina J: **Exercise and antioxidant supplements in the elderly.** *Journal of Sport and Health Science* 2013, **2:**94–100.
30. Padayatty SJ, Levine M: **New insights into the physiology and pharmacology of vitamin C.** *CMAJ* 2001, **164:**353–355.
31. Lodge JK: **Vitamin E bioavailability in humans.** *J Plant Physiol* 2005, **162:**790–796.
32. Padayatty SJ, Sun H, Wang Y, Riordan HD, Hewitt SM, Katz A, Wesley RA, Levine M: **Vitamin C pharmacokinetics: implications for oral and intravenous use.** *Ann Intern Med* 2004, **140:**533–537.
33. Black AE, Goldberg GR, Jebb SA, Livingstone MB, Cole TJ, Prentice AM: **Critical evaluation of energy intake data using fundamental principles of energy physiology: 2. Evaluating the results of published surveys.** *Eur J Clin Nutr* 1991, **45:**583–599.
34. Andersen LF, Pollestad ML, Jacobs DR Jr, Lovo A, Hustvedt BE: **Validation of a pre-coded food diary used among 13-year-olds: comparison of energy intake with energy expenditure.** *Public Health Nutr* 2005, **8:**1315–1321.
35. Borg G: **Perceived exertion as an indicator of somatic stress.** *Scand J Rehabil Med* 1970, **2:**92–98.
36. Anderson LJ, Erceg DN, Schroeder ET: **Utility of multifrequency bioelectrical impedance compared with dual-energy x-ray absorptiometry for**

assessment of total and regional body composition varies between men and women. *Nutr Res* 2012, **32:**479–485.

37. Berntsen S, Hageberg R, Aandstad A, Mowinckel P, Anderssen SA, Carlsen KH, Andersen LB: **Validity of physical activity monitors in adults participating in free-living activities.** *Br J Sports Med* 2010, **44:**657–664.
38. Paulsen G, Vissing K, Kalhovde JM, Ugelstad I, Bayer ML, Kadi F, Schjerling P, Hallen J, Raastad T: **Maximal eccentric exercise induces a rapid accumulation of small heat shock proteins on myofibrils and a delayed HSP70 response in humans.** *Am J Physiol Regul Integr Comp Physiol* 2007, **293:**R844–R853.
39. Hanssen KE, Kvamme NH, Nilsen TS, Ronnestad B, Ambjornsen IK, Norheim F, Kadi F, Hallen J, Drevon CA, Raastad T: **The effect of strength training volume on satellite cells, myogenic regulatory factors, and growth factors.** *Scand J Med Sci Sports* 2012, **23:**728–739.
40. Mackey AL, Kjaer M, Charifi N, Henriksson J, Bojsen-Moller J, Holm L, Kadi F: **Assessment of satellite cell number and activity status in human skeletal muscle biopsies.** *Muscle Nerve* 2009, **40:**455–465.
41. Paulsen G, Lauritzen F, Bayer ML, Kalhovde JM, Ugelstad I, Owe SG, Hallen J, Bergersen LH, Raastad T: **Subcellular movement and expression of HSP27, alphaB-crystallin, and HSP70 after two bouts of eccentric exercise in humans.** *J Appl Physiol* 2009, **107:**570–582.
42. Sakhi AK, Russnes KM, Smeland S, Blomhoff R, Gundersen TE: **Simultaneous quantification of reduced and oxidized glutathione in plasma using a two-dimensional chromatographic system with parallel porous graphitized carbon columns coupled with fluorescence and coulometric electrochemical detection.** *J Chromatogr A* 2006, **1104:**179–189.
43. Zhang XJ, Chinkes DL, Wolfe RR: **Measurement of muscle protein fractional synthesis and breakdown rates from a pulse tracer injection.** *Am J Physiol Endocrinol Metab* 2002, **283:**E753–E764.
44. Niess AM, Simon P: **Response and adaptation of skeletal muscle to exercise–the role of reactive oxygen species.** *Front Biosci* 2007, **12:**4826–4838.
45. Powers SK, Lennon SL: **Analysis of cellular responses to free radicals: focus on exercise and skeletal muscle.** *Proc Nutr Soc* 1999, **58:**1025–1033.
46. Diplock AT: **Safety of antioxidant vitamins and beta-carotene.** *Am J Clin Nutr* 1995, **62:**1510S–1516S.
47. Garewal HS, Diplock AT: **How 'safe' are antioxidant vitamins?** *Drug Saf* 1995, **13:**8–14.
48. Novotny JA, Fadel JG, Holstege DM, Furr HC, Clifford AJ: **This kinetic, bioavailability, and metabolism study of RRR-alpha-tocopherol in healthy adults suggests lower intake requirements than previous estimates.** *J Nutr* 2012, **142:**2105–2111.
49. Yfanti C, Akerstrom T, Nielsen S, Nielsen AR, Mounier R, Mortensen OH, Lykkesfeldt J, Rose AJ, Fischer CP, Pedersen BK: **Antioxidant supplementation does not alter endurance training adaptation.** *Med Sci Sports Exerc* 2010, **42:**1388–1395.
50. Roberts LA, Beattie K, Close GL, Morton JP: **Vitamin C consumption does not impair training-induced improvements in exercise performance.** *Int J Sports Physiol Perform* 2011, **6:**58–69.
51. Ristow M, Zarse K, Oberbach A, Kloting N, Birringer M, Kiehntopf M, Stumvoll M, Kahn CR, Bluher M: **Antioxidants prevent health-promoting effects of physical exercise in humans.** *Proc Natl Acad Sci U S A* 2009, **106:**8665–8670.
52. Aguilo A, Tauler P, Sureda A, Cases N, Tur J, Pons A: **Antioxidant diet supplementation enhances aerobic performance in amateur sportsmen.** *J Sports Sci* 2007, **25:**1203–1210.
53. Gomez-Cabrera MC, Domenech E, Romagnoli M, Arduini A, Borras C, Pallardo FV, Sastre J, Vina J: **Oral administration of vitamin C decreases muscle mitochondrial biogenesis and hampers training-induced adaptations in endurance performance.** *Am J Clin Nutr* 2008, **87:**142–149.
54. Zoppi CC, Hohl R, Silva FC, Lazarim FL, Neto JM, Stancanneli M, Macedo DV: **Vitamin C and e supplementation effects in professional soccer players under regular training.** *J Int Soc Sports Nutr* 2006, **3:**37–44.
55. Hunter GR, McCarthy JP, Bamman MM: **Effects of resistance training on older adults.** *Sports Med* 2004, **34:**329–348.
56. Kosek DJ, Kim JS, Petrella JK, Cross JM, Bamman MM: **Efficacy of 3 days/wk resistance training on myofiber hypertrophy and myogenic mechanisms in young vs. older adults.** *J Appl Physiol* 2006, **101:**531–544.
57. Kraemer WJ, Fleck SJ, Evans WJ: **Strength and power training: physiological mechanisms of adaptation.** *Exerc Sport Sci Rev* 1996, **24:**363–397.
58. Seynnes OR, De Boer M, Narici MV: **Early skeletal muscle hypertrophy and architectural changes in response to high-intensity resistance training.** *J Appl Physiol* 2007, **102:**368–373.
59. Lorenz DS, Reiman MP, Walker JC: **Periodization: current review and suggested implementation for athletic rehabilitation.** *Sports Health* 2010, **2:**509–518.
60. Fleck SJ: **Periodized strength training: a critical review.** *J Strength Cond Res* 1999, **13:**82–89.
61. Burton GW, Traber MG, Acuff RV, Walters DN, Kayden H, Hughes L, Ingold KU: **Human plasma and tissue alpha-tocopherol concentrations in response to supplementation with deuterated natural and synthetic vitamin E.** *Am J Clin Nutr* 1998, **67:**669–684.
62. Traber MG, Ramakrishnan R, Kayden HJ: **Human plasma vitamin E kinetics demonstrate rapid recycling of plasma RRR-alpha-tocopherol.** *Proc Natl Acad Sci U S A* 1994, **91:**10005–10008.
63. Mazzetti SA, Kraemer WJ, Volek JS, Duncan ND, Ratamess NA, Gomez AL, Newton RU, Hakkinen K, Fleck SJ: **The influence of direct supervision of resistance training on strength performance.** *Med Sci Sports Exerc* 2000, **32:**1175–1184.
64. Staron RS, Karapondo DL, Kraemer WJ, Fry AC, Gordon SE, Falkel JE, Hagerman FC, Hikida RS: **Skeletal muscle adaptations during early phase of heavy-resistance training in men and women.** *J Appl Physiol* 1994, **76:**1247–1255.
65. Wretman C, Lionikas A, Widegren U, Lannergren J, Westerblad H, Henriksson J: **Effects of concentric and eccentric contractions on phosphorylation of MAPK(erk1/2) and MAPK(p38) in isolated rat skeletal muscle.** *J Physiol* 2001, **535:**155–164.
66. Maughan RJ, Depiesse F, Geyer H: **The use of dietary supplements by athletes.** *J Sports Sci* 2007, **25**(Suppl 1):S103–S113.
67. Sobal J, Marquart LF: **Vitamin/mineral supplement use among athletes: a review of the literature.** *Int J Sport Nutr* 1994, **4:**320–334.
68. Kennedy ET, Luo H, Houser RF: **Dietary supplement use pattern of U.S. adult population in the 2007–2008 National Health and Nutrition Examination Survey (NHANES).** *Ecol Food Nutr* 2013, **2013**(52):76–84.
69. Stewart ML, McDonald JT, Levy AS, Schucker RE, Henderson DP: **Vitamin/mineral supplement use: a telephone survey of adults in the United States.** *J Am Diet Assoc* 1985, **85:**1585–1590.
70. Braun H, Koehler K, Geyer H, Kleiner J, Mester J, Schanzer W: **Dietary supplement use among elite young German athletes.** *Int J Sport Nutr Exerc Metab* 2009, **19:**97–109.
71. Maughan RJ, Greenhaff PL, Hespel P: **Dietary supplements for athletes: emerging trends and recurring themes.** *J Sports Sci* 2011, **29**(Suppl 1):S57–S66.
72. Hemila H, Chalker E: **Vitamin C for preventing and treating the common cold.** *Cochrane Database Syst Rev* 2013, **1:**CD000980.
73. Wintergerst ES, Maggini S, Hornig DH: **Contribution of selected vitamins and trace elements to immune function.** *Ann Nutr Metab* 2007, **51:**301–323.
74. Sebastian RS, Cleveland LE, Goldman JD, Moshfegh AJ: **Older adults who use vitamin/mineral supplements differ from nonusers in nutrient intake adequacy and dietary attitudes.** *J Am Diet Assoc* 2007, **107:**1322–1332.
75. Bloomer RJ: **The role of nutritional supplements in the prevention and treatment of resistance exercise-induced skeletal muscle injury.** *Sports Med* 2007, **37:**519–532.
76. Evans WJ: **Vitamin E, vitamin C, and exercise.** *Am J Clin Nutr* 2000, **72:**647S–652S.

7

A pilot study on biomarkers for tendinopathy: lower levels of serum TNF-α and other cytokines in females but not males with Achilles tendinopathy

James E. Gaida[1,2,3,4*], Håkan Alfredson[5,6], Sture Forsgren[4] and Jill L. Cook[7]

Abstract

Background: Achilles tendinopathy is a painful musculoskeletal condition that is common among athletes, and which limits training capacity and competitive performance. The lack of biomarkers for tendinopathy limits research into risk factors and also the evaluation of new treatments. Cytokines and growth factors involved in regulating the response of tendon cells to mechanical load have potential as biomarkers for tendinopathy.

Methods: This case–control study compared serum concentration of cytokines and growth factors (TNF-α, IL-1β, bFGF, PDFG-BB, IFN-γ, VEGF) between individuals with chronic Achilles tendinopathy and controls. These were measured in fasting serum from 22 individuals with chronic Achilles tendinopathy and 10 healthy controls. Results were analysed in relation to gender and physical activity pattern.

Results: TNF-α concentration was lower in the entire tendinopathy group compared with the entire control group; none of the other cytokines were significantly different. TNF-α levels were nevertheless highly correlated with the other cytokines measured, in most of the subgroups. Analysed by gender, TNF-α and PDGF-BB concentrations were lower in the female tendinopathy group but not the male tendinopathy group. A trend was seen for lower IL-1β in the female tendinopathy group. Physical activity was correlated with TNF-α, PDGF-BB and IL-1β to varying extents for control subgroups, but not for the female tendinopathy group. No correlations were seen with BMI or duration of symptoms.

Conclusions: This pilot study indicates a lower level of TNF-α and PDGF-BB, and to some extent IL-1β among females, but not males, in the chronic phase of Achilles tendinopathy. It is suggested that future studies on tendinopathy biomarkers analyse male and female data separately. The lack of correlation between cytokine level and physical activity in the female tendinopathy group warrants further study.

Keywords: Cytokines, Tumor necrosis factor alpha, Biomarkers, Musculoskeletal pain

What is known about the subject

Tendinopathy has a lifetime incidence of more than 50 % in middle distance runners and presents a significant barrier to optimal performance in many elite sports. Much work has focussed on cytokine and growth factor expression at the tissue level, however, this approach is not suitable for longitudinal studies with multiple data collection points due to the trauma induced by the biopsy. Serum levels of cytokine expression overcomes this limitation but has received little research attention.

What this study adds to existing knowledge

In this study, we found lower levels of TNF-α and PDGF-BB among females with chronic Achilles tendinopathy. Curiously, the association between physical activity and cytokine levels seen in the female control group was absent in the female tendinopathy group. These

* Correspondence: Jamie.Gaida@canberra.edu.au
[1]University of Canberra Research Institute for Sport and Exercise (UCRISE), Canberra, Australia
[2]Discipline of Physiotherapy, University of Canberra, ACT 2601 Canberra, Australia
Full list of author information is available at the end of the article

results should be seen as preliminary due to the low subject numbers, however, they provide direction and justification for further studies in this area.

Clinical relevance

Potential biomarkers for chronic Achilles tendinopathy include TNF-α and PDGF-BB. These findings require verification in larger samples and should be extended to populations with recently developed tendinopathy.

Background

Achilles tendinopathy is commonly seen in sports medicine and general practice. The cumulative lifetime incidence is 6 % in the non-athletic general population and 52 % in middle distance runners [1]. Contributing factors among athletes can include a sudden increase in loading [2, 3], a hard training surface [4], lower limb biomechanics [5] and calf muscle weakness [6]. Among non-athletic individuals, systemic factors such as diabetes [7] and blood lipids [8] may decrease the capacity of the tendon to tolerate everyday loads and contribute to tendinopathy in the absence of high tendon loading.

Serum biomarkers such as tumour necrosis factor alpha (TNF-α) are useful for monitoring disease severity and can even help to confirm a suspected diagnosis. For example, certain markers discriminate persons with bipolar disorder from controls [9]. In addition, an association between TNF-α and objective measures of depression and fatigue is shown in studies of chronic obstructive pulmonary disease (COPD) [10]. The TNF-α system is also strongly involved in inflammatory disorders such as inflammatory bowel disease and rheumatoid arthritis. Blood levels of both TNF-α and the soluble form of tumour necrosis factor receptor 1 (sTNFR1) [11] are increased among inflammatory bowel disease patients. sTNFR1 is generated when transmembrane TNFR1 is cleaved and the extracelluar receptor fragment is released [12]. At low concentrations, sTNFR1 stabilises the structure of TNF-α and slows its decay, while at higher concentrations it acts as a competitive antagonist for TNF-α action [13]. TNF receptor levels also correlate with disease activity for inflammatory bowel disease patients [14], and in rheumatoid arthritis TNF-α levels are increased in the synovial fluid of affected joints [15] and serum sTNFR1 levels are also elevated [16]. The presence of TNF-α and its two receptors has been confirmed in human Achilles tendon [17].

There is very little information on the effects of marked exercise on levels of TNF-α. In one study, in which the effects of heavy resistance exercise was evaluated for 30 resistance trained men, an initial increase but later, at recovery, a decrease in blood TNF-α levels was noted [18]. These authors also concluded that neuromuscular electrical stimulation appeared to prevent the decline in the circulating TNF-α that was observed during recovery [18]. In a study by Andersson and co-workers, it was found that the levels of TNF-α significantly increased after endurance physical exercise in non-athletes [19]. Likewise, it was found that there were increases in levels of TNF-α and other cytokines directly after 90-min soccer games in elite female players but that the levels were normalized within 21 h [20]. In a study on horses it was noted that the TNF-α blood level did not change in response to exercise competition but the authors concluded that circulating cytokines may after all be predictive of athletic performance [21]. In another study the mechanisms underlying overtraining syndrome for men was discussed and it was suggested that increased cytokine productions might be involved in this syndrome [22].

Only two human studies have investigated serum biomarkers for tendinopathy. In one study, serum levels of sTNFR1 and brain-derived neurotropic factor (BDNF) were no different between groups with and without tendinopathy [23]. However, gender-dependent correlations with physical activity levels were seen in the tendinopathy group but not in the control group. The other study investigated serum levels of oxidative derivatives of an omega-6 fatty acid (linoleic acid), which are known as oxylipins [24]. Other potentially interesting biomarkers for musculoskeletal diseases [25], such as tendinopathy, include TNF-α, interleukin 1 beta (IL-1), basic fibroblast growth factor (bFGF), interferon gamma (IFN-), platelet derived growth factor BB (PDGF-BB) and vascular endothelial growth factor (VEGF).

It is a drawback that there is so little information concerning serum biomarkers in tendinopathy, as this condition is so frequently occurring among sports active individuals. Therefore, the aim of this study was to compare concentrations in serum of the cytokines referred to above between patients with Achilles tendinopathy and healthy controls. As the pattern of physical activity of patients with Achilles tendinopathy can influence biomarker concentrations [23], correlations with physical activity level were explored, as were correlations with two other factors [body mass index (BMI) and pain symptom length]. The hypothesis was that certain biomarker/s might show a special pattern for tendinopathy patients as compared with control persons.

Methods

This project was approved by the Committee of Ethics at the Faculty of Medicine, Umeå University, and by the Regional Ethical Review Board in Umeå (04–157 M). All procedures were conducted according to the principles of the declaration of Helsinki. All participants gave written, informed consent.

Twenty-two individuals referred to the Sports Medicine Unit at Umeå University for management of chronic Achilles tendon pain were included in this study. All individuals had a diagnosis of mid-portion Achilles tendinopathy established by an experienced orthopaedic surgeon (HA). Diagnostic criteria included exercise-related pain in the Achilles tendon, localised 2 to 6 cm proximal to the calcaneal attachment. Only individuals with gradual onset of pain were included to avoid the possibility of including cases of partial rupture. The included patients had been referred to the Sports Medicine Unit following unsuccessful treatment of their condition with their local clinician (e.g. GP, physiotherapist). Previous treatments reported by these patients were rest from aggravating activities and heavy-load eccentric training. Ten control individuals with no history of Achilles tendon pain were recruited from the local community.

Both patients and controls had an ultrasound examination by the same orthopaedic surgeon (HA) using an Acuson Sequoia 512 (Siemens AG, Berlin, Germany) fitted with 8–13 MHz linear array transducer. From the prone position with both feet hanging off the end of the bed, the right and left Achilles tendons were examined using grey-scale and colour Doppler ultrasound. Characteristic features of tendinopathy were present in the patient group (increased anterior-posterior diameter, hypoechoic regions, and the loss of the clear demarcation between the anterior border of the tendon and Kager's fat pad). Colour Doppler showed increased vascularity in the affected region of the painful tendon. All control participants had normal ultrasound examination findings.

Blood samples were collected in an identical manner for the tendinopathy and control groups. Blood was collected in the morning following an overnight fast in a serum separating tube, which was clotted at room temperature for 30 min and then centrifuged at 1300 × g for 10 min. Serum aliquots were stored at −80 °C awaiting analysis and did not undergo repeated freeze-thaw cycles.

Serum aliquots were thawed on ice immediately prior to analysis. Cytokine concentrations (TNF-α, IL-1 , bFGF, IFN- , PDGF-BB, and VEGF) were quantified using the Human Cytokine Group 1, 6-plex assay (catalogue number: X50007Z13H) on a Bio-Plex 200 Suspension Array System (Bio-Rad, Hercules, California, USA), according to the manufacturers instructions. Measurements were made in duplicate wells and all samples were tested on a single 96-well plate, which eliminated the possibility of plate-to-plate variation.

The limit of detection, defined as 2 standard deviations (SD) above the mean background fluorescence, is provided by the manufacturer based on measurement of 10 replicate wells containing all reagents except the cytokine of interest. The limit of detection for TNF-α is 3.0 pg/mL, for IL-1 0.8 pg/mL, for bFGF 6.8 pg/mL, for IFN- 19.3 pg/mL, for PDGF-BB 1.0 pg/mL, and for VEGF 0.5 pg/mL.

The physical activity level of all participants was quantified using the Past Year Physical Activity Questionnaire (PYT-PAQ). The questionnaire prompts participants to estimate the frequency (months/year, days/week), duration (hours/day) and perceived intensity (sedentary, light, moderate, heavy) of occupational, household, and recreational activities over the past 12-months. These questionnaires are coded according to the typical metabolic cost of each activity to yield a metabolic equivalent (MET) of physical activity that is expressed in MET-hours/week.

The reproducibility of the MET-hours/week estimates from questionnaires completed 9-week apart is 0.70 (Spearman's rank correlation coefficient) for occupational activity, 0.65 for household activitity, 0.73 for recreational activity and 0.64 for total activity [26]. This questionnaire has also been validated using 4 × 7-day physical activity diaries and 4 × 7-day accelerometer data, with the 4-time points in different weather seasons. Questionnaire validity against physical activity logs (intraclass correlation coefficient (ICC) = 0.42, 95 % CI = 0.28 to 0.54)) and against accelerometer data (ICC = 0.18 (95 % CI = 0.03 to 0.32) is comparable to other physical activity questionnaires.

Due to the relatively small and uneven group numbers, all analyses were conducted using non-parametric statistics. Continuous variables were tested using the Mann–Whitney U test. Significance level was set at $p < 0.05$ and Bonferroni adjustment was not used due to the pilot nature of this study.

The analysis was conducted first using all data points and then repeated following removal of any cytokine analysis result with a coefficient of variation (CV) greater than 15 %. Results are reported as mean (SD) throughout the manuscript unless otherwise indicated. Analysis was performed using STATA/IC 13.1.

Results

Individuals with Achilles tendinopathy were well matched to the control participants according to key demographic variables (Table 1). There was a similar ratio of men to women, with 60 and 68 % of the patient and control group being male. Symptom data indicated that all patients had chronic tendinopathy as the shortest duration was 3.5 months.

Serum concentration of TNF-α was significantly lower in individuals with Achilles tendinopathy, when females and males were grouped together, compared with the entire control group (Table 2). No differences were

Table 1 Participant demographics

	Achilles tendon status		
	Normal ($n = 10$)	Tendinopathy ($n = 22$)	p
Sex (male:female)	6:4	15:7	0.652
Age (years)	54.5 (8.4)	53.0 (10.8)	0.475
Height (cm)	172.1 (11.3)	175.2 (7.1)	0.416
Weight (kg)	82.5 (18.8)	86.9 (16.4)	0.490
BMI (kg/m^2)	27.6 (3.8)	28.2 (4.2)	0.968
Physical activity (MET-hours/week)[a]	137.2 (29.1)	151.2 (54.2)	0.637
Pain: symptom duration (months)	N/A	24 (IQR 8 to 24) Range 3.5 to 120	

Data reported as mean (standard deviation (SD)) except symptom duration, which is given as median and interquartile range (IQR). [a]Physical activity data missing for 1 individual in control group and 2 individuals in tendinopathy group

detected between the two groups for the other cytokines that were analysed. The findings were unchanged when the analysis was repeated after excluding data with CV >15 % (Table 3).

The mean CV for the cytokines analysis was 7.8 % (TNF-α), 5.3 % (IL-1), 8.5 % (bFGF), 6.9 % (IFN-), 1.1 % (PDGF-BB), and 5.9 % (VEGF). Sixteen data points were removed due to a CV >15 %, which left 176 of the original 192 data points. As described above, repeating the analysis after removal of these data did not affect the results.

When separated by gender, serum TNF-α and PDGF-BB levels were lower in women with tendinopathy compared to women in the control group (Table 4). There was a non-significant trend for IL-1 to be lower in women with tendinopathy ($p = 0.059$). In contrast, no group differences were seen for men ($p > 0.5$ for all cytokines). After excluding data with CV >15 % there was a clear trend towards significance for a difference in TNF-α levels between women with and without tendinopathy ($p = 0.053$, Table 5). Significance testing for PDGF-BB ($p = 0.023$) and IL-1 ($p = 0.059$) levels between women with and without tendinopathy remained unchanged. The results for the men were unaffected by removal of data with CV >15 % (p > 0.3 for all cytokines).

As TNF-α was different between the tendinopathy and control group, correlations with potential confounding factors (physical activity, BMI, pain symptom duration) were determined to further explore this finding (Table 6). A significant correlation was seen between TNF-α and physical activity level for all men, however, when examined by subgroup there was a correlation for the men of the control group but not those of the tendinopathy group. No other correlations were seen for physical activity, BMI or pain symptom duration.

Analysis of potential confounding factors was repeated for PDGF-BB (Table 7) and IL-1 (Table 8). There was no correlation between PDGF-BB and physical activity for all men, however, when examined by subgroup there was a negative correlation for the men of the tendinopathy group but not those of the control group. There was no correlation between PDGF-BB and physical activity for all women, however, when examined by subgroup there was a positive correlation for the women of the control group but not the tendinopathy group. There was no correlation between IL-1 and physical activity for all men, however, when examined by subgroup there was a positive correlation for the men of the control group but not the tendinopathy group. No correlations were seen for PDGF-BB or IL-1 with BMI or pain symptom duration.

A further question of interest was whether a systematic pattern of cytokine expression existed. Therefore, bivariate correlations between pairs of cytokines were examined using Spearmans rho ( ) with TNF-α as the reference cytokine (Table 9). Strong correlations were observed between TNF-α and IFN- among all subgroups of men and women. Strong correlations were observed between TNF-α and bFGF, and between TNF-α and VEGF in men but not women. Finally, correlations between TNF-α and IL-1 , and between TNF-α and

Table 2 Serum cytokine concentrations (all data points)

	Achilles tendon status		
Analyte (pg/mL)	Normal ($n = 10$)	Tendinopathy ($n = 22$)	p-value
TNF-α	173.58 (64.98)	114.40 (45.17)	0.018
IL-1β	13.08 (3.38)	11.18 (2.99)	0.193
bFGF	67.72 (26.60)	66.34 (26.53)	0.968
INF-γ	180.70 (74.90)	141.89 (46.94)	0.371
PDGF-BB	12041.49 (2813.68)	11062.68 (3447.73)	0.088
VEGF	203.21 (129.25)	217.05 (123.28)	0.626

Table 3 Serum cytokine concentrations (excluding observations with CV >15 %)

	Achilles tendon status				
Analyte (pg/mL)	n	Normal	n	Tendinopathy	*p*-value
TNF-α	8	179.52 (62.30)	18	119.93 (47.35)	0.030
IL-1β	10	13.08 (3.38)	22	11.18 (2.99)	0.193
bFGF	9	68.42 (28.11)	18	70.12 (27.89)	0.643
INF-γ	9	171.65 (73.43)	21	147.58 (39.57)	0.769
PDGF-BB	10	12041.49 (2813.68)	22	11062.68 (3447.73)	0.088
VEGF	9	211.36 (134.34)	20	232.60 (117.48)	0.5093

PDGF-BB were seen for all women but not when control and tendinopathy groups were examined separately. A limitation for this analysis was small group numbers.

Discussion

This study of serum biomarkers for Achilles tendinopathy has three key findings. First, TNF-α levels were lower in women with tendinopathy than women without tendinopathy. Second, contrasting findings were seen for men and women across a number of outcomes. For example, PDGF levels were lower in women with tendinopathy but not in males with tendinopathy, and IL-1 showed a non-significant trend toward being lower in the female tendinopathy group as well. Third, the physical activity level correlated with TNF-α only for control men but not for any of the other groups. The finding for TNF-α was an unexpected finding as previous research mainly points toward an increased activation of the TNF-α system in tendinopathy and tendon overuse [17, 23, 27]. However, consistent with the findings in the present study, Pingel and collaborators [28] found decreased TNF-α mRNA levels in the most abnormal part of the affected tendon in comparison to 3 cm proximal in the same tendon. Together these data indicate that although the TNF-α system appears to be involved in tendinopathy, whether it is up or down regulated appears to depend on several factors. These factors appear to include whether measurement is made 1) at the mRNA or protein level, 2) in the tissue or blood, 3) of the cytokine itself, of its two receptors, or of the soluble receptor fragments. Importantly, it also appears as if the situation varies according to gender.

The influence of potential confounding factors on TNF-α levels was explored with correlation analysis in the various subgroups. The data showed a strong relationship between physical activity and TNF-α in the male control group. The same relationship was not seen in the male tendinopathy, the female control or female tendinopathy groups. It is well known that plasma TNF-α (and also sTNFR1 and sTNFR2) rises following strenuous and prolonged exercise (i.e. marathon running), and that the peak is seen during the first hour after the race [29]. In a study on the effects of 14-days of endurance physical activity (cross-country skiing) it was found that the levels of TNF-α increased significantly at week-1 and week-2 of the exercise but that they returned to baseline values during the recovery period [19]. The source of this increase is unclear, although it has been shown that neither blood mononuclear cells [30] nor skeletal muscle [31] is the source. It has been suggested that prolonged strenuous exercise causes gastrointestinal ischaemia, which leads to endotoxin leakage into the circulation and a secondary increase in TNF-α [32]. This is supported by evidence of no increase in serum or muscle TNF-α during prolonged but non-exhaustive exercise [33]. In contrast to exhaustive exercise, the transition to habitual aerobic exercise reduces plasma TNF-α in mildly overweight healthy women [34] whereas no effect is seen following 12-weeks of strength training in obese men [35] or obese hypertensive men and women [36],

Table 4 Serum cytokine concentrations analysed by sex and tendon status (all data points)

	Male			Female		
Analyte (pg/mL)	Normal (*n* = 6)	Tendinopathy (*n* = 15)	*p*	Normal (*n* = 4)	Tendinopathy (*n* = 7)	*p*
TNF-α	153.25 (65.81)	132.02 (30.06)	0.586	204.09 (58.13)	76.65 (50.93)	0.014
IL-1β	12.23 (3.79)	11.68 (2.08)	0.938	14.35 (2.60)	10.12 (4.37)	0.059
bFGF	76.64 (29.83)	72.54 (24.76)	0.815	54.35 (15.56)	53.049 (27.06)	0.850
INF-γ	168.99 (72.33)	150.93 (42.14)	0.876	198.26 (86.17)	122.53 (54.10)	0.257
PDGF-BB	11108.4 (3378.3)	11181.3 (2857.4)	0.640	13441.1 (613.2)	10808.5 (4737.1)	0.023
VEGF	238.97(155.33)	240.2367 (130.653	0.876	149.57 (59.24)	167.4 (95.6)	0.571

Table 5 Serum cytokine concentrations analysed by sex and tendon status (excluding observations with CV >15 %)

	Male			Female		
Analyte (pg/mL)	Normal	Tendinopathy	*p*	Normal	Tendinopathy	*p*
TNF-α	167.65 (62.11)	135.77 (30.36)	0.301	199.29 (70.22)	78.72 (61.85)	0.053
	5	13		3	5	
IL-1β	12.23 (3.79)	11.68 (2.08)	0.938	14.35 (2.60)	10.12 (4.37)	0.059
	6	15		4	7	
bFGF	79.67 (32.30)	75.56 (25.30)	0.883	54.35 (15.56)	56.00 (2.26)	0.807
	5	13		4	5	
INF-γ	168.99 (72.33)	150.92 (42.14)	0.876	176.99 (91.78)	139.22 (34.25)	0.796
	6	15		3	6	
PDGF-BB	11108.4 (3378.3)	11181.3 (2857.4)	0.640	13441.1 (613.2)	10808.5 (4737.3)	0.023
	6	15		4	7	
VEGF	238.97 (155.33)	240.24 (130.65)	0.876	156.12 (70.7)	209.69 (70.28)	0.297
	6	15		4	5	

despite improvements in insulin sensitivity. Thus, the effect of exercise on serum TNF-α is dependent upon the intensity of exercise, whether it is a single bout or habitual and also to some extent on the obesity level of the participants. Of interest, several studies in this area note a relationship between plasma TNF-α and VO2max [37]. It is reasonable to draw a parallel between VO2max and physical activity (as measured in this study), as VO2max and the questionnaire used in this study have previously been shown to be moderately correlated (Spearman's rank correlation = 0.37) [26]. However, it is unclear why the correlation between physical activity and TNF-α seen in control men was not detected in the tendinopathy group. It can be speculated that patients with tendinopathy experience pain with physical activities such as running and brisk walking, and therefore avoid these activities. The level of total physical activity did not differ between the tendinopathy and control group, however, the questionnaire used does not indicate the proportion of physical activity that is taken at high, moderate and low intensity. Notwithstanding this limitation, avoidance of painful activities might explain why there was the difference in TNF-α level between females with and without tendinopathy.

The association of potential confounders (physical activity, BMI, pain symptom duration) with PDGF-BB and IL-1 was also examined. Associations were only found for physical activity (tendinopathy males and control females for PDGF-BB, control males for IL-1), but interestingly no associations were found for the most noteworthy group – females with tendinopathy. The explanation for this finding may be an interesting topic for future research.

In studies such as the one we conducted, it is important to clarify the potential influence of confounding factors. In contrast to physical activity (for control men),

Table 6 Spearman's rank correlation between serum TNF-α and physical activity, BMI, and symptom duration

		Achilles tendon status (grouped by gender)					
		Total M	AT M	Control M	Total F	AT F	Control F
Physical Activity[a]	rho	0.5105	0.3846	0.9000	−0.2242	−0.6000	0.4000
	p	0.025519	0.1745	0.0374	0.5334	0.2080	0.6000
	n	19	14	5	10	6	4
BMI[b]	rho	−0.1338	−0.1607	−0.1429	0.2545	0.6071	0.2000
	p	0.5632	0.5672	0.7872	0.4500	0.1482	0.8000
	n	19	14	5	10	6	4
Pain: symptom duration[c]	rho		0.033514			−0.67737	
	p		0.9094			0.0946	
	n		14			7	

[a]Measured in MET-hours/week, [b]measured in kg/m^2, [c]measured in months
Note: *M* male, *F* female, *AT* Achilles tendinopathy
Physical activity score was missing for 2 men and 1 woman, symptom duration was missing for 1 man with tendinopathy

Table 7 Spearman's rank correlation between serum PDGF-BB and physical activity, BMI, and symptom duration

		Achilles tendon status (grouped by gender)					
		Total M	AT M	Control M	Total F	AT F	Control F
Physical Activity[a]	rho	−0.1895	−0.5868	0.7000	−0.0545	−0.4857	1.0000
	p	0.4372	0.0274	0.1881	0.8810	0.3287	0.0000
	n	19	14	5	10	6	4
BMI[b]	rho	−0.0831	−0.0536	−0.1429	0.2455	0.3214	0.0000
	p	0.7202	0.8496	0.7872	0.4669	0.4821	1.000
	n	21	15	6	11	7	4
Pain: symptom duration[c]	rho		0.2995			−0.4383	
	p		0.2982			0.3253	
	n		14			7	

[a]Measured in MET-hours/week, [b]measured in kg/m^2, [c]measured in months
Note: *M* male, *F* female, *AT* Achilles tendinopathy
Physical activity score was missing for 2 men and 1 woman, symptom duration was missing for 1 man with tendinopathy

neither BMI nor duration of pain symptoms demonstrated a relationship with serum TNF-α, PDGF-BB or IL-1 . Therefore, in this study these do not appear to be important confounding factors. It is also worthwhile noting that the mean BMI of the participants was within the overweight category (25 – 30 kg/m^2) but also that the two groups were well matched. Some previous studies in tendinopathy have shown that pain symptom duration is relevant, with one study finding that patellar tendinopathy biopsies showing VEGF protein expression were from individuals that had a shorter duration of symptoms than biopsies without VEGF expression [38]. In this case, neither BMI nor symptoms duration appear to be confounding factors for the cytokines and growth factors measured.

Very little is known regarding the role of TNF-α signalling in tendinopathy, necessitating a broader view across other research fields. The importance of the TNF-α system in chronic pain diseases has been recently shown in studies on humans and mice with arthritis; anti-TNF treatment leads to a rapid inhibition of pain responses in the central nervous system, with the effect occurring much more rapidly than the anti-inflammatory effect of TNF-α blockade [39]. In addition, it is known that preconditioning with a short ischaemic event reduces the severity of cerebral damage by a subsequent severe ischaemic event, and that this effect is induced by upregulation of sTNFR1 by TNF-α signalling [40]. Transient activity of the TNF-α system may result in a sustained increase in sTNFR1 expression [40]. Therefore, increased sTNFR1 expression, as is seen in Achilles tendon biopsies [17], may increase sensitivity to TNF-α stimulation as has been shown in other tissues [41]. Therefore, it remains of interest to examine TNF-α levels, as well as other cytokines, in the very early stages of tendinopathy, which will be the focus of future research endeavours.

A key finding was the contrast in results between men and women. This included finding lower levels of TNF-α (and a lower level in PDGF-BB and a trend for a

Table 8 Spearman's rank correlation between serum IL-1β and physical activity, BMI, and symptom duration

		Achilles tendon status (grouped by gender)					
		Total M	AT M	Control M	Total F	AT F	Control F
Physical Activity[a]	rho	0.0018	−0.4154	0.9000	0.1152	−0.2571	0.8000
	p	0.9943	0.1397	0.0374	0.7514	0.6228	0.2000
	n	19	14	5	10	6	4
BMI[b]	rho	−0.0026	−0.0107	−0.1429	−0.0091	0.0357	0.4000
	p	0.9911	0.9698	0.7872	0.9788	0.9394	0.6000
	n	21	15	6	11	7	4
Pain: symptom duration[c]	rho		0.2704			−0.4383	
	p		0.3497			0.3253	
	n		14			7	

[a]Measured in MET-hours/week, [b]measured in kg/m^2, [c]measured in months
Note: *M* male, *F* female, *AT* Achilles tendinopathy
Physical activity score was missing for 2 men and 1 woman, symptom duration was missing for 1 man with tendinopathy

Table 9 Spearman correlations between TNF-α and other cytokines

		Spearman's correlations with TNF-α (grouped by gender and tendon status)					
Analyte (pg/mL)		Total M ($n = 21$)	AT M ($n = 15$)	Control M ($n = 6$)	Total F ($n = 11$)	AT F ($n = 7$)	Control F ($n = 4$)
TNF-α	rho	1	1	1	1	1	1
	p						
IL-1β	rho	0.5182	0.2321	1.0000	0.7182	0.3571	0.8000
	p	0.0161	0.4051	0.0000	0.0128	0.4316	0.2000
bFGF	rho	0.6442	0.5286	0.9429	0.2091	0.3214	0.2000
	p	0.0016	0.0428	0.0048	0.5372	0.4821	0.8000
INF-γ	rho	0.7067	0.6416	0.8857	0.7182	0.6786	1.0000
	p	0.0003	0.0099	0.0188	0.0128	0.0938	0.0000
PDGF-BB	rho	0.1312	−0.2536	0.7143	0.7182	0.4286	0.4000
	p	0.5709	0.3618	0.1108	0.0128	0.3374	0.6000
VEGF	rho	0.6844	0.5786	1.0000	0.1455	0.3929	0.4000
	p	0.0006	0.0238	0.0000	0.6696	0.3833	0.6000

decrease in IL-1) in the female tendinopathy group, as compared to the control female group. Such a difference was not seen for males with tendinopathy compared to control males. Similarly, the correlation between TNF-α and physical activity that was seen in the male control group was not seen for the female control group. Finally, correlations between pairs of cytokines that were highly correlated for men (TNF-α & bFGF, TNF-α & VEFG) were not correlated among the female groups. This suggests that separate analyses for men and women are important for future research on tendinopathy biomarkers. This should be taken into consideration when doing future studies on levels of cytokines and closely related substances in relation to not only tendinopathy but also various sports related activities and complaints (see [42] for an overview of biomarkers in upper extremity musculoskeletal disorders).

There are several limitations of this study that should be acknowledged. First, this study had relatively small cohorts of tendinopathy patients and controls, and therefore may not have been adequately powered to detect changes in the cytokines studied. Second, this clinical cohort was heterogenous in terms of age, BMI and duration of symptoms, however, the groups means were actually well matched. Nevertheless, it is certainly possible that potential confounding factors not considered may have influenced the results. This might for example include menstrual cycle phases for women, which was not measured in this study. Third, cytokine levels were measured in serum and it is feasible that during processing, activated platelets affected the cytokine profile in the sample. It is also unknown to what extent serum levels of cytokines reflect intratendinous or paratendinous cytokine levels. While healthy tendons have a low vascular supply, there is a markedly increased vascular supply in chronic tendinopathy [43], and so the relationship between tendon and serum cytokine levels may be non-linear. However, all samples were taken at the same time of day and processed identically. Fourth, all the participants presented with chronic tendinopathy so at this stage we don't know anything about serum cytokine levels in recently developed tendinopathy. Furthermore, the details concerning the physical activity pattern the days just before the day for the taking of the blood sample was not clarified; it was the general physical activity pattern that was taken into consideration. Identifying biomarkers of recently developed tendinopathy and in relation to the physical activity pattern just before the sample is taken are questions to be addressed in future research projects.

Conclusion

This study identified lower serum TNF-α as a potential tendinopathy biomarker among females but not males. A lowering in PDGF-BB and a trend for a decrease in IL-1 was also seen in the female tendinopathy group, when compared to the female control group. A strong correlation between physical activity level and serum TNF-α was seen in the male control group but not the male tendinopathy group, nor in any of the female groups. Physical activity was also correlated with PDGF and IL-1 for certain subgroups. BMI and pain symptom duration were not associated with TNF-α, PDGF or IL-1 for any of the groups, and therefore do not appear to be confounding factors for these biomarkers in this study. The findings suggest that various cytokine systems, including the TNF-α system, are related to the presence of chronic Achilles tendinopathy. Further research on biomarkers of tendinopathy should analyse data for men and women separately and also extensively measure physical activity levels both short and long term.

Abbreviations

BDNF: brain-derived neurotropic factor; bFGF: basic fibroblast growth factor; BMI: body mass index; COPD: chronic obstructive pulmonary disease; CV: coefficient of variation; ICC: intraclass correlation coefficient; IFN-γ: interferon gamma; IL-1β: interleukin 1 beta; MET: metabolic equivalent; PDGF-BB: platelet derived growth factor BB; PYT-PAQ: past year physical activity questionnaire; sTNFR2: soluble tumour necrosis factor receptor 2; sTNFR1: soluble tumour necrosis factor receptor 1; TNF-α: tumour necrosis factor alpha; VEGF: vascular endothelial growth factor.

Competing interests

The authors declare that they have no competing interests.

Authors' contributions

JEG was involved in study design, subject recruitment, data collection, data analysis, data interpretation, and manuscript preparation. HA was involved in study design, subject recruitment, data collection, and manuscript preparation. SF was involved in study design, cytokine analysis, data analysis, data interpretation, and manuscript preparation. JLC was involved in study design, data interpretation, and manuscript preparation. All authors read and approved the final manuscript.

Acknowledgements

Professor Anders Sjöstedt, Department of Clinical Microbiology, Umeå University for kind assistance with cytokine analysis.
Lotta Alfredson, Sports Medicine Unit, Umeå University for valuable assistance with collection of blood samples.

Funding

Support was obtained from the Swedish National Centre for Research in Sports (CIF) and the Faculty of Medicine, Umeå University.
This paper was supported by the Australian Centre for Research into Sports Injury and its Prevention, which is one of the International Research Centres for Prevention of Injury and Protection of Athlete Health supported by the International Olympic Committee.
Prof Jill Cook is a NHMRC practitioner fellow (ID 1058493).

Author details

[1]University of Canberra Research Institute for Sport and Exercise (UCRISE), Canberra, Australia. [2]Discipline of Physiotherapy, University of Canberra, ACT 2601 Canberra, Australia. [3]Department of Surgical and Perioperative Sciences, Sports Medicine, Umeå University, Umeå, Sweden. [4]Department of Integrative Medical Biology, Anatomy Section, Umeå University, Umeå, Sweden. [5]Department of Community Medicine and Rehabilitation, Umeå University, S-901 87 Umeå, Sweden. [6]Institute of Sport Exercise and Health, University College Hospital London, London, UK. [7]La Trobe University Sport and Exercise Medicine Research Centre, Melbourne, Australia.

References

1. Kujala UM, Sarna S, Kaprio J. Cumulative incidence of achilles tendon rupture and tendinopathy in male former elite athletes. Clin J Sport Med. 2005;15(3):133–5.
2. Kvist M. Achilles tendon injuries in athletes. Ann Chir Gynaecol. 1991;80(2):188–201.
3. Van Ginckel A, Thijs Y, Hesar NG, Mahieu N, De Clercq D, Roosen P, et al. Intrinsic gait-related risk factors for Achilles tendinopathy in novice runners: a prospective study. Gait Posture. 2009;29(3):387–91. doi:10.1016/j.gaitpost.2008.10.058.
4. Fernandez-Palazzi F, Rivas S, Mujica P. Achilles tendinitis in ballet dancers. Clin Orthop Relat Res. 1990;257:257–61.
5. Reule CA, Alt WW, Lohrer H, Hochwald H. Spatial orientation of the subtalar joint axis is different in subjects with and without Achilles tendon disorders. Br J Sports Med. 2011;45(13):1029–34. doi:10.1136/bjsm.2010.080119.
6. Mahieu NN, Witvrouw E, Stevens V, Van Tiggelen D, Roget P. Intrinsic risk factors for the development of achilles tendon overuse injury: a prospective study. Am J Sports Med. 2006;34(2):226–35. doi:10.1177/0363546505279918.
7. Ranger TA, Wong AMY, Cook JL, Gaida JE. Is there an association between tendinopathy and diabetes mellitus? A systematic review with meta-analysis. Br J Sports Med. 2015:in press. doi:10.1136/bjsports-2015-094735.
8. Tilley BJ, Cook JL, Docking SI, Gaida JE. Is higher serum cholesterol associated with altered tendon structure or tendon pain? A systematic review. Br J Sports Med. 2015;49(23):1504–9.
9. Kapczinski F, Dal-Pizzol F, Teixeira AL, Magalhaes PV, Kauer-Sant'Anna M, Klamt F, et al. Peripheral biomarkers and illness activity in bipolar disorder. J Psychiatr Res. 2011;45(2):156–61. doi:10.1016/j.jpsychires.2010.05.015.
10. Al-shair K, Kolsum U, Dockry R, Morris J, Singh D, Vestbo J. Biomarkers of systemic inflammation and depression and fatigue in moderate clinically stable COPD. Respir Res. 2011;12:3. doi:10.1186/1465-9921-12-3.
11. Spoettl T, Hausmann M, Klebl F, Dirmeier A, Klump B, Hoffmann J, et al. Serum soluble TNF receptor I and II levels correlate with disease activity in IBD patients. Inflamm Bowel Dis. 2007;13(6):727–32. doi:10.1002/ibd.20107.
12. Black RA, Rauch CT, Kozlosky CJ, Peschon JJ, Slack JL, Wolfson MF, et al. A metalloproteinase disintegrin that releases tumour-necrosis factor-alpha from cells. Nature. 1997;385(6618):729–33. doi:10.1038/385729a0.
13. Aderka D, Engelmann H, Maor Y, Brakebusch C, Wallach D. Stabilization of the bioactivity of tumor necrosis factor by its soluble receptors. J Exp Med. 1992;175(2):323–9.
14. Hanai H, Watanabe F, Yamada M, Sato Y, Takeuchi K, Iida T, et al. Correlation of serum soluble TNF-alpha receptors I and II levels with disease activity in patients with ulcerative colitis. Am J Gastroenterol. 2004;99(8):1532–8. doi:10.1111/j.1572-0241.2004.30432.x.
15. Saxne T, Palladino Jr MA, Heinegard D, Talal N, Wollheim FA. Detection of tumor necrosis factor alpha but not tumor necrosis factor beta in rheumatoid arthritis synovial fluid and serum. Arthritis Rheum. 1988;31(8):1041–5.
16. Barrera P, Boerbooms AM, Janssen EM, Sauerwein RW, Gallati H, Mulder J, et al. Circulating soluble tumor necrosis factor receptors, interleukin-2 receptors, tumor necrosis factor alpha, and interleukin-6 levels in rheumatoid arthritis. Longitudinal evaluation during methotrexate and azathioprine therapy. Arthritis Rheum. 1993;36(8):1070–9.
17. Gaida JE, Bagge J, Purdam C, Cook J, Alfredson H, Forsgren S. Evidence of the TNF-alpha system in the human Achilles tendon: expression of TNF-alpha and TNF receptor at both protein and mRNA levels in the tenocytes. Cells Tissues Organs. 2012;196(4):339–52. doi:10.1159/000335475.
18. Townsend JR, Hoffman JR, Fragala MS, Jajtner AR, Gonzalez AM, Wells AJ, et al. TNF-alpha and TNFR1 responses to recovery therapies following acute resistance exercise. Front Physiol. 2015;6:48. doi:10.3389/fphys.2015.00048.
19. Andersson J, Jansson JH, Hellsten G, Nilsson TK, Hallmans G, Boman K. Effects of heavy endurance physical exercise on inflammatory markers in non-athletes. Atherosclerosis. 2010;209(2):601–5. doi:10.1016/j.atherosclerosis.2009.10.025.
20. Andersson H, Bohn SK, Raastad T, Paulsen G, Blomhoff R, Kadi F. Differences in the inflammatory plasma cytokine response following two elite female soccer games separated by a 72-h recovery. Scand J Med Sci Sports. 2010;20(5):740–7. doi:10.1111/j.1600-0838.2009.00989.x.
21. Holbrook TC, McFarlane D, Schott II HC. Neuroendocrine and non-neuroendocrine markers of inflammation associated with performance in endurance horses. Equine Vet J Suppl. 2010;38:123–8. doi:10.1111/j.2042-3306.2010.00256.x.
22. MacKinnon LT. Special feature for the Olympics: effects of exercise on the immune system: overtraining effects on immunity and performance in athletes. Immunol Cell Biol. 2000;78(5):502–9. doi:10.1111/j.1440-1711.2000.t01-7-.x.
23. Bagge J, Gaida JE, Danielson P, Alfredson H, Forsgren S. Physical activity level in Achilles tendinosis is associated with blood levels of pain-related factors: a pilot study. Scand J Med Sci Sports. 2011;21(6):e430–8. doi:10.1111/j.1600-0838.2011.01358.x.
24. Gouveia-Figueira S, Nording ML, Gaida JE, Forsgren S, Alfredson H, Fowler CJ. Serum levels of oxylipins in achilles tendinopathy: an exploratory study. PLoS ONE. 2015;10(4), e0123114. doi:10.1371/journal.pone.0123114.
25. Carp SJ, Barr AE, Barbe MF. Serum biomarkers as signals for risk and severity of work-related musculoskeletal injury. Biomark Med. 2008;2(1):67–79. doi:10.2217/17520363.2.1.67.

26. Friedenreich CM, Courneya KS, Neilson HK, Matthews CE, Willis G, Irwin M, et al. Reliability and validity of the past year total physical activity questionnaire. Am J Epidemiol. 2006;163(10):959–70. doi:10.1093/aje/kwj112.
27. Gold JE, Mohamed FB, Ali S, Barbe MF. Serum and MRI biomarkers in mobile device texting: a pilot study. Hum Factors. 2014;56(5):864–72. doi:10.1177/0018720813507953.
28. Pingel J, Fredberg U, Mikkelsen LR, Schjerling P, Heinemeier KM, Kjaer M, et al. No inflammatory gene-expression response to acute exercise in human Achilles tendinopathy. Eur J Appl Physiol. 2013;113(8):2101–9. doi:10.1007/s00421-013-2638-3.
29. Ostrowski K, Rohde T, Asp S, Schjerling P, Pedersen BK. Pro- and anti-inflammatory cytokine balance in strenuous exercise in humans. J Physiol. 1999;515(Pt 1):287–91.
30. Moldoveanu AI, Shephard RJ, Shek PN. Exercise elevates plasma levels but not gene expression of IL-1beta, IL-6, and TNF-alpha in blood mononuclear cells. J Appl Physiol. 2000;89(4):1499–504.
31. Steensberg A, Keller C, Starkie RL, Osada T, Febbraio MA, Pedersen BK. IL-6 and TNF-alpha expression in, and release from, contracting human skeletal muscle. Am J Physiol Endocrinol Metab. 2002;283(6):E1272–8. doi:10.1152/ajpendo.00255.2002.
32. Jeukendrup AE, Vet-Joop K, Sturk A, Stegen JH, Senden J, Saris WH, et al. Relationship between gastro-intestinal complaints and endotoxaemia, cytokine release and the acute-phase reaction during and after a long-distance triathlon in highly trained men. Clin Sci (Lond). 2000;98(1):47–55.
33. Febbraio MA, Steensberg A, Starkie RL, McConell GK, Kingwell BA. Skeletal muscle interleukin-6 and tumor necrosis factor-alpha release in healthy subjects and patients with type 2 diabetes at rest and during exercise. Metabolism. 2003;52(7):939–44.
34. Straczkowski M, Kowalska I, Dzienis-Straczkowska S, Stepien A, Skibinska E, Szelachowska M, et al. Changes in tumor necrosis factor-alpha system and insulin sensitivity during an exercise training program in obese women with normal and impaired glucose tolerance. Eur J Endocrinol. 2001;145(3):273–80.
35. Klimcakova E, Polak J, Moro C, Hejnova J, Majercik M, Viguerie N, et al. Dynamic strength training improves insulin sensitivity without altering plasma levels and gene expression of adipokines in subcutaneous adipose tissue in obese men. J Clin Endocrinol Metab. 2006;91(12):5107–12. doi:10.1210/jc.2006-0382.
36. Reynolds TH, Supiano MA, Dengel DR. Resistance training enhances insulin-mediated glucose disposal with minimal effect on the tumor necrosis factor-alpha system in older hypertensives. Metabolism. 2004;53(3):397–402.
37. Ho SS, Dhaliwal SS, Hills AP, Pal S. Effects of chronic exercise training on inflammatory markers in Australian overweight and obese individuals in a randomized controlled trial. Inflammation. 2013;36(3):625–32. doi:10.1007/s10753-012-9584-9.
38. Scott A, Lian O, Bahr R, Hart DA, Duronio V. VEGF expression in patellar tendinopathy: a preliminary study. Clin Orthop Relat Res. 2008;466(7):1598–604. doi:10.1007/s11999-008-0272-x.
39. Hess A, Axmann R, Rech J, Finzel S, Heindl C, Kreitz S, et al. Blockade of TNF-alpha rapidly inhibits pain responses in the central nervous system. Proc Natl Acad Sci U S A. 2011;108(9):3731–6. doi:10.1073/pnas.1011774108.
40. Pradillo JM, Romera C, Hurtado O, Cardenas A, Moro MA, Leza JC, et al. TNFR1 upregulation mediates tolerance after brain ischemic preconditioning. J Cereb Blood Flow Metab. 2005;25(2):193–203. doi:10.1038/sj.jcbfm.9600019.
41. Cook EB, Stahl JL, Graziano FM, Barney NP. Regulation of the receptor for TNFalpha, TNFR1, in human conjunctival epithelial cells. Invest Ophthalmol Vis Sci. 2008;49(9):3992–8. doi:10.1167/iovs.08-1873.
42. Gold JE, Hallman DM, Hellstrom F, Bjorklund M, Crenshaw AG, Djupsjobacka M, et al. Systematic review of biochemical biomarkers for neck and upper-extremity musculoskeletal disorders. Scand J Work Environ Health. 2015. doi:10.5271/sjweh.3533.
43. Ohberg L, Lorentzon R, Alfredson H. Neovascularisation in Achilles tendons with painful tendinosis but not in normal tendons: an ultrasonographic investigation. Knee Surg Sports Traumatol Arthrosc. 2001;9(4):233–8.

8

Is a threshold-based model a superior method to the relative percent concept for establishing individual exercise intensity? a randomized controlled trial

Ali E. Wolpern[1], Dara J. Burgos[1], Jeffrey M. Janot[2] and Lance C. Dalleck[1*]

Abstract

Background: Exercise intensity is arguably the most critical component of the exercise prescription model. It has been suggested that a threshold based model for establishing exercise intensity might better identify the lowest effective training stimulus for all individuals with varying fitness levels; however, experimental evidence is lacking. The purpose of this study was to compare the effectiveness of two exercise training programs for improving cardiorespiratory fitness: threshold based model vs. relative percent concept (i.e., % heart rate reserve – HRR).

Methods: Apparently healthy, but sedentary men and women ($n = 42$) were randomized to a non-exercise control group or one of two exercise training groups. Exercise training was performed 30 min/day on 5 days/week for 12weeks according to one of two exercise intensity regimens: 1) a relative percent method was used in which intensity was prescribed according to percentages of heart rate reserve (HRR group), or 2) a threshold based method (ACE-3ZM) was used in which intensity was prescribed according to the first ventilatory threshold (VT1) and second ventilatory threshold (VT2).

Results: Thirty-six men and women completed the study. After 12weeks, VO_2max increased significantly ($p < 0.05$ vs. controls) in both HRR (1.76 ± 1.93 mL/kg/min) and ACE-3ZM (3.93 ± 0.96 mL/kg/min) groups. Repeated measures ANOVA identified a significant interaction between exercise intensity method and change in VO_2max values ($F = 9.06$, $p < 0.05$) indicating that VO_2max responded differently to the method of exercise intensity prescription. In the HRR group 41.7 % (5/12) of individuals experienced a favorable change in relative VO_2max ($\Delta > 5.9$ %) and were categorized as responders. Alternatively, exercise training in the ACE-3ZM group elicited a positive improvement in relative VO_2max ($\Delta > 5.9$ %) in 100 % (12/12) of the individuals.

Conclusions: A threshold based exercise intensity prescription: 1). elicited significantly ($p < 0.05$) greater improvements in VO_2max, and 2). attenuated the individual variation in VO_2max training responses when compared to relative percent exercise training. These novel findings are encouraging and provide important preliminary data for the design of individualized exercise prescriptions that will enhance training efficacy and limit training unresponsiveness.

Trial registration: ClinicalTrials.gov Identifier: ID NCT02351713 Registered 30 January 2015.

Keywords: Cardiorespiratory fitness, Cardiovascular Disease, Exercise prescription, Primary prevention, VO_2max

* Correspondence: ldalleck@western.edu
[1]Recreation, Exercise, and Sport Science Department, Western State Colorado University, 600 N. Adams St., Gunnison, CO 81230, USA
Full list of author information is available at the end of the article

Background

Cardiorespiratory fitness, typically determined by maximal oxygen uptake (VO_2max), is a fundamental measurement for the exercise physiologist and other health professionals. The magnitude of an individual's cardiorespiratory fitness has been viewed as representative of overall health and studies have consistently demonstrated an inverse relationship between VO_2max values and risk of cardiovascular disease and all-cause mortality [1, 2]. The "F.I.T.T." principle is an acronym for the four components for exercise prescription: frequency, intensity, time (length), and type of exercise. Exercise intensity is arguably the most critical component of the exercise prescription model. Failure to meet minimal threshold values may result in lack of a training effect, while too high of an exercise intensity could lead to overtraining and negatively impact adherence to an exercise program. The traditional reference standard for prescribing exercise intensity is expressed in terms of percentages of heart rate reserve (%HRR) or oxygen uptake reserve (%VO_2R). This is considered the *'relative percent method'*. The American College of Sports Medicine (ACSM) currently recommends an exercise intensity of 40-59 % HRR/VO_2R for improving and maintaining cardiorespiratory fitness [3].

Nevertheless, despite the large base of Category A evidence [4] supporting the ACSM relative percent concept recommendation for prescribing exercise intensity, there is concern that the relative percent concept approach consists of a very large range of acceptable percentages [5] and also fails to take into account individual metabolic responses (e.g., blood lactate) to exercises [6]. For example, it has been demonstrated [7–9] that there is considerable individual variation in the blood lactate response to exercise when intensity is anchored to relative percent concepts (e.g., %HRR, %VO_2max). In turn, it has been suggested that this heterogeneous variation in the metabolic strain of each exercise session may ultimately yield individual variation in training adaptations; thus resulting in positive responders and non-responders to chronic exercise training [10].

Alternatively, it has been suggested that a *'threshold based model'* for establishing exercise intensity might better identify the lowest effective training stimulus and elicit comparable relative metabolic strain across individuals with varying fitness levels [5, 6, 9]. Indeed, the American Council on Exercise (ACE) [11] recommends a *'threshold based model'* approach to prescribing exercise intensity in its *ACE three-zone training model*. However, it has been acknowledged elsewhere that the experimental evidence supporting a *'threshold based model'* approach to exercise training is lacking [11]. Moreover, it remains to be determined if a threshold based training model will attenuate individual variation in training responses when compared to exercise training prescription anchored to relative percent methods [10].

Therefore, the purpose of this study was to compare the effectiveness of two exercise training programs for improving cardiorespiratory fitness: a threshold based training model vs. the relative percent method (i.e., %HRR).

It was hypothesized that:

1. The threshold based training model would elicit greater mean changes in cardiorespiratory fitness (as measured by VO_2max) when compared to the relative percent method.
2. Participants in the threshold based training model group would be more likely to have favorable VO_2max responses; while comparatively, participants in the relative percent method group would be more likely to experience a VO_2max nonresponse to exercise training.

Methods

Participants

Forty-two nonsmoking men and women (18 to 54 years) were recruited from the student and faculty population of a local university, as well as the surrounding community, via advertisement through the university website, local community newspaper, and word-of-mouth. Participants were eligible for inclusion into the study if they were low-to-moderate risk as defined by the ACSM and sedentary. Participants were considered sedentary if they reported not participating in at least 30 min of moderate intensity physical activity on at least three days of the week for at least three months [3]. Participants were also eligible for inclusion into the study if they verbally agreed to continue previous dietary habits and not perform additional exercise beyond that required for the present study. Exclusionary criteria included evidence of cardiovascular pulmonary, and/or metabolic disease as determined by medical history questionnaire. This study was approved by the Human Research Committee at Western State Colorado University. Each participant signed an informed consent form prior to participation.

Baseline, midpoint, and post-program experimental testing procedures

Measurements of all primary and secondary outcome variables were obtained both before and after the exercise training intervention. Additionally, a measure of the primary outcome variable (maximal oxygen uptake – VO_2max) was also obtained at midpoint. Secondary outcome variables consisted of resting heart rate and blood pressure, and basic anthropometric measures including height, weight, waist circumference, and skinfolds. Fasting blood lipid and blood glucose measurements were also performed. All measurements were obtained by following standardized procedures as outlined elsewhere [3]. Procedures for each measurement are also briefly described below. Prior to testing participants refrained from all food and drink other than water for 12 h. Participants were also instructed to refrain from strenuous exertion 12 h prior to testing. All post-program testing took place within 1 to 4 days of the last exercise training session.

Resting heart rate and blood pressure measurement

The procedures for assessment of resting heart rate and blood pressure outlined elsewhere were followed [3]. Briefly, participants were seated quietly for 5 min in a chair with a back support with feet on the floor and arm supported at heart level. Resting heart rate was obtained via manual palpation of radial artery in the left wrist and recording the number of beats for 60 s. The left arm brachial artery blood pressure was measured using a sphygmomanometer in duplicate and separated by 1-min. The mean of the two measurements was reported for baseline and post-program values.

Anthropometric measurements

Participants were weighed to the nearest 0.1 kg on a medical grade scale and measured for height to the nearest 0.5 cm using a stadiometer. Percent body fat was determined via skinfolds [3]. Skinfold thickness was measured to the nearest ± 0.5 mm using a Lange caliper (Cambridge Scientific Industries, Columbia, MD). All measurements were taken on the right side of the body using standardized anatomical sites (three-site) for men and women. These measurements were performed until two were within 10 % of each other. Waist circumference measurements were obtained using a cloth tape measure with a spring loaded-handle (Creative Health Products, Ann Arbor, MI). A horizontal measurement was taken at the narrowest point of the torso (below the xiphoid process and above the umbilicus). These measurements were taken until two were within 0.5 mm of each other.

Fasting blood lipid and blood glucose measurement

All fasting lipid and blood glucose analyses were collected in duplicate and performed at room temperature. The mean of the two measurements was reported for baseline and post-program values. Participants' hands were washed with soap and rinsed thoroughly with water, then cleaned with alcohol swabs and allowed to dry. Skin was punctured using lancets and a fingerstick sample was collected into heparin-coated 40 μl capillary tube. Blood was allowed to flow freely from the fingerstick into the capillary tube without milking of the finger. Samples were then dispensed immediately onto commercially available test cassettes for analysis in a Cholestech LDX System (Alere Inc., Waltham, MA) according to strict standardized operating procedures. The LDX Cholestech measured total cholesterol, high density lipoprotein (HDL) cholesterol, low density lipoprotein (LDL) cholesterol, triglycerides, and blood glucose in fingerstick blood. A daily optics check was performed on the LDX Cholestech analyzer used for the study. Independent studies have provided data to indicate that the Cholestech LDX system has excellent reproducibility with standard clinical laboratory measurement of plasma lipids and lipoproteins [12, 13] and meets the National Cholesterol Education Program Adult Treatment Panel III (NCEP-ATP) criteria for accuracy and reproducibility [14].

Maximal exercise testing

Participants completed a modified-Balke, pseudo-ramp graded exercise test (GXT) on a power treadmill (Powerjog GX200, Maine). Participants walked or jogged at a self-selected pace. Treadmill incline was increased by 1 % every minute until the participant reached volitional fatigue. Participant HR was continuously recorded during the GXT via a chest strap and radio-telemetric receiver (Polar Electro, Woodbury, NY, USA). Expired air and gas exchange data were recorded continuously during the GXT using a metabolic analyzer (Parvo Medics TrueOne 2.0, Salt Lake City, UT, USA). Before each exercise test, the metabolic analyzer was calibrated with gases of known concentrations (14.01 ± 0.07 % O_2, 6.00 ± 0.03 % CO_2) and with room air (20.93%O_2 and 0.03 % CO_2) as per the instruction manual. Volume calibration of the pneumotachometer was done via a 3-Litre calibration syringe system (Hans-Rudolph, Kansas City, MO, USA). The last 15 s of the GXT were averaged – this was considered the final data point. The closest neighbouring data point was calculated by averaging the data collected 15 s immediately before the last 15 s of the test. The mean of the two processed data points represented VO_2max. Maximal HR was considered to be the highest recorded HR in beats per minute (bpm) during the GXT. Participant heart rate reserve (HRR) was determined by taking the difference between maximal HR and resting HR.

Determination of ventilatory thresholds

Determination of both the first ventilatory threshold (VT1) and second ventilatory threshold (VT2) were made by visual inspection of graphs of time plotted against each relevant respiratory variable (according to 15 s time-averaging). The criteria for VT1 was an increase in VE/VO_2 with no concurrent increase in VE/VCO_2 and departure from the linearity of VE. The criteria for VT2 was a simultaneous increase in both VE/VO_2 and VE/VCO_2 [15]. All assessments were done by two experienced exercise physiologists. In the event of conflicting results, the original assessments were reevaluated and collectively a consensus was agreed upon.

Randomization and exercise intervention

After the completion of baseline testing, participants were randomized to a non-exercise control group or one of two exercise training groups according to a computer generated sequence of random numbers that was stratified by sex (Fig. 1). This was a double-blind research design in that participants were unaware of the group to which they had been assigned. Likewise, the researchers specifically responsible for testing and supervision of exercise sessions were unaware of the group to which participants had been allocated. Participants randomized to the exercise training groups performed 12weeks of exercise training according to one of two exercise intensity regimens: 1) a relative percent method was used in which intensity was prescribed according to percentages of HRR (HRR group), or 2) a threshold-based method (ACE-3ZM) was used in which intensity was prescribed according to VT1 and VT2 as recommended by ACE in its three-zone model [11]. The exercise prescription details for each training group over the course of the 12weeks training period is presented in Fig. 1.

Each group performed a similar frequency and duration of exercise training. All exercise training sessions for each treatment group were performed on a treadmill. Overall, the exercise prescription was intended to fulfill the consensus recommendation of 150 min/week [4]. The exercise prescription for exercise intensity method differed between treatment groups. The HRR group was prescribed exercise intensity according to a percentage of HRR. Conversely, the ACE-3ZM group was prescribed exercise intensity according to ventilatory

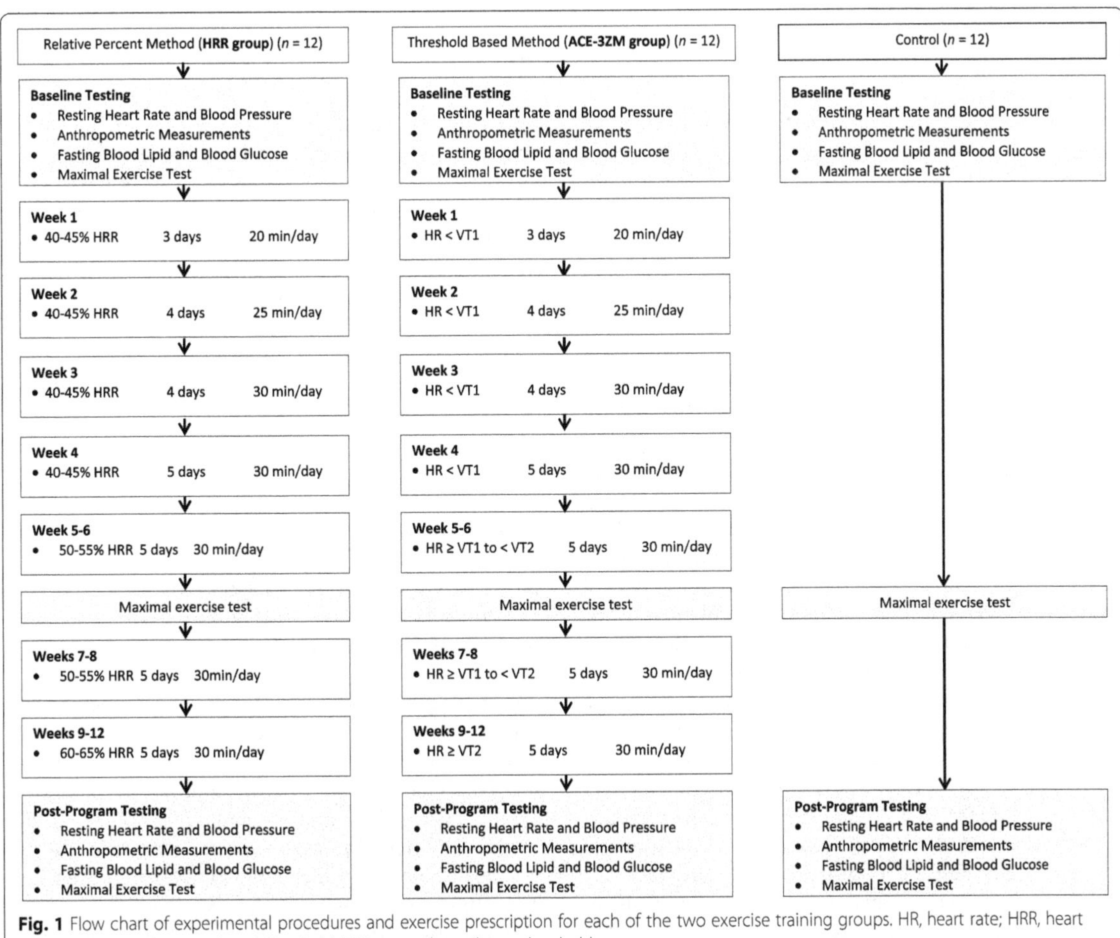

Fig. 1 Flow chart of experimental procedures and exercise prescription for each of the two exercise training groups. HR, heart rate; HRR, heart rate reserve; VT1, first ventilatory threshold; VT2, second ventilatory threshold

threshold. In both exercise training groups a target heart rate (HR) coinciding with either the prescribed HRR or prescribed VT (Fig. 1) was used to establish a specific exercise training intensity for each exercise session. In the ACE-3ZM group target HR for each training zone (Fig. 1) was established in the following manner:

- Wk 1–4 (HR < VT1): target HR = HR range of 10–15 bpm just below VT1
- Wk 5–8 (HR ≥ VT1 to < VT2): target HR = HR range of 10–20 bpm above VT1 and below VT2
- Wk 9–12 (HR ≥ VT2): target HR = HR range of 10–15 bpm just above VT2

Exercise training was progressed according to recommendations made elsewhere by the ACSM [3] and ACE [11]. Polar HR monitors (Polar Electro Inc., Woodbury, NY) were used to monitor HR during all exercise sessions. Researchers adjusted treadmill workload accordingly during each exercise session to ensure actual HR responses aligned with target HR.

Statistical analyses

All analyses were performed using SPSS Version 22.0 (Chicago, IL) and GraphPad Prism 6.0. (San Diego, CA). Sample size was projected with change in VO_2max as the main outcome variable. The means and standard deviation of a previous study [16] were examined and the effect size of this study was calculated. Assuming that a power of 0.90 was needed and the calculated effect size for change in VO_2max was 0.8, it was determined that approximately 12 subjects would be needed for each of the three groups [17]. Further, we assumed there would be an approximate 20 % dropout rate based on findings from one of our previous exercise training studies [18]. Accordingly, we recruited and randomized an additional three participants to each of the exercise training groups to account for potential attrition.

Measures of centrality and spread are presented as mean ± standard deviation (SD). All baseline-dependent variables were compared using general linear model (GLM) ANOVA and, where appropriate, Tukey post hoc tests. Within-group comparisons were made using paired *t*-tests. Because baseline, 6weeks, and post-program data were available, the effect of exercise training on cardiorespiratory fitness (VO_2max) was determined using repeated-measures GLM-ANOVA with exercise intensity method (HRR or ACE-3ZM) as the between-subjects factor. All other between-group 12weeks changes were analyzed using GLM-ANOVA and, where appropriate, Tukey post hoc tests. The assumption of normality was tested by examining normal plots of the residuals in ANOVA models. Residuals were regarded as normally distributed if Shapiro-Wilk tests were not significant [17].

Delta values (Δ) were calculated (post-program minus baseline value divided by baseline value) for percent change in relative VO_2max (%) and participants were categorized as: '1' = responders (% $\Delta > 5.9$ %) or '0' = non-responders ($\Delta \leq 5.9$ %) to exercise training using a day-to-day variability, within subject coefficient of variation (CV) criterion applied previously in the literature [6, 19]. Chi-square (χ^2) tests were subsequently used to analyze the point prevalence of responders and non-responders to exercise training separated by exercise intensity group (i.e., HRR and ACE-3ZM) between baseline and post-program. The probability of making a Type I error was set at $p \leq 0.05$ for all statistical analyses.

Results

All analyses and data presented in the results are for those participants who completed the investigation. At baseline, treatment (HRR and ACE-3ZM) and non-exercise control groups did not differ significantly in physical or physiological characteristics. The physical and physiological characteristics for participants are shown in Table 1.

The exercise prescription in both treatment groups was well tolerated for the 24 of 30 participants who completed the study. Six participants were unable to complete the study for the following reasons: injury outside the study ($n = 2$), illness ($n = 2$), out-of-town move ($n = 1$), and personal reasons (n = 1). Dropout was similar in both treatment groups. Overall, there was excellent adherence to the total number of prescribed training sessions: HRR group – mean, 90.6 % (range, 76.8-100 %) and ACE-3ZM group – mean, 89.3 % (range, 78.6-100 %). Additionally, adherence to the prescribed exercise intensity for both treatment groups throughout the duration of the intervention was excellent (Table 2).

After 12 week, changes in body mass, waist circumference, resting HR, systolic and diastolic blood pressure, total cholesterol, LDL cholesterol, triglycerides, and blood glucose were not significantly different ($p > 0.05$) in either the HRR or ACE-3ZM groups when compared with the control group. In contrast, changes in VO_2max from baseline to 12weeks in the HRR group were significantly greater ($p < 0.05$) when compared with the control group. Moreover, changes in body fat percentage, VO_2max, and HDL cholesterol in the ACE-3ZM group were significantly more favorable ($p < 0.05$) when compared to both the HRR and control groups. After 12weeks, VO_2max increased significantly ($p < 0.05$ vs. controls) in both HRR (1.76 ± 1.93 $mL \cdot kg^{-1} \cdot min^{-1}$) and ACE-3ZM ($3.93 \pm 0.96$ $mL \cdot kg^{-1} \cdot min^{-1}$) groups. Repeated measures ANOVA identified a significant interaction between exercise intensity method and change in VO_2max values ($F = 9.06$, $p < 0.05$) indicating that VO_2max responded differently to the method of exercise intensity prescription (Fig. 2).

Table 1 Physical and physiological characteristics at baseline and 12weeks for control, HRR, and ACE-3ZM groups. (Values are mean ± SD)

Parameter	Control group (*n* = 12; women = 7, men = 5)		HRR group (*n* = 12; women = 6, men = 6)		ACE-3ZM group (*n* = 12; women = 6, men = 6)	
	Baseline	12weeks	Baseline	12weeks	Baseline	12weeks
Age (yr)	33.5 ± 7.0	____	33.0 ± 9.8	____	31.7 ± 9.6	____
Height (cm)	165.5 ± 9.6	____	170.3 ± 7.1	____	169.3 ± 12.7	____
Body mass (kg)	72.1 ± 9.6	72.2 ± 9.2	73.3 ± 12.4	73.8 ± 12.2*	72.8 ± 15.7	72.8 ± 15.5
Waist circumference (cm)	81.8 ± 8.4	82.0 ± 8.2	81.7 ± 8.3	82.5 ± 8.4*	80.1 ± 11.3	79.8 ± 10.8
Body fat (%)	19.8 ± 5.9	20.6 ± 5.4*	16.1 ± 5.1	16.6 ± 5.2*	19.5 ± 6.4	18.7 ± 6.2*‡
Resting HR (b·min^{-1})	64.6 ± 12.2	65.2 ± 8.9	59.4 ± 11.6	59.3 ± 7.6	69.1 ± 7.4	65.1 ± 3.7
Maximal HR (b·min^{-1})	179.0 ± 14.0	180.6 ± 12.3	180.9 ± 14.3	182.3 ± 12.0	182.4 ± 12.8	184.5 ± 12.9*
VO_2max (mL·kg^{-1}·min^{-1})	30.4 ± 6.4	29.9 ± 6.0	34.9 ± 5.3	36.6 ± 5.4*†	34.3 ± 9.0	38.3 ± 9.2*‡
Systolic BP (mmHg)	118.4 ± 9.7	120.0 ± 8.9	117.4 ± 6.8	119.3 ± 5.3	117.9 ± 9.8	115.9 ± 7.1
Diastolic BP (mmHg)	78.4 ± 8.9	80.5 ± 4.9	79.4 ± 3.7	78.6 ± 4.8	73.7 ± 11.2	74.0 ± 9.1
Total cholesterol (mg·dL^{-1})	192.1 ± 32.9	194.4 ± 28.0	188.4 ± 23.8	188.9 ± 23.8	179.0 ± 47.1	168.3 ± 30.0
HDL cholesterol (mg·dL^{-1})	52.0 ± 21.9	50.5 ± 19.1	53.3 ± 14.5	55.0 ± 14.7	51.8 ± 20.9	60.2 ± 20.3*‡
LDL cholesterol (mg·dL^{-1})	111.0 ± 29.2	113.1 ± 25.8	110.2 ± 25.6	109.7 ± 22.4	92.2 ± 28.8	85.9 ± 27.7*
Triglycerides (mg·dL^{-1})	115.4 ± 41.5	123.2 ± 40.8	118.2 ± 70.4	120.3 ± 57.5	94.8 ± 45.9	97.5 ± 33.0
Blood Glucose (mg·dL^{-1})	88.5 ± 5.5	89.8 ± 7.1	90.1 ± 5.1	89.8 ± 5.1	92.4 ± 10.2	90.1 ± 4.9

*Within-group change is significantly different from baseline, $p < 0.05$; † Change from baseline is significantly different than control group, $p < 0.05$; ‡ Change from baseline is significantly different than control and HRR groups, $p < 0.05$

Prevalence of VO_2max non-responders and responders

The point prevalence of responders and non-responders to exercise training in both the HRR and ACE-3ZM groups are shown in Fig. 2. In the HRR group 41.7 % (5/12) of individuals experienced a favorable change in VO_2max ($\Delta > 5.9$ %) and were categorized as responders. Alternatively, 58.3 % (7/12) of individuals in the HRR group experienced an undesirable change in VO_2max ($\Delta \leq 5.9$ %) and were categorized as non-responders to exercise training. There were no significant differences ($p < 0.05$) in several potential influencing factors of responder/non-responder, including age, baseline VO_2max, exercise adherence, and sex. In the ACE-3ZM group the prevalence of individuals who experienced a favorable change in VO_2max was significantly ($p < 0.05$) greater when compared to the HRR group. Indeed, exercise training in the ACE-3ZM group elicited a positive improvement in VO_2max ($\Delta > 5.9$ %) in 100 % (12/12) of the individuals.

Discussion

The major findings from the present study were as follows: 1) threshold based exercise intensity prescription elicited significantly ($p < 0.05$) greater improvements in VO_2max when compared to a relative percent exercise intensity prescription following 12weeks of exercise training, and 2) threshold based exercise training attenuated the individual variation in VO_2max training responses when compared to relative percent exercise training as evidenced by the significantly reduced ($p < 0.05$) point prevalence of exercise training non-responders in the ACE-3ZM treatment group. Therefore, these current

Table 2 Prescribed and actual exercise intensity for HRR and ACE-3ZM groups throughout the 12weeks exercise intervention

Week	HRR Group (*n* = 12)			ACE-3ZM Group (*n* = 12)		
	Prescribed intensity	*THR*	*Actual HR*	*Prescribed intensity*	*THR*	*Actual HR*
1	40-45 % HRR	109 ± 15 to 116 ± 15	113 ± 15	HR < VT1	126 ± 13 to 136 ± 13	131 ± 16
2	40-45 % HRR	109 ± 15 to 116 ± 15	115 ± 13	HR < VT1	126 ± 13 to 136 ± 13	133 ± 12
3	40-45 % HRR	109 ± 15 to 116 ± 15	113 ± 15	HR < VT1	126 ± 13 to 136 ± 13	131 ± 13
4	40-45 % HRR	109 ± 15 to 116 ± 15	112 ± 13	HR < VT1	126 ± 13 to 136 ± 13	135 ± 12
5-6	50-55 % HRR	116 ± 14 to 121 ± 15	118 ± 14	HR ≥ VT1 to < VT2	137 ± 12 to 147 ± 15	141 ± 9
7-8	50-55 % HRR	117 ± 16 to 125 ± 16	123 ± 16	HR ≥ VT1 to < VT2	140 ± 14 to 151 ± 13	145 ± 14
9-12	60-65 % HRR	127 ± 16 to 133 ± 16	132 ± 16	HR ≥ VT2	153 ± 9 to 161 ± 10	155 ± 11

Values are mean ± SD. *HR* heart rate, *HRR* heart rate reserve, *THR* target heart rate, *VT1* first ventilatory threshold, *VT2* second ventilatory threshold

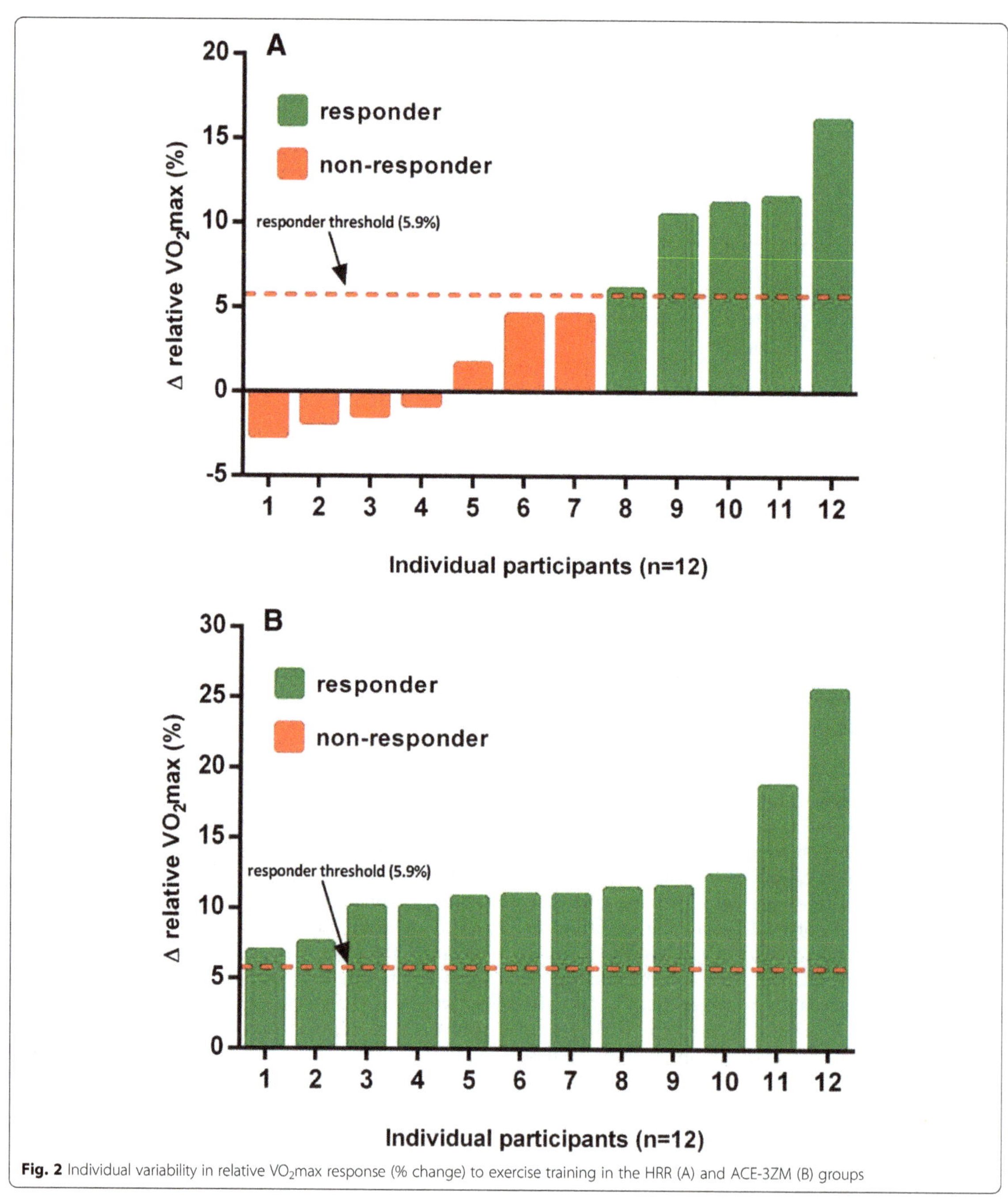

Fig. 2 Individual variability in relative VO_2max response (% change) to exercise training in the HRR (A) and ACE-3ZM (B) groups

results support both our research hypotheses and underscores the importance of establishing exercise training intensity relative to threshold measurements. To our knowledge, this is the first prospective, randomized, controlled trial to compare individual variation in VO_2max training responses following threshold-related training versus training at a %HRR [10].

Heterogeneity in VO_2 Response to Exercise Training

Although it is well accepted that regular exercise has positive effects on cardiorespiratory fitness and numerous other health outcomes related to cardiovascular morbidity and mortality [4], it has also been recently highlighted that considerable heterogeneity exists with respect to the magnitude of VO_2 response to chronic exercise training [20]. Indeed, wide variability (−33.2 % to +58 %) in the individual VO_2 response to exercise training has been previously described in the literature [18, 21–23]. It has been reported that age, sex, race, and initial VO_2max do not influence the heterogeneity in the individual VO_2 response to exercise training [21, 23]. Results from the present study corroborate these earlier findings as the potential influencing factors of age, baseline VO_2max, exercise adherence, and sex were not significantly different between VO_2max responders and non-responders. In contrast, it has been reported that genetics is responsible for 47 % of the change in VO_2max [24]. Additionally, it has previously been demonstrated that one of the most important predictors of a positive VO_2 response to exercise training is a greater volume of exercise [25].

Recently, it has been suggested that the method of exercise intensity prescription may underpin the inter-individual variation in VO_2 response to exercise training [10]. Those previous studies [21–23, 25] that have reported wide variability in the individual VO_2 response to exercise training have used one of several relative exercise intensity methods, including %HRmax, %HRR, or $\%VO_2max$. However, it has been demonstrated that these exercise intensity prescription methods elicit large inter-individual variation in the metabolic responses to exercise training [10, 26]. On this basis, it has been postulated that the individual variation in metabolic response will subsequently lead to differences in the overall homeostatic stress from each training session which will ultimately result in heterogeneity in the exercise training response (i.e., change in VO_2max). Alternatively, it has been suggested that use of a threshold based method for establishing exercise intensity might better normalize the metabolic stimulus for individuals with varying fitness levels [5, 11]. Results from the present study provide experimental evidence to support the merits of a threshold based method for prescription of exercise intensity. Consistent with previous studies [6, 26], this current study found considerable heterogeneity in terms of VO_2max responders (41.7 %) and non-responders (58.3 %) when exercise intensity was prescribed in relative terms as a %HRR. In contrast, we demonstrated a consistent positive VO_2max response to exercise training (100 % responders) when a threshold based exercise intensity prescription method was employed. Taken together, the results of this novel study are encouraging and provide important preliminary data for the design of individualized exercise prescriptions that will enhance training efficacy and limit training unresponsiveness [27].

Primary prevention of chronic disease perspective

In the past decade low cardiorespiratory fitness has garnered considerable attention as an independent and powerful predictor of CVD risk and premature mortality. For example, Williams [2] showed in a meta-analysis that there was a marked increase in relative risk for CVD in the lowest quartile of cardiorespiratory fitness. More recently Blair [28] estimated that low cardiorespiratory fitness accounted for more overall deaths when compared to deaths which could be attributed to traditional CVD risk factors, such as obesity, smoking, hypertension, high cholesterol, and diabetes. Accordingly, the ACE-3ZM change in VO_2max results from the current study have novel clinical and public health relevance, as a large number of adults fall into clinically-defined low cardiorespiratory fitness categories and therefore demonstrate increased CVD risk [29]. Importantly, exercise training in the ACE-3ZM group elicited a positive improvement in VO_2max in 100 % (12/12) of the individuals. Overall, VO_2max was improved on average by 1.1 METs (range +0.65 to +1.63 METs) in the ACE-3ZM group following 12weeks of exercise training. These improvements likely have important long-term prevention implications as a recent study reported a 1 MET increase in VO_2max was associated with an 18 % reduction in deaths due to CVD [30].

Methodological considerations

There are several limitations to the present study that warrant further discussion. First, overall sample size in our study is lower than other major training studies in the literature [16, 25]. However, advantages of a smaller sample size were the ability to better supervise the exercise program and more closely interact with participants on a daily basis during exercise sessions [31]. In particular, the adherence to the prescribed exercise intensity and program was excellent for both exercise treatment groups (Table 2). Second, the present study (12weeks) was also relatively modest in duration compared to previous training investigations [16, 25, 31]. Nevertheless, the significant improvements in VO_2max found in the present study indicate that a 12weeks exercise training period is a sufficient timeframe to demonstrate significant training effects. Future research is needed to confirm the possibility of additional improvements in VO_2max following an exercise training program similar in characteristics to the present study but for prolonged durations. Third, while participants were instructed to maintain their regular dietary intake during the 12weeks intervention, diet intake was not strictly controlled for in this study. Moreover, physical activity outside of the training program was not monitored and thus may have influenced the current findings.

Conclusion

There is a wealth of previous research demonstrating an independent, inverse, dose–response relationship between cardiorespiratory fitness and all-cause and CVD mortality [1, 3, 32, 33]. Moreover, cardiorespiratory fitness has been called the ultimate marker for risk stratification and health outcomes [34]. In the present study a threshold based exercise intensity prescription elicited significantly greater improvements in VO_2max and attenuated the individual variation in VO_2max training responses when compared to relative percent exercise training. These novel findings are encouraging and provide important preliminary data for the design of individualized exercise prescriptions that will enhance training efficacy and limit training unresponsiveness.

Competing interests
This investigation was supported financially by the American Council on Exercise. The American Council on Exercise was not involved in development of the study design, data collection and analysis, or preparation of the manuscript. There are no other potential conflicts of interest related to this article.

Authors' contributions
Conception and design of the experiment: LD, JJ. Performance of the experiment: LD, AW, DB. Analyses of the data: LD, AW, DB, JJ. Preparation of the manuscript: LD, AW, DB, JJ. All authors read and approved the final manuscript.

Acknowledgements
This study was supported by a research grant from the American Council on Exercise (to LD).

Author details
[1]Recreation, Exercise, and Sport Science Department, Western State Colorado University, 600 N. Adams St., Gunnison, CO 81230, USA. [2]Department of Kinesiology, University of Wisconsin – Eau Claire, 105 Garfield Ave, PO Box 4004, Eau Claire, WI 54702, USA.

References

1. Blair SN, Kampert JB, Kohl 3rd HW, Barlow CE, Macera CA, Paffenbarger Jr RS, et al. Influences of cardiorespiratory fitness and other precursors on cardiovascular disease and all-cause mortality in men and women. JAMA. 1996;276:205–10.
2. Williams PT. Physical fitness and activity as separate heart disease risk factors: A meta-analysis. Med Sci Sports Exerc. 2001;33:754–61.
3. Pescatello LS, editor. ACSM's Guidelines for Exercise Testing and Prescription. 9th ed. Baltimore, MD: Lippincott Williams & Wilkins; 2014.
4. Garber CE, Blissmer B, Deschenes MR, Franklin BA, Lamonte MJ, Lee I, et al. Quantity and quality of exercise for developing and maintaining cardiorespiratory, musculoskeletal, and neuromotor fitness in apparently healthy adults: guidance for prescribing exercise. Med Sci Sports Exerc. 2011;43:1334–59.
5. Katch V, Weltman A, Sady S, Freedson P. Validity of the relative percent concept for equating training intensity. Eur J Appl Physiol Occup Physiol. 1978;39:219–27.
6. Scharhag-Rosenberger F, Walitzek S, Kindermann W, Meyer T. Differences in adaptations to 1 year of aerobic endurance training: individual patterns of nonresponse. Scand J Med Sci Sports. 2012;22:113–8.
7. Weltman A, Weltman J, Rutt R, Seip R, Levine S, Snead D, et al. Percentages of maximal heart rate, heart rate reserve, and VO_2max for determining endurance training intensity in sedentary women. Int J Sports Med. 1989;10:212–6.
8. Weltman A, Snead D, Seip R, Schurrer R, Weltman J, Rutt R, et al. Percentages of maximal heart rate, heart rate reserve and VO_2max for determining endurance training intensity in male runners. Int J Sports Med. 1990;11:218–22.
9. Meyer T, Gabriel HH, Kindermann W. Is determination of exercise intensities as percentages of VO_2max or HRmax adequate? Med Sci Sports Exerc. 1999;31:1342–5.
10. Mann TN, Lamberts RP, Lambert MI. High responders and low responders: factors associated with individual variation in response to standardized training. Sports Med. 2014;44:1113–24.
11. Bryant CX, Green DJ. ACE personal trainer manual. San Diego, CA: American Council on Exercise; 2010.
12. Shephard MD, Mazzachi BC, Shephard AK. Comparative performance of two point-of-care analysers for lipid testing. Clin Lab. 2007;53:561–6.
13. Dale RA, Jensen LH, Krantz MJ. Comparison of two point-of-care lipid analyzers for use in global cardiovascular risk assessments. Ann Pharmacother. 2008;42:633–9.
14. Bachorik PS, Ross JW. National cholesterol education program recommendations for measurement of low-density lipoprotein cholesterol: Executive summary. The national cholesterol education program working group on lipoprotein measurement. Clin Chem. 1995;41:1414–20.
15. Wasserman K, McIlroy MB. Detecting the threshold of anaerobic metabolism in cardiac patients during exercise. Am J Cardiol. 1964;14:844–52.
16. Skinner JS, Jaskolski A, Jaskolska A, Krasnoff J, Gagnon J, Leon AS, et al. Age, sex, race, initial fitness, and response to training: the HERITAGE Family Study. J Appl Physiol. 2001;90:1770–6.
17. Cohen J. Statistical power analysis for the behavioral sciences (2nd ed.). New Jersey: Lawrence Erlbaum Associates, Publishers; 1988.
18. Dalleck LC, Allen BA, Hanson BA, Borresen EC, Erickson ME, De Lap SL. Dose–response relationship between moderate-intensity exercise duration and coronary heart disease risk factors in postmenopausal women. J Womens Health (Larchmt). 2009;18:105–13.
19. Katch VL, Sady SS, Freedson P. Biological variability in maximum aerobic power. Med Sci Sports Exerc. 1982;14:21–5.
20. Astorino TA, Schubert MM. Individual responses to completion of short-term and chronic interval training: a retrospective study. PLoS One. 2014;9:e97638. doi:10.1371/journal.pone.0097638.
21. Kohrt WM, Malley MT, Coggan AR, Spina RJ, Ogawa T, Ehsani AA, et al. Effects of gender, age, and fitness level on response of VO_2max to training in 60–71 year olds. J Appl Physiol (1985). 1991;71:2004–11.
22. Skinner JS, Wilmore KM, Krasnoff JB, Jaskólski A, Jaskólska A, Gagnon J, et al. Adaptation to a standardized training program and changes in fitness in a large, heterogeneous population: the HERITAGE Family Study. Med Sci Sports Exerc. 2000;32:157–61.
23. Bouchard C, Rankinen T. Individual differences in response to regular physical activity. Med Sci Sports Exerc. 2001;33(6 Suppl):S446–51.
24. Bouchard C, An P, Rice T, Skinner JS, Wilmore JH, Gagnon J, et al. Familial aggregation of VO(2max) response to exercise training: results from the HERITAGE Family Study. J Appl Physiol (1985). 1999;87:1003–8.
25. Sisson SB, Katzmarzyk PT, Earnest CP, Bouchard C, Blair SN, Church TS. Volume of exercise and fitness nonresponse in sedentary, postmenopausal women. Med Sci Sports Exerc. 2009;41:539–45.
26. Scharhag-Rosenberger F, Meyer T, Gässler N, Faude O, Kindermann W. Exercise at given percentages of VO2max: heterogeneous metabolic responses between individuals. J Sci Med Sport. 2010;13:74–9.
27. Buford TW, Roberts MD, Church TS. Toward exercise as personalized medicine. Sports Med. 2013;43:157–65.
28. Blair SN. Physical inactivity: the biggest public health problem of the 21st century. Br J Sports Med. 2009;43:1–2.
29. Lobelo F, Pate R, Dowda M, Liese A, Daniels S. Cardiorespiratory fitness and clustered cardiovascular disease risk in U.S. adolescents. J Adolesc Health. 2010;47:352–9.
30. Barlow CE, Defina LF, Radford NB, Berry JD, Cooper KH, Haskell WL, et al. Cardiorespiratory fitness and long-term survival in "low-risk" adults. J Am Heart Assoc. 2012;1:e001354.
31. Kraus WE, Torgan CE, Duscha BD, Norris J, Brown SA, Cobb FR, et al. Studies of a targeted risk reduction intervention through defined exercise (STRRIDE). Med Sci Sports Exerc. 2001;33:1774–84.
32. Blair SN, Kohl III HW, Paffenbarger RS, Clark DG, Cooper KH, Gibbons LW. Physical fitness and all-cause mortality: a prospective study of healthy men and women. JAMA. 1989;262:2395–401.
33. Gulati M, Pandey DK, Arnsdorf MF, Lauderdale DS, Thisted RA, Wicklund RH, et al. Exercise capacity and the risk of death in women: the St James Women Take Heart Project. Circulation. 2003;108:1554–9.
34. Franklin BA. Fitness: the ultimate marker for risk stratification and health outcomes? Prev Cardiol. 2007;10:42–6.

9

Comparison of three activity monitors for estimating sedentary time among children

Jarle Stålesen[1], Frøydis Nordgård Vik[1], Bjørge Herman Hansen[2] and Sveinung Berntsen[1*]

Abstract

Background: Time spent sedentary appears to be associated with several health outcomes in adults, but findings are inconsistent in children. Further, the assessment of sedentary time represents a major challenge. The objectives of the present study were to determine whether 1) ActiGraph GT3X+, ActivPAL and SenseWear Armband Pro3 (SWA) provide comparable estimates of sedentary time in 9–12-year-old children, 2) these devices are valid compared with direct observation, and 3) ActivPAL discriminates between sitting and standing behavior.

Methods: The sample was 67 children. Data were collected during three consecutive days in November 2012. To test the activity monitors in contexts related to physical and sedentary activities commonly performed by children, the children participated in sessions of activity while sitting (watching television, playing video games and tossing a ball while sitting) and standing (musical chairs, active video gaming and tossing a ball) while wearing three different activity monitors at the same time. All activity sessions were observed by two researchers. Differences between monitors were determined using Friedman's two-way analysis of variance by rank order.

Results: Minutes of estimated sedentary time differed across device brands during combined sitting activities: SWA vs. ActiGraph GT3X+ ($P = 0.048$), SWA vs. ActivPAL, ($P < 0.001$) and ActiGraph GT3X+ vs. ActivPAL ($P = 0.002$). Out of 12 min in total of combined recorded sitting activity, SWA reported a median of 6 min (95 % Confidence Interval [CI] = 5.0, 7.0), ActiGraph GT3X+ 7 min (7.0, 8.0) and ActivPAL 10 min (8.6, 10.8) as sedentary time. ActivPAL recorded 3.7 (2.4, 4.0) minutes of the non-sitting activities 'musical chairs', 4.0 (4.0, 4.0) minutes in 'standing ball toss'; and 4.0 (2.7, 4.0) minutes in 'active video gaming' as sitting time.

Conclusion: Recorded sedentary time varied among the monitors GT3X+, SWA and ActivPAL, and misclassification of standing activities as sitting activities were apparent for ActivPAL in certain activities.

Keywords: Accelerometer, ActiGraph, ActivPAL, Inclinometer, Indirect calorimetry, SenseWear

Background

The word "sedentary" comes from the Latin *sedentarius*, meaning sitting or remaining in one place. Sedentary time is associated with detrimental health outcomes in adults [1], but whether this is the case in children is uncertain [2]. Sedentary time has been inversely associated with high-density lipoprotein cholesterol in overweight and obese children [3] and self-reported screen time has been associated with pediatric obesity and cardio metabolic disease [4].

* Correspondence: sveinung.berntsen@uia.no
[1]Department of Public Health, Sport and Nutrition, Faculty of Health and Sport Sciences, University of Agder, P.O. Box 422, NO-4604 Kristiansand, Norway
Full list of author information is available at the end of the article

Previously, screen time has often been used to quantify sedentary time [5–7]. However, this may be inadequate, given that sedentary time includes more than screen-based activities [8]. In other studies in which accelerometers are used, associations are not always found between objectively recorded sedentary time and health risks [8–10], especially when adjusting for moderate- to vigorous intensity physical activity [10]. Thus, the relation between sedentary time and health risk may not be as clear as it is between physical activity and health. Findings are also complicated by researchers' use of different definitions of sedentary [8]. Further understanding the objective relations between sedentary time and health risks in children is therefore dependent on the use of valid assessment methods. Accelerometers and inclinometers are now commonly used to objectively record total sedentary time [8, 11, 12]. ActiGraph GT3X+ (ActiGraph, Pensacola, FL, USA), a hip-worn accelerometer, ActivPAL™ (ActivPAL Technologies Ltd., Glasgow, UK), an inclinometer worn on the leg between the knee and hip, and SenseWear Armband Pro3 (SWA, BodyMedia Inc., Pittsburgh, PA, USA), a multisensor activity monitor worn on the arm, are three commonly used activity monitors that have been used previously to record sedentary time in children [13–15].

To our knowledge there are no published comparisons of GT3X+, ActivPAL and SWA for recording sedentary time in children. In a study comparing reports of sedentary time with ActivPAL and GT3X+ over a seven-day period in preschool children, a correlation between these monitors of $r = 0.66$ ($P = 0.001$) was reported [16]. GT3X+ and ActivPAL have also been compared with direct observation in 15–18-year-old females [17]. The overall agreements with direct observation were 67 % for GT3X+ and 99 % for ActivPAL across sitting, standing and slow walking (3.6 km/h) [17].

In several studies comparing older generations of SWA with indirect calorimetry, SWA underestimated energy expenditure during sedentary time in children [12, 18]. Calabro et al. [19] compared SWA with indirect calorimetry in 21 children during various activities including coloring and computer games and found no significant differences between SWA and indirect calorimetry [19].

When evaluating the validity and reliability of activity monitors, it is essential to assess relevant activities in a free-living setting. Although few studies have evaluated the validity of activity monitors during activities out of a laboratory [13] or during both out and in a laboratory [20], the majority have been laboratory based [21–23].

The objective of the present study were to 1) determine whether the GT3X+, ActivPAL and SWA provided comparable estimates of sedentary time in 9–12-year-old children, 2) evaluate the validity of these device estimates against direct observation and 3) investigate whether ActivPAL could discriminate between sitting and standing activities.

Methods

Design

Data were collected during three consecutive days in November 2012. To test the activity monitors in contexts related to physical and sedentary activities commonly performed by children, 67 children participated in sitting and standing activities in random order while simultaneously wearing all three activity monitors. Two researchers observed each activity. Written informed consent was obtained from the participating children and their parents or guardians. Application was sent to the Norwegian regional committee for medical and health research ethics South East (2012/1803) and the committee advised running the study without further approval. The specificity of activities the children participated in was carefully arranged, and the purpose of the observers was to write down any deviation to the pre-determined activity on a time sheet.

Subjects

In the present study, 35 boys and 32 girls were recruited from an elementary school in Kristiansand, Norway. The total number of children asked to participate was 27 in 5th grade, 26 in 6th grade and 24 7th grade, respectively. No children declined to participate, and the reason for those that did not participate was absence from school during the days of testing. Eligible participants were between the ages of 9 and 12 years. Due to technical errors when downloading data, 13 children were excluded (five with GT3X+, four with ActivPAL and four with SWA). This resulted in a total sample of 54 children (27 boys and 27 girls).

Procedures

The researchers followed the participants in groups of two and recorded their age, gender, body mass and time intervals for each activity on a standardized form. The test location was a classroom. Each child's body mass was measured to the nearest 0.1 kg using a Seca Optima (Seca, Hamburg, Germany). Prior to testing, observers' watches were synchronized with the computer clock. The total duration of collection of data per child was approximately 1 hour. Physical activity data was collected in a consecutive way while participating in the following activity stations.

The ActiGraph GT3X+ is an activity monitor with a triaxial accelerometer that has previously been described in detail [24]. Data were collected at a sampling rate of 100 Hz, and analyzed in 60-s epochs. When analyzing the data, we derived counts per minute and minutes of intensity-specific physical activity from the vertical axis data using the youth-specific cutoffs proposed by Evenson et al. [21] of less than 100 counts per minute defined as sedentary time. ActiLife v.6.8.0 (Pensacola, FL, USA) software was used for analyses.

The ActivPAL™ physical activity logger is an inclinometer that can discriminate between and record time spent in different postures over a 7-day period.

The ActivPAL has previously been described in detail [25, 26]. Date were collected in 15-s epochs with a sampling frequency of 10 Hz and analyzed in 60-s epochs. When comparing ActivPAL with GT3X+ and SWA, time registered as sitting was categorized as sedentary time, while standing and stepping time was categorized as other activities. ActivPAL™ data were processed and analyzed using Research Edition v6.5.1 (Glasgow, UK).

Table 1 Summary of the six activity stations

Station 1: Standing Ball- toss	Two children stood upright in the same spot for the duration of the test and threw a rubber ball back and forth over a distance of approximately 2.5 m.
Station 2: Sitting Ball- toss	Two children performed this exercise in a sitting position facing each other, and threw a rubber ball over a distance of approximately 2 m.
Station 3: Musical chairs	The test group prepared a round table, 1.5 m in diameter. Then added one chair, made the children walk in circles around the table, at a low pace with a fixed distance between. The children sat down and stood up again when the test leader notified. The children were sitting no more than 10 s in each interval.
Station 4: Television viewing	The children watched television sitting.
Station 5: Sedentary gaming	The children were sitting in front of a television and played a video game using a handheld controller.
Station 6: Active Video gaming	The children were standing upright in front of a television, playing a video game with a motion controller.

The SenseWear Armband Pro_3 (SWA) is a multisensor activity monitor worn over the triceps of the right arm. The SWA has been described in detail previously [13, 27]. The sampling frequency was 1-min epochs. Time spent sedentary was defined as metabolic equivalents (METs) below 1.5 and time spent in other activities as 1.5 METS or above for the SWA. The SenseWear Professional 6.1 software was used to analyze raw data.

ActivPAL, SWA and GT3X+ were initialized and attached to the child according to the manufacturers' instructions.

To quantify time spent in a wide range of physical activities, including light intensity and sedentary time, six activities were used: standing ball toss, sitting ball toss, musical chairs, television viewing, sedentary video gaming and active video gaming. The individual activities are described more in detail in Table 1. Activities were further divided into those performed sitting or standing. Standing activities included ball toss, musical chairs and active video gaming. Television viewing, sitting ball toss and sedentary gaming were sitting activities. Each activity lasted 6 min and was performed in a randomized order.

Statistical analysis

Descriptive data are presented as mean and standard deviation (SD). Results are presented as medians and 95 % confidence intervals (CIs). Due to skewness, non-parametric tests (related-samples Friedman's two-way analysis of variance by rank order) were performed. The first and last minutes of each session were excluded, leaving the middle 4 minutes of each session for analyses. The criterion for statistical significance was $P \leq 0.05$. Analyses were conducted using SPSS® (Statistical Package for Social Sciences, Version 22 for Windows. SPSS Inc., Chicago, USA).

Results

A total of 54 children (27 boys, 11.1 ± 0.7 years) with a mean body mass of 41.9 ± 9.6 kg were included. Median sedentary times recorded by each of the three monitors during activities are summarized in Table 2. ActivPAL recorded significantly more sedentary time ($P < 0.001$) during four of the six activities compared with both SWA and GT3X+. Out of the possible 4 min, ActivPAL recorded 3.7 (95 % CI 2.4, 4.0) minutes as sedentary time during musical chairs, 4.0 (2.7, 4.0) minutes during active video gaming and during standing ball toss 4.0 (4.0, 4.0). As shown in Table 2, SWA and GT3X+ were significantly different ($P = 0.018$) from each other for sitting ball toss, during which SWA recorded 0.0 min (0.0, 1.0) and GT3X+ recorded 0.5 min (0.0, 1.0) as sedentary time. ActivPAL was also significantly different from each of the other monitors ($P < 0.001$), recording 4.0 min (3.3, 4.0) as sedentary time in sitting ball toss.

When stratified into standing activities (Fig. 1), ActivPAL recorded significantly different sedentary time ($P < 0.001$) to that recorded by SWA or GT3X+. In the standing activities ActivPAL recorded that the children were sedentary with a median of 8.9 (8.4, 9.8) out of 12 min in total. During the sitting activities (Fig. 1), there were significant differences between all three monitors (SWA vs. GT3X+, $P = 0.048$; SWA vs. ActivPAL, $P < 0.001$; GT3X+ vs. ActivPAL, $P = 0.002$). ActivPAL recorded 10 min (8.6, 10.8) of sedentary time while SWA

Table 2 Median (95 % confidence intervals) of minutes spent sedentary for SWA, GT3X+ and ActivPAL (APAL) ($n = 54$)

	Standing ball- toss	Sitting ball- toss	Musical chairs	Television viewing	Sedentary gaming	Active video gaming
SWA	0.0 (0.0, 0.0)	0.0 (0.0, 0.0)*	0.0 (0.0, 0.0)	4.0 (2.0, 4.0)	4.0 (3.0, 4.0)	0.0 (0.0, 0.0)
GT3X+	0.0 (0.0, 0.0)	0.5 (0.0, 1.0)*	0.0 (0.0, 0.0)	3.0 (2.0, 4.0)	4.0 (4.0, 4.0)	0.0 (0.0, 0.0)
APAL	4.0 (4.0, 4.0)**	4.0 (3.3, 4.0)**	3.7 (2.4, 4.0)	4.0 (3.2, 4.0)	4.0 (4.0, 4.0)**	4.0 (2.7, 4.0)**

*Significantly different compared to the other monitors ($P < 0.05$)
**Significantly different compared to the other monitors ($P < 0.001$)
The activities lasted 4 min in total

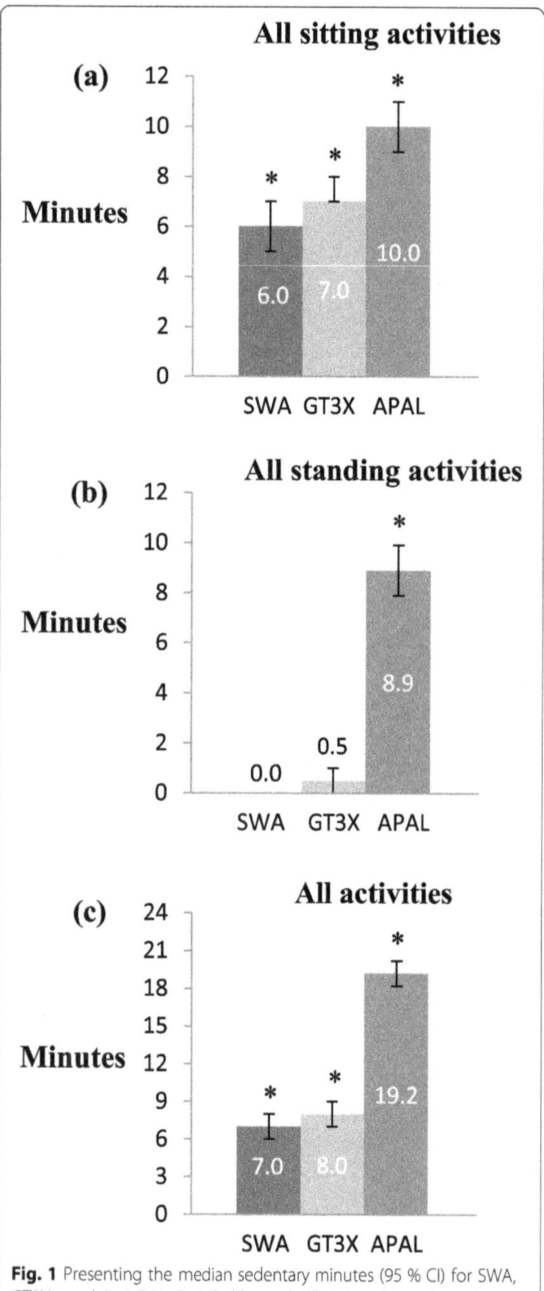

Fig. 1 Presenting the median sedentary minutes (95 % CI) for SWA, GT3X+ and ActivPAL. Detailed legend: All sitting- (**a**) and standing (**b**) activities were compared, with a total of 12 min. All activities (**c**) were compared with a total of 24 min. In these figures $n = 54$

recorded 6 min (5.0, 7.0) and GT3X+ 7 min (7.0, 8.0) out of a possible 12 min during the sitting activities (Fig. 1).

Table 3 presents the amount of time recorded by ActivPAL as sitting, standing and stepping in all activity stations. For standing ball toss, musical chairs, and active video gaming, ActivPAL recorded 4 min (4.0, 4.0), 3.7 min (2.4, 4.0) and 4 min (2.7, 4.0) respectively, out of 4 min in total as sitting

Discussion

We found that activity monitors differed in their recordings of sedentary time. All three activity monitors recorded sedentary time significantly different during sitting activities. ActivPAL recorded sedentary time more accurately compared with SWA and GT3X+. However, in our study ActivPAL seemed to have difficulty discriminating between sitting activities and standing or moving exercises, and therefore misclassified standing or moving exercises as time spent sitting.

Our findings differ somewhat from previous reports indicating that ActivPAL is valid for discriminating between sedentary, standing and walking activities [17, 22, 25]. Davis et al. [25] reported that ActivPAL misclassified posture in a few individuals, most often recording sitting as standing activities, although they did not state the number of participants to which this applied. It was reported that occasionally standing was misidentified by ActivPAL as sitting, for example if a child stood with one leg straight and one leg bent at the knee with the foot resting on top of the other foot, thereby altering the angle [25]. These findings resembles ours; however, it is unlikely any child in the present study rested one foot on top of the other in the standing activity where we tested the inclinometer, as that most likely would compromise the balance required to throw a ball in standing ball toss, confirmed by direct observation. The angle of the leg; however, may explain some of the misclassifications by the ActivPAL. When comparing ActivPAL's ability to record sitting time compared with direct observation, it accurately recorded sitting ball toss, television viewing and sedentary gaming as sedentary activities.

Similar to ActivPAL's reported occasional misidentification when a child stood with one leg straight and one leg resting on top of the other [25]; SWA recorded 0 min as sedentary time, in sitting ball toss activity, a station involving marked arm movement. This may be explained by the location of activity monitor on the arm and the arm movement. Similar explanation was reported in a previous study as a possible cause of overestimation of energy expenditure by SWA [28].

It has been argued that using various ActiGraph cut-offs provides distinct estimates of sedentary time [16]. This is a challenge when comparing our results with those of previous studies of GT3X+. For instance, Martin et al. [16] defined sedentary cut-offs as <1100 counts per minute, while in the present study we used <100 counts per minute as recommended in studies

Table 3 Median (95 % confidence intervals) of minutes spent sitting, standing and stepping for AcitvPAL ($n = 54$)

	Standing ball- toss	Sitting ball- toss	Musical chairs	Television viewing	Sedentary gaming	Active video gaming
Sitting	4.0 (4.0, 4.0)	4.0 (3.3, 4.0)	3.7 (2.4, 4.0)	4.0 (3.2, 4.0)	4.0 (4.0, 4.0)	4.0 (2.7, 4.0)
Standing	0.0 (0.0, 0.0)	0.0 (0.0, 0.6)	0.3 (0.0, 1.4)	0.0 (0.0, 0.6)	0.0 (0.0, 0.0)	0.0 (0.0, 0.9)
Stepping	0.0 (0.0, 0.0)	0.0 (0.0, 0.1)	0.0 (0.0, 0.2)	0.0 (0.0, 0.1)	0.0 (0.0, 0.0)	0.0 (0.0, 0.2)

The activities lasted 4 min in total

comparing various cut-offs for GT3X+ [29, 30] . In a study examining the validity of seven child-specific ActiGraph cut-offs using indirect calorimetry as the criterion, the majority overestimated sedentary time and underestimated moderate to vigorous physical activity in children [20].

In two studies comparing GT3X+ and ActivPAL, ActivPAL was more valid for both recording sedentary time [16, 17] and distinguishing between sitting and standing [17]. The results of the present study support the accuracy of ActivPAL in recording sitting time but show that it may overestimate sedentary time and partly misclassify standing activities as sitting.

Inclinometers and accelerometers may be promising tools in lifestyle intervention studies. However, due to the observed differences in how monitors record sedentary and sitting time, we recommend additional research. A more comprehensive exploration of the strengths and weaknesses of different activity monitors in both laboratory and natural settings may provide a better understanding of the relation between sedentary time and health.

Study strengths were the inclusion of multiple monitors to record sedentary time and the fact that activities were conducted in a natural rather than a laboratory-based setting. Our study included activities such as watching television and sedentary gaming, both of which are common leisure-time activities that contribute significantly to children's total sedentary time. The activities were also presented in a randomized order. Furthermore, the use of direct observation to verify the children's adherence to the study protocol and the ways in which they performed the activity strengthened the study.

A primary study limitation was definition of sedentary time for ActivPAL versus SWA and GT3X+. When comparing ActivPAL with SWA and GT3X+, we did not include standing without movement as part of sedentary time. However, consideration should be given to the different definitions of sedentary time upon which the three monitors are based, i.e. ActivPAL records sitting, standing without movement and walking or stepping, while GT3X + and SWA primarily record movements of various body parts. Standing without movement in the definition of sedentary time for ActivPAL could have been included based on that SWA and GT3X+ were designed to record movement, as in previous research comparing ActivPAL with GT3X+ [16]. However, ActivPAL was designed to record posture, and including standing without movement as sedentary time would have been to take away ActivPAL's purpose. To further investigate whether ActivPAL discriminates between sitting, standing and stepping activities, ActivPAL was individually compared with direct observation.

Conclusion

In conclusion, children's sedentary time recorded simultaneously by GT3X+, SWA and ActivPAL differed significantly. Recorded sedentary time varied among the monitors GT3X+, SWA and ActivPAL and misclassification of standing activities as sitting activities were apparent for ActivPAL in certain activities.

Competing interests

The authors declare that they do not have competing interests.

Authors' contributions

JS and SB contributed to the concept and design and conducted the acquisition of data, statistical analysis, and interpretation of data and drafting of the manuscript. FNV contributed to the concept and design and conducted the acquisition and interpretation of data, and editing of the manuscript. BHH contributed to the interpretation of data and to the editing of the manuscript. All authors have read and approved the final manuscript.

Acknowledgments

We thank children of Karuss Elementary School in Kristiansand, Norway, for participating in the study and teachers for making available the testing location. The present study was funded by the University of Agder.

Author details

[1]Department of Public Health, Sport and Nutrition, Faculty of Health and Sport Sciences, University of Agder, P.O. Box 422, NO-4604 Kristiansand, Norway. [2]Department of Sports Medicine, Norwegian School of Sport Sciences, Oslo, Norway.

References

1. Healy GN, Dunstan DW, Salmon J, Cerin E, Shaw JE, Zimmet PZ, et al. Breaks in sedentary time: Beneficial associations with metabolic risk. Diabetes Care. 2008;31(4):661–6.
2. Chinapaw MJM, Proper KI, Brug J, van Mechelen W, Singh AS. Relationship between young peoples' sedentary behaviour and biomedical health indicators : a systematic review of prospective studies. Obes Rev. 2011;12(7): e621.
3. Cliff D, Okely T, Burrows T, Morgan P, Collins C, Jones R, et al. Levels and bouts of sedentary behaviour and physical activity : Associations with cardio - metabolic health in overweight and obese children. J Sci Med Sport. 2012; 15(supplement):S42.
4. Tremblay MS, Leblanc AG, Kho ME, Saunders TJ, Larouche R, Colley RC, et al. Systematic review of sedentary behaviour and health indicators in school - aged children and youth. Int J Behav Nutr Phys Act. 2011;8(1):98.

5. Ford ES, Kohl 3rd HW, Mokdad AH, Ajani UA. Sedentary behavior, physical activity, and the metabolic syndrome among U.S. adults. Obes Res. 2005;13(3):608–14.
6. Schmitz KH, Harnack L, Fulton JE, Jacobs DR Jr, Gao S, Lytle LA, et al. Reliability and validity of a brief questionnaire to assess television viewing and computer use by middle school children. J Sch Health. 2004;74(9):370–7.
7. Robinson TN. Reducing children's television viewing to prevent obesity: a randomized controlled trial. JAMA. 1999;282(16):1561–7.
8. Colley RC, Garriguet D, Janssen I, Wong SL, Saunders TJ, Carson V et al. The association between accelerometer - measured patterns of sedentary time and health risk in children and youth : results from the Canadian health measures survey. BMC Public Health. 2013;13(1):1.
9. Carson V, Janssen I. Volume, patterns, and types of sedentary behavior and cardio - metabolic health in children and adolescents : a cross - sectional study. BMC Public Health. 2011;11(1):274.
10. Froberg A, Raustorp A. Objectively measured sedentary behaviour and cardio-metabolic risk in youth: a review of evidence. Eur J Pediatr. 2014;173(7):845–60.
11. Bouten CV, Westerterp KR, Verduin M, Janssen JD. Assessment of energy expenditure for physical activity using a triaxial accelerometer. Med Sci Sports Exerc. 1994;26(12):1516.
12. Arvidsson D, Slinde F, Larsson S, Hulthén L. Energy cost of physical activities in children: validation of SenseWear Armband. Med Sci Sports Exerc. 2007;39(11):2076–84.
13. Calabró MA, Stewart JM, Welk GJ. Validation of pattern - recognition monitors in children using doubly labeled water. Med Sci Sports Exerc. 2013.
14. Rosenkranz RR, Lubans DR, Peralta LR, Bennie A, Sanders T, Lonsdale C. A cluster-randomized controlled trial of strategies to increase adolescents' physical activity and motivation during physical education lessons: the Motivating Active Learning in Physical Education (MALP) trial. BMC Public Health. 2012;12(1):834.
15. Hinckson EA, Aminian S, Ikeda E, Stewart T, Oliver M, Duncan S, et al. Acceptability of standing workstations in elementary schools: a pilot study. Prev Med. 2013;56(1):82–5.
16. Martin A, McNeill M, Penpraze V, Dall P, Granat M, Paton JY, et al. Objective measurement of habitual sedentary behavior in pre-school children: comparison of activPAL With Actigraph monitors. Pediatr Exerc Sci. 2011; 23(4):468–76.
17. Dowd KP, Harrington DM, Donnelly AE. Criterion and concurrent validity of the activPAL™ professional physical activity monitor in adolescent females. PLoS One. 2012;7(10):e47633.
18. Arvidsson D, Slinde F, Larsson S, Hulthén L. Energy cost in children assessed by multisensor activity monitors. Med Sci Sports Exerc. 2009;41(3):603–11.
19. Calabro MA, Welk GJ, Eisenmann JC. Validation of the SenseWear Pro Armband algorithms in children. Med Sci Sports Exerc. 2009;41(9):1714–20.
20. Crouter SE, Horton M, Bassett Jr DR. Validity of ActiGraph child - specific equations during various physical activities. Med Sci Sports Exerc. 2013;45:1403–9.
21. Evenson KR, Catellier DJ, Gill K, Ondrak KS, McMurray RG. Calibration of two objective measures of physical activity for children. J Sports Sci. 2008;26(14): 1557–65.
22. Aminian S, Hinckson EA. Examining the validity of the ActivPAL monitor in measuring posture and ambulatory movement in children. Int J Behav Nutr Phys Act. 2012;9:119.
23. Harrington DM, Dowd KP, Tudor-Locke C, Donnelly AE. A steps/minute value for moderate intensity physical activity in adolescent females. Pediatr Exerc Sci. 2012;24(3):399–408.
24. Hänggi JM, Phillips LR, Rowlands AV. Original research : Validation of the GT3X ActiGraph in children and comparison with the GT1M ActiGraph. J Sci Med Sport. 2012;16(1):40.
25. Davies G, Reilly JJ, McGowan AJ, Dall PM, Granat MH, Paton JY. Validity, practical utility, and reliability of the acfiVPAL™ in preschool children. Med Sci Sports Exerc. 2012;44(4):761–9.
26. Harrington DM, Welk GJ, Donnelly AE. Validation of MET estimates and step measurement using the ActivPAL physical activity logger. J Sports Sci. 2011;29(6):627–33.
27. Soric M, Turkalj M, Kucic D, Marusic I, Plavec D, Misigoj-Durakovic M. Validation of a multi-sensor activity monitor for assessing sleep in children and adolescents. Sleep Med. 2013;14(2):201–5.
28. Dorminy CA, Choi L, Akohoue SA, Chen KY, Buchowski MS. Validity of a multisensor armband in estimating 24-h energy expenditure in children. Med Sci Sports Exerc. 2008;40(4):699–706.
29. Trost SGWR, Okely AD. Predictive validity of three actigraph energy expenditure equations for children. Med Sci Sports Exerc. 2006;38(2):380.
30. Kim Y, Lee JM, Peters BP, Gaesser GA, Welk GJ. Examination of different accelerometer cut-points for assessing sedentary behaviors in children. PLoS One. 2014;9(4):e90630.

10

Associations between poor oral health and reinjuries in male elite soccer players: a cross-sectional self-report study

Henny Solleveld[1], Arnold Goedhart[1*] and Luc Vanden Bossche[2]

Abstract

Background: Although it is well known that oral pathogens can enter the systemic circulation and cause disease, it is largely unknown if poor oral health increases the risk of sports injuries. The purpose of this study is to investigate the association between poor oral health and reinjuries in male elite soccer players, adjusted for psychosocial problems and player characteristics.

Methods: 184 Players in premier league soccer clubs and 31 elite, junior soccer players in the Netherlands, Belgium and England, were enrolled in a retrospective cross-sectional study. The Sports Injury Risk Indicator, a self assessed questionnaire, was used to obtain information on reinjuries, age and player position, oral health and psychosocial problems. The number of different types of oral health problems was used as an indicator of poor oral health. (SumDental, range 0–2: 0 = no oral health problems, 1 = one type of oral health problem and 2 = two or more types of oral health problems). Multivariable logistic regression was used to investigate whether SumDental was associated with reinjuries, after adjustment for psychosocial problems and player characteristics.

Results: 37% of the players reported no oral health problems, 43% reported one type of oral health problem and 20% reported two or more types of oral health problems. After full adjustment for age, player position and psychosocial problems (i.e. injury anxiety, psychophysical stress, unhealthy eating habits and dissatisfaction with trainer/team), poor oral health (SumDental) was positively associated with all kind of reinjuries whether analyzed as a continuous variable or as a categorical variable. The fully adjusted odds ratios for SumDental analyzed as a continuous variable were: in relation to repeated exercise-associated muscle cramps: 1.82 (95% confidence interval (CI): 1.07, 3.12), in relation to muscle or tendon reinjury 1.57 (95% CI: 1.01, 2.45) and in relation to multiple types of reinjury 1.88 (95% CI: 1.19, 2.97).

Conclusion: The results from this study justify a thorough examination of the effects of oral health problems on the injury risk of playing elite soccer.

Keywords: Sports injuries, Soccer, Oral health, Gingival diseases, Dental caries, Dental plaque, Psychosocial factors

Background

Injuries in male elite soccer players are common, with muscle and tendon injuries comprising almost half of all injuries [1]. On average, one injury occurs every 106 hours of sport-related activity and 65 - 95% of players have at least one injury every year [1-3]. The injury model of Bahr and Krosshaug states that intrinsic and extrinsic risk factors and the interaction between them make players susceptible to an injury caused by events such as jumping, tackling and shooting [4]. The intrinsic risk factors proposed by Bahr and Krosshaug comprise health, including previous injury, age, physical fitness and psychological factors. Poor oral health is not included as an intrinsic risk factor in the injury causation model. This is noteworthy because it is widely accepted that good oral health is essential for good general health [5]. Many studies have shown that dental diseases are associated with systemic illness including cardiovascular diseases (CVDs) and various other pathologies [6]. The well-known MilanLab of AC Milan includes an assessment of oral health in the injury prevention program. However, we are aware of only one study that has investigated the

* Correspondence: goedhart@ub4m.nl
[1]SportsInjuryLab, Box 3141, 3760 DC Soest, The Netherlands
Full list of author information is available at the end of the article

possible impact of dental and occlusal problems on sports injuries. Gay-Escoda et al. found in their study of 30 professional soccer players of F.C. Barcelona, that the Plaque Index and periodontal pocket depth were associated with muscle injuries [7].

The most prevalent oral diseases in humans, periodontitis and dental caries, are dental plaque related diseases [8]. Dental plaque is a microbial biofilm formed by microorganisms tightly bound to a tooth surface and each other. The microbial composition is diverse and remains relatively stable over time. However, when this microbial homeostasis breaks down oral disease can occur [8,9]. Oral disease cause elevated levels of cytokines, especially tumour necrosis factor (TNF-a) and interleukin-6 (IL-6). These cytokines play an important role in the origin of muscle fatigue during exercise and oxidative stress after exercise [10-13]. Muscle fatigue may cause exercise-associated muscle cramps and leads to a reduction in its energy-absorbing capabilities, making the muscle more susceptible to strain injury [14,15]. In addition, muscle fatigue increases the possibility of proprioceptive errors and disturbances in the interactions between limb segments [16,17]. Therefore, oral disease is a potential risk factor for sports injury and reinjuries.

Risk factors associated with oral disease include poor oral hygiene, cigarette smoking, systemic conditions such as diabetes mellitus, rheumatoid arthritis, possibly obesity, stress and poor coping behaviours [18,19]. Stress and poor coping behaviours are also risk factors for sports injuries. Many studies have found evidence for the stress-injury model of Williams and Andersen [20]. This model suggests that stress is associated with a increased risk of injury and is directly, as well as indirectly, influenced by personality traits and coping resources. As these psychosocial factors are related to both sports injuries and poor oral health, associations between poor oral health and sports (re)injuries are compounded by these factors.

Stress has been etiologically linked to occlusal and temporomandibular joint (TMJ) problems [21,22]. Individuals with high levels of stress display muscular tension and parafunctional habits like bruxism that give rise to jaw joint problems. Occlusal and TMJ problems may therefore be regarded as physical signs of stress.

This study focuses on reinjury because of the stability of oral conditions [8,9] and because previous sports reinjuries will probably be more accurately reported than previous sports injuries. The aim of this retrospective cross-sectional study is (1) to assess the association of poor oral health with sports reinjuries and repeated exercise-associated muscle cramps (REAMC) in male elite soccer players; and (2) to determine whether the association of poor oral health with sports reinjuries and REAMC persisted after adjustment for other possible risk factors.

Methods

Procedure

The study was conducted between September 2011 and December 2012. Five Dutch clubs, four Belgian clubs and one British premier league club were invited to participate in this study using medical staff known to two of the researchers (HS and LvdB) and via acquaintances of these acquaintances. The clubs were asked to present a questionnaire to all players from the first team squads (there were no eligibility criteria). In addition, one Belgian and one Dutch club were also asked to present the questionnaire to their elite junior squads. Two Dutch clubs refused to participate with their elite squad. The average number of players of first team squads is about 30 for Belgian and Dutch elite soccer clubs and about 40 for British elite soccer clubs. The Belgian and Dutch elite junior squads have about 20 players each. This makes a total of about 290 soccer players potentially in the study.

The participating clubs were visited by the first author to explain the aims and procedures of the project, to gather information on the number of players and the language they spoke and to make arrangements with regard to the presentation and administration of the questionnaires. Anonymous questionnaires were presented to the players by a staff member of each participating club as a survey on a diversity of health aspects. The staff member made it clear that everyone was free to participate and to stop answering the questions at any time.

The self-report questionnaire consisted of 71 questions on reinjuries, age and player position, oral health and psychosocial problems. To prevent low response rates typically associated with questionnaires, we kept it short, with simple, straightforward questions, of which most were answered on a 4-point Likert scale. The questionnaire was tested with 12 amateur soccer players to check understanding and response time (below 30 minutes). The Dutch questionnaire was professionally translated into 9 languages (English, French, Spanish, German, Italian, Danish, Portuguese, Russian and Estonian) and then translated back into Dutch to ensure accuracy.

Ethical approval was not sought for this study which used an anonymous questionnaire. In general, ethical protection is required for research on human participants which includes identifiable human material or identifiable data [23]. In the Netherlands, research requires ethical approval only if respondents are "subjected to procedures" or required to follow "rules of behaviour", [24]. The Belgian Advisory Committee on Bioethics states that ethical approval is not required if the conditions of "experiment" are not met, e.g. if the researchers have had no direct influence on the observed situation [25]. We concluded after a detailed review of the guidance given by the National Research Ethics Service: "Does my project require review by a Research Ethics Committee?", that ethical approval was not required in the United Kingdom [26]. The players could read the anonymous questionnaire before starting to respond and were free to stop responding at any time. Completion of the questionnaire constituted consent to participate in the study.

Assessment of reinjuries

The questionnaire item: "Which of the following types of injury have you had more than once (more responses possible)?" was used to assess the dependent variables *repeated exercise-associated muscle cramps (REAMC), muscle or tendon reinjury (MTR) and multiple types of reinjury (MR).* Respondents could mark 'none' or mark one or more of the following 11 types of reinjuries: groin, hamstring, quadriceps, Achilles tendon, muscle cramps, other muscle injuries, fracture, knee, ankle, sprain/ligament or other reinjury. The reinjury variable REAMC was scored 1 (present) if the reinjury type muscle cramps was checked and 0 otherwise. MTR was scored 1 (present) if one or more of the following types of reinjury was indicated: groin, hamstring, quadriceps, Achilles tendon and other muscle reinjuries, else MTR was scored 0 (absent). MR was scored 1 (present) if two or more types of reinjury were checked and 0 otherwise. It may be noted that in this study repeated exercise-associated muscle cramps were not included in the category muscle or tendon reinjuries.

Assessment of oral health

Three types of oral health problems: *Gum problems, Restorations* and *Apex resections* were assessed using questionnaire items and scored as 1 = present or 0 = absent.

Gum problems was scored present if the respondent answered either "always" or "often" on the question "Have you gum problems (bleeding, swelling or recession)" or "no" on the question "Are your wisdom teeth removed?" (presence of wisdom teeth is a well known risk factor for periodontitis in adults because these teeth are in a area where periodontal pathogens accumulate due to the difficulty of keeping this relatively inaccessible area clean and to the qualitatively poorer soft tissue) [27].

Restorations was deemed present if participant answered "yes" on the question "Have you had one or more restorations (crowns and bridges included)". We used a question about restorations instead of a question about caries as questions on utilization of dental care have been found valid in previous research [28].

Apex resections were scored present if participant reported one or more apex resections or endodontic microsurgeries. We used these questions instead of questions on endodontic disease because questions on endodontic therapy have been found valid in previous research [29]. A three-level ordered categorical variable, SumDental indicating poor oral health, was created by summing the three types of oral health problems. SumDental was coded as 0 if no oral health problems were present, as 1 if one type of oral health problems was present, and as 2 if two or three types of oral health problems were present.

Assessment of other covariates

Injury anxiety

The injury anxiety scale assess worries and concerns about injuries resulting from soccer training activities. The scale consists of five items derived from the Tampa Scale for Kinesiophobia [30], e.g. "I am afraid that an injury will occur during training", "Pain lets me know when to stop the training so that I don't injure myself.". Each item was answered on a 4-point Likert scale (1–4). The scale score was obtained by calculating the mean across the five (equal weighted) items, with higher scores indicating higher levels of injury anxiety. Cronbach's alpha = 0.54.

Psychophysical stress

A measure of psychophysical stress was used to assess psychological and physical manifestations of psychological stress related to competitive sports, e.g. fear of performance failure. Items of this scale were drawn from the Sports Anxiety Scale (e.g. "I'm concerned about choking under pressure", "I'm concerned about performing poorly") and the Langner index (e.g. "How often are you bothered by your heart beating fast?", "How often are you troubled with headaches or pains in the head?" [31,32] and three items asked about malocclusion and TMJ problems, i.e. "Have you lockjaw or popping?", "Have you toothache of unknown origin?" and "Are you grinding your teeth?". Each item was answered on a 4-point Likert scale (1–4). The scale score was obtained by averaging the responses of the twelve (equal weighted) scale items, and higher scores corresponded to higher levels of psychophysical stress. Cronbach's alpha = 0.61.

Dissatisfaction with trainer/team

This scale measures the level of acceptance and satisfaction with the role in the team and the level of perceived support from the coach. The items were taken from the Athlete Satisfaction Questionnaire (ASQ) [33], e.g. "I am satisfied with my social status on the team"; "I am satisfied with the extent to which the trainer is behind me". Each item was answered on a 4-point Likert scale (1–4); the positively worded items were reverse scored (e.g. the response 'always' as 1, and 'never' as 4) so that higher scores indicate dissatisfaction. The scale score was obtained by by calculating the mean across the six (equal weighted) items; Cronbach's alpha = 0.78.

Unhealthy eating habits

This scale consists of two items, "How often do you eat unhealthy food?" and "How often are you looking for products with sugar", scored from 1, 'never' to 4, 'always'. The scale score was obtained by by calculating the mean across the two (equal weighted) items, with higher scores indicating unhealthy eating habits.

Player Position is a dichotomized variable with the positions external defenders (full backs), external midfielders, attacking midfielders and forwards scored as 1 and the remaining positions scored as 0, based on findings of previous studies that players on the positions scored as 1 performed significantly more sprints or covered more sprint distance than the other players [34,35]. Of the respondents, 88 (41%) played on less high-intensity positions (scored 0), 127 (59%) played on high-intensity positions (scored 1).

Age was categorized into five age groups: 16–20, 21–23, 24–26, 27–30 and ≥31.

Data analysis

Frequencies and percentages were used to summarize categorical study variables; mean item scores and standard deviations were computed for the scales. Data distributions were examined for normality with the Lilliefors modification of the Kolmogorov–Smirnov test. Significant non-normality was found for all continuous covariates and SumDental. Therefore, Spearman rank correlations were used to examine relations between the covariates injury anxiety, psychophysical stress, unhealthy eating habits, dissatisfaction with trainer/team, age and SumDental. Point biserial correlations were used to examine relations between the dichotomous covariate player position and the other covariates.

Univariate logistic regression was used to assess the associations of the reinjury variables (i.e. REAMC, MTR, MR) with SumDental and with the other covariates. In univariate and multivariable logistic regression analyses the continuous covariates were analyzed as categorical variables, after division into quartiles, to avoid assumptions of linearity in the log odds and to minimize the effect of outlying values. The first quartile served as reference category in the logistic regression analyses, the other quartiles were entered as dummy variables. We analyzed SumDental as continuous variable and as categorical variable with the lowest score (0) as reference category and the other scores (1 and 2) entered as dummy variables. Multivariable logistic regression analysis was used to estimate the adjusted odds ratios for the association of SumDental with the reinjury variables, controlling for the effects of the other covariates. P-values less than 0.05 were considered statistically significant. Analyses were performed using SPSS Version 18.0 for Windows.

Results

Out of 290 potential participants, 232 soccer players were given questionnaires and asked to fully complete it. Seventeen questionnaires were discarded because the respondent did not answer all items, leaving a final sample of 215 elite soccer players, which represents a response of about 75%.

The frequencies and percentages of ordered categorical study variables are presented in Table 1, the mean item scores and standard deviation of the scales in Table 2. As shown in Table 1, gum problems and apex resections were reported by a small minority (16% and 13%, respectively), most respondents (56%) reported one or more restorations.

Spearman rank correlations and point biserial correlations are given in Table 3. Positive associations were found between SumDental and age (e.g. older respondents reported more types of oral health problems), between psychophysical stress and dissatisfaction with trainer/team and between injury anxiety and unhealthy eating habits. Playing position showed a weak positive correlation with injury anxiety (e.g. slightly higher levels of injury anxiety were reported by external defenders, external and attacking midfielders and forwards).

Table 4 present the crude odds ratio's of the other covariates in relation to the reinjury variables. The odds of having a REAMC was higher for external defenders,

Table 1 Characteristics of the participants; categorical variables (n = 215)

Characteristic	n	%
Age, years		
16 - 20 y	51	24
21 -23 y	69	32
24 - 26 y	37	17
27 - 30 y	33	15
31+ y	25	12
Playing position: High intensity position[1]	127	59
Gum problems present	34	16
Restorations present	121	56
Apex resections present	27	13
SumDental		
no type of oral health problems present (score 0)	80	37
one type of oral health problems present (score 1)	93	43
two or more types of oral health problems present (score 2)	42	20
Repeated exercise-associated muscle cramps (REAMC) present	43	20
Muscle or tendon reinjury (MTR) present	97	45
Multiple types of reinjury (MR) present	99	46

Legend: [1]High intensity positions are: external defender (n = 34), central) attacking midfielder (n = 40), external midfielder (n = 29) and forward (n = 24); Lower intensity positions are: goalkeeper (n = 26), central defender (n = 34) and central defending midfielder (n = 26).

Table 2 Characteristics of the participants; means, standard deviations and observed ranges of scale scores (n = 215)

Scale	Mean	Standard deviation	Observed range
Injury anxiety	2.0	0.4	1.00 - 3.40
Psychophysical stress	1.4	0.2	1.00 - 2.25
Unhealthy eating habits	2.4	0.7	1.00 - 4.00
Dissatisfaction with trainer/team	1.7	0.5	1.00 - 3.83

Note: Scale scores are mean item score; all items were answered on a 4-point Likert scale (1–4); for all scales higher scores indicate higher levels of the construct.

external and attacking midfielders and forwards (OR 4.6, 95% CI 1.93-10.85) than for soccer players at other positions (reference category). Compared to soccer players with an injury anxiety score of 1–1.60 (first quartile, reference category), the odds of having a MTR were higher for soccer players with an injury anxiety score of 1.81 – 2.20 (third quartile, OR 3.41, 95% CI 1.58-7.34) and for players with scores above 2.20 (fourth quartile, OR 2.41, 95% CI 1.03-5.68). Similarly, higher odds of having a MR were found for soccer players with an injury anxiety score of 1.61 – 1.80 (OR 3.72, 95% CI 1.63-8.50), for players with scores of 1.81 – 2.20 (OR 3.67, 95% CI 1.67- 8.07) and for players with scores above 2.20 (OR 2.93, 95% CI 1.22-7.03) than those soccer players who reported an injury anxiety score of 1–1.6 (reference category). Compared to soccer players with a psychophysical stress score of 1–1.25 (first quartile, reference category), the odds of having a MR were higher for soccer players with a psychophysical stress score above 1.50 (fourth quartile, OR 3.45, 95% CI 1.47-8.09). There were no statistical significant associations observed between

Table 3 Spearman rank and point-biserial correlations (n = 215)

Variable	Injury anxiety[1]	Psyphy. stress[1]	Age[1]	Unh. eating h[1]	Dissatis- fact. t/t[1]	Playing position[2]
SumDental	.07	.13	.33**	.13	.13	.03
Injury anxiety		.11	-.04	.20**	.03	.15*
Psyphy. stress			.08	.06	.31**	.02
Age				.03	.15*	.02
Unh. eating h.					.00	.01
Dissatisfact. t/t						-.07

Legend: Psyphy. stress = Psychophysical stress; Unh. eating h. = Unhealthy eating habits, Dissatisfact. t/t = Dissatisfaction with trainer/team; [1]: correlations in the column are Spearman correlations; [2]: correlations in the column are point-biserial correlations; *:p < 0.05 (2-tailed); **p < 0.01 (2-tailed).

dissatisfaction with trainer/team, unhealthy eating habits, age categories and the reinjury variables.

The crude and adjusted odds ratios for SumDental in relation to the reinjury variables were similar (see Table 5). SumDental showed statistically significant associations with all reinjury variables when analyzed as a continuous variable (adjusted odds ratios above 1.5). Players with two or all three types of oral health problems had higher odds of having REAMC, of having MTR and of having MT (adjusted odds ranging from 2.48 to 3.40) when compared to players without any of the oral health problems (reference category).

Discussion

The results of this preliminary study indicate that poor oral health is associated with repeated exercise-associated muscle cramps, muscle or tendon reinjury and multiple types of reinjury. These associations persisted after adjustment for age, player position, injury anxiety, psychophysical stress, unhealthy eating habits and dissatisfaction with trainer/team.

Our findings using self-report to assess oral health are consistent with the study by Gay-Escoda et al. [7] which reported that two objective clinical indicators of oral health, the plaque index and the probing pocket depth, were associated with muscle injury in professional male soccer players. On the basis of these results it is tempting to suggest that poor oral health may belong to the class of intrinsic risk factors for sports injuries labeled 'health problems' by Bahr and Krosshaug [4]. Support for this suggestion comes from studies showing that (1) poor oral health is also associated with chronically higher levels of IL-6 and other cytokines [10-13], that (2) chronically higher levels of IL-6 and other cytokines are associated with fatique [12,13] and that (3) fatique is a serious risk factor for (re)injuries [14,15].

According to the neuromuscular theory of exercise-associated muscle cramps, muscular fatigue is not only a risk factor but is a requirement for cramping [14]. Therefore, our finding that REAMC was associated with player position and with SumDental, indicates that both physical effort and poor oral health are associated with the development of muscular fatigue.

Our finding that injury anxiety was associated with past muscle or tendon reinjuries and with multiple types of past reinjuries, but not with repeated muscle cramps, is consistent with findings of previous studies, indicating a higher level of perceived risk of injury after an injury [36,37]. In accordance with the stress-injury model of Williams and Andersen [38], we found that psychophysical stress was associated with multiple types of past reinjuries.

Table 4 Univariate logistic regression analysis of other covariates with reinjury variables (n = 215)

	REAMC	MTR	MR
	OR (95% CI)	OR (95% CI)	OR (95% CI)
Injury anxiety			
1st Q (1.00 - 1.60)	reference category	reference category	reference category
2nd Q (1.61 - 1.80)	1.65 (0.61- 4.43)	1.94 (0.87- 4.36)	3.72**(1.63- 8.50)
3rd Q (1.81 - 2.20)	1.59 (0.62- 4.10)	3.41**(1.58-7.34)	3.67**(1.67- 8.07)
4th Q (2.21 - 3.40)	1.36 (0.46- 4.01)	2.41*(1.03- 5.68)	2.93*(1.22- 7.03)
Psychophysical stress			
1st Q (1.00 - 1.25)	reference category	reference category	reference category
2nd Q (1.26 - 1.42)	0.43 (0.16- 1.13)	0.49 (0.23- 1.03)	0.57 (0.27- 1.22)
3rd Q (1.43 - 1.50)	0.55 (0.22- 1.36)	0.74 (0.36- 1.52)	1.26 (0.62- 2.59)
4th Q (1.51 - 2.25)	0.99 (0.40- 2.46)	1.90 (0.84- 4.28)	3.45**(1.47- 8.09)
Dissatisfaction with t/t			
1st Q (1.00 - 1.17)	reference category	reference category	reference category
2nd Q (1.18 - 1.67)	0.87 (0.36- 2.10)	0.82 (0.39- 1.73)	1.17 (0.55- 2.49)
3rd Q (1.68 - 2.00)	0.43 (0.15- 1.29)	1.01 (0.45- 2.24)	1.22 (0.54- 2.76)
4th Q (2.01 - 3.83)	0.92 (0.35- 2.39)	0.82 (0.38- 1.84)	2.26 (0.99- 5.13)
Unhealthy eating habits			
1st Q (1.00 - 1.50)	reference category	reference category	reference category
2nd Q (1.51 - 2.00)	0.95 (0.34- 2.64)	1.59 (0.70- 3.59)	1.68 (0.75- 3.81)
3rd Q (2.01 - 2.50)	1.11 (0.36- 3.41)	1.73 (0.70- 4.27)	1.90 (0.77- 4.71)
4th Q (2.51 - 4.00)	1.49 (0.55- 4.03)	2.19 (0.96- 5.00)	2.19 (0.96- 5.00)
Age			
16-20 years	reference category	reference category	reference category
21-23 years	0.69 (0.27- 1.74	0.80 (0.39- 1.65)	0.71 (0.34- 1.47)
24-26 years	0.85 (0.29- 2.45)	0.50 (0.21- 1.20)	0.71 (0.30- 1.67)
27 years and older	1.16 (0.47- 2.84)	1.11 (0.52- 2.37)	1.19 (0.56- 2.54)
Playing position[a]	4.58***(1.93-10.85)	1.69 (0.97- 2.95)	1.31 (0.76- 2.27)

Legend: REAMC = Repeated Exercise-Associated Muscle Cramps; MTR = Muscle or Tendon Reinjury; MR = Multiple types of Reinjury; Dissatisfaction with t/t = Dissatisfaction with trainer/team; Q = quartile; *p < 0.05; **p < 0.01;. ***p < 0.001.
[a]reference qroup: lower intensity positions (goalkeeper, central defender and central defending midfielder).

Table 5 Crude and adjusted odds ratios for SumDental in relation to reinjury variables (n = 215)

Sum dental	REAMC		MTR		MR	
	Crude OR (95% CI)	Adj. OR[a] (95% CI)	Crude OR (95% CI)	Adj. OR[a] (95% CI)	Crude OR (95% CI)	Adj. OR[a] (95% CI)
As continuous variable	1.77* (1.12- 2.81)	1.82* (1.07- 3.12)	1.59* (1.10- 2.32)	1.57* (1.01- 2.45)	1.87** (1.28- 2.75)	1.88** (1.19- 2.97)
As ordered categorical variable						
0 = no oral health problems present	reference category	reference category	reference category	reference category	reference category	reference category
1 = one type of o.h.p. present	1.92 (0.84- 4.38)	2.39 (0.92- 6.22)	1.51 (0.82- 2.79)	1.56 (0.78- 3.13)	1.84 (0.99- 3.41)	2.16* (1.06- 4.39)
2 = two or more types of o.h.p. present	3.14* (1.24- 7.96)	3.33* (1.11- 9.96)	2.59* (1.20- 5.57)	2.48* (1.01- 6.09)	3.53** (1.61- 7.73)	3.40** (1.35- 8.59)

Legend: REAMC = Repeated Exercise-Associated Muscle Cramps, MTR = Muscle or Tendon Reinjury, MR = Multiple types of Reinjury; o.h.p. = oral health problems.
[a]adjusted by the covariates injury anxiety, psychophysical stress, unhealthy eating habits, dissatisfaction with trainer/team, age and player position, all these covariates were analyzed as categorical variables; *p < 0.05, **p < 0.01.

Strength and limitations of this study

This study is unique in that it is the first to examine the associations between poor oral health and reinjury risk of male elite soccer player, after adjusting for other covariates related to injury variables, i.e. injury anxiety, psychophysical stress, playing position and unhealthy eating habits. However, there are some important limitations of this study that deserve consideration.

Firstly, this study used self-reports on gum problems, restorations and apex resections. Clinical assessment of gum problems offers a much more reliable estimation than self-reports, but many researchers have argued that self- reports of gum problems are accurate enough for epidemiological studies [39]. With regard to the self-reported restorations and apex resections, it may be noted that self-reports of these dental services have been found valid [28]. Because of the chronic nature of dental diseases due to the ongoing presence of risk factors, we think that the likelihood of caries or apical periodontitis is higher in players with restorations or apex resections.

Secondly, self-reports on reinjuries were used. The reliability of these reports may be restricted due to response bias (i.e. denial of vulnerability), careless response and lack of insight into the type of reinjury. However, as lower identification and reporting generally results in lower associations, the associations found in this study can be regarded as conservative.

Thirdly, the scales of the questionnaire used in this study, the Sports Injury Risk Indicator, were not validated in previous studies. However, the items of the scales were extracted from previously validated scales, including the Tampa Scale for Kinesiophobia, the Sport Anxiety Scale, the Langner Index and the Athlete Satisfaction Questionnaire. In this study we assessed whether the selected items contributed to the reliability of the scales in our sample; items that lowered Cronbach's alpha were removed. In addition we presented the associations between the scales in the results section.

Fourthly, the respondents were not randomly selected from all professional soccer players. They were recruited from eight premier league clubs with a medical staff that had a positive attitude towards this functional approach. Moreover, because players from different clubs from only three countries were enrolled, generalization of the results may be further restricted.

Finally, as we used a retrospective cross-sectional design, the results offer only preliminary evidence for dental and psychosocial problems as intrinsic risk factors for reinjury. In addition, the generalization of our findings on reinjuries to injuries may be limited because of a more structural character of reinjuries compared with injuries. The relationships of sports injuries with dental and psychosocial problems may be somewhat weaker than the comparable relationships of sports reinjuries. Hence, the results of this study should be confirmed in a prospective study, in which self-reports of dental problems are substantiated by examination of orthopantomograms (OPTs), and injury and injury severity are recorded by teams' medical staff. Also recommended is research into the effects of improving or treating dental and occlusal problems on (re)injury risk in the longer term.

Conclusions

Our study found associations between poor oral health and the kinds of reinjury examined in this study, i.e. repeated exercise-associated muscle cramps, muscle or tendon reinjury and multiple types of reinjury. These associations persisted after adjusting for the other covariates, i.e. injury anxiety, psychophysical stress, unhealthy eating habits, dissatisfaction with trainer/team, age and player position. These results justify a more thorough examination of the impact of poor oral health on the reinjury risk of playing elite soccer.

Although this study is preliminary, the findings may stimulate the organisation of comprehensive dental and occlusal examination before the beginning of the soccer season, first as a contribution to the prevention of oral pathologies and a stimulation for oral hygiene, but also as a possible contribution to the prevention of reinjuries.

Abbreviations

REAMC: Repeated Exercise-Associated Muscle Cramps; MTR: Muscle or Tendon Reinjury; MR: Multiple types of Reinjury.

Competing interests

The authors declare that they have no competing interests.

Authors' contributions

HS was involved in original study design, data collection, manuscript preparation. AG was responsible for the analysis and interpretation of the study data, and contributed to all parts of the work of this study. LvdB was involved in the theoretical conceptualization and in the interpretation of the study data. All authors commented on the draft, read and approved the final manuscript.

Acknowledgements

We thank the clubs, coaches, medical staffs and players for their cooperation and Dr John Flutter, BDS for his valuable advice. Finally, we wish to thank the reviewers of this journal for their valuable insights and helpful suggestions.

Author details

[1]SportsInjuryLab, Box 3141, 3760 DC Soest, The Netherlands. [2]Physical Rehabilitation and Sports Medicine, Ghent University Hospital, De Pintelaan 185, 9000 Ghent, Belgium.

References

1. Ekstrand J. Playing too many matches is negative for both performance and player availability – results from the on-going UEFA injury study. Dtsch Z Sportmed. 2013;64:5–9.
2. Waldén M, Hägglund M, Ekstrand J. UEFA champions league study: a prospective study of injuries in professional football during the 2001–2002 season. Br J Sports Med. 2005;39:542–6.

3. Hawkins RD, Hulse MA, Wilkinson C, Hodson A, Gibson M. The association football medical research programme: an audit of injuries in professional football. Br J Sports Med. 2001;35:43–7.
4. Bahr R, Krosshaug T. Understanding injury mechanisms: a key component of preventing injuries in sport. Br J Sports Med. 2005;39:324–9.
5. Sheiham A. Oral health, general health and quality of life. Bull World Health Organ. 2005;83:644–4.
6. Ford PJ, Raphael SL, Cullinan MP, Jenkins AJ, West MJ, Seymour GJ. Why should a doctor be interested in oral disease? Expert Rev Cardiovasc Ther. 2010;2010(8):1483–93.
7. Gay-Escoda G, Vieira-Duarte-Perreira DM, Ardèvol J, Pruna R, Fernandez J, Valmaseda-Castellón E. Study of the effect of oral health on the physical condition of professional soccer players of Football Club Barcelona. Med Oral Patol. 2011;16:e436–9.
8. Sbordone L, Bortolaia C. Oral microbial biofilms and plaquerelated diseases: microbial communities and their role in the shift from oral health to disease. Clin Oral Investig. 2003;7:181–8.
9. Marsh PD. Dental plaque as a biofilm and a microbial community–implications for health and disease. BMC Oral Health. 2006;6 Suppl 1:S14.
10. Silva TA, Garlet GP, Fukada SY, Silva JS, Cunha FQ. Chemokines in oral inflammatory diseases: apical periodontitis and periodontal disease. J Dent Res. 2007;86:306–19.
11. Gornowicz A, Bielawska A, Bielawski K, Grabowska SZ, Wójcicka A, Zalewska M, et al. Pro-inflammatory cytokines in saliva of adolescents with dental caries disease. Ann Agric Environ Med. 2011;19:711–6.
12. Robson-Ansley PJ, de Milander L, Collins M, Noakes TD. Acute interleukin-6 administration impairs athletic performance in healthy, trained male runners. Can J Appl Physiol. 2004;29:411–8.
13. Ament W, Verkerke GJ. Exercise and fatigue. Sports Med. 2009;39:389–422.
14. Miller KC, Stone MS, Huxel KC, Edwards JE. Exercise-associated muscle cramps causes, treatment, and prevention. Sports Health. 2010;2:279–83.
15. Mair SD, Seaber AV, Glisson RR, Garrett Jr WE. The role of fatigue in susceptibility to acute muscle strain injury. Am J Sports Med. 1996;24:137–43.
16. Allen TJ, Leung M, Proske U. The effect of fatigue from exercise on human limb position sense. J Physiol. 2010;588:1369–77.
17. Reilly T, Drust B, Clarke N. Muscle fatigue during football match-play. Sports Med. 2008;38:357–67.
18. Borrell LN, Papapanou P. Analytical epidemiology of periodontitis. J Clin Periodontol. 2005;32 suppl 6:132–58.
19. Pihlstrom BL, Michalowicz BS, Johnson NW. Periodontal diseases. Lancet. 2005;366:1809–20.
20. Johnson U. Psychosocial antecedents to sport injury, prevention and intervention: an overview on theoretical approaches and empirical findings. Int J Sport Exerc Psychol. 2007;5:352–69.
21. Manfredini D, Castroflorio T, Perinetti G, Guarda-Nardini L. Dental occlusion, body posture and temporomandibular disorders: where we are now and where we are heading for. J Oral Rehabil. 2012;39:463–71.
22. Benoliel R. TMD: taxonomic mix-up beyond description. Quintessence Int. 2010;41:183.
23. Schroter S, Plowman R, Hutchings A, Gonzalez A. Reporting ethics committee approval and patient consent by study design in five general medical journals. J Med Ethics. 2006;32:718–23.
24. Centrale Commissie voor Mensgebonden Onderzoek, CCMO voor onderzoekers (Central Committee on Research involving Human Subjects, CCMO for researchers). [http://www.ccmo.nl/nl/help-mij-op-weg]
25. Raadgevend Comité voor Bio-ethiek: Advies nr. 40 van 12 februari 2007 betreffende het toepassingsgebied van de wet van 7 mei 2004 inzake experimenten op de menselijke persoon (Advisory Committee on Bioethics: Opinion no. 40 dated 12 February 2007 concerning the area of application of the law dated 7 May 2004 regarding experiments on the human person). [http://www.health.belgium.be/eportal/Healthcare/Consultativebodies/Commitees/Bioethics/Opinions/index.htm]
26. National Research Ethics Service. Does my project require review by a Research Ethics Committee? [http://www.hra.nhs.uk/research-community/before-you-apply/determine-which-review-body-approvals-are-required/]
27. Raymond P, White Jr RP, Madianos PN, Offenbacher S, Phillips C, Blakey GH, et al. Microbial complexes detected in the second/third molar region in patients with asymptomatic third molars. J Oral Maxillofac Surg. 2002;60:1234–40.
28. Gilbert GH, Rose JS, Shelton BJ. A prospective study of the validity of self-reported use of specific types of dental services. Public Health Rep. 2003;118:18–26.
29. Caplan DJ, Pankow JS, Cai J, Offenbacher S, Beck JD. The relationship between self-reported history of endodontic therapy and coronary heart disease in the atherosclerosis risk in communities study. J Am Dent Assoc. 2009;140:1004–12.
30. Roelofs J, Sluiter J, Frings-Dresen MHW, Goossens M, Thibault P, Boersma K, et al. Fear of movement and (re)injury in chronic musculoskeletal pain: evidence for an invariant two-factor model of the Tampa scale for Kinesiophobia across pain diagnoses and Dutch, Swedish, and Canadian samples. Pain. 2007;131:181–90.
31. Johnson DR, Meile RL. Does dimensionality bias in Langner's 22-item index affect the validity of social status comparisons? An empirical investigation. J Health Soc Behav. 1981;22:415–33.
32. Smith RE, Smoll FL, Schutz RW. Measurement and correlates of sportspecific cognitive and somatic trait anxiety: the sport anxiety scale. Anxiety Res. 1990;2:263–80.
33. Riemer HA, Chellandurai P. Development of the Athlete Satisfaction Questionnaire (ASQ). J Sport Exerc Psychol. 1998;20:127–56.
34. Di Salvo V, Baron R, Tschan H, Calferon Montero FJ, Bachl N, Pigozzi F. Performance characteristics according to playing position in elite soccer. Int J Sports Med. 2007;28:222–7.
35. Dellal A, Chamari C, Wong DP, Ahmaidi S, Keller D, Barros MLR, et al. Comparison of physical and technical performance in European professional soccer match-play: the FA premier league and La LIGA. Eur J Sport Sci. 2011;11:51–9.
36. Deroche T, Stephan Y, Woodman T, Le Scanff C. Psychological mediators of the sport injury—perceived risk relationship. Risk Anal. 2012;32:113–21.
37. Short SE, Reuter J, Brandt J, Short MW, Kontos AP. The relationships among three components of perceived risk of injury, previous injuries and gender in contact sport athletes. Athletic Insight. 2004;6:78–85.
38. Andersen MB, Williams JM. A model of stress and athletic injury: prediction and prevention. J Sport Exercise Psychol. 1988;10:294–306.
39. Bahekar AA, Singh S, Saha S, Molnar J, Arora R. The prevalence and incidence of coronary heart disease is significantly increased in periodontitis: a meta-analysis. Am Heart J. 2007;154:830–7.

11

The child and adolescent athlete: a review of three potentially serious injuries

Dennis Caine[1*], Laura Purcell[2] and Nicola Maffulli[3]

Abstract

The increased participation of children and adolescents in organized sports worldwide is a welcome trend given evidence of lower physical fitness and increased prevalence of overweight in this population. However, the increased sports activity of children from an early age and continued through the years of growth, against a background of their unique vulnerability to injury, gives rise to concern about the risk and severity of injury. Three types of injury–anterior cruciate ligament (ACL) injury, concussion, and physeal injury – are considered potentially serious given their frequency, potential for adverse long-term health outcomes, and escalating healthcare costs. Concussion is probably the hottest topic in sports injury currently with voracious media coverage and exploding research interest. Given the negative cognitive effects of concussion, it has the potential to have a great impact on children and adolescents during their formative years and potentially impair school achievement and, if concussion management is not managed appropriately, there can be long term negative impact on cognitive development and ability to resume sports participation. Sudden and gradual onset physeal injury is a unique injury to the pediatric population which can adversely affect growth if not managed correctly. Although data are lacking, the frequency of stress-related physeal injury appears to be increasing. If mismanaged, physeal injuries can also lead to long-term complications which could negatively affect ability to participate in sports. Management of ACL injuries is an area of controversy and if not managed appropriately, can affect long-term growth and recovery as well as the ability to participate in sports. This article considers the young athlete's vulnerability to injury, with special reference to ACL injury, concussion, and physeal injury, and reviews current research on epidemiology, diagnosis, treatment, and prevention of these injury types. This article is intended as an overview of these injury types for medical students, healthcare professionals and researchers.

Keywords: Anterior Cruciate Ligament (ACL) Tear, Concussion, Physeal injury, Children and adolescents

Introduction

Participation of children and adolescents aged 5–18 years in organized sports is increasingly popular and widespread in Western countries. It is not uncommon for teens to train 20 or more hours each week at regional training centers, or for youngsters as young as six to eight to play organized sports and travel with select teams to compete against other teams of similar caliber [1]. Regular physical activity during childhood and adolescence improves overall health and fitness and reduces risk for many chronic diseases [2]. While physical activity prevents all-cause morbidity associated with a sedentary lifestyle, injuries can become a barrier to participation in physical activity [3].

The increased involvement of children and adolescents in organized sports beginning at an early age raises concern regarding risk and severity of sport injury. Inevitably, with increased participation and training come increasing numbers of sports injuries. Sports and recreational injuries are the leading cause of injury in youth in many countries [3]. Three types of youth sports injury–anterior cruciate ligament (ACL) injury, concussion, and physeal injury–are the focus of much recent media and scholarly attention given their frequency, potential for adverse long-term health outcomes, and escalating healthcare costs [4-7]. If not managed appropriately, they can also lead to long term complications which could negatively affect ability to continue to participate in exercise and sports as well as

* Correspondence: dennis.caine@email.und.edu
[1]Department of Kinesiology and Public Health Education, University of North Dakota, Grand Forks, ND, USA
Full list of author information is available at the end of the article

threaten general health maintenance and contribute to obesity [8]. For example, more than 50% of patients show early signs of irreversible osteoarthritis within 10 years of ACL reconstruction [9].

Concussion is probably the hottest topic in sports injury currently [5,10] with voracious media coverage and exploding research interest. Given the negative cognitive effects of concussion, it has the potential to have a great impact on children and adolescents during their formative years and potentially impair school achievement and, if concussion management is not managed appropriately, there can be long term negative impact on cognitive development and ability to resume sports participation. Sudden and gradual onset growth plate injury is a unique injury to the pediatric population which can adversely affect growth if not managed correctly [6]. Although data are lacking, overuse injury of the physis is believed to be a growing problem among young athletes [11]. If mismanaged, epiphyseal injuries can also lead to long-term complications which could negatively affect ability to participate in sports [12]. Management of ACL injuries is an area of controversy and if not managed appropriately, can affect long-term growth and recovery as well as the ability to participate in sports [13].

This article considers the vulnerability of children and youth to injury, three types of injuries sustained by pediatric athletes which have the potential for long-term negative impact if not managed appropriately – ACL injuries, concussions, and growth plate injuries – and discusses the epidemiology, diagnosis, treatment, and prevention of these injury types. This article is intended as an overview of these injury types for medical students, healthcare professionals and researchers.

Epidemiology

Analysis of youth sport injury studies indicates that most injuries involve the knee and ankle [14]. For example, in a representative sample of 100 United States high schools involved in 9 sports during 2005–2007, ankle injury was most common (20.9%), followed by the knee (15.2%) [15]. However, the knee was the most common severely injured (more than 21 days' time loss) location (29%), accounting for 44.6% of all surgeries [16]. The most common knee injuries were ligament tears (45.4%), contusions (15.2%), and torn menisci (8.0%) [16]. A focus on ACL injuries is important, as these injuries may increase the risk of osteoarthritis in the future [12]. Notably, among 102 Swedish female soccer players injured before the age of 20 years, the prevalence of radiographic OA was 51% compared with 8% in the uninjured knee, 12 years later [17].

Although gridiron football was associated with the highest rate of ACL injuries among high school athletes, of particular interest are the higher rates of ACL injury seen in adolescent female athletes compared to males in sports like soccer, basketball and baseball/softball [4]. For example, Rechel et al. [18] reported that U.S. high school girls sustained more than twice as many complete ligament sprains than boys.

As a result of their frequency of occurrence and potential for catastrophic injury, pediatric concussions are viewed as a public health concern [19,20]. It is estimated that as many as 3.8 million concussions occur in the US per year during competitive sports; however, as many as 50% of concussions may go unreported [10]. More than 250,000 patients aged 8–19 years presented to emergency departments in the U.S. for sport-related concussions between 2001 and 2005 [21]. Gesell et al. [22], using data from the High School Reporting Information Online (RIO), reported that concussions represented 8.9%, or almost one out of ten of all high school injuries. A Canadian emergency department (ED) study of head injuries involving five EDs in Edmonton, Alberta found that the majority of sport-related head injuries occurred to individuals less than 20 years of age (66%). It also found that 53.4% of head injuries in children 10–14 years of age were sport-related [23].

Incidence rates for U.S. high school concussions during the 2008–2010 years were estimated to be 2.5 per 10,000 Athletic-Exposures (AE's) [24]. Football had the highest concussion rate (6.4), followed by boy's ice hockey (5.4) and lacrosse (4.0). In gender comparable sports, girls had a higher concussion rate (1.7) than boys (1.0).

Physeal injuries account for between 15% and 30% of all emergency room skeletal injuries in children [25]. A systematic review of the case series literature on growth plate injuries revealed that 38.3% of 826 acute cases were sport-related, and among these 45 (14.2%) were associated with some degree of growth disturbance [6]. These injuries occur in a variety of sports, although gridiron football is most often reported [6].

Most cohort studies reporting on the nature and incidence of pediatric sports injuries do not specify the frequency or severity of physeal fractures. Among cohort studies which do report acute physeal injuries, a range of from 1 to 30 percent of injuries are reported as physeal fractures [6]. Tabulation of the number of injuries (n = 3762) and number of acute physeal injuries (n = 536) in these studies reveals that 14.3% of all injuries were acute physeal injuries. However, these studies report injuries as a percentage of all injuries and do not provide incidence data based on participant exposure. Thus, knowledge of the incidence rate of acute physeal injuries is lacking and awaits the results of cohort studies where exposure data is meticulously monitored.

Although incidence data are lacking, there is evidence of the existence of stress-related physeal injury affecting young athletes participating in a variety of sports including baseball (proximal humerus), basketball (distal femur/ proximal tibia) climbing (phalanages), distance running (proximal tibia, first metatarsal growth plate), rugby (proximal tibia), gymnastics (clavicle, distal radius, proximal humerus), soccer (distal tibia/fibula), and tennis (proximal tibia) [6]. Most of these injuries resolved without growth complication during short-term follow-up. However, there are also reports of partial and complete epiphyseal closure in athletes representing basketball, baseball, dance, gymnastics, football, rugby and tennis [26-34]. These data are consistent with results from animal studies where prolonged intense physical training may precipitate pathological changes in the physis and, in extreme cases, produce growth disturbance [6].

Vulnerability to injury

The young athlete may be particularly vulnerable to sport injury because of the physical and physiological processes of growth. Injury risk factors unique to the young athlete and related to the three injury types considered in the present article include growth plate vulnerability, possible differences between biological and chronological age, the adolescent growth spurt, and differential growth [35]. Young athletes might also be at increased risk of injury because of immature or underdeveloped coordination, skills, and perception [36].

Growth plate vulnerability

Skeletally immature athletes are at risk for unique injuries not seen in adults, including growth plate fractures, apophysitis, apophyseal avulsion fractures, and greenstick fractures [35,37]. These unique injuries result from differences in the structure of growing bone compared to mature adult bone.

The differences between growing bone and mature bone include vulnerability of growth plates to shearing injury (at the epiphyseal-metaphyseal junction) resulting in growth plate fractures; vulnerability of apophyses to traction and strong muscle contractions resulting in apophysitis or avulsion injuries; and increased elasticity and resiliency of the metaphysis of long bones which, coupled with the thick periosteum typical of this age group, can result in greenstick or incomplete fractures [1,35,37,38]. Because of these differences, children and adolescents are more likely to injure bone or avulse an apophysis than to sprain a ligament or tear a muscle or tendon. However, it is also possible that the injury mechanism may be of sufficient magnitude and orientation to sprain a ligament or tear a muscle or tendon. Notably, ACL reconstruction in younger patients with significant growth remaining carries a risk of growth plate injury and growth disruption [39].

Adolescent growth spurt

The adolescent growth spurt appears to be a time of increased risk for sports injury. Some studies of the frequency of growth plate and other sports- and recreation-related injuries indicate an increased occurrence of injury during pubescence [40-42] and a noteworthy association between peak height velocity and peak fracture rate [43]. Peak adolescent fracture incidence at the distal end of the radius coincides with a decline in size-corrected bone mineral density (BMD) in both boys and girls. Peak gains in bone area preceded peak gains in bone mineral content (BMC) in a longitudinal sample of boys and girls, supporting the theory that the dissociation between skeletal expansion and skeletal mineralization results in a period of relative bone weakness [44]. Overuse or repetitive microtrauma can strain the musculotendinous units which may also occur more frequently during growth spurts [37,45].

The results of recent research suggests that increased quadriceps strength, combined with increased knee laxity and no accompanying hamstring strength development during the adolescent growth spurt in girls, might contribute to a decrease in their knee joint stability during landing tasks. These musculoskeletal changes could potentially increase anterior cruciate ligament injury risk at a time of rapid height and lower limb growth [46].

Sensorimotor function is not fully mature by the time children reach adolescence and some mechanisms may actually regress during this period [47]. Deficits in a variety of these same sensorimotor mechanisms have been correlated with increased ACL injury risk [48-50]. Notably, three studies reported that neuromuscular control of knee motion and landing forces is significantly worse in females than in males during the transition from prepubertal to pubertal stages, with females showing regressions in control abilities [51-53].

Differences between biological and chronological age

The structural, functional, and performance advantages of early-maturing boys in sports requiring size, strength, and power are well known. Children of the same chronological age may vary considerably in biological maturity status, particularly during adolescence, and individual differences in maturity status influence growth and performance during this period [54]. Bone age, which can be determined using standardized radiographs of the wrist, is one of the ways to assess biological age. Bone age does reflect the degree of maturity of the child, but it should be kept in mind that the appearance of bone can change between various ethnic groups.

Chronological age may add yet another dimension of individual variation, as most youth sports are categorized by chronological age. The fear is that an unbalanced competition between early- and late-maturing and/or older and younger boys in contact sports such as football and wrestling contributes to at least some of the serious injuries in these sports. For example, in a study of injury incidence in elite French youth football players, late-maturing boys sustained a significantly greater incidence rate of major injuries than early-maturing boys [55]. There were also differences between maturity groups when patterns of injury location, type, severity and re-injury were analyzed [55].

Differential growth

The normal growth pattern is nonlinear: differential growth of the body segments (head, trunk, and lower extremities) occurs throughout growth and influences body proportions accordingly [54]. At birth, the relative contribution of head and trunk to total stature is highest, and this declines through childhood into adolescence. Thus, the child is characterized by a proportionately larger head and trunk, and shorter legs compared with an adult. This "top-heavy" characteristic could predispose the young athlete to increased risk of injuries [35]. Although data are lacking it seems logical to presume, for example, that a young 'top-heavy' child would be at increased risk of falling in sports which involve riding on top of animals such as sheep (mutton-busting), camels (camel-racing), horses, or on top of various vehicles, including bicycles; or at increased risk of overuse injury in sport activities involving substantial running activity.

Child and adolescent athletes may have a more prolonged recovery and are more susceptible to concussion accompanied by catastrophic injury [5,10]. Children's greater head-to-body ratio and weaker neck muscles, combined with their relative nervous system immaturity, lesser myelinization, and thinner frontal and temporal bones, may predispose them to increased risk of head injury and concussion [56]. Concussion in the young athlete is also of specific concern because of their continuing cognitive maturation. Whereas the adult brain has achieved its operational skills for everyday life, the child's brain is still developing in areas of concentration, establishing memory patterns, reasoning, problem-solving, and other cognitive skills [56].

Diagnosis and management

ACL Tear

A focus on ACL injuries is important, as these injuries may increase the risk of osteoarthritis in the future [12]. The most common mechanism of ACL injury is a non-contact pivoting motion on a fixed foot or a trauma with the knee in hyperextension [57]. If a hemarthrosis develops within a few hours after the trauma in the absence of a bony injury there is a 70% chance of ACL injury [58]. The examiner should assess gait and alignment, range of motion, and assess the affected joint and compare it with the contralateral joint, taking into account that most children may have hyperlaxity which decreases with maturity [59]. Radiographs should be examined for bony injuries. Magnetic resonance imaging (MRI) can be useful in very experienced hands [60], but may be no better than accurate clinical examination [60].

The management of ACL deficiency in skeletally mature children is still controversial, especially in terms of operative timing and surgical technique [61]. Conservative management is not recommended, as it is accompanied by marked reduction in activity, decline in functional performance, and development of early osteoarthritis [62,63]. Historically, delayed anatomic ACL reconstructions were preferred [64], recommending extensive rehabilitation and return to activities with a brace to skeletal maturity and growth plate closure, to allow an anatomical adult-like reconstruction [65]. The present trend favours early reconstruction, using either extra physeal techniques in very young athletes, or anatomical reconstruction technique placing the tibial and femoral tunnels close to the centre on the growth plate of the tibia and femur in young athletes closer to skeletal maturity.

More anatomic physeal-sparing reconstruction techniques seems to be promising, but these techniques are technically challenging. Partial transphyseal techniques avoid the distal lateral femoral physis, providing more isometric tibial graft positioning and over the top reconstructions, provide excellent stability and return to sporting activities. Complete transphyseal ACL reconstruction is very similar to adult ACL reconstructions [66]. This procedure allows ideal tunnel placement and improves graft longevity and knee function, but the incidence of growth disturbance may increase, especially in very skeletally immature children [67-70].

In Tanner stage III or IV patients receiving transphyseal quadrupled hamstring autogenous ACL reconstruction, graft fixation to the femur with a suspension device and tibial fixation with interference screw have been promising [69]. Transphyseal reconstruction is recommended for patients with Tanner II and III stages, but the evidence in Tanner stage I patients is insufficient [70].

In general, Tanner stage IV-V children are considered adolescents without substantial growth remaining, and can be treated like adults. Tanner stage III children are considered "adolescents with substantial growth remaining" and a modified transphyseal reconstruction with soft tissue graft (hamstrings) small tunnels and avoiding fixatioin across the physis can be undertaken with little risk of physeal injury. Tanner stage I and II patients have significant growth remaining. In these children, management options are (1) brace and activity followed by delayed reconstruction when older; (2) extra-physeal reconstruction; or (3) partial/complete transphyseal, but this carries the risk of significant growth arrest. Complications of ACL reconstruction are rare, and most of the documented growth complications are secondary to surgeon errors such as placement of a fixation device across a growth plate [71,72]. With careful attention to surgical technique, paediatric ACL reconstruction can be safe and effective.

Concussion

Any direct blow to the head/face or a blow to the body that transmits a force to the brain can cause a concussion [5]. Signs and symptoms of concussion can be subtle and easily overlooked. These may include headache, nausea, dizziness, difficulty concentrating or remembering, confusion and emotional lability. Younger children may present with even more subtle signs, such as abdominal pain or behavioral changes [73]. Symptoms typically last for 7–10 days [5], although they may be prolonged for weeks to months [74-76]. In younger children, recovery may take longer [77,78]. Cognitive sequelae of concussion, including impaired memory, poor attention and lack of concentration, may negatively impact on a child's ability to learn and attend to schoolwork [74,75,78,79].

Management of concussions in pediatric athletes generally adheres to adult guidelines outlined in the Zurich Consensus Statement [5], but should be more cautious [80,81]. Children and adolescents take longer than adults to recover after a concussion, which underscores the need for a more conservative approach to management and return to play [56]. Any child or adolescent suspected to have sustained a concussion should be immediately removed from play and not allowed to return until cleared by a physician [5,80,81]. A concussion can be evaluated on the sideline by a coach or athletic trainer using a concussion tool such as the SCAT3 or Child SCAT 3 [5,80,81]. Assessment should include a neurological exam and assessment of attention and memory.

A physician should evaluate any athlete who has sustained a concussion as soon as possible after the injury to ensure proper diagnosis. Diagnostic imaging, such as CT or MRI, is generally not required.

Studies of concussion management in paediatric patients are sparse. One study of high school and college student athletes found that cognitive and physical rest immediately after injury, as well as later during recovery, resulted in improved symptoms and increased performance on computerized neuropsychological tests [82].

Consensus agreement is that rest, both physical and mental, is the keystone of concussion management [5,80]. Physical activities, including sports and exercise, and mental activities, including video games, TV, computer work, and reading, should be limited to allow symptoms to improve. Mental rest may require that a concussed athlete abstain from school or modify assignments/tests for a period of time to allow symptoms to decrease [5,81]. As symptoms improve, students can gradually increase cognitive tasks and social activities, including school, as long as symptoms are not exacerbated [5,83].

Return to learn is a vital component of concussion management in children and adolescents [84-86]. Mental rest can be challenging for students. Recovery may be prolonged if students participate in cognitive tasks that exacerbate symptoms, known as "cognitive overexertion" [84]. Students may need to abstain from school for a day or two until symptoms improve, and then gradually return (e.g., attending half-days or only certain courses), until they are able to attend full-time without exacerbating symptoms [75,81,84-86].

Students do not need to be symptom-free to return to school. However, students may require accommodation or modifications to their schedule to allow school participation without worsening symptoms [75,81,83,84,86]. Academic accommodations/modifications may include taking frequent breaks during the day, having a quiet area they can go to; shortened assignments, more time to complete assignments; limiting tests/exams to one per day, etc. [75,80,81,83,84,86]. Full return to academics must precede return to sports. If a prolonged absence from school (more than a couple of weeks) is necessary due to persistent symptoms, referral to a specialist with expertise in concussion, as well as a neuropsychologist, may be required.

Return to play decisions for pediatric athletes following a concussion can be difficult. Because of the different physiological response and longer recovery after concussion during childhood and adolescence, a more conservative return to play approach is recommended [5,80]. No athlete should return to sport/activity until all symptoms have resolved and medical clearance has been obtained. Pediatric athletes should be symptom-free for several days [80] prior to starting a gradual return to activity following a stepwise exertion protocol [5]. Each step should take a minimum of 24 hours [5,80,87]. If any symptoms return, the athlete should rest until symptoms resolve and then try going back to the previous asymptomatic step and be reassessed by a physician.

Specific factors may require modification of concussion management [5]. These modifying factors may include medications; a history of multiple prior concussions; younger age; and co-morbid conditions such as mental illness, attention deficit hyperactivity disorder, headache disorder, and learning disabilities. The presence of modifying factors may predict the potential for prolonged recovery and require additional management considerations, including formal neuropsychological testing and diagnostic imaging [5].

Governments are becoming increasingly cognizant of the importance of concussion awareness and are taking steps to improve concussion education. In the United States, the Lystedt Law was passed in 2009 recommending concussion education for athletes, parents and coaches [88]. In Canada, the Ontario Ministry of Education has mandated that all school boards in the province develop and enforce concussion policies [89].

Physeal injury

Disturbed physeal growth as a result of acute growth plate injury can result in limb length discrepancy, angular deformity, or altered joint mechanics [90]. Osteoarthritis may result from chondral damage at the time of growth plate injury, articular incongruity, or joint malalignment [91,92].

Epiphyseal injury may present with persistent or severe pain, visible deformity, or an inability to move or put pressure on a limb [93,94]. Swelling near a joint with focal tenderness over the physis may also be present. Lower extremity injuries may present as an inability to bear weight on the injured side; upper extremity injuries present with complaints of impaired function and reduced range of motion [95]. X-rays are typically used to determine whether a growth plate fracture has occurred. However, other diagnostic tests such as magnetic resonance imaging (MRI) or ultrasound, are also useful [96,97].

Management of acute epiphyseal plate injury depends on type of fracture. The system most widely used to describe acute growth plate injuries was developed by Salter and Harris (SH) and includes five types of injury [98]. In minimally displaced SH I and II injuries only symptomatic treatment may be necessary. However, if there is a wide displacement manipulation under anaesthesia with immobilization is indicated. The child is instructed to limit activities that impose pressure on the injured area. These injury types may be associated with growth impairment [99]. SH III and IV injuries are intraarticular, and operative anatomical reduction most often with internal fixation is necessary depending on patient age, fracture location, intra-articular displacement, and angulation. In these instances, the child needs to be followed up to skeletal maturity. Sometimes a growth arrest line may appear as a marker of the injury. SH V physeal injuries often result in partial or complete growth arrest. As a result, physeal bar resection may be required or other surgical procedures may be necessary to prevent or correct deformity [100].

Young athletes are also vulnerable to stress-related physeal injuries [6]. Symptoms of chronic epiphyseal plate injuries include pain on weight-bearing and decreased function. These injuries may not show evidence of abnormalities during early radiographs; however, growth arrest and/or angular malalignment may follow.

Physeal stress injuries are thought to develop when repetitive loading of the extremity disrupts metaphyseal perfusion which in turn inhibits ossification of the chondrocytes in the zone of provisional calcification [101]. The hypertrophic zone continues to widen as the chondrocytes continue to transition from the germinal layer to the proliferative zone [102]. Widening of the physis may be seen radiographically, whereas physeal cartilage extension into the metaphysis has been shown with magnetic resonance imaging [102,103].

Treatment for physeal stress injury is straightforward: rest from loading of the extremity [6,11,101]. However, in cases involving growth disturbance, corrective surgery may be required [29,30].

Physeal injury may also arise from ACL surgery. The current literature now supports the trend toward early operative treatment of ACL injury to restore knee stability and prevent progressive meniscal and/or articular cartilage damage, but the optimal approach to ACL reconstruction in this age group remains controversial [104]. Despite the reported clinical success of transphyseal reconstruction, iatrogenic growth disturbance secondary to physeal damage remains a genuine concern [104].

Injury prevention

ACL injury, concussion, and growth plate injury may cause significant discomfort and disability. Unfortunately, these injuries may also result temporarily or even permanently in reduced levels of physical activity, thus negating the potential benefits of sports participation for children and adolescents. Although it is impossible to eliminate these injuries, attempts to reduce them are obviously warranted. Unfortunately, the level of evidence regarding the prevention of these injuries is quite variable. Whereas, there has been considerable research to test preventive measures for ACL injury, there is a dearth of data available related to the prevention of concussion and physeal injury.

ACL injury

Preliminary data reveal that integrative neuromuscular training protocols implemented in pre-adolescent and early adolescent stages may artificially induce the neuromuscular spurt [105,106] and have the potential to reduce the risk of sports-related injury in young athlete [105-107]. Noyes & Barber-Westin [108] conducted a systematic review of studies which attempted to prevent ACL injuries in female athletes under the age of 19 years. Only 8 studies met inclusion criteria and of these, only three ACL intervention programs (Sportsmetrics, Prevent Injury and Enhance Performance, and Knee Injury Prevention) successfully reduced noncontact ACL injury incidence rates in female adolescent athletes. Ladenhauf et al. [109] recommend that young athletes should be encouraged to partake in preseason training programs focused on strengthening, neuromuscular and proprioceptive training units under the appropriate supervision of qualified personnel [109].

Concussion

Surprisingly, little research has tested interventions specifically related to concussion prevention. Modification of sporting rules, including padding of soccer posts and banning of spearing in American football have reduced concussive injuries [73]. There is also evidence that helmet use reduces head injury risk in skiing, snowboarding and bicycling, but the effect on concussion risk is inconclusive [110]. It is important to recognize that helmets are not concussion-proof [80,81].

Elimination of checking in youth hockey has also been shown to reduce the frequency of concussions [111]. For example, comparison of hockey leagues in Canada for 11–12 year old players finds that compared with leagues that do not allow body checking, those that do have an associated 3-fold increased risk of game-related injuries, including severe injuries and severe concussions [111].

Research indicates knowledge regarding concussion among youth sports coaches and athletes is limited [112,113], and that nearly half of concussions that occur each year go unreported [10]. Education programs designed to increase awareness of concussive symptoms are believed to reduce the incidence and reoccurrence of concussions, but have not been tested [56]. It is believed that concussion education initiatives should focus on improving attitudes and beliefs among athletes, coaches and parents to promote better care-seeking behaviors among young athletes [114]. Notably, three years after the passage of a concussion law in Washington State in the United States, high school football and soccer coaches are receiving substantial concussion education and have good concussion knowledge [88].

Coaches, athletic trainers, parents and athletes and anyone involved in youth sports should be educated about concussion and how to recognize and manage concussions. Encouraging fair play, respect for opponents and eliminating violence can help reduce the incidence of concussions. In addition, advising children to participate in non-contact sports, such as volleyball and swimming, or in non-contact leagues may also reduce concussions [80].

Physeal injury

Given the frequency of growth plate injury it is also surprising that little research has tested interventions specifically related to physeal injury prevention, including both acute and overuse injury. However, several preventive measures are worthy of consideration [6]. First, given the elevated susceptibility of the growth plate to injury during pubescence, coaches should reduce training loads and delay skill progressions for young athletes experiencing periods of rapid growth. Second, coaches should utilize a variety of drills or activities during practice to avoid excessively repetitive movements that may result in physeal overuse injury. Emphasis should be on quality and individualization of workouts rather than training volume. There should also be avoidance of single sports and year round sports prior to skeletal maturity, multi-game tournaments, and mandatory months off for recovery. Finally, clinicians need to educate parents and coaches as to the existence of overuse physeal injury and the need for rest to ensure proper recovery and return to sport participation.

Conclusion

The increased organized sports involvement of children from an early age, against a background of their unique characteristics and vulnerability to injury, raises concern about the risk and severity of sports-related injury in this population. Three types of injury–ACL tear, concussion, and physeal injury (both acute and overuse)–have become the focus of much recent attention due to their frequency, potential for adverse long-term health outcomes, and the financial burden of medical care. This paper provides an up-to-date review of current concepts and developments related to the epidemiology, diagnosis, management and prevention of these injuries.

Competing interests

The authors declare that they have no competing interests.

Authors' contributions

All three authors made substantive contributions to this review, including feedback on sections developed by the other co-authors. All authors contributed equally to the section on 'Vulnerability to Injury' and 'Epidemiology of Injury'. DC wrote the subsections related to 'Growth Plate Injury' as well as developing the first draft of the 'Introduction' and 'Conclusion' sections. LP wrote the subsections related to 'Concussion'. NM wrote the subsections related to 'ACL Tear'. All authors read and approved the final manuscript.

Author details

[1]Department of Kinesiology and Public Health Education, University of North Dakota, Grand Forks, ND, USA. [2]Department of Pediatrics, David Braley Sport Medicine and Rehabilitation Centre, McMaster University, Hamilton, ON, Canada. [3]Sports and Exercise Medicine, Queen Mary University of London, Barts and The London School of Medicine and Dentistry, William Harvey Research Institute, Centre for Sports and Exercise Medicine, Mile End Hospital, 275 Bancroft Road, London E1 4DG, UK.

References

1. Maffulli N, Caine D: **The epidemiology of children's team sports injuries.** In *Epidemiology of Pediatric Sports Injuries: Team Sports*, Med Sport Sci, Volume 49. Edited by Maffuli N, Caine D. Basel: Karger; 2005:1–8.
2. U.S. Department of Health and Human Services: *Physical Activity Guidelines Advisory Committee Report.* Washington, DC: U.S. Department of Health and Human Services; 2008.
3. Emery CA: **Injury prevention in paediatric sport-related injuries: A scientific approach.** *Br J Sports Med* 2010, **44:**64–69.
4. Shea KG, Grimm NL, Ewing CK, Aoki SK: **Youth sports anterior cruciate ligament and knee injury epidemiology: Who is getting injured? In what sports? When?** *Clin Sports Med* 2011, **30:**691–706.
5. McCrory P, Meewisse WH, Aubry M, Cantu B, Dvorak J, Echemendia RJ, Engebretsen L, Johnston K, Kutcher JS, Raftery M, Sills A, Benson B, Davis GA, Ellenbogen RG, Guskiewicz K, Herring ST, Iverson GL, Jordan BD, Kissick J, McCrea M, McIntosh AS, Maddocks D, Makdissi M, Purcell L, Putukian M, Schneider K, Tator CH, Turner M: **Concensus statement on concussion in**

sport: the 4th International Conference on Concussion in Sport held in Zurich, November 2012. *Br J Sports Med* 2013, **47**:250–258.

6. Caine D, DiFiori J, Maffulli N: **Physeal injuries in children's and youth sports: Reasons for concern?** *Br J Sports Med* 2006, **40**:749–760.
7. Nierenberg C: *Knee Injuries on the Rise in Young Athletes. WebMD Health News, October 17, 2011.* http://www.webmd.com/children/news/20111017/knee-injuries-on-the-rise-in-young-athletes.
8. Schub D, Saluan P: **Anterior cruciate ligament injuries in the young athlete: evaluation and treatment.** *Sports Med Arthrosc* 2011, **19**:34–43.
9. Hewett TE, Johnson DL: **ACL prevention programs: fact or fiction.** *Orthop* 2010, **33**:36–39.
10. Harmon KG, Drezner J, Gammons M, Guskiewicz K, Halstead M, Herring S, Kutcher J, Pana A, Putukian M, Roberts W: **American Medical Society for Sports Medicine Position Statement: concussion in sport.** *Clin J Sport Med* 2013, **23**:1–18.
11. DiFiori JP: **Overuse injury of the physis: a "growing" problem.** *Clin J Sport Med* 2010, **20**:336–337.
12. Caine DJ, Golightly YM: **Osteoarthritis as an outcome of paediatric sport: an epidemiological perspective.** *Br J Sports Med* 2011, **45**:52–56.
13. Frank JS, Gambacorta PL: **Anterior cruciate ligament injuries in the skeletally immature athlete: diagnosis and management.** *J Am Acad Orthop Surg* 2013, **21**:78–87.
14. Caine D, Caine C, Maffulli N: **Incidence and distribution of pediatric sport-related injuries.** *Clin J Sport Med* 2006, **16**:501–514.
15. Ingram JG, Fields SK, Yard EE: **Epidemiology of knee injuries among boys and girls in US High School Athletes.** *Am J Sports Med* 2008, **36**:1116–1122.
16. Darrow CJ, Collins CL, Yard EE, Comstock RD: **Epidemiology of severe injures among United States high school athletes, 2005–2007.** *Am J Sports Med* 2009, **37**:1798–1805.
17. Lohmander LS, Ostenberg A, Englund M, Roos H: **High prevalence of knee osteoarthritis, pain, and functional limitations in female soccer players twelvey ears after anterior cruciate ligament injury.** *Arthritis Rheum* 2004, **50**:3145–3152.
18. Rechel JA, Collins CL, Comstock RD: **Epidemiology of injuries requiring surgery among high school athletes in the United States, 2005 to 2010.** *J Trauma* 2011, **71**:982–989.
19. Wiebe DJ, Comstock RD, Nance ML: **Concussion research: a public health priority.** *Inj Prev* 2011, **17**:69–70.
20. MeehanWP III: **High school concussions in the 2008–2009 academic year.** *Am J Sports Med* 2010, **38**:2405–2409.
21. Bakhos LL, Lockhart GR, Myers R, Linakis JG: **Emergency department visits for concussion in young child athletes.** *Pediatrics* 2010, **126**:e550–e556.
22. Gessel LM, Fields SK, Collins CL, Dick RW, Comstock RD: **Concussions among United States high school and collegiate athletes.** *J Athl Tr* 2007, **42**:495–503.
23. Kelly KD, Liseeel HL, Rowe BH, Vincenten JA, Voaklander DC: **Sport and recreation-related head injuries treated in the emergency department.** *Clin J Sport Med* 2001, **11**:77–81.
24. Marar M, McIlvain NM, Fields SK, Comstock SD: **Incidence rates for U.S. high school concussions during the 2008–2010 academic years.** *Am J Sports Med* 2012, **40**:747–755.
25. Perron AD, Miller MD, Brady WJ: **Orthopedic pitfalls in the ED: pediatric growth plate injuries.** *Am J Emerg Med* 2002, **20**:50–54.
26. Albanese SA, Palmer AK, Kerr DR, Carpenter CN, Lisi D, Levinsohn EM: **Wrist pain and distal growth plate closure of the radius in gymnasts.** *J Ped Orthop* 1989, **9**:23–28.
27. Bak K, Boeckstyns M: **Epiphysiodesis for bilateral irregular closure of the distal radial physis in a gymnast.** *Scand J Med Sci Sports* 1997, **7**:363–366.
28. Ejnisman B, Andreoli CV, Pochini ADC, Monteiro GC, Faloppa F, Cohen M, Skaf AY: **Proximal humeral epiphysiolysis in a gymnast.** *Acta Ortop Bras* 2007, **15**:290–291.
29. Howe WB, Caine D, Bergman GD, Ross W: **Wrist pain-gymnastics.** *Med Sc Sports Exerc* 1997, **29**:S151.
30. Laor T, Wall EJ, Vu LP: **Physeal widening in the knee due to stress injury in child athletes.** *Am J Roentgenol* 2006, **186**:1260–1264.
31. Nanni M, Butt S, Mansour R, Cassar-Pullicino VN, Roberts A: **Stress-induced Salter–Harris I growth plate injury of the proximal tibia: first report.** *Skeletal Radiol* 2005, **34**:405–410.
32. Sato T, Shinozaki T, Fukudo T, Watanabe H, Aoki J, Yanagawa T, Takagishi K: **Atypical growth plate closure: a possible chronic Salter and Harris Type V injury.** *J Pediatr Orthop* 2002, **11**:155–158.
33. Shih C, Chang CY, Penn IW: **Chronically stressed wrists in adolescent gymnasts: MR imaging appearance.** *Radiol* 1995, **195**:855–859.
34. Shybut TB, Rose DJ, Strongwater AM: **Second metatarsal physeal arrest in an adolescent flamenco dancer: a case report.** *Foot Ankle Int* 2008, **29**:859–862.
35. Maffulli N, Caine D: **The Younger Athlete.** In *Clinical Sports Medicine.* 4th edition. Edited by Brukner P, Khan K. McGraw-Hill: Sydney; 2012.
36. National Center for Injury Prevention and Control: *CDC Injury Research Agenda 2009–2018.* Atlanta (GA): Centers for Disease Control and Prevention; http://www.cdc.gov/injury/researchagenda/.
37. Frank JB, Jarit GJ, Bravman JT, Rosen JE: **Lower extremity injuries in the skeletally immature athlete.** *J Am Acad Orthop Surg* 2007, **15**:356–366.
38. Demorest RA, Landry GL: **Training issues in elite young athletes.** *Curr Sport Med Reports* 2004, **3**:167–172.
39. AlHardy SW: **Anterior cruciate ligament injuries in growing skeleton.** *Int J Health Sci* 2010, **4**:71–79.
40. Flaschsmann R, Broom ND, Hardy AE, Moltschaniwyskyi G: **Why is the adolescent joint particularly susceptible to osteochondral shear fracture?** *Clin Orthop Relat Res* 2000, **381**:212–221.
41. Schuch T, Hanson C, Goodwin BJ, Romanick M, Caine D: **A hospital-based study of pediatric sport and recreational injuries.** *Med Sci Sports Exerc* 2012, **44**:S629.
42. Alexander CJ: **Effect of growth rate on the strength of the growth plate-shaft function.** *Skeletal Radiol* 1976, **1**:67–76.
43. Bailey DA, Wedge JH, McCulloch RG, Martin AD, Bernhardson SC: **Epidemiology of fractures of the distal end of the radius in children as associated with growth.** *J Bone Joint Surg Am* 1989, **71**:1225–1231.
44. Faulkner RA, Davison KS, Bailey DA, Mirwald RL, Baxter-Jones AD: **Size-corrected BMD decreases during peak linear growth: implications for fracture incidence during adolescence.** *J Bone Mineral Res* 2006, **21**:1864–1870.
45. Brenner JS: **Overuse injuries, overtraining and burnout in child and adolescent athletes.** *Pediatr* 2007, **119**:1242–1245.
46. Wild CY, Steele JR, Munro BJ: **Musculoskeletal and estrogen changes during the adolescent growth spurt in girls.** *Med Sci Sports Exerc* 2013, **45**:138–145.
47. Quatman-Yates CC, Quatman CE, Meszaros AJ, Paterno MV, Hewett TE: **A systematic review of sensorimotor function during adolescence: a developmental state of increased motor awkwardness?** *Brit J Sports Med* 2012, **46**:649–655.
48. Paterno MV, Schmitt LC, Ford KR, Rauh MJ, Myer GD, Huang B, Hewett TE: **Biomechanical measures during landing and postural stability predict second anterior cruciate ligament injury after anterior cruciate ligament reconstruction and return to sport.** *Am J Sports Med* 2010, **38**:1968–1978.
49. Hewett TE, Myer GD, Ford KR, Heidt RS Jr, Colosimo AJ, McLean SG, van den Bogert AJ, Paterno MV, Succop P: **Biomechanical measures of neuromuscular control and valgus loading of the knee predict anterior cruciate ligament injury risk in female athletes: a prospective study.** *Am J Sports Med* 2005, **33**:492–501.
50. Swanik CB, Covassin T, Stearne DJ, Schatz P: **The relationship between neurocognitive function and noncontact anterior cruciate ligament injuries.** *Am J Sports Med* 2007, **35**:943–948.
51. Ford KR, Myer GD, Hewett TE: **Longitudinal effects of maturation on lower extremity joint stiffness in adolescent athletes.** *Am J Sports Med* 2010, **38**:1829–1837.
52. Hewett TE, Myer GD, Ford KR: **Decrease in neuromuscular control about the knee with maturation in female athletes.** *J Bone Jt Surg Am* 2004, **86-A**:1601–1608.
53. Quatman CE, Ford KR, Myer GD, Hewett TE: **Maturation leads to gender differences in landing force and vertical jump performance: a longitudinal study.** *Am J Sports Med* 2006, **34**:806–813.
54. Malina RM, Bouchard C, Bar-Or O: *Growth, maturation and physical activity.* 2nd edition. Champaign: Human Kinetics; 2004.
55. Le Gall F, Carling C, Reilly T: **Biological maturity and injury in elite youth football.** *Scand J Med Sci Sports* 2007, **17**:564–572.

56. Guskiewicz KW, Valovich McLeod TC: **Pediatric sports-related concussion.** *PM&R* 2011, **3:**353–364.
57. Boden BP, Dean GS, Feagin JA Jr, Garrett WE Jr: **Mechanisms of anterior cruciate ligament injury.** *Orthopedics* 2000, **23:**573–578.
58. Luhmann SJ: **Acute traumatic knee effusions in children and adolescents.** *J Pediatr Orthop* 2003, **23:**199–202.
59. Hinton RY, Rivera VR, Pautz MJ, Sponseller PD: **Ligamentous laxity of the knee during childhood and adolescence.** *J Pediatr Orthop* 2008, **28:**184–187.
60. Kocabey Y, Tetik O, Isbell WM, Atay OA, Johnson DL: **The value of clinical examination versus magnetic resonance imaging in the diagnosis of meniscal tears and anterior cruciate ligament rupture.** *Arthroscopy* 2004, **20:**696–700.
61. Maffulli N, Del Buono A: **Anterior ligament tears in children.** *Surgeon* 2013, **11:**59–62.
62. Aichroth PM, Patel DV, Zorrilla P: **The natural history and treatment of rupture of the anterior cruciate ligament in children and adolescents. A prospective review.** *J Bone Joint Surg (Br)* 2002, **84:**38–41.
63. Pressman AE, Letts RM, Jarvis JG: **Anterior cruciate ligament tears in children: an analysis of operative versus nonoperative treatment.** *J Pediatr Orthop* 1997, **17:**505–511.
64. Woods GW, O'Connor DP: **Delayed anterior cruciate ligament reconstruction in adolescents with open physes.** *Am J Sports Med* 2004, **32:**201–210.
65. Moksnes H, Engebretsen L, Risberg MA: **Performance-based functional outcome for children 12 years or younger following anterior cruciate ligament injury: a two to nine-year follow-up study.** *Knee Surg Sports Traumatol Arthrosc* 2008, **16:**214–223.
66. Andrews M, Noyes FR, Barber-Westin SD: **Anterior cruciate ligament allograft reconstruction in the skeletally immature athlete.** *Am J Sports Med* 1994, **22:**48–54.
67. Cohen M, Ferretti M, Quarteiro M, Marcondes FB, de Hollanda JP, Amaro JT, Abdalla RJ: **Transphyseal anterior cruciate ligament reconstruction in patients with open physes.** *Arthroscopy* 2009, **25:**831–838.
68. Courvoisier A, Grimaldi M, Plaweski S: **Good surgical outcome of transphyseal ACL reconstruction in skeletally immature patients using four-strand hamstring graft.** *Knee Surg Sports Traumatol Arthrosc* 2011, **19:**588–591. Epub 2010 Oct 2.
69. Kocher MS, Smith JT, Zoric BJ, Lee B, Micheli LJ: **Transphyseal anterior cruciate ligament reconstruction in skeletally immature pubescent adolescents.** *J Bone Joint Surg Am* 2007, **89:**2632–2639.
70. Kaeding CC, Flanigan D, Donaldson C: **Surgical techniques and outcomes after anterior cruciate ligament reconstruction in preadolescent patients.** *Arthroscopy* 2010, **26:**1530–1538.
71. Kocher MS, Saxon HS, Hovis WD, Hawkins RJ: **Management and complications of anterior cruciate ligament injuries in skeletally immature patients: survey of the Herodicus Society and The ACL Study Group.** *J Pediatr Orthop* 2002, **22:**452–457.
72. Barber FA: **Anterior cruciate ligament reconstruction in the skeletally immature high-performance athlete: what to do and when to do it?** *Arthroscopy* 2000, **16:**391–392.
73. Lovell MR, Fazio V: **Concussion management in the child and adolescent athlete.** *Curr Sports Med Rep* 2008, **7:**12–15.
74. Iverson GL, Brooks BL, Collins MW, Lovell MR: **Tracking neuropsychological recovery following concussion in sport.** *Brain Inj* 2006, **20:**245–252.
75. Kirkwood MW, Yeates KO, Taylor HG, Randolph C, McCrea M, Anderson VA: **Management of pediatric mild traumatic brain injury: A neuropsychological review from injury through recovery.** *Clin Neuropsychol* 2008, **22:**769–800.
76. Sim A, Terryberry-Spohr L, Wilson KR: **Prolonged recovery of memory functioning after mild traumatic brain injury in adolescent athletes.** *J Neurosurg* 2008, **108:**511–516.
77. Fazio VC, Lovell MR, Pardini JE, Collins MW: **The relation between post concussion symptoms and neurocognitive performance in concussed athletes.** *Neuro Rehabilitation* 2007, **22:**207–216.
78. Kirkwood MW, Yeates KO, Wilson PE: **Pediatric sport-related concussion: A review of the clinical management of an oft-neglected population.** *Pediatr* 2006, **117:**1359–1371.
79. McCrory P, Collie A, Anderson V, Davis G: **Can we manage sport-related concussion in children the same as in adults?** *Br J Sports Med* 2004, **38:**516–519.
80. Purcell L, Canadian Paediatric Society, Healthy Active Living and Sport Medicine Committee: **Sport-related concussion: Evaluation and management.** *Paediatr Child Health* 2014, **19:**153–158.
81. Halstead ME, Walter KD, The American Academy of Pediatrics, Council on Sports Medicine and Fitness: **Clinical Report – Sport-related concussion in children and adolescents.** *Pediatr* 2010, **126:**597–611.
82. Moser RS, Glatts C, Schatz P: **Efficacy of immediate and delayed cognitive and physical rest for treatment of sports-related concussion.** *J Pediatr* 2012, **161:**922–926.
83. Davis GA, Purcell LK: **The evaluation and management of acute concussion differs in young children.** *Brit J Sports Med* 2013, **48**(2):98–101.
84. Sady MD, Vaughan CG, Bioia GA: **School and the concussed youth: Recommendations for concussion education and management.** *Phys Med Rehabil Clin N Am* 2011, **22:**701–719.
85. McGrath N: **Supporting the student-athlete's return to the classroom after sport-related concussion.** *J Athl Train* 2010, **45:**492–498.
86. Centers for Disease Control and Prevention: *Heads up to schools: Know your concussion ABC's.* 2010. http://www.cdc.gov/concussion/HeadsUp/high_school.html accessed 11 June 2014.
87. Purcell L: **What are the most appropriate return-to-play guidelines for concussed child athletes?** *Br J Sports Med* 2009, **43**(Suppl 1):i51–i55.
88. Chrisman SP, Schiff MA, Chung SK, Herring SA, Rivera F: **Implementation of concussion legislation and extent of concussion education for athletes, parents, and coaches in Washington State.** *Am J Sports Med.* doi:10.1177/0363546513519073.
89. Ontario Ministry of Education: *Policy/Program Memorandum No. 158: School Board Policies on Concussion.* Ontario, Canada; http://www.edu.gov.on.ca/extra/eng/ppm/158.pdf *(Accessed on 27 May 2014).*
90. Ogden JA: *Skeletal injury in the child.* New York: Springer-Verlag; 2000.
91. Bible JE, Smith BG: **Ankle fractures in children and adolescent.** *Techn Orthop* 2009, **24:**211–219.
92. Peterson HE: *Epiphyseal growth plate fractures.* Berlin: Spring-Verlag; 2007.
93. American Academy of Orthopedic Physicians: *Growth Plate Injuries.* http://orthoinfo.aaos.org/topic.cfm?topic=A00040.
94. National Institute of Arthritis and Musculoskeletal and Skin Diseases (NIAMS): *Growth Plate Injuries: Questions and Answers about Growth Plate Injuries 2011.* http://www.niams.nih.gov/Health_info/Growth_Plate_Injuries/default.asp#1.
95. Mehlman CT, Koepplinger ME: *Growth plate (physeal) fractures,* Medscape. http://emedicine.medscape.com/article/1260663-overview#showall.
96. Cutler L, Molloy A, Dhukuram V, Bass A: **Do CT scans aid assessment of distal tibial physeal fractures?** *J Bone Joint Surg Br* 2004, **86:**239–243.
97. Boutis K, Narayanan UG, Dong FF, Mackenzie H, Yan H, Chew D, Babyn P: **Magnetic resonance imaging of clinically suspected Salter-Harris I fracture of the distal fibula.** *Injury* 2010, **41:**852–856.
98. Salter RB, Harris WR: **Injuries involving the epiphyseal plate.** *J Bone Jt Surg (USA)* 1963, **45:**587–622.
99. Barmeda A, Gaynor T, Mubarek SJ: **Premature closure following distal tibia physeal fractures.** *J Pediatr Orthop* 2003, **33:**733–739.
100. Lee SH, Lee DH, Baek JR: **Proximal humerus Salter type III physeal injury with posterior dislocation.** *Arch Orthop Trauma Surg* 2007, **127:**143–146.
101. DiFiori J, Caine D, Malina R: **Wrist pain, distal radial growth plate injury, and ulnar variance in the young gymnast.** *Am J Sports Med* 2006, **34:**840–849.
102. Jaramillo D, Laor T, Zaleske DJ: **Indirect trauma to the growth plate: results of MR imaging after episphyseal and metaphyseal injury in rabbits.** *Radiology* 1993, **187:**171–178.
103. Dwek JR, Cardoso F, Chung CR: **MR imaging of overuse injuries in the skeletally immature gymnast: spectrum of soft-tissue and osseous lesions in the hand and wrist.** *Pediatr Radiol* 2009, **39:**1310–1316.
104. Fabricant PD, Jones KJ, Delos D, Cordasco FA, Marx RG, Pearle AD, Warren RF, Green DW: **Reconstruction of the anterior cruciate ligament in the skeletally immature athlete: a review of current concepts: AAOP exhibit selection.** *J Bone Joint Surg Am* 2013, **e28:**1–13. doi:10.2106/JBJS.L.00772.
105. Hewett TE, Lindenfeld TN, Riccobene JV, Noyes FR: **The effect of neuromuscular training on the incidence of knee injury in female athletes: A prospective study.** *Am J Sports Med* 1999, **27:**699–706.
106. Myer GD, Brunner HI, Melson PG, Paterno MY, Ford KR, Hewett TE: **Specialized neuromuscular training to improve neuromuscular function and biomechanics in a patient with quiescent juvenile rheumatoid arthritis.** *Phys Ther* 2005, **85:**791–802.

107. Myer GD, Ford KR, Barber Foss KD, Liu C, Nick TG, Hewett TE: **The relationship of hamstrings and quadriceps strength to anterior cruciate ligament injury in female athletes.** *Clin J Sport Med* 2009, **19**:3–8.
108. Noyes FR, Barber-Westin SD: **Neuromuscular retraining intervention programs: do they reduce noncontact anterior cruciate ligament injury rates in adolescent females?** *Arthroscop* 2014, **30**:245–255.
109. Ladenhauf HN, Graziano J, Robert G, Marx RG: **Anterior cruciate ligament prevention strategies: are they effective in young athletes – current concepts and review of literature.** *Curr Opin Pediatr* 2013, **25**:64–71.
110. Schiff M, Caine D, O'Halleron R: **Injury prevention in sports.** *Am J Lifestyle Med* 2010, **4**:42–64.
111. Emery CA, Kang J, Shrier I, Goulet C, Hagel BE, Benson BW, Nettel-Aguirre JR, McAllister JR: **Risk of injury associated with body checking among Youth Ice Hockey Players.** *JAMA* 2010, **303**:2265. doi: 10.1001/jama.2010.755.
112. McCrea M, Hammeke T, Olsen G, Leo P, Guskiewicz K: **Unreported concussion in high school football players: Implication for injury prevention.** *Clin J Sport Med* 2004, **14**:13–17.
113. Valovich McLeod TC, Schwartz CD, Bay RC: **Sport-related concussion misunderstanding among youth coaches.** *Clin J Sport Med* 2007, **17**:140–142.
114. Register-Mihalik JK, Linnan LA, Marshall SW, Valovich McLeod TC, Mueller FO, Guskiewicz KM: **Using theory to understand high school aged athletes' intentions to report sport-related concussion: implications for concussion education initiatives.** *Brain Inj* 2013, **27**:878–886.

12

Reliability of the Q Force; a mobile instrument for measuring isometric quadriceps muscle strength

K. W. Douma[1,2*], G. R. H. Regterschot[3], W.P. Krijnen[1], G. E. C. Slager[4], C. P. van der Schans[1,2] and W. Zijlstra[5]

Abstract

Background: The ability to generate muscle strength is a pre-requisite for all human movement. Decreased quadriceps muscle strength is frequently observed in older adults and is associated with a decreased performance and activity limitations. To quantify the quadriceps muscle strength and to monitor changes over time, instruments and procedures with a sufficient reliability are needed. The Q Force is an innovative mobile muscle strength measurement instrument suitable to measure in various degrees of extension. Measurements between 110 and 130° extension present the highest values and the most significant increase after training.
The objective of this study is to determine the test-retest reliability of muscle strength measurements by the Q Force in older adults in 110° extension.

Methods: Forty-one healthy older adults, 13 males and 28 females were included in the study. Mean (SD) age was 81.9 (4.89) years. Isometric muscle strength of the Quadriceps muscle was assessed with the Q Force at 110° of knee extension. Participants were measured at two sessions with a three to eight day interval between sessions. To determine relative reliability, the intraclass correlation coefficient (ICC) was calculated. To determine absolute reliability, Bland and Altman Limits of Agreement (LOA) were calculated and t-tests were performed.

Results: Relative reliability of the Q Force is good to excellent as all ICC coefficients are higher than 0.75. Generally a large 95 % LOA, reflecting only moderate absolute reliability, is found as exemplified for the peak torque left leg of −18.6 N to 33.8 N and the right leg of −9.2 N to 26.4 N was between 15.7 and 23.6 Newton representing 25.2 % to 39.9 % of the size of the mean. Small systematic differences in mean were found between measurement session 1 and 2.

Conclusion: The present study shows that the Q Force has excellent relative test-retest reliability, but limited absolute test-retest reliability. Since the Q Force is relatively cheap and mobile it is suitable for application in various clinical settings, however, its capability to detect changes in muscle force over time is limited but comparable to existing instruments.

Keywords: Quadriceps, Isometric muscle strength, Q force, Elderly

* Correspondence: k.w.douma@pl.hanze.nl
[1]Research and Innovation Group in Healthy Aging, Allied Health Care and Nursing, Hanze University of Applied Sciences Groningen, Groningen, The Netherlands
[2]Department of Rehabilitation Medicine, University of Groningen, University Medical Center Groningen, Groningen, The Netherlands
Full list of author information is available at the end of the article

Background

Muscle strength is essential for all physical activities such as activities of daily living, work, sports and maintaining posture [1–4]. Reduced muscle strength is frequently apparent in older participants and creates a potential risk for a decline of activities. It may induce balance deficits, a risk of falling [3–10], and predisposition for disability, premature nursing home admission, and ultimately premature mortality [5, 11]. Also functional walking tests and rising tests, such as the timed up and go test, are used to predict the occurrence of future falls. Retrospective studies show that these tests are associated to a history of falls, the predictive capability however is limited [8, 11–13].

The quadriceps muscle is prominently important due to its major contribution to activities such as walking stairs, rising from a chair, and walking [3, 4, 7].

To quantify Quadriceps muscle strength and to monitor changes over a period of time, a muscle strength measurement with high reliability is required. Several viable quantitative muscle strength measurement methods are available. The Medical Research Counsel Scale (MRC) is the most commonly and clinically used method. The MRC scale ranges over 6 grades, 0 to 5. Unfortunately, this scale is inaccurate and inefficient in detecting changes over a period of time [14–18]. MRC grade 4 covers a wide range from 4 up to 99 % of the generated strength [19]. More precise measurements are possible with handheld dynamometry allowing muscle strength to be measured on a continuous scale. Handheld dynamometry has been demonstrated to have good reliability according to the intra class correlation coefficient of 0.8 or higher [19–22]. Measurements with a handheld dynamometer, however, are required to be performed in a reproducible joint position of 90° flexion [23–25]. Joint positions other than 90° flexion however, have exhibited greater maximal muscle strength values [26–28], as well as more extensive sensitivity when detecting changes over time [27]. For the knee the highest values were recorded by measurements at 110 and 130° extension and the most significant increase after training was determined in a knee angle position between 110 and 130° extension [28]. Another possible limitation of handheld dynamometry is the variance induced by different observers, i.e., certain patients restrain their efforts when working with presumed weaker observers. Consequently, fixation during measurement in healthy participants might be difficult [22, 23, 29]. The fixation possibilities of the observers are limited when using handheld dynamometry and this may negatively influence reliability and validity of muscle strength measurements [22, 23, 30]. An additional relevant aspect in any non-computerized type of muscle strength measurement is that it does not provide insight into coordination, slope, or duration of the contraction. Sustainable and repetitive contractions, however, are required in sports, and activities of daily living.

Another type of muscle strength measurement is isokinetic muscle strength measurement. Isokinetic equipment is capable of measuring from different body positions and angles, presenting an abundance of graphical, numerical, and derivative information which are considered to be the gold standard. The equipment, however, is expensive and immobile, and the procedure is time consuming.

The Q Force chair has been recently developed as a successor of the Quadriso Tester [31] to measure isometric muscle strength of the Quadriceps muscle in different joint angles. Advantages of the Q Force compared to other instrumentation is that it is transportable and can be employed easily in a clinical setting as for example a hand held dynamometer. It provides however as isokinetic instrumentation, relevant graphical, numerical and derivative information about the contraction besides measured peak values.

However, the test-retest reliability of the Q Force in older adults is unclear. Therefore the purpose of this study was to determine the test retest reliability of muscle strength measurements with the Q Force in older adults.

Methods

The Medical Ethics Committee of the University Hospital Groningen approved this study.

All participants gave written informed consent before data collection began.

Participants

In this study, inclusion criteria were:

*At least 70 years of age, being able to walk ≥10 m without support, and rise from a chair without resources or assistance;

*Absence of cardiovascular/respiratory or neurological disorders;

*No comorbidity or cognitive disorders that influence mobility, understanding, or execution of measurements. No current or recent participation in exercise programs or any other physical intervention;

*No orthopedic surgery or stroke within the last six months;

Participants were included after providing and signing informed consent. The Medical Ethics Committee of the University Medical Center Groningen, The Netherlands, approved the study protocol.

Design

Muscle strength was assessed on two occasions within three to eight days. Four trials were performed on each occasion at approximately the same time of the day. If the participant was unable to perform four trials for any reason, fewer repetitions were performed and used for analysis

Device

The Q Force (Fig. 1) has been constructed for measuring isometric Quadriceps muscle strength. It consists of a chair with an attached, adjustable fixed leg brace at the front (Fig. 2). Three sensors are located in the brace to determine the generated force (Newton); the angle between the horizontal chair surface and the brace and the distance between the force transducer and the rotation axle of the brace (millimeter). All three signals pass through an analog-digital converter, are read and saved on a laptop.

The chair incorporates a solid frame, base, back support, and a seat. Bars are fitted at both sides of the seat for manual fixation. The height of the sitting surface is fully adjustable. At the left and right bottom of the seat, in an anterior posterior direction, rails are attached to which the brace is connected so that both the left and right leg can be tested. The fixed brace consists of a

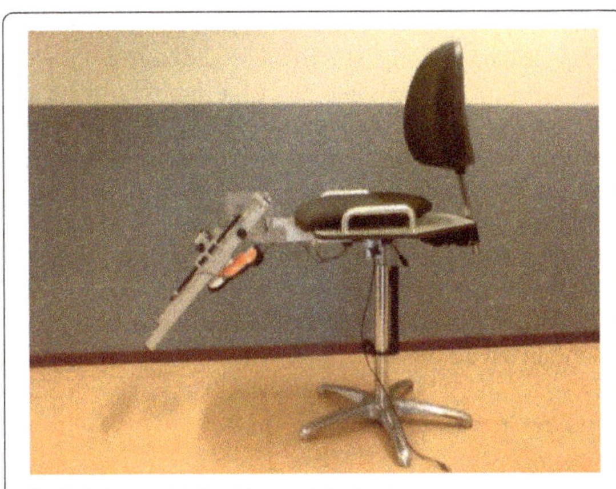

Fig. 2 Q Force with fixed brace at the front

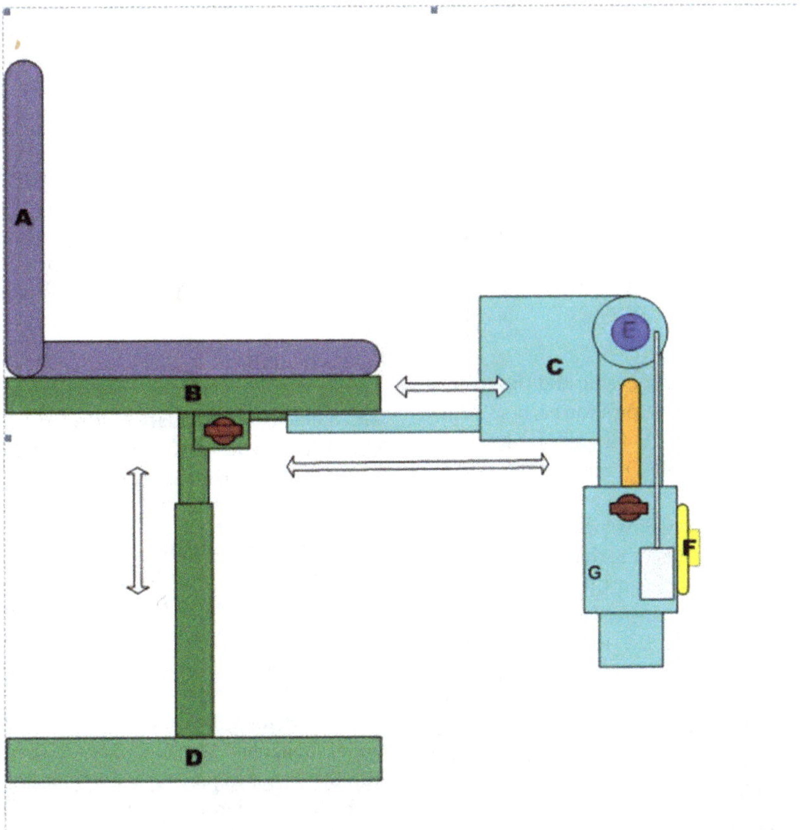

Fig. 1 Schematic view, Q Force. **a** = Back support, **b** = Seat, **c** = Fixed brace, **d** = Base, **e** = Astrolabe/Goniometer, **f** = Force transducer, **g** = Distance transducer

fixed horizontal and an adjustable distal component with a hinge in between; the brace can be slid horizontally via rails. The brace is adjustable to fit the subject's upper leg dimensions. This affords placing the rotation axle of the brace in the same position as the rotation axle of the knee for that specific angle (Fig. 3). The measuring angle of the fixed brace is adjustable between 90° and 180°. The force transducer is covered with a pad to minimize pressure on the subject's lower leg. The position of the pad is adjustable in vertical and horizontal directions in accordance with the subject's dimensions.

Computer and control

Hardware

The hardware consists of an analog-digital converter, a force, and a distance and angle transducer. The ADC is an NI-9219 4Ch Universal Analog input module. As an interface, the NI USB-9162 converter is utilized for establishing a USB connection between the ADC and the laptop. National Instruments Corporation Austin. The force transducer is an LLB400 Loadcell which is capable of measuring force up to 1100 Newton with a break load of 1650 Newton (Futek, Irvine). The distance transducer is a CLS1321 Linear potentiometer (Active Sensors Indianapolis). The angle is measured by a single strike potentiometer.

Software

The accompanying software is developed by the ICT Software Development Laboratory of the Faculty of Medical Sciences from the University of Groningen and the University Medical Center Groningen in the Netherlands.

Outcome measures

We measured and calculated a peak value and three different average torque operationalization's for each separated measurement; Peak Torque (PT), Filtered Peak Torque (FPT), Median Peak Torque (MPT) and Average Plateau Peak Torque (APT).

PT is the actually measured peak value and is calculated as Fmax * r + fixation torque. Fmax is the registered maximal force; r is the distance between the knee joint rotation point and the sensor on the lower leg; fixation torque is the torque required keeping the lower leg stabilized against gravity. Arrow 2 in Fig. 3 illustrates the PT value.

Filtered Peak Torque is the average peak torque of the sample that recorded the PT value [1] with the sample before (−1) and the sample after (+1) this sample and is calculated as $\mathrm{FPT} = \left(\frac{total\ torque\ (i-1)+total\ torque\ (i)+totaltorque\ (i+1))}{3}\right.$.

Arrow 1 and 3 in Fig. 3 indicate FPT.

MPT is defined as the median of the total torque above the level of 0.5 * PT. This is calculated as: median total torque = median (total torque (a:b)) whereby *a* is defined as the moment where total torque is greater than 0.5 * PT for the first time, and *b* is defined as the moment where total torque is smaller than 0.5 * PT for the first time. Line a-b in Fig. 4 represents 50 % of the PT level. Line c-d represents the MPT.

APT is the value above 50 % of the PT level. It is the average peak torque over the plateau phase. It is calculated as: average (total torque (c : d)) *c* is defined as the initial sample following sample *a* when the absolute difference with sample c −1 is less than 4 Nm. Sample *d* is defined as the sample following sample *a* where the absolute difference with sample d −1 is smaller than 4 Newtonmeter (Nm). Point *e* in Fig. 4 represents the first sample where the increase of the generated force is less than 4 Nm, and point *f* represents the last sample where the decline of the generated force *f* is less than 4 Nm. Line *e-f* represents the calculated value. This signifies that a plateau phase between samples c and d can be recognized in which the absolute differences between the sequential samples during this plateau are less than 4 Nm. This was considered a reliable contraction [30] representing the maximum generated torque. The level of elevation of this plateau corresponds with the generated torque. The mass and center of gravity of the lower leg were calculated according to Winter 1979 [32]. The sample ratio which recorded the generated forces was 2Hz.

Fig. 3 represents a graphic interpretation of the outcome measures. The vertical axis represents the generated torque while the horizontal axis represents the time. The letters g and h correspond with the start and the end of the contraction, a-b represents 05 * PT level, c-d represents the MPT and e-f represents the APT.

Data acquisition

All algorithms for data acquisition were programmed and collected in Matlab Mathworks 7, Nathick, USA. The collected data were transferred to Microsoft Excel 2010 files for statistical analysis.

Measurement procedure

The angle of the fixed leg brace was positioned at 110°, and the subject was subsequently positioned in the chair without back support and with the back of their knee positioned against the seat. The lateral condyle of the femur was aligned with the rotation point of the Q Force. The force transducer was positioned 3 cm above lateral malleolus. The tuberosity of the tibiae was aligned with the sensor to prevent adduction, abduction, or rotation in the knee or hip in the starting position. The computer program was initiated as the subject was instructed to elevate the leg to minimize pressure on the force transducer in order to calibrate the system. The distance between the

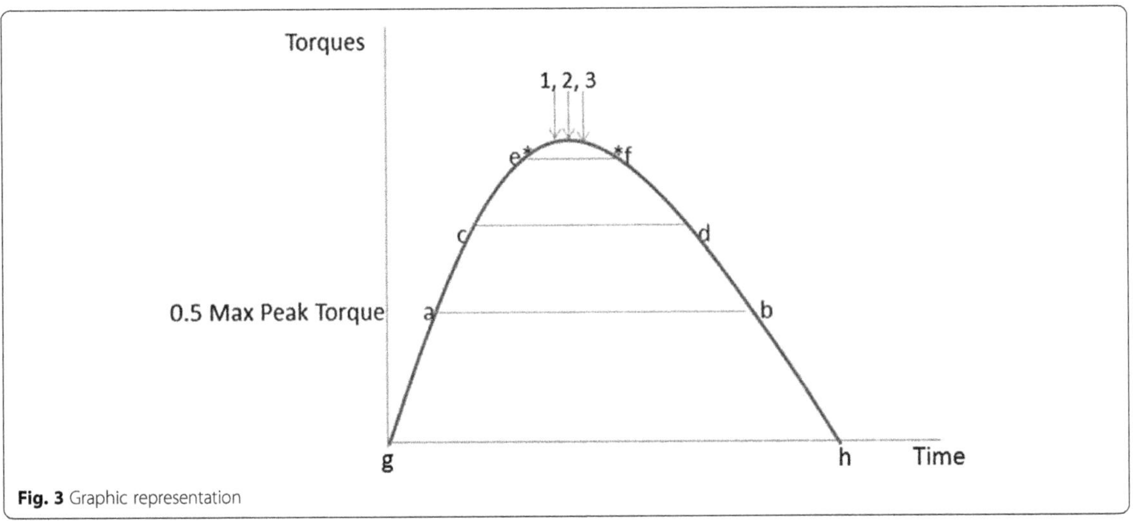

Fig. 3 Graphic representation

transducer and the rotation point was determined to calculate the generated torque and the average knee angle. Additionally, the average distance from the rotation axle to the force transducer was measured to determine whether the current angle was actually 110°. Following the calibration, the actual measurement began whereby the left leg was tested first. Participants were allowed to fixate themselves to the sidebars using their hands. Four trials were performed for each leg. If the subject was not capable of performing four trials for any reason, fewer repetitions were performed and applied to the analysis. A 1 min break was administered between the successive trials. Following each trial, it was evaluated if the contraction had been maximal by asking, "Was this a maximal effort?" If the contraction had not been maximal, it was excluded.

Instruction of the participant

The participants were instructed as follows: "Extend your knee as forceful as possible. I will measure the strength you will generate. You are allowed to fixate yourself to the side bars using your hands. Each leg is tested four times each with a one minute break in between. I will encourage you and tell you when to start and when to stop. The maximal contraction has to endure for three seconds. Build up your contraction gradually and let go slowly.

Statistical analyses

All data were analyzed with the statistical programming language string R version 3.1.2 2014.

To determine relative reliability, the two-way absolute agreement variant of the intraclass correlation coefficient (ICC) was calculated. To determine absolute reliability the Bland and Altman limits of agreement (LOA) were calculated according to 1.96 * SD of the mean difference [33]. The LOA were calculated for each pair of measurements and were interpreted with regard to the clinical relevance to their size.

Bland and Altman plots were constructed with the difference and the mean of the of the two measurements for each subject. Means, standard deviation, mean difference, and standard deviations were calculated for descriptive purposes. The paired t-test was used to test for systematic differences in mean between session 1 and session2. ICCs were interpreted as: ICC < 0.25 low; 0.25 < ICC < 0.50 moderate; 0.50 < ICC < 0.75 moderate to good; and ICC > 0.75 is excellent reliability [34–36]. A level of 0.05 was considered significant.

Results

Participants

Forty-one healthy older adults were included in the study comprised of 13 males and 28 females. Mean (SD) of age was 81.9 (4.89) years; of body weight was 78.5 (13.0) kg; and of body height 165.3 (5.8) cm.

Outcome measures

Table 1 presents the reliability results of session1 and session 2 for the left and right leg.

All differences between Session1 and Session2 are significant according to the Paired T-Test. It can be observed from Table 1 that the ICC coefficients are higher for the right than for the left leg and all ICC coefficients are greater than 0.75. The LOA's are smaller for the right leg compared to the left and are in general relatively large, 17.6 to 26.5 Newton, and represent values between 25.2 % to 39.9 % of the mean measured values of session 1 and session2. The LOAs are smaller for the right than for the left leg.

Figures 4, 5, 6, 7, 8, 9, 10 and 11 present Bland and Altman plots of the limits of agreement between session1 and session2 measurements of the mean Peak Torque; the

Table 1 Shows the intraclass correlations, the t-test outcomes and the LOA's for the left and right leg

		Session 1	Session 2	diff		*P* value			
		Mean (SD)	Mean (SD)	Mean (SD)	t-test	ICC	L. Loa	U. Loa	Loa % Mean
PT	left	63.1 (27.2)	70.7 (29.2)	7.6 (13.4)	0.0078	0.89	−18.6	33.8	39.1
PT	right	66.1 (30.4)	74.8 (34.2)	8.6 (9.1)	0.0001	0.96	−9.2	26.4	25.1
FPT	left	62.5 (27.0)	70.2 (29.1)	7.7 (13.5)	0.0077	0.88	−18.8	34.2	39.9
FTP	right	65.6 (30.3)	74.0 (34.1)	8.4 (9.1)	0.0001	0.96	−9.4	26.2	25.5
MPT	left	58.5 (26.0)	66.4 (28.5)	7.9 (12.5)	0.0037	0.89	−16.6	32.4	39.2
MPT	right	62.0 (29.1)	69.9 (32.9)	7.9 (9.0)	0.0001	0.96	−9.7	25.5	26.7
APT	left	58.3 (26.2)	65.9 (28.6)	7.6 (12.9)	0.0058	0.80	−17.6	32.8	38.7
APT	right	61.8 (29.6)	70.2 (33.5)	8.4 (9.1)	0.0001	0.96	−9.4	26.2	26.9

PTL Peak Torque, *FTP* Filtered Peak Torque, *MPT* Median Peak Torque, *APT* Average Plateau Peak Torque, expressed in Newton, * *Significant level; ≤ 0.01, ICC; Intraclass Correlation Coefficient, L.LOA; Lower Limits of Agreement, U. LOA upper Limits of Agreement. LOA as percentage of mean of session1 and session 2*

mean Median Peak Torque; the mean Plateau Peak Torque; and the mean Filtered Peak Torque of the left and right leg, respectively.

The uninterrupted horizontal line is located above zero in all cases due to the systematic difference between Session1 and Session2. The variation of all of the measurements is not increasing with increasing Q Force torque, and there are only minimal outlying points observed. The right leg measurements result in smaller LOA than those for the left.

Discussion

The outcomes of this study indicate that muscle strength measurements with the Q Force at 110° flexion of the knee are reliable according to the ICC coefficients. The ICC coefficients exceed 0.75 which indicate excellent relative test-retest reliability [34–36]. However, the obtained LOA's are substantial indicating moderate absolute reliability. The mean values at the second measurement are significantly higher than those at the first measurement. The encountered ICC and LOA presented are consistently better for the right leg compared to the left.

The obtained ICC coefficients indicate that the Q Force is capable of reliably measuring muscle strength on group level [34–36]. The encountered ICC coefficients are between 0.80 and 0.95 and therefore consistent with coefficients determined in other muscle strength measurement reliability studies [20–23, 29, 37, 38, 40, 41]. The

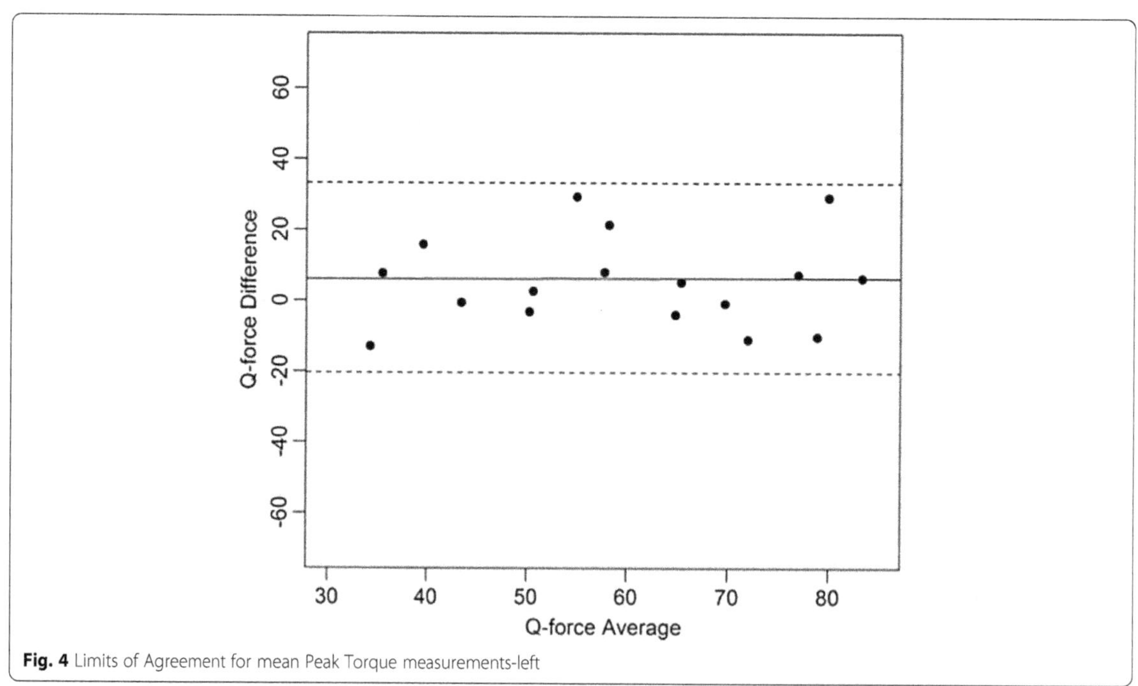

Fig. 4 Limits of Agreement for mean Peak Torque measurements-left

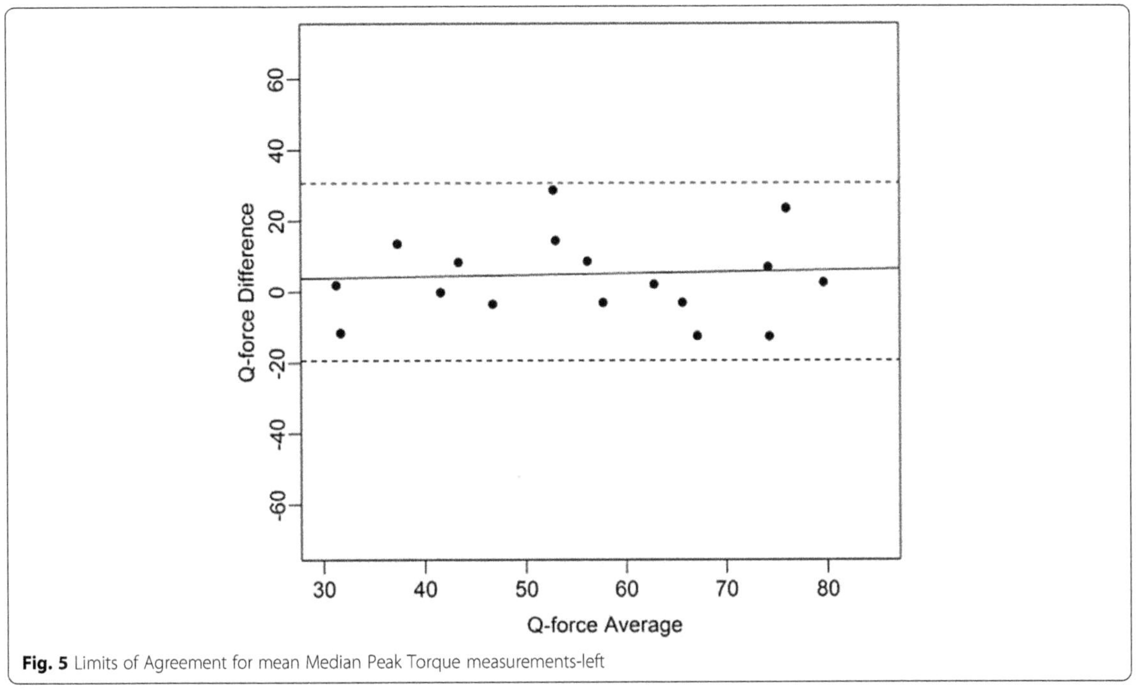

Fig. 5 Limits of Agreement for mean Median Peak Torque measurements-left

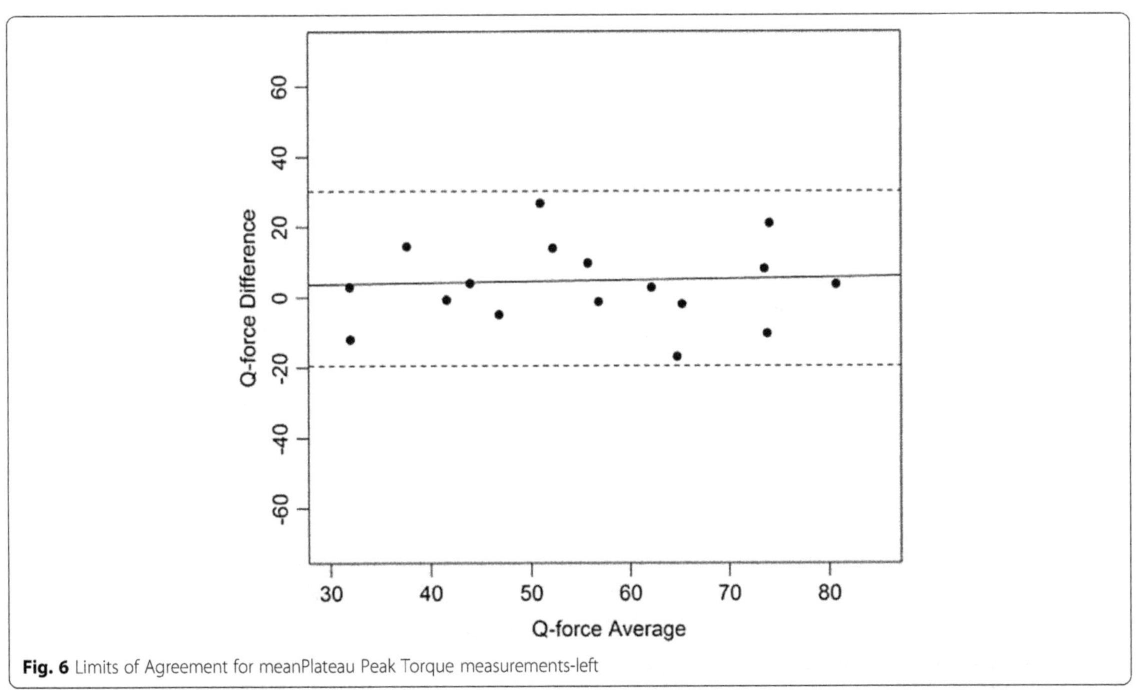

Fig. 6 Limits of Agreement for meanPlateau Peak Torque measurements-left

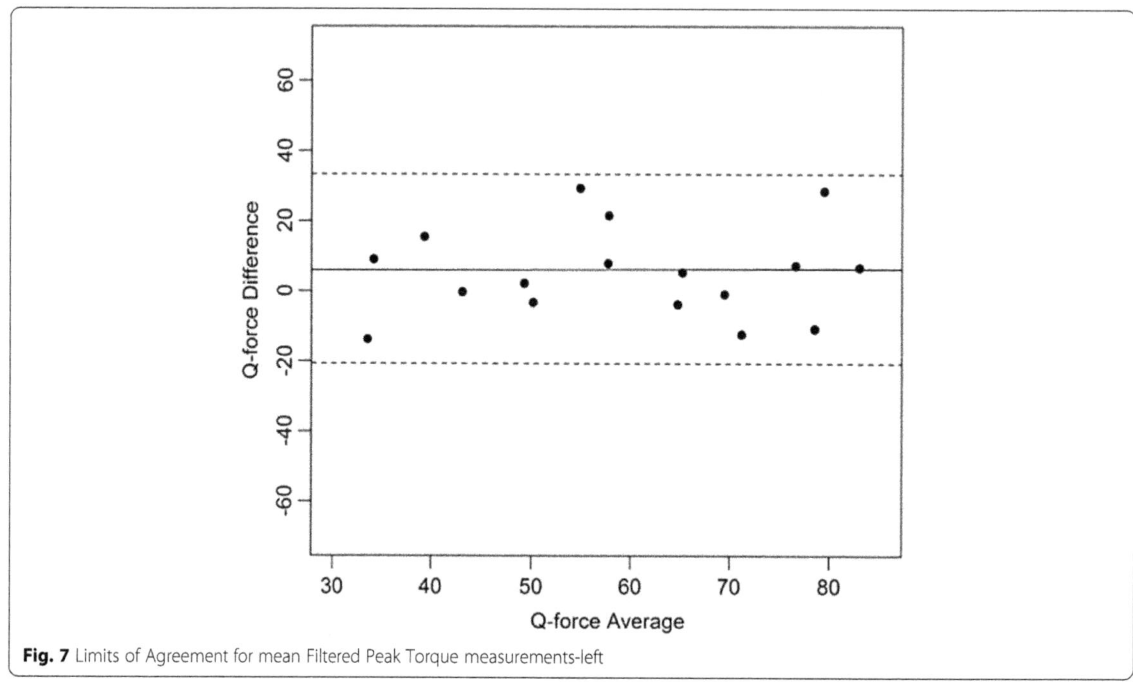

Fig. 7 Limits of Agreement for mean Filtered Peak Torque measurements-left

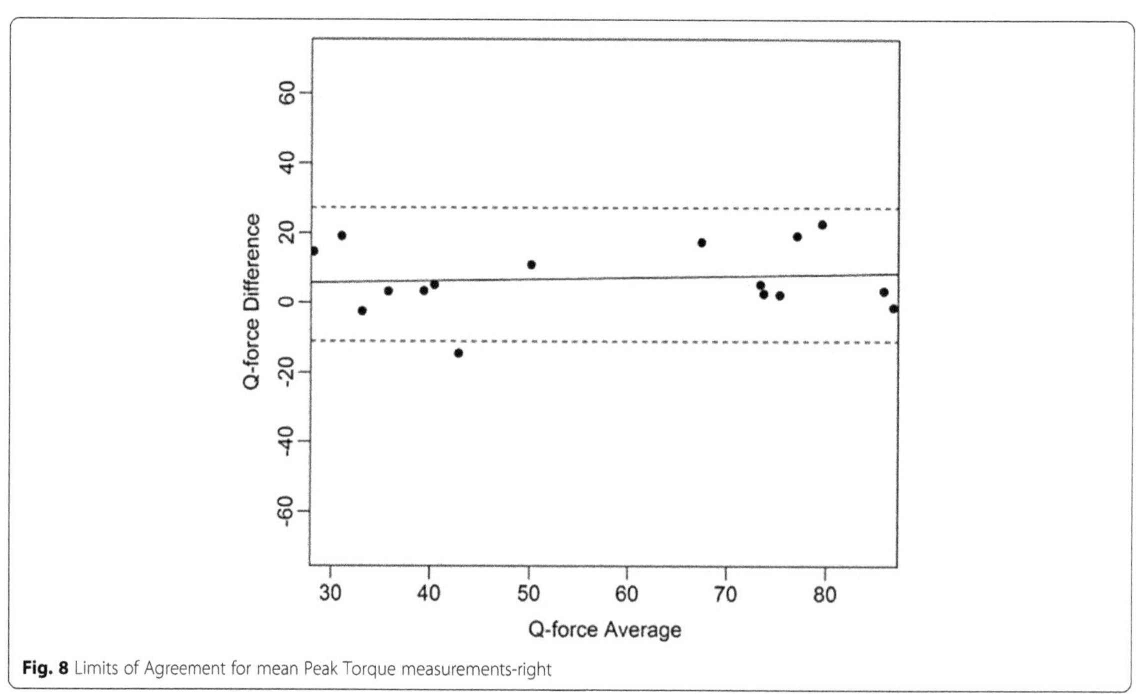

Fig. 8 Limits of Agreement for mean Peak Torque measurements-right

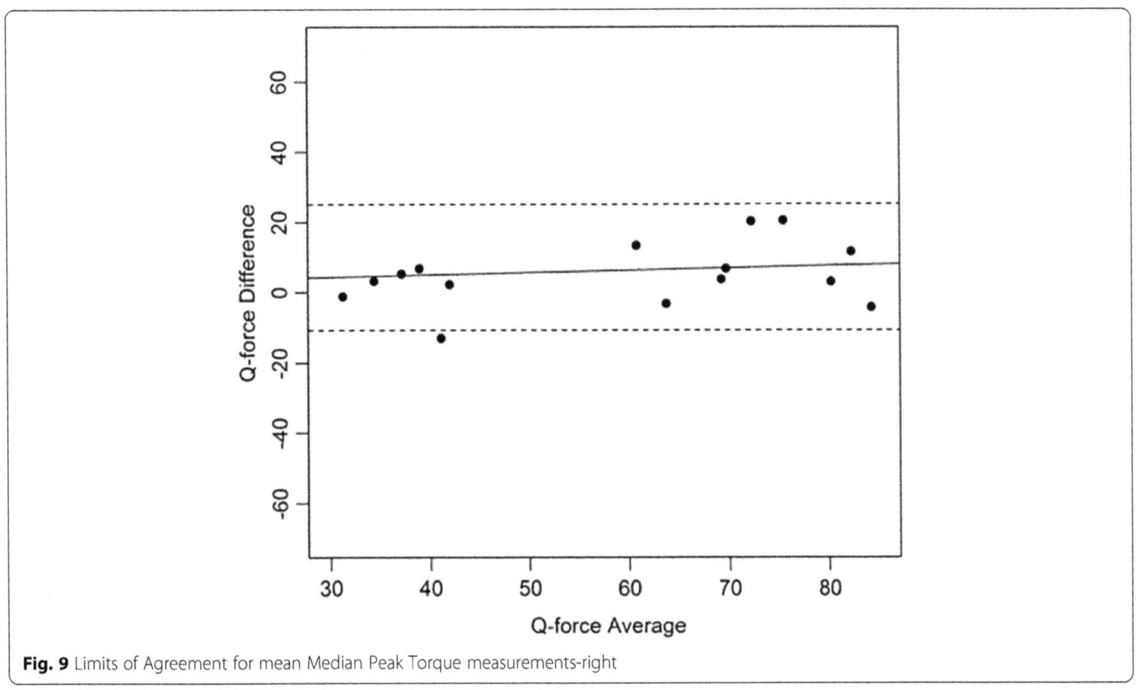

Fig. 9 Limits of Agreement for mean Median Peak Torque measurements-right

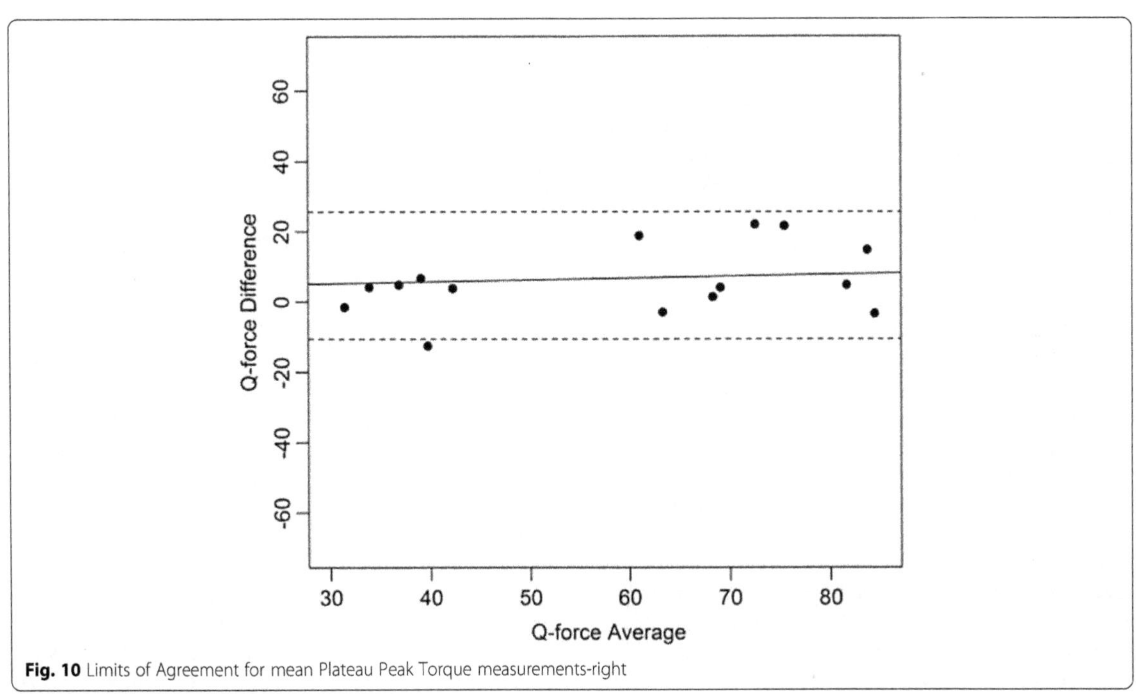

Fig. 10 Limits of Agreement for mean Plateau Peak Torque measurements-right

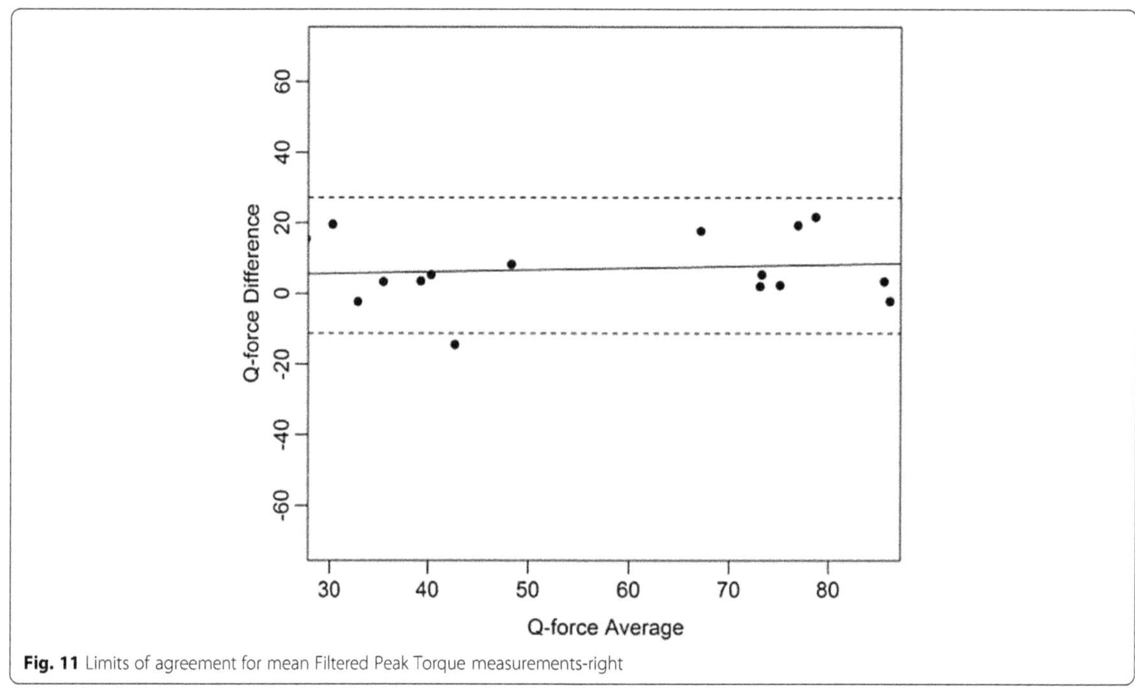

Fig. 11 Limits of agreement for mean Filtered Peak Torque measurements-right

ICC coefficients computed over the outcome measures, Peak 8Torque (PT), Filtered Peak Torque (FPT), Median peak Torque (MPT) and Average Plateau Peak Torque (APT) are very comparable, indicating that the relative reliability can be generalized over different types of muscle strength measures. We measured muscle strength at 110° knee extension. Studies based on different degrees of extension ascertained ICC coefficients between 0.87 and 0. 99 and are in accordance with our findings [20–23, 29, 37–41] This suggests that the reliability of Q Force measurements can be generalized to measurements other than 110° extension.

ICC coefficients provide information regarding relative test-retest reliability of the instrument. The ICC coefficients do however not provide information on the magnitude of the intra individual variation between two observations [42]. These intra individual variations are represented by the absolute reliability as expressed by the limitis of agreement (LOA) . The overall variation summarized in the LOA can be influenced by several sources of variation such as the time of the day, type of measurement, subject, observer, and protocol. The LOAs we found are substantial and vary between 15.7 and 23.6 Nm which corresponds to 22.5 % and 36 % of the mean. This magnitude of the LOA's is consequential for clinical or research practice since a true change after training, for example, can only be detected if it is at least 22.5 % in magnitude. Other studies with different type of instrumentation and different populations also describe a limited absolute reliability [20, 32, 38, 43, 44]. This indicates that though the clinical usefulness of the Q Force for measuring muscle strength, the ability to detect changes over time is limited, although quite comparable with other instruments. In addition, the measurements outcomes for the right leg presents smaller LOA than the left. The different LOA size between the left and right leg can possibly be explained by differences in individual variation due to the fact that the majority of a population is right-side dominant [44]. Right dominance might result in a increased neural drive to the dominant right leg resulting in more consistent values. However differences in ICC and LOA values between left and right are not always found in comparable studies.

By the results of the paired T-test we found systematic differences between the first and second session in the sense that means on the second are approximately ten percent higher compared to the first session. Other studies using isokinetic devices or pre trials prior to the actual measurement also present systematic differences or a tendency to higher values at the second measurement session [45–50]. Several studies suggest that fear, a distinct learning effect or increased muscle recruitment may be responsible for systematic differences [20, 28, 46–50].

In our study we tested a population of healthy older adults. It does not provide any information about measurements reliably for example a chronically ill population or healthy working adults. We did not register if people were left or right dominant. This limits de insight in the origin of the observed difference in ICC, LOA between left and right. We did not perform pre trials at session 1 which might contribute to the observed differences between the measured values during session 1 and 2. Though strength measurements reflect the quadriceps muscle force however no reliable procedures are available translating muscle strength into function. Therefore interpretation of strength measurement should be performed with caution.

Though muscle strength is often decreased in older subjects and associated with balance deficits and risk of falling, it is probably insufficient to use only muscle strength measurements in the predicting of fall incidents. A combination of measurements of muscle strength and functional rising and walking tests may increase the predictive capacity considerably.

Conclusion

Q Force measurements in 110° extension have excellent absolute reliability (ICC), but only moderate absolute reliability (LOA). The size of the latter indicates a limited capability to detect changes in muscle force over time. Since the Q Force is relatively cheap and mobile it seems suitable for application in various clinical settings. Future studies should investigate the degree in which its discriminative ability can be improved especially in older adults.

Abbreviations

APT: average plateau peak torque; FPT: filtered peak torque; ICC: intraclass correlation coefficient; LOA: limits of agreement; MPT: median peak torque; MRC: medical research council scale; PT: peak torque.

Competing interests

The authors declare that they have no competing interests.

Authors' contributions

KWD Made substantial intellectual contributions the draft of the manuscript design and analysis and interpretation of the data and wrote the manuscript. GRHR Made substantial intellectual contributions the draft of the manuscript and to the conception and design and analysis and interpretation of the data. Contributed to the development of the Q force. Contributed to the development of the software and collected the original data. WPK Made substantial intellectual contributions the draft of the manuscript and design and analysis and interpretation of the data. Supervised the statistical analysis and interpretation. GECS Made substantial intellectual contributions the draft of the manuscript and interpretation of the data. CPS Made substantial intellectual contributions the draft of the manuscript design and analysis and interpretation of the data and supervised the development of the manuscript process. WZ Made substantial intellectual contributions the draft of the manuscript and to the conception and design and analysis and interpretation of the data. Contributed to original concept of the Q force and further development of the Q force. Contributed to the development of the software and to the collection the original data. Authors give final approval of the version to be submitted and any revised version.

Acknowledgements

None

Author details

[1]Research and Innovation Group in Healthy Aging, Allied Health Care and Nursing, Hanze University of Applied Sciences Groningen, Groningen, The Netherlands. [2]Department of Rehabilitation Medicine, University of Groningen, University Medical Center Groningen, Groningen, The Netherlands. [3]University of Groningen, University Medical Center Groningen, Center for Human Movement Sciences Groningen, Groningen, The Netherlands. [4]School of Health Care Studies Hanze University of Applied Science Groningen, Groningen, The Netherlands. [5]Institute of Movement and Sport Gerontology, German Sport University, Cologne, Germany.

References

1. Muehlbauer T, Besemer C, Wehrle A, Gollhofer A, Granacher A. Relationship between strength, power and balance performance in seniors. Gerontology. 2012;58:504–12.
2. Daubney ME, Culham GE. Lower-extremity muscle force and balance performance in adults aged 65 years and older. Phys Ther. 1999;79:1177–85.
3. Brooks SV, Faulkner JA. Skeletal muscle weakness in old age; underlying mechanisms. Med Sci Sports Exe. 1994;26:432–9.
4. Guralnik JM, Simonsick EM, Ferrucci L, Glynn RJ, Berkman LF, Blazer DG, et al. A short physical performance battery assessing lower extremity functio:association with self-reported disability and prediction of mortality and nursing home admission. J Geront. 1994;49:85–94.
5. Howe TE, Rochester L, Neil F, Skelton DA, Ballinger C. Exercise for improving balance in older people. Cochrane Database Syst Rev. 2011;11. doi:10.1002/14651858.
6. Ciciliot S, Rossi A, Dyar KA, Blaauw B, Schiaffino S. Muscle type and fiber type specificity in muscle wasting. Int J Biochem Cell Biol. 2013;45(10):2191–9.
7. Horlings CGC, van Engelen BGM, Allum JHJ, Bloem BR. A weak balance: the contribution of muscle weakness to postural instability and falls. Nat Rev Neurol. 2008;4:504–15.
8. Zasadzka E, Borowicz AM, Roszak M, Pawlaczyk M. Assessment of the risk of falling with the use of timed up and go test in the elderly with lower extremity osteoarthritis. Clin Interv Aging. 2015;10:1289–98.
9. YY Cheng YY, Wei SH, Chen PY, Tsai MW, Cheng IC. Can sit-to-stand lower limb muscle power predict fall status? Gait Posture. 2014;40(3):403–7.
10. Pijnappels M, Van der Burg JCE. Identification of elderly fallers by muscle strength measures. Eur J Appl Physiol. 2008;201:585–92.
11. Evans D, Pester J, Vera L, Jeanmonod D, Jeanmonod R. Elderly fall patients triaged to the trauma bay: age, injury patterns, and mortality risk. Am J Emerg Med. 2015;11(33):1635–8.
12. Beauchet O, Fantino B, Allali G, Muir SW, Montero-Odasso M, Annweiler C. Timed up and go test and risk of falls in older adults: a systematic review. J Nutr Health Aging. 2011;15(10):933–8.
13. de Souza Moreira B, Barroso CM, Cavalcanti Furtado CR, Ferreira Sampaio R, das Chagas Vallone MLD, Kirkwood RN. Clinical functional tests help identify elderly women highly concerned about falls. Exp Aging Res. 2015;41(1):89–103.
14. Andres PL, Skeny LM, Munsat TL. Measurement of strength in neuromuscular diseases. In: Munsat TL, editor. Quantification of neurologic deficit. Boston: Butterworths; 1989. p. 87–100.
15. Beasley WC. Influence of method on estimates of normal knee extensor force among normal and postpolio children. Phys Ther. 1956;36:21–41.
16. Van der Ploeg RJO, Oosterhuis HJGH, Reuvekamp J. Measuring muscle strength. J Neurol. 1984;231:200–3.
17. Schwartz S, Cohen ME, Herbison GJ, Shah A. Relationship between two measures of upper extremity strength: manual muscle test compared to hand-held myometry. Arch Phys Med Rehabil. 1992;73(11):1063–8.
18. MacAvoy MC, Green DP. Critical reappraisal of medical research council muscle testing for elbow flexion. J Hand Surg. 2007;32(2):149–53.
19. Dunn JC, Iversen MD. Interrater reliability of knee muscle forces obtained by hand-held dynamometer from elderly subjects with degenerative back pain. J Geriatr Phys Ther. 2003;26:23–9.
20. Wang CY, Olson SL, Protas EJ. Test-retest strength reliability: hand-held dynamometry in community dwelling elderly fallers. Arch Phys Med Rehabil. 2002;83:811–5.
21. Gilles Roy MA, Doherty TJ. Reliability of hand-held dynamometry in assessment of knee extensor strength after hip fracture. Am J Phys Med Rehab. 2004;83:813–8.
22. Bohannon RW, Andrews AW. Interrater reliability of hand-held dynamometry. Phys Ther. 1987;67:931–3.
23. Andrews AW, Thomas MW, Bohannon RW. Normative values for muscle strength obtained by hand-held dynamometry. Phys Ther. 1996;76:248–59.
24. Bohannon RW. Comparability of force measurements obtained with different strain gauge hand-held dynamometers. J Orthop Sports Phys Ther. 1993;18:564–7.

25. Bohannon RW. Comparability of force measurements obtained with different hand-held dynamometers from older adults. Isokinet Exerc Sci. 1993;3:148–51.
26. Ullrich B, Brueggemann GP. Moment-knee angle relation inWell trained athletes. Int J Sports Med. 2008;29(8):639–45.
27. Sosnoff JJ, Voudrie SJ, Ebersole KT. The effect of knee joint angle on torque control, journal of motor behavior. J Mot Behav. 2009;42(1):5–10.
28. Narici MV, Hoppeler H, Kayser BL, Landoni H, Claassen C, Gavardi G, et al. Human quadriceps cross-sectional area, torque and neural activation during 6 months strength training. Acta Physiol Scand. 1996;157:175–86.
29. Phillips BA, Lo SK, Frank L, Mastaglia MD. Muscle force measured using "break" testing with a hand-held myometer in normal subjects aged 20 to 69 years. Arch Phys Med Rehabil. 2000;81(5):653–61.
30. Wikholm JB, Bohannon RW. Hand-held dynamometer measurements: tester strength makes a difference. J Orthop Sports Ther. 1991;13:191–8.
31. Verkerke GJ, Lemmink KAPM, Slagers AJ, Westhof MA, van Riet JA, Rakhorst G. Precision, comfort and mechanical performance of the Quadriso-tester, a quadriceps force measuring device. Med Biol Eng Comput. 2003;41:283–9.
32. Winter DA. Biomechanics of human movement. New York: Wiley; 1979.
33. Bland JM, Altman DG. Statistical methods for assessing agreement between two methods of clinical measuring. The Lancet. 1986;1(8476):307–10.
34. McGraw KO, Wong SP. Forming inferences about some intraclass correlation coefficients. Psych Meth. 1996;1:30–46.
35. Shrout PE, Fleiss JL. Intraclass correlations: uses in assessing rater reliability. Psychol Bull. 1979;86:420–8.
36. Fleiss JL. Chapter 1: reliability of measurement. The design and analysis of clinical experiments. London: Wiley; 1986. p. 1–33.
37. Janssen JC, Le-Ngoc L. Intratester reliability and validity of concentric measurements using a New hand-held dynamometer. Arch Phys Med Rehabil. 2009;90(9):1541–7.
38. Douma KW, Soer R, Krijnen WP, Reneman M, van der Schans CP. Reference values for isometric muscle force among workers for the Netherlands: a comparison of reference values. BMC Sports Sci Med Rehabil. 2014;6:10.
39. Buckinx F, Croisier JL, Reginster JY, Dardenne N, Beaudart C, Slomian J, et al. Reliability of muscle strength measures obtained with a hand-held dynamometer in an elderly population. Clin Physiol Funct Imaging. 2015;30: 10.1111.
40. Cadogan A, Laslett M, Hing W, McNair P, Williams M. Reliability of a new hand-held dynamometer in measuring shoulder range of motion and strength. Manual Therapy. 2011;16:97–101.
41. Reuter SE, Massy-Westropp N, Evans AM. Reliability and validity of indices of hand-grip strength and endurance. Aust Occup Ther J. 2011;58:82–7.
42. Evans WJ, Cayten CG, Green PA. Determining the generalizability of rating scales in clinical settings. Med Care. 1981;14:1211–20.
43. Bardis C, Kalamara G, Loucaides G, Michaelides M, Tsaklis P. Intramachine and intermachine reproducibility of concentric performance: A study of the Con-Trex MJ and the Cybex Norm dynamometers. Isokinet Exerc Sci. 2004;12:91–7.
44. Porac S, Coren S. Lateral preferences and human behavior. New York: Springer; 1981.
45. O'Shea SD, Taylor NF, Paratz JD. Measuring muscle strength for people with chronic obstructive pulmonary disease: retest reliability of hand-held dynamometry. Arch Phys Med Rehabil. 2007;88(1):32–8.
46. Ritti-Dias RM, Basyches M, Câmara L, Puech-Leao P, Battistella L, Nelson Wolosker N. Test-retest reliability of isokinetic strength and endurance tests in patients with intermittent claudication. Vasc Med. 2010;15(4):275–8.
47. Barden HL, Nott MT, Baguley IJ, Heard R, Chapparo C. Test–retest reliability of computerized hand dynamometry in adults with acquired brain injury. Aust Occup Ther J. 2012;59:319–27.
48. Scott DA, Quin Bond E, Ann Sisto S, Nadler SF. The intra- and interrater reliability of Hip muscle strength assessments using a handheld versus a portable dynamometer anchoring station. Arch Phys Med Rehabil. 2004;85(4):598–603.
49. Almosnino S, Stevenson JM, Bardana DD, Diaconescu ED, Dvirb Z. Reproducibility of isokinetic knee eccentric and concentric strength indices in asymptomatic young adults. Phys Ther Sport. 2012;13(3):156–62.
50. Wadsworth CT, Krishnan R, Sear M, Harrold J, Nielsen DH. Intrarater reliability of manual and hand held muscle testing. Phys Ther. 1987;67:1342–7.

13

Biomechanical symmetry in elite rugby union players during dynamic tasks: an investigation using discrete and continuous data analysis techniques

Brendan Marshall[1,2,5*], Andrew Franklyn-Miller[1,4], Kieran Moran[2,5], Enda King[1], Chris Richter[1,2,5], Shane Gore[1,2,5], Siobhán Strike[3] and Éanna Falvey[1,4,6]

Abstract

Background: While measures of asymmetry may provide a means of identifying individuals predisposed to injury, normative asymmetry values for challenging sport specific movements in elite athletes are currently lacking in the literature. In addition, previous studies have typically investigated symmetry using discrete point analyses alone. This study examined biomechanical symmetry in elite rugby union players using both discrete point and continuous data analysis techniques.

Methods: Twenty elite injury free international rugby union players (mean ± SD: age 20.4 ± 1.0 years; height 1.86 ± 0.08 m; mass 98.4 ± 9.9 kg) underwent biomechanical assessment. A single leg drop landing, a single leg hurdle hop, and a running cut were analysed. Peak joint angles and moments were examined in the discrete point analysis while analysis of characterising phases (ACP) techniques were used to examine the continuous data. Dominant side was compared to non-dominant side using dependent t-tests for normally distributed data or Wilcoxon signed-rank test for non-normally distributed data. The significance level was set at $\alpha = 0.05$.

Results: The majority of variables were found to be symmetrical with a total of 57/60 variables displaying symmetry in the discrete point analysis and 55/60 in the ACP. The five variables that were found to be asymmetrical were hip abductor moment in the drop landing ($p = 0.02$), pelvis lift/drop in the drop landing ($p = 0.04$) and hurdle hop ($p = 0.02$), ankle internal rotation moment in the cut ($p = 0.04$) and ankle dorsiflexion angle also in the cut ($p = 0.01$). The ACP identified two additional asymmetries not identified in the discrete point analysis.

Conclusions: Elite injury free rugby union players tended to exhibit bi-lateral symmetry across a range of biomechanical variables in a drop landing, hurdle hop and cut. This study provides useful normative values for inter-limb symmetry in these movement tests. When examining symmetry it is recommended to incorporate continuous data analysis techniques rather than a discrete point analysis alone; a discrete point analysis was unable to detect two of the five asymmetries identified.

Keywords: Landing, Cutting, Dominant versus non-dominant, Kinetics, Kinematics

* Correspondence: brendanmarshall@sportssurgeryclinic.com
[1]Sports Medicine Department, Sports Surgery Clinic, Santry Demesne, Dublin, Ireland
[2]School of Health and Human Performance, Dublin City University, Dublin, Ireland
Full list of author information is available at the end of the article

Background

The assessment of movement control and inter-limb symmetry during functional tasks is increasingly popular as a means of screening for predisposition to injury, in the evaluation of athletic performance and in the assessment of rehabilitation following injury [1–3]. A number of research studies provide support for these practises, and in turn, the premise that functional asymmetry (side to side differences in kinetics or kinematics) [4] may provide an insight into future injury risk [5–7].

Various studies have identified kinetic and kinematic asymmetry as an underlying risk factor for injury. Hewett and colleagues [7] found significantly greater asymmetries in landing knee abduction moments (6.4 times greater) in individuals who went on to injure their anterior cruciate ligament. In another prospective study, Paterno and colleagues [8] found that individuals who suffered a second anterior cruciate ligament injury had 4.1 times greater asymmetry in knee extensor moments on landing.

Asymmetry as an injury risk factor is not confined to a single joint, variable or injury type. Angle and moment variables at the ankle [9, 10], knee [7, 11], hip [8, 12], pelvis [13] and torso [14], as well as ground reaction forces [15] and ground contact times [16] have all been implicated in the development of lower extremity injury. Such injuries include ankle ligament injury [10], tibial stress fracture [11], knee ligament injury [8] and patello-femoral pain syndrome [17]. It is suggested that a notable asymmetry in these biomechanical factors may increase the risk of lower extremity injury in one limb over the other [7, 6].

In order to use measures of asymmetry as a means of identifying individuals predisposed to injury it is extremely important to establish normative values for uninjured individuals on a number of biomechanical measures. Normative values across multiple joints are not only required due to the numerous factors associated with injury, but also because poor movement control and excessive force at a proximal/distal joint can influence moments and forces at another joint [13, 18]. Zazulak and colleagues [14], for example, found that deficits in neuromuscular control at the trunk could prospectively predict knee injury risk. This phenomenon arises due to the inter-linked nature of the body's segments and the presence of bi-articular muscles (intersegmental movement constraint).

While some normative values of asymmetry exist for straight line running [6, 19], and bilateral landing [20], a full range of three dimensional measures on more specific multi-directional tasks, such as uni-lateral landing, hopping and cutting, are lacking in the literature. These more dynamic tasks are commonly associated with injury [5, 21–23]. In addition, there is a need for normative symmetry values for elite athletic populations as the majority of previous work in this area has been carried out with sub-elite athletes [6, 24, 25]. Elite athletes may develop asymmetries due to the preferential use of a dominant limb in training. Vittasalo and colleagues [26], for example, highlighted that training history influences the timing and magnitude of lower extremity muscle activation on landing in a jump.

Previous studies investigating biomechanical symmetry in dynamic movements have typically done so using discrete points (e.g. peak values) [20, 24, 25]. There are a number of limitations with this type of analysis however: (a) asymmetry may occur over phases that are not captured in a single data point, (b) the timing of discrete points can differ between limbs, and (c) the discrete points utilised typically vary between studies [27]. Continuous data analysis techniques [28], such as Analysis of Characterising Phases (ACP) [27], have been developed to overcome these issues but it appears that a comparison of symmetry findings from both continuous and discrete analyses has yet to be undertaken for dynamic sporting movements. Such an examination is warranted as the use of a discrete point analysis alone may not detect all significant asymmetries.

The primary aim of this study was to examine biomechanical symmetry during multi directional neuromuscular challenge tests in a cohort of elite injury free rugby union players. It was hypothesised that there would be a general trend toward inter-limb symmetry but that some biomechanical variables would display asymmetry due to the preferential use of a dominant limb in training. A secondary aim was to compare the findings of both discrete point and ACP analyses techniques. It was hypothesised that the results of these distinct analyses would differ due to the utilisation of discrete point and continuous data, respectively. In an attempt to adequately simulate movements that are associated with injury in field sport play [5], a single-leg landing [29], a single-leg lateral hop [5], and a change-of-direction cut [21] were examined.

Methods

Participants

Prior to the commencement of the rugby season, twenty elite rugby union players (mean ± SD: age 20.4 ± 1.0 years; height 1.86 ± 0.08 m; mass 98.4 ± 9.9 kg) were recruited to undergo three dimensional (3D) biomechanical assessment. All participants were professional academy players ($n = 11$ had made senior club appearances), and all had international caps at an age-group level. Both forward ($n = 11$) and back ($n = 9$) players were selected and all were injury free for three months at the time of testing and had no history of chronic lower extremity injury or surgery in the previous two years (self-report). The study was approved by the Sport Surgery Clinic Hospital Ethics Committee and all subjects signed informed consent.

Experimental protocol

Prior to testing, participants' mass and height was recorded using an electronic scale (Seca 876) and stadiometer (Seca 213) and their dominant leg was identified (the leg one would use to kick a ball for distance). A warm-up consisting of a three minute treadmill jog at 8 km/h followed by five body weight bilateral squats was then undertaken. Testing involved three trials of: (1) a single leg drop landing, (2) a single leg hurdle hop, and (3) a running cut. The 3D Biomechanics Laboratory is equipped with an artificial grass surface (polyethylene mono filament, Condor Grass, Holland) which is permanently and firmly fixed to the force plates (Sanctuary Synthetic Adhesive, Ireland). Participants wore their own molded football boots.

The drop landing was initiated from a 30 cm step where participants stood upright with their hands across their chest and their non-weight bearing foot behind with an approximate 90° knee bend. They then dropped off the step, made a uni-lateral landing on the force platform and held the landing position for 2 s [30]. An additional movie file shows this in more detail [see Additional file 1]. Participants were instructed to drop directly from the 30 cm height rather than jump vertically. The hurdle hop consisted of a lateral hop over a 15 cm hurdle and an immediate hop back to the initial starting position. The distance between foot contacts was approximately 40 cm; the distance between force plate centres. Participants undertook the hop as quickly as possible, and while the free leg was in the same orientation as described for the drop landing, the arms were free to move [see Additional file 2]. The landing from the first hop over the hurdle was analysed. For the cut, participants ran as fast as possible toward a marker placed on the floor, made a single complete foot contact on the force plate, and performed a 75° cut before running maximally to the finish (Fig. 1). An additional movie file shows the cut in greater detail [see Additional file 3]. Time to complete the cut was recorded using the Hotspot timing system (Games Education - Hotspot, UK).

Testing was carried out in the order of drop landing, hurdle hop and cut and all trials of one movement were completed on one leg (the choice of leg was randomised) before moving to the other leg. Participants undertook two practice trials of each movement (submaximal practice trials for the cut) before capture. Recovery of 30s was allocated between repetitions of the drop landing and hop with 1 min allocated between trials of the cut. To facilitate an assessment of the test-retest reliability of measures, fifteen players were re-tested one week after their initial testing session.

Data acquisition and analysis

An eight camera 3D motion analysis system (Vicon - Bonita B10, UK), synchronized with two 40x60cm force platforms (AMTI – BP400600, USA), was used to collect movement data. The force platforms had force ranges in the Fx, Fy and Fz directions of 2224 N, 2224 N and 4448 N, respectively and were zeroed at the start of every new data capture session. Force plate calibration was checked by placing a known weight on the plates and examining the subsequent data. Reflective markers (1.4 cm diameter) were placed at bony landmarks on the lower limbs, pelvis and trunk according to Plug in Gait marker locations [31]. Vicon Nexus software controlled simultaneous collection of motion and force data at 200Hz and 1,000Hz, respectively and both were filtered using a fourth order Butterworth filter with a cut-off frequency of 15Hz to avoid impact artefacts [32, 33]. The Vicon Plug in Gait modelling routine defined rigid body segments (foot, shank, thigh, pelvis and torso) and used standard inverse dynamics techniques [34] to calculate segmental and joint kinematics and kinetics.

Ankle, knee, hip, pelvis and thorax angles were calculated as well as internal joint moments at the hip, knee and ankle during foot contact with the force plate. Peak ground reaction forces and ground contact time in the cut were also examined. These variables were chosen as they have previously been associated with the development of numerous lower extremity injuries [7–16].

Angles were normalised to a standing static trial [35] and thorax angles were calculated relative to the pelvis as opposed to the global axis. It was not possible to measure thorax angles in the drop landing due to upper body marker occlusion. Transverse plane angles and moments for the single leg drop landing and hurdle hop were calculated but for brevity are not reported. The drop landing and hurdle hop involve movement primarily in the sagital and frontal plane, and no significant inter-limb differences in transverse plane variables were observed in these tasks. Similarly, medial/lateral and longitudinal ground reaction forces in the hurdle hop and drop landing were captured but are not reported; these measures displayed no inter-limb asymmetries.

For the discrete point analysis, peak variable values were calculated during nominal eccentric and concentric phases (eccentric phase only in the drop landing). Initial contact with the force platform marked the start of the eccentric phase in all movements. The minimum vertical height of the centre-of-mass marked the end of the eccentric phase in the drop landing while the maximal lateral/anterior position of the centre-of-mass was used to identify the end of the eccentric/start of the concentric

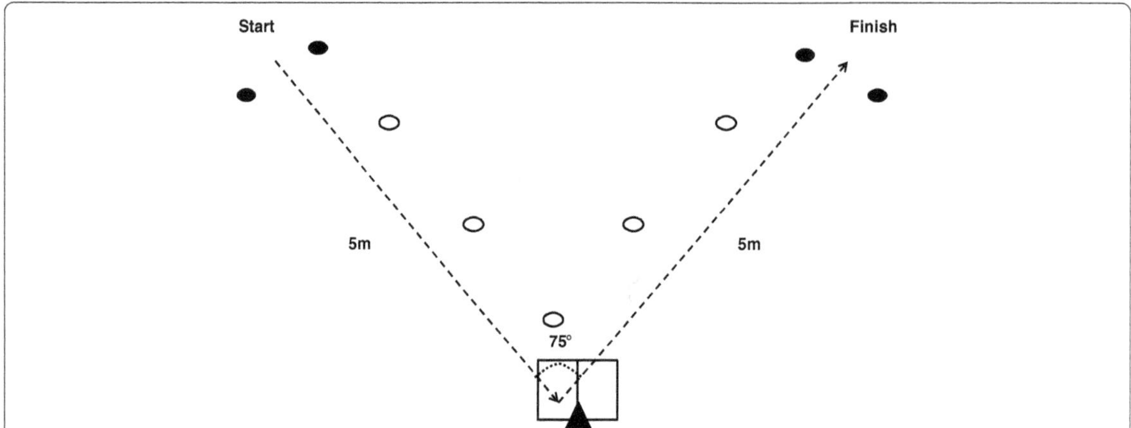

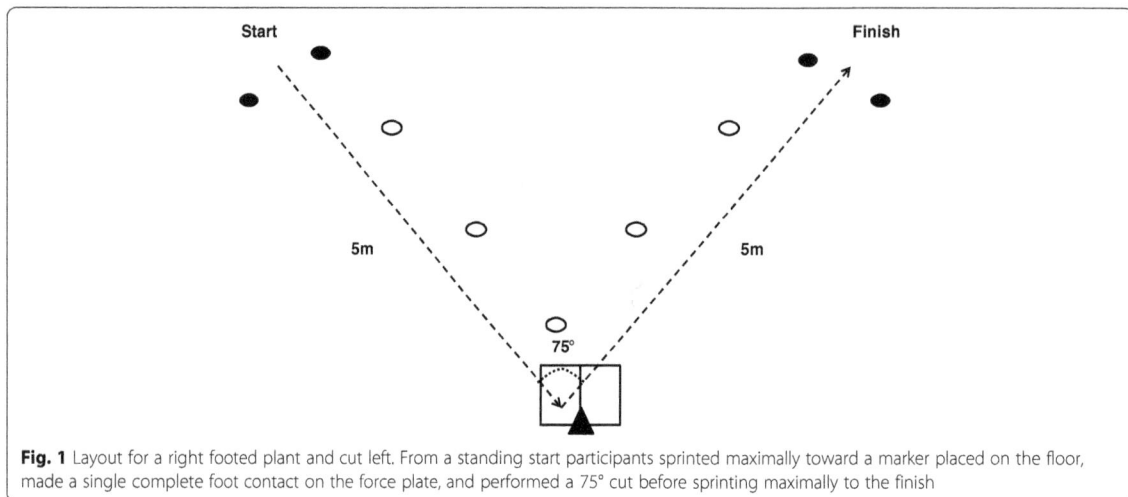

Fig. 1 Layout for a right footed plant and cut left. From a standing start participants sprinted maximally toward a marker placed on the floor, made a single complete foot contact on the force plate, and performed a 75° cut before sprinting maximally to the finish

phase in the hop and cut, respectively. The end of the concentric phase in the hop and cut occurred at toe-off from the force platform. Discrete-point data from the eccentric phase, which is more typically associated with injury development [6, 36], is presented herein while data for the concentric phase of the hurdle hop and drop landing is presented as additional data [see Additional file 4: Table S1 and Additional file 5: Table S2, respectively]. The mean of each participant's three trials for each limb was utilised in further analysis.

For the continuous waveform analysis, Analysis of Characterising Phases (ACP) was utilised; ACP has previously been shown to be effective at identifying additional features in biomechanical data to those identified in a discrete point analysis [27]. ACP was performed as described in Richter and colleagues [37] and landmark registration was applied to reduce phase shift intra subject variability [37]. As with the discrete point analysis, the mean of each participant's three trials was utilised for further analysis.

Statistical analysis

For both the discrete point analysis and ACP a Levene's test and a Kolmogorov-Smirnov test was used to examine equality of variance and normality of distribution, respectively. If data were parametric a paired Student's *t*-test was used to examine differences between the dominant and non-dominant sides [20], while a Wilcoxon signed-rank test was otherwise performed. It was assumed that an asymmetry existed when a significant between limb difference was found [20].

As a further measure of asymmetry an absolute asymmetry index was also calculated as per Karaminidis and colleagues [19] [Eq. 1] for the discrete point data. The asymmetry index is a popular measure that is often cited in the literature [38] but its ability to provide a standardised score across variables of different magnitudes has been questioned [24].

$$\text{Asymmetry Index }\% = \frac{|X_D\text{-}X_{ND}|}{0.5(X_D + X_{ND})} * 100 \tag{1}$$

where X_D is the measure of the dominant side; X_{ND} is the measure of the non-dominant side.

The authors deemed it inappropriate to calculate an asymmetry index for the continuous data; the use of a single value to represent differences between two continuous data sets would be subject to the limitations of a discrete analysis that we were attempting to avoid.

An intraclass correlation coefficient (ICC (3,k)) was used to examine the test-retest reliability of peak values for each variable. The ICC classifications of Ford and colleagues [39] (<0.4 poor, 0.4–0.75 fair to good, >0.75 excellent) were employed to describe the range of values obtained.

The significance level was set at $\alpha = 0.05$. Data processing and statistical analyses were performed using MATLAB (R2012a, MathWorks Inc., USA).

Results

Discrete point findings for the drop landing, hurdle hop and cut are displayed in Tables 1, 2 and 3, respectively. Peak variable magnitudes, asymmetry index and the findings of tests of significant difference between dominant and non-dominant sides (with effect sizes) are presented. The vast majority of variables displayed no statistically significant asymmetries ($p > 0.05$) in the drop landing (14/15), hurdle hop (16/17) and cut (27/28). Asymmetry indexes for these variables however ranged

Table 1 Drop landing discrete point findings – inter-limb differences in peak variable magnitudes during the eccentric phase

Variable	Dominant	Non-dominant	Diff	AI%	p value	Effect size
Ankle angles (deg)						
DorsiF (+)/PlantF(−)	18.4 ± 2.8	19.4 ± 3.8	1.0	5	0.46	0.28
Ever(+)/ Inv(−)	5.7 ± 2.4	5.0 ± 2.2	0.7	17	0.39	−0.32
Ankle moments (Nm/kg)						
PlantF(+)/DorsiF(−)	2.7 ± 0.4	2.8 ± 0.6	0.1	4	0.39	0.32
Ever(+)/ Inv(−)	−0.1 ± 0.2	−0.2 ± 0.2	0.1	67	0.52	−0.24
Knee angles (deg)						
Flex(+)/Ext(−)	66.6 ± 8.8	66.3 ± 8.0	0.3	1	0.93	−0.03
Var(+)/Valg(−)	4.3 ± 5.6	7.6 ± 8.5	3.3	143	0.22	0.46
Knee moments (Nm/kg)						
Ext (+)/Flex(−)	3.1 ± 0.4	3.1 ± 0.3	0.0	0	0.95	0.02
Valg(+)/Var(−)	1.9 ± 0.4	2.0 ± 0.5	0.1	5	0.56	0.22
Hip angles (deg)						
Flex(+)/Ext(−)	59.3 ± 10.9	59.4 ± 9.1	0.1	0	0.98	0.01
Add(+)/ Ab(−)	9.3 ± 5.6	10.0 ± 3.0	0.7	19	0.70	0.15
Hip moments (Nm/kg)						
Ext (+)/Flex(−)	5.4 ± 2.0	5.0 ± 1.3	0.4	8	0.47	−0.27
Ab(+)/Add(−)	2.7 ± 0.7	2.2 ± 0.8	0.5	20	0.09	−0.63
Pelvis angles (deg)						
AntT(+)/PostT(−)	13.8 ± 8.0	14.5 ± 7.5	0.7	8	0.79	0.10
Contra Drop(+)/Contra Lift(−)	−12.1 ± 4.0	−8.9 ± 3.4*	3.2	31	0.02	0.80
Ground reaction force (N/kg)						
Vertical	43.7 ± 5.1	44.8 ± 6.6	1.1	3	0.61	0.19

*Significant inter-limb difference ($p < 0.05$)
Diff: difference; AI: asymmetry index; Sig: significance
DorsiF: dorsiflexion; PlantF: plantarflexion; Ever: eversion; Inv: inversion; Flex: flexion; Ext: extension; Var: varus; Val: valgus; Add: adduction; Ab: abduction; AntT: anterior tilt; PostT: posterior tilt; Contra: contralateral

from 0 to 143 % in the drop landing, 1–264 % in the hurdle hop and 1–49 % in the cut.

Table 4 summarises the three variables that did display statistically significant ($p < 0.05$) asymmetries in the discrete point analysis. Two differences were associated with the pelvis, one in the drop landing and one in the hurdle hop. There was significantly greater pelvis contralateral hip lift ($p < 0.05$) when landing on the dominant leg during the drop landing. When landing on the non-dominant leg during the hurdle hop, there was significantly ($p < 0.05$) greater pelvis contralateral drop. In the cut, ankle internal rotation moments were significantly ($p < 0.05$) greater on the non-dominant side during the eccentric phase.

For the ACP, Figs. 2, 3, 4 and 5 display group mean wave-forms for all variables in the drop landing, hurdle hop and cut, respectively. Areas of the wave-form that displayed significant differences between dominant and non-dominant leg are highlighted. The majority of variables under examination displayed no significant asymmetries in the drop landing (13/15), hurdle hop (16/17) or cut (26/28). Those variables that did display significant differences ($p < 0.05$) are summarised in Table 5. For the drop landing on the dominant leg there was significantly greater hip abductor moments early in the eccentric phase ($p = 0.02$, effect size = 0.62) and more pelvis contralateral lift from 52 % of the movement onwards ($p = 0.04$, effect size = 0.66). There was significantly greater contralateral pelvic drop on the non-dominant side throughout the hop test ($p = 0.01$ - 0.02, effect size = 0.88). In the cut, ankle internal rotation moments were significantly greater in the non-dominant ankle ($p =$ 0.02 – 0.04, effect size = 0.52) from 23-38 % of the movement. The ankle joint was also significantly more dorsiflexed on the non-dominant side during the latter stages (78–94 %) of the cut push-off ($p = 0.011$, effect size = 0.57).

The test-retest reliability findings for variables in the drop landing, hurdle hop and cut are detailed in Additional file 6: Table S3. There were no significant differences in reliability scores between limbs so the values provided in Additional file 6: Table S3 are the mean ICC values of the dominant and non-dominant sides. All

Table 2 Hurdle hop discrete point findings – inter-limb differences in peak variable magnitudes during the eccentric phase

Variable	Dominant	Non-dominant	Diff	AI%	*p* value	Effect size
Ankle angles (deg)						
DorsiF (+)/PlantF(−)	16.8 ± 4.2	17.8 ± 4.4	1.0	5	0.58	0.21
Ever(+)/ Inv(−)	4.5 ± 2.4	4.2 ± 2.6	0.3	8	0.73	−0.13
Ankle moments (Nm/kg)						
PlantF(+)/DorsiF(−)	3.4 ± 0.5	3.4 ± 0.5	0.0	0	0.86	0.07
Ever(+)/ Inv(−)	0.4 ± 0.2	0.4 ± 0.2	0.0	0	0.93	0.04
Knee angles (deg)						
Flex(+)/Ext(−)	42.3 ± 10.3	43.3 ± 8.8	1.0	2	0.79	0.10
Var(+)/Valg(−)	−3.1 ± 5.6	−0.6 ± 5.7	2.5	132	0.25	0.44
Knee moments (Nm/kg)						
Ext (+)/Flex(−)	2.6 ± 0.7	2.8 ± 0.5	0.2	7	0.50	0.26
Valg(+)/Var(−)	1.9 ± 0.6	2.1 ± 0.6	0.2	10	0.23	0.46
Hip angles (deg)						
Flex(+)/Ext(−)	34.0 ± 6.5	33.3 ± 7.2	0.7	2	0.79	−0.10
Add(+)/ Ab(−)	−8.1 ± 5.3	−5.9 ± 4.0	2.2	31	0.24	0.45
Hip moments (Nm/kg)						
Ext (+)/Flex(−)	2.9 ± 1.0	2.9 ± 0.9	0.0	0	1.00	0.00
Ab(+)/Add(−)	1.5 ± 0.3	1.5 ± 0.4	0.0	0	0.55	0.23
Pelvis angles (deg)						
AntT(+)/PostT(−)	11.9 ± 4.4	11.7 ± 4.3	0.2	2	0.91	−0.05
Contra Drop(+)/Contra Lift(−)	−1.4 ± 4.7	3.1 ± 4.1*	4.5	264	0.01	0.92
Thorax angles (deg)						
Flex(+)/Ext(−)	6.8 ± 7.9	4.7 ± 7.4	2.1	38	0.46	0.29
LatFlex(+)/MedFlex(−)	7.9 ± 5.9	8.7 ± 4.0	0.8	10	0.68	0.16
Ground reaction force (N/kg)						
Vertical	29.2 ± 4.0	28.6 ± 2.6	0.6	2	0.67	0.16

*Significant inter-limb difference ($p < 0.05$)
Diff: difference; AI: asymmetry index; Sig: significance
DorsiF: dorsiflexion; PlantF: plantarflexion; Ever: eversion; Inv: inversion; Flex: flexion; Ext: extension; Var: varus; Val: valgus; Add: adduction; Ab: abduction; AntT: anterior tilt; PostT: posterior tilt; Contra: contralateral; LatFlex: lateral flexion; MedFlex: medial flexion

variables displayed good to excellent reliability (ICC > 0.60) in the drop landing (mean ICC [95 % confidence intervals (CI)]: 0.89 [0.90, 0.88]), hurdle hop (0.88 [0.89, 0.87]), and cut (0.85 [0.86, 0.84]).

Discussion

Our findings highlighted a clear tendency toward biomechanical inter-limb symmetry during multi directional neuromuscular challenge tests in a cohort of elite, injury free, rugby union players. Asymmetries that were identified were limited to frontal plane pelvis angles and moments in the drop landing and hurdle hop, alongside ankle sagittal plane angle and internal rotation moment in the cut. The analysis of characterising phases (ACP) identified two additional asymmetries not identified in the discrete point analysis. Previous investigations of symmetry in elite athletes have utilised tests such as isokinetic dynamometry [40] but these are uni-planar assessments of a single joint, which do not have immediate relevance to athletic movement. Conversely, studies that have examined more dynamic tasks like running have done so only in linear running at a submaximal pace or with sub-elite athletes [6].

Hip eccentric abductor moment in the drop landing and ankle dorsiflexion angle in the cut (Tables 4 and 5) were found to be asymmetrical in the ACP, but not in the discrete point analysis. It would appear that these asymmetries were missed in the discrete analysis because the phase of the movement where the difference lay did not coincide with their peak magnitude (Figs. 2 and 4). Similar to work by Richter and colleagues [37] and Shorter and colleagues [41], our findings highlight the benefit of using continuous movement plane analysis techniques when examining biomechanical data as they do not require *a priori* knowledge of which event/phase to analyse.

Table 3 Running cut discrete point findings – inter-limb differences in peak variable magnitudes during the eccentric phase

Variable	Dominant	Non-dominant	Diff	AI%	p value	Effect size
Ankle angles (deg)						
DorsiF (+)/PlantF(−)	11.1 ± 7.6	12.0 ± 7.3	0.9	8	0.28	0.41
Ever(+)/ Inv(−)	5.4 ± 2.4	4.5 ± 2.7	0.9	17	0.39	0.33
IntR(+)/ExtR(−)	−33.5 ± 13.2	−29.1 ± 12.4	4.4	14	0.37	0.35
Ankle moments (Nm/kg)						
PlantF(+)/DorsiF(−)	1.9 ± 0.4	2.0 ± 0.4	0.1	5	0.59	0.21
Ever(+)/ Inv(−)	0.7 ± 0.2	0.7 ± 0.1	0.0	0	0.91	0.04
IntR(+)/ExtR(−)	0.1 ± 0.1	0.2 ± 0.1 *	0.1	67	0.04	0.74
Knee angles (deg)						
Flex(+)/Ext(−)	57.4 ± 6.0	60.3 ± 10.2	2.9	5	0.37	0.35
Var(+)/Valg(−)	−7.5 ± 5.0	−6.1 ± 7.1	1.4	21	0.54	0.23
IntR(+)/ ExtR(−)	21.2 ± 9.4	24.7 ± 10.5	3.5	15	0.36	0.35
Knee moments (Nm/kg)						
Ext (+)/Flex(−)	2.6 ± 0.5	2.5 ± 0.6	0.1	4	0.84	0.08
Valg(+)/Var(−)	−2.5 ± 1.0	−2.3 ± 0.8	0.2	8	0.55	0.23
IntR(+)/ExtR(−)	0.4 ± 0.1	0.3 ± 0.2	0.1	29	0.23	0.46
Hip angles (deg)						
Flex(+)/Ext(−)	45.1 ± 11.9	49.4 ± 15.9	4.3	9	0.42	0.31
Add(+)/ Ab(−)	−17.9 ± 6.7	−18.0 ± 7.6	0.1	1	0.96	0.02
IntR(+)/ExtR(−)	22.4 ± 10.1	27.2 ± 12.5	4.8	20	0.27	0.42
Hip moments (Nm/kg)						
Ext (+)/Flex(−)	4.0 ± 1.4	4.5 ± 1.6	0.5	12	0.34	0.37
Ab(+)/Add(−)	−3.6 ± 1.4	−3.3 ± 1.3	0.3	9	0.61	0.20
IntR(+)/ExtR(−)	1.3 ± 0.5	1.2 ± 0.5	0.1	8	0.91	0.04
Pelvis angles (deg)						
AntT(+)/PostT(−)	2.2 ± 5.1	3.7 ± 7.5	1.5	49	0.56	0.23
Contra Drop(+)/Contra Lift(−)	15.0 ± 5.9	14.4 ± 7.8	0.6	4	0.81	0.09
IntR(+)/ExtR(−)	−11.1 ± 13.1	−11.2 ± 12.3	0.1	1	0.98	0.01
Thorax angles (deg)						
Flex(+)/Ext(−)	30.5 ± 5.8	28.5 ± 6.4	2.0	7	0.41	0.32
LatFlex(+)/MedFlex(−)	21.0 ± 7.9	21.8 ± 5.5	0.8	4	0.75	0.12
ExtR(+)/ IntR(−)	−11.8 ± 6.6	−11.6 ± 5.6	0.2	2	0.93	0.03
Ground reaction forces (N/kg)						
Vertical	15.1 ± 2.9	16.9 ± 4.4	1.8	11	0.21	0.48
Medial/lateral	1.3 ± 0.8	1.5 ± 1.1	0.2	14	0.52	0.25
Longitudinal	9.5 ± 1.7	10.2 ± 2.7	0.7	7	0.42	0.31
Timing (s)						
Ground contact time	0.32 ± 0.04	0.35 ± 0.06	0.03	9	0.11	0.6

*Significant inter-limb difference ($p < 0.05$)
Diff: difference; AI: asymmetry index; Sig: significance
DorsiF: dorsiflexion; PlantF: plantarflexion; Ever: eversion; Inv: inversion; IntR: internal rotation; ExtR: external rotation; Flex: flexion; Ext: extension; Var: varus; Val: valgus; Add: adduction; Ab: abduction; AntT: anterior tilt; PostT: posterior tilt; Contra: contralateral; LatFlex: lateral flexion; MedFlex: medial flexion

While the majority of variables exhibited no significant asymmetry, several exhibited a large asymmetry index (AI) in the discrete point analysis; AI ranges for symmetrical variables in the drop, hop and cut were 0–143 %, 0–264 % and 0–49 %, respectively (Tables 1–3). These differences are likely due to the AI calculation being

Table 4 Significant inter-limb differences ($p < 0.05$) as identified in the discrete point analysis

	Dominant Mean (±SD)	Non-dominant Mean (±SD)	Difference	*p* value	Effect size	AI%
Drop landing						
Pelvis contralateral drop(+)/lift(−) (deg)	−12.1 (4.0)	−8.9 (3.4)	3.2 (D > ND)	0.02	0.80	31
Hurdle Hop						
Pelvis contralateral drop(+)/lift(−) (deg)	−1.4 (4.7)	3.1 (4.1)	4.5 (ND > D)	0.01	0.92	264
Cut						
Ankle internal rotation moment (Nm/kg)	0.1(0.1)	0.2 (0.1)	0.1 (ND > D)	0.04	0.74	67

AI: asymmetry index; D: dominant; ND: non-dominant

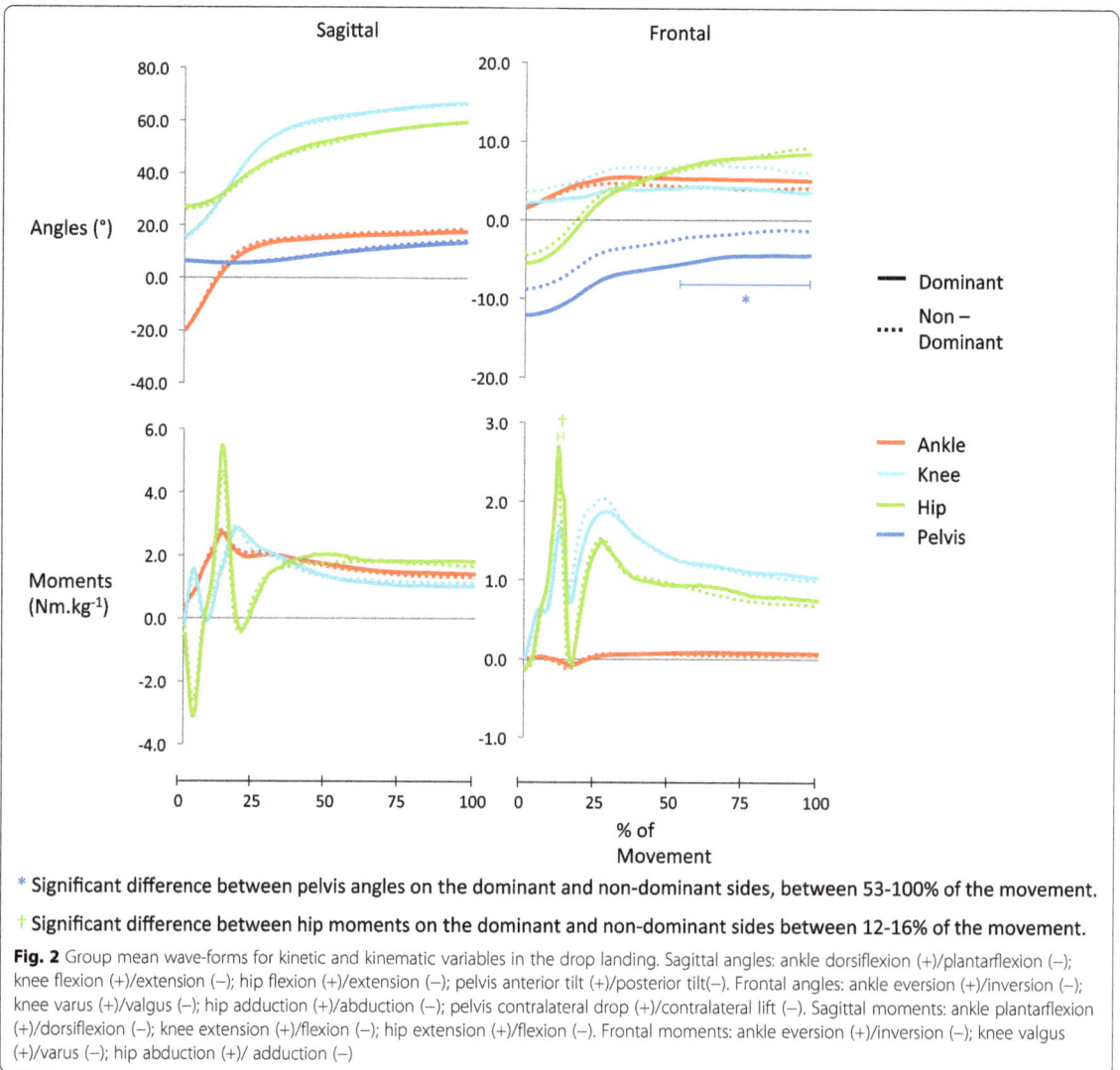

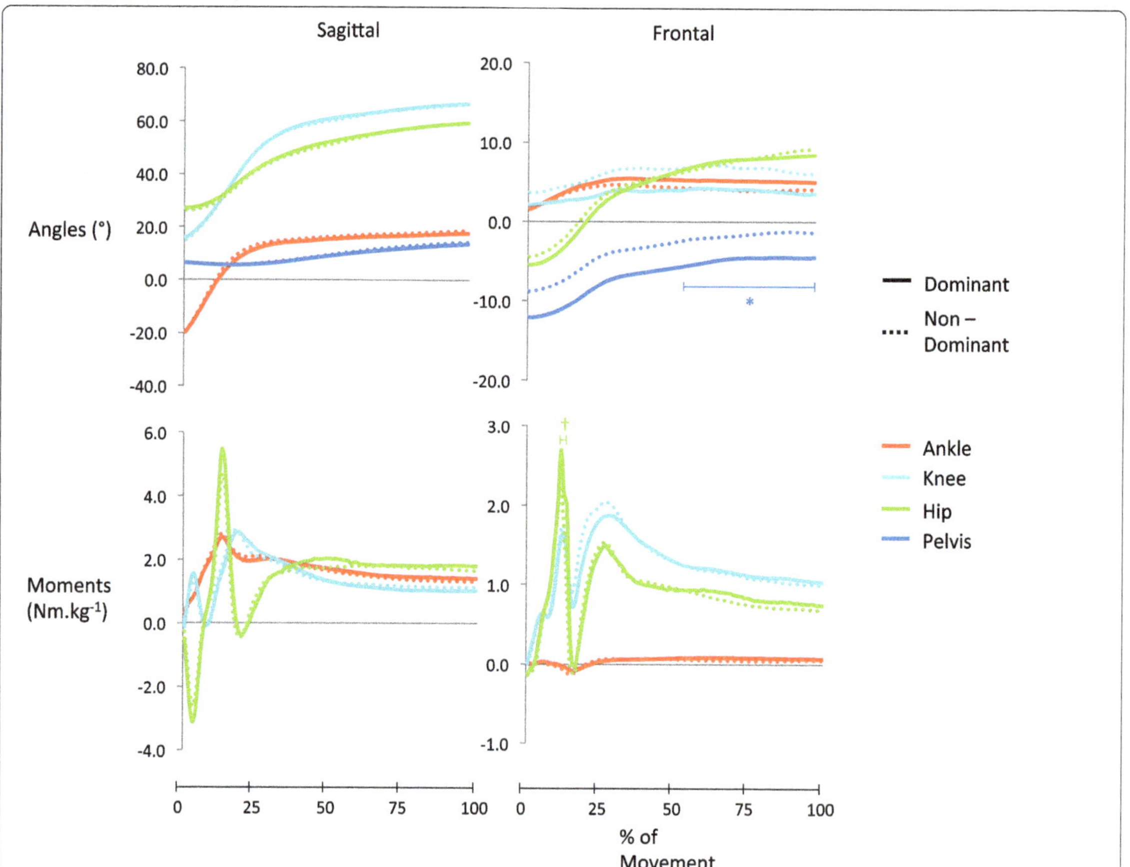

* Significant difference between pelvis angles on the dominant and non-dominant sides, between 53-100% of the movement.

† Significant difference between hip moments on the dominant and non-dominant sides between 12-16% of the movement.

Fig. 2 Group mean wave-forms for kinetic and kinematic variables in the drop landing. Sagittal angles: ankle dorsiflexion (+)/plantarflexion (−); knee flexion (+)/extension (−); hip flexion (+)/extension (−); pelvis anterior tilt (+)/posterior tilt(−). Frontal angles: ankle eversion (+)/inversion (−); knee varus (+)/valgus (−); hip adduction (+)/abduction (−); pelvis contralateral drop (+)/contralateral lift (−). Sagittal moments: ankle plantarflexion (+)/dorsiflexion (−); knee extension (+)/flexion (−); hip extension (+)/flexion (−). Frontal moments: ankle eversion (+)/inversion (−); knee valgus (+)/varus (−); hip abduction (+)/ adduction (−)

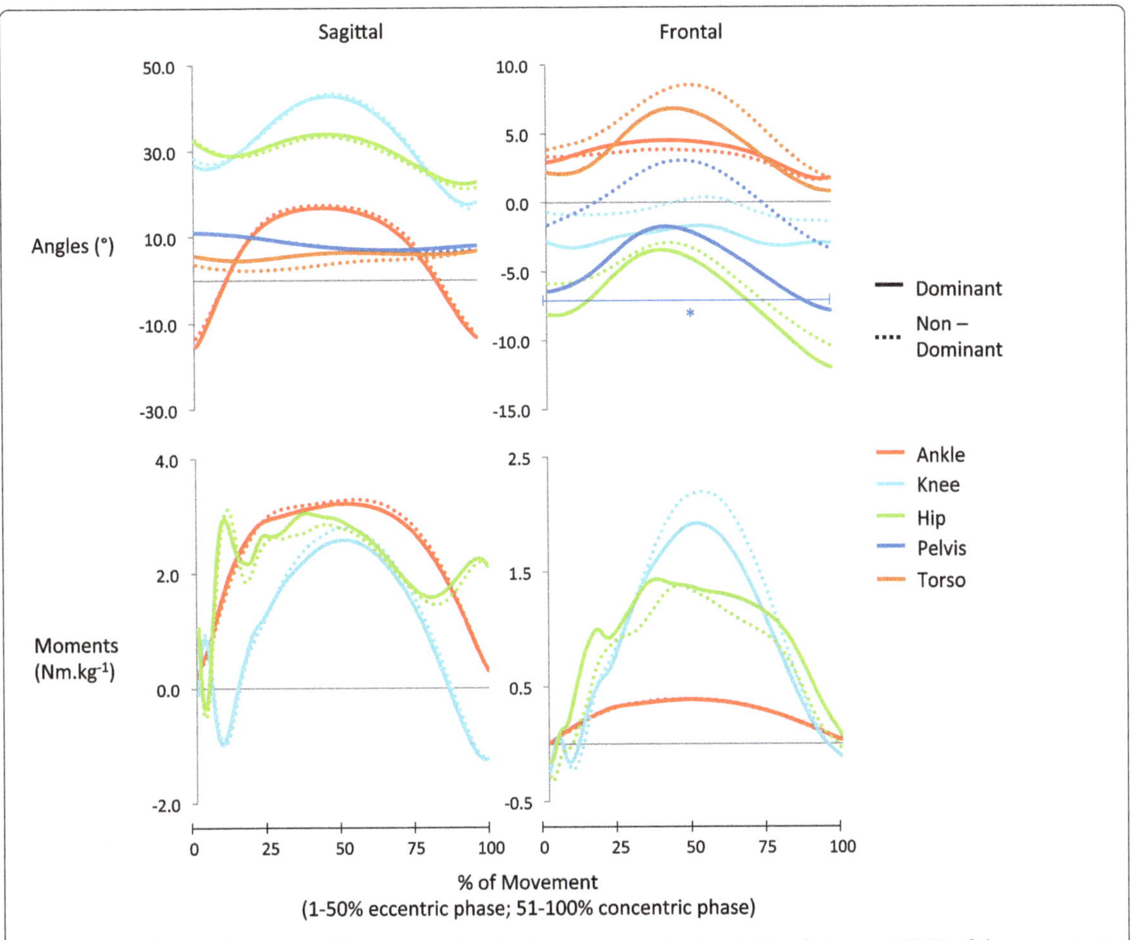

* **Significant difference between pelvis angles on the dominant and non-dominant sides, between 1-100% of the movement.**

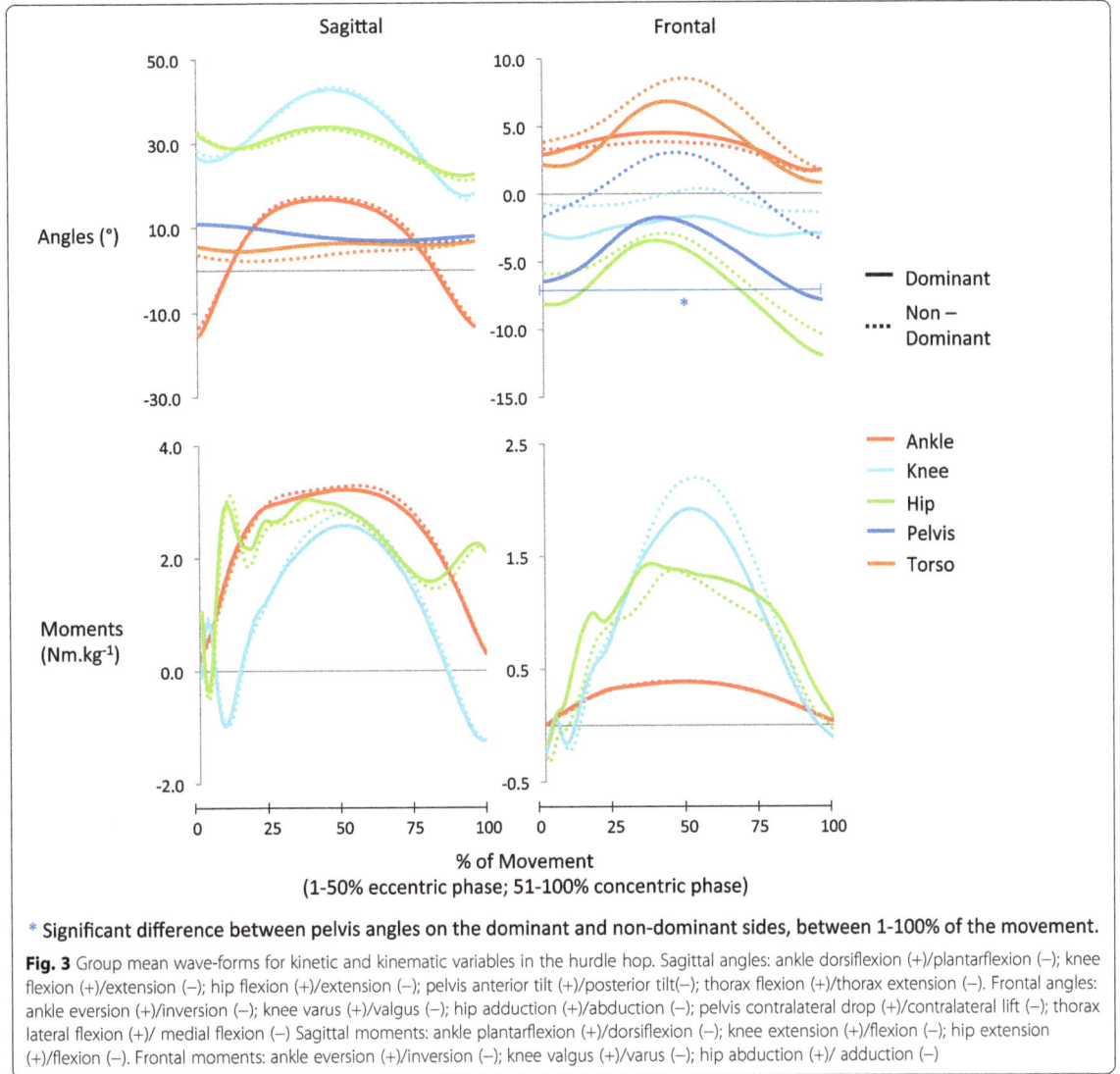

Fig. 3 Group mean wave-forms for kinetic and kinematic variables in the hurdle hop. Sagittal angles: ankle dorsiflexion (+)/plantarflexion (–); knee flexion (+)/extension (–); hip flexion (+)/extension (–); pelvis anterior tilt (+)/posterior tilt(–); thorax flexion (+)/thorax extension (–). Frontal angles: ankle eversion (+)/inversion (–); knee varus (+)/valgus (–); hip adduction (+)/abduction (–); pelvis contralateral drop (+)/contralateral lift (–); thorax lateral flexion (+)/ medial flexion (–) Sagittal moments: ankle plantarflexion (+)/dorsiflexion (–); knee extension (+)/flexion (–); hip extension (+)/flexion (–). Frontal moments: ankle eversion (+)/inversion (–); knee valgus (+)/varus (–); hip abduction (+)/ adduction (–)

overly sensitive to variables with small magnitudes and tending to inflate their score as a result [24]. In the drop landing, for example, knee varus angle and knee flexion angle differed by similar amounts between dominant and non-dominant legs (3° and 2°, respectively), but the AIs for these variables were notably different (143 % and 3 %, respectively). This is due to the magnitudes of knee varus being approximately ten times smaller than the magnitudes of knee flexion (Table 1). It appears that frontal plane variables in the drop and hop are particularly affected by the inflation of AI scores due to small variable magnitudes (Tables 1 and 2). If frontal plane variables are excluded, ranges of AI fall to 0–31 % in the drop landing and 0–7 % in the hurdle hop which are closer to the 0–49 % in the cut and the 3–50 % found in studies of straight line running [6]. These findings, which are similar to those of Herzog and colleagues [24] in gait analysis, suggest that the use of AIs to provide normative symmetry values for biomechanical variables of small magnitude (e.g. knee varus/valgus) is questionable. As an alternative it may be more appropriate to simply examine magnitude differences between limbs for each variable of interest. To this end the results presented in Tables 1–3 for discrete points, and in Figs. 2–4 for the complete movement phase, provide useful normative values for rehabilitation specialists who are undertaking injury screening testing or monitoring rehabilitation progress in similar population groups.

In total, five variables were found to display significant inter-limb asymmetries. Pelvis contralateral lift and hip eccentric abductor moment in the drop landing were

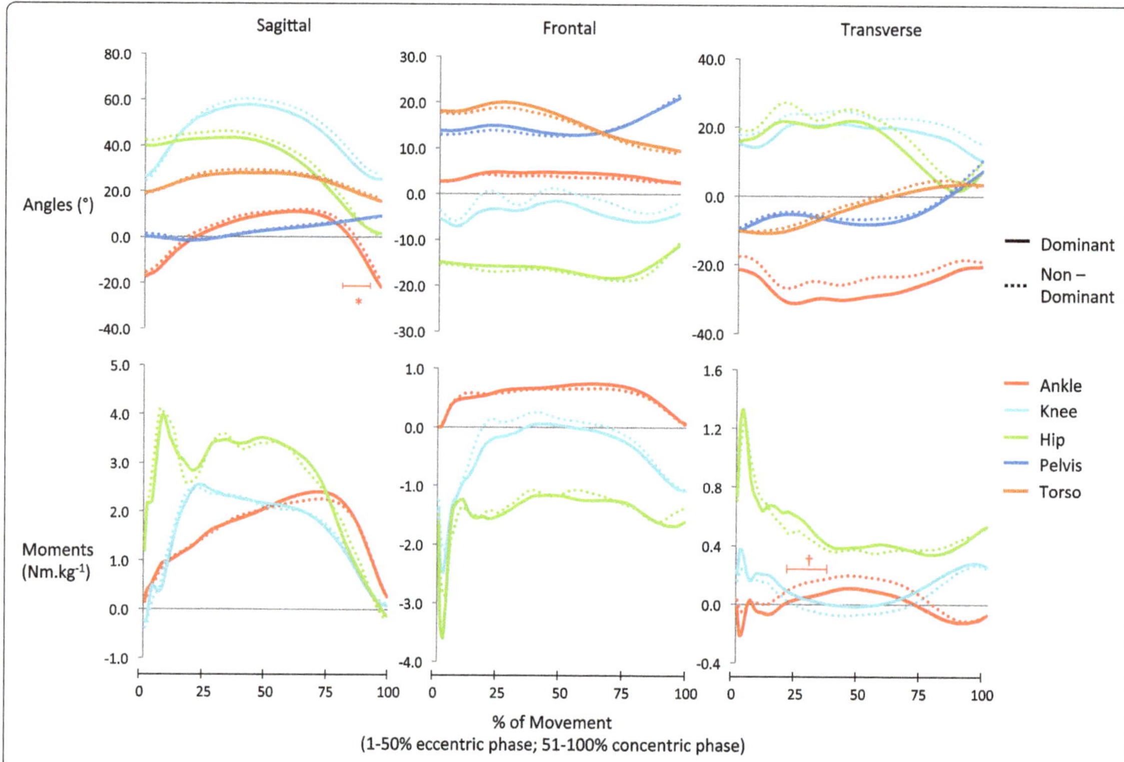

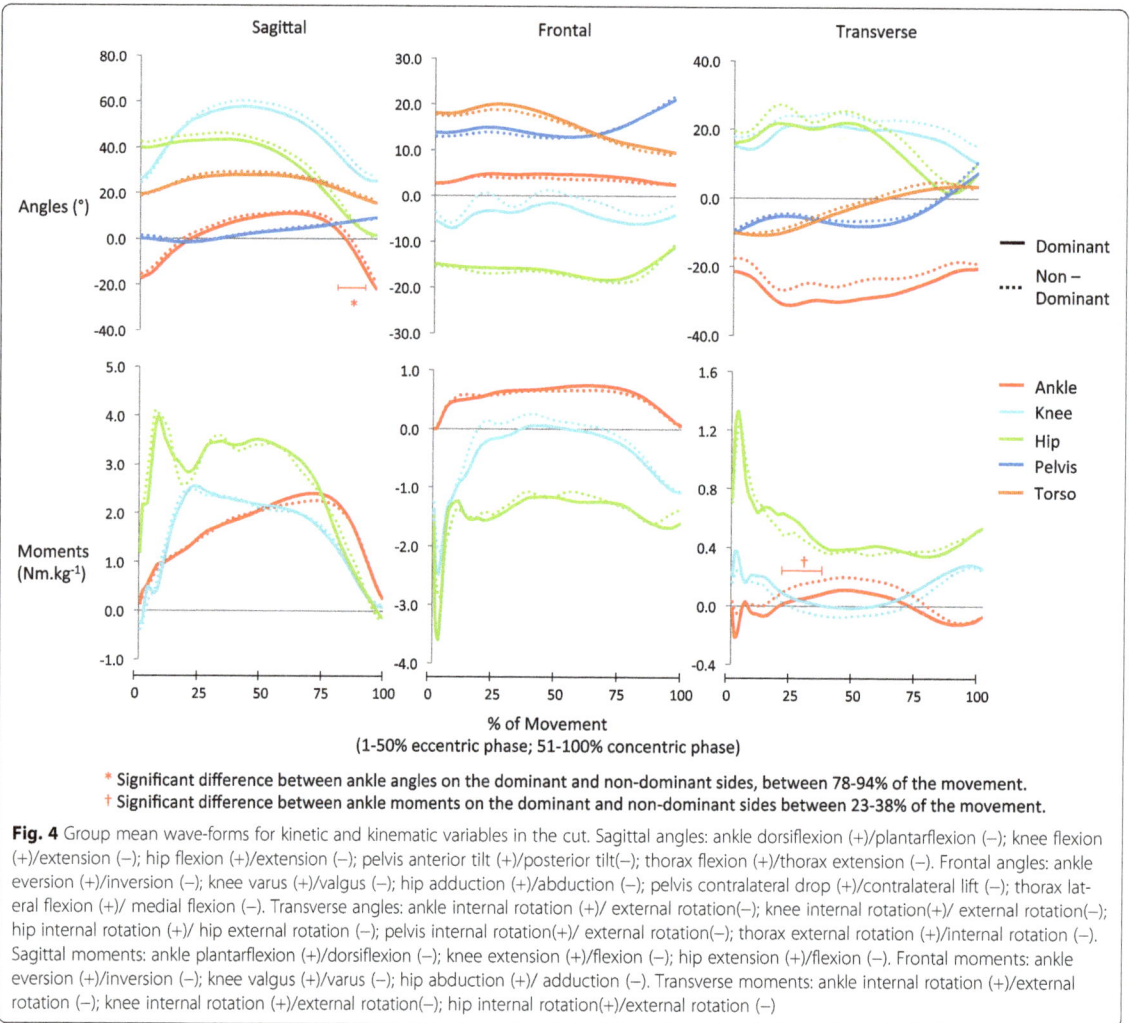

* Significant difference between ankle angles on the dominant and non-dominant sides, between 78-94% of the movement.

† Significant difference between ankle moments on the dominant and non-dominant sides between 23-38% of the movement.

Fig. 4 Group mean wave-forms for kinetic and kinematic variables in the cut. Sagittal angles: ankle dorsiflexion (+)/plantarflexion (–); knee flexion (+)/extension (–); hip flexion (+)/extension (–); pelvis anterior tilt (+)/posterior tilt(–); thorax flexion (+)/thorax extension (–). Frontal angles: ankle eversion (+)/inversion (–); knee varus (+)/valgus (–); hip adduction (+)/abduction (–); pelvis contralateral drop (+)/contralateral lift (–); thorax lateral flexion (+)/ medial flexion (–). Transverse angles: ankle internal rotation (+)/ external rotation(–); knee internal rotation(+)/ external rotation(–); hip internal rotation (+)/ hip external rotation (–); pelvis internal rotation(+)/ external rotation(–); thorax external rotation (+)/internal rotation (–). Sagittal moments: ankle plantarflexion (+)/dorsiflexion (–); knee extension (+)/flexion (–); hip extension (+)/flexion (–). Frontal moments: ankle eversion (+)/inversion (–); knee valgus (+)/varus (–); hip abduction (+)/ adduction (–). Transverse moments: ankle internal rotation (+)/external rotation (–); knee internal rotation (+)/external rotation(–); hip internal rotation(+)/external rotation (–)

greater on the dominant side, while pelvis contralateral drop in the hurdle hop, ankle eccentric internal rotation moment and ankle dorsiflexion angle in the cut were all greater on the non-dominant side (Tables 4 and 5). It would appear that in the drop landing, participants were able to generate larger eccentric hip abductor moments on the dominant leg early in the landing (Table 5) which allowed them to achieve a greater contralateral pelvis lift later in the movement (Table 5). This may be as a result of a different landing strategy on the dominant side as a result of preferential use in training [26, 42]. Vittasalo and colleagues [26] found that training history influences the timing and magnitude of lower extremity muscle activation on landing in a jump. They found that trained athletes activated their lower extremity muscles earlier and to a greater extent than physically active controls [26].

Preferential use of the dominant limb during training may also explain, at least in part, the asymmetries observed in the hurdle hop, a movement which places an emphasis on frontal plane movement control. Participants exhibited a significant contralateral pelvis drop on the non-dominant limb but in contrast maintained a contralateral lift throughout the movement on the dominant limb (Fig. 3). This particular asymmetry had the largest effect size of all significant findings (discrete analysis = 0.93; ACP = 0.88), and was present throughout the entire movement phase (Table 5 and Fig. 3). A contralateral pelvis drop on the non-dominant leg may be as a result of poorer neuromuscular control produced by the hip abductors (e.g. gluteus medius) [43–46] and may indicate a reduced ability to protect the knee from the excessive frontal plane moments associated with injury [13].

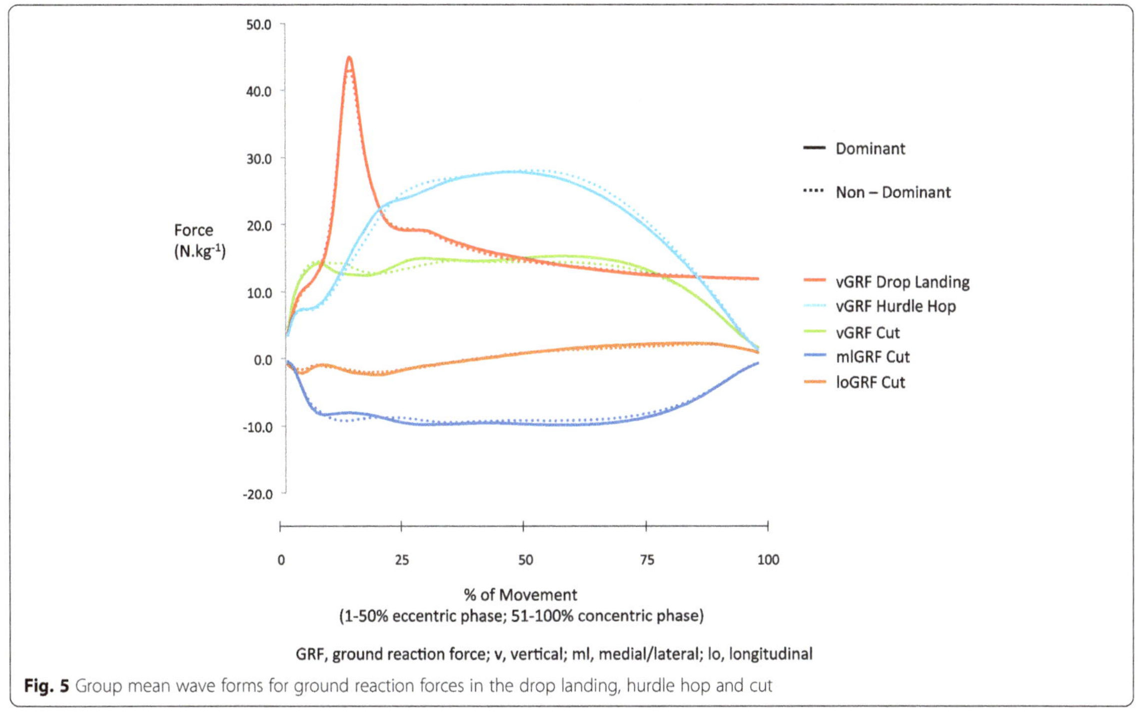

Fig. 5 Group mean wave forms for ground reaction forces in the drop landing, hurdle hop and cut

In the cut, the non-dominant side exhibited significantly greater ankle eccentric internal rotation moments early in the movement (Tables 5) and a more dorsiflexed/less plantar flexed ankle during the later phase of the movement (Table 5 and Fig. 4). Further examination of the data identified a highly significant correlation ($r = 0.86$, $p < 0.01$) between these variables indicating that the greater ankle internal rotation moments are related to the greater ankle dorsiflexion/less plantarflexion. The actual relevance of these asymmetries in elite athletes from an injury development standpoint, as with all of the asymmetries discussed here, requires further investigation with prospective studies. In addition, it is important to emphasise that while our findings illustrate that in an uninjured group of elite players some dominant versus non-dominant asymmetries may exist, the vast majority of variables exhibited no significant asymmetries. This provides a very valuable set of normative data with which to examine whether asymmetries in individuals are indicative of a predisposition to injury.

While the current study provides useful normative data for the movements examined, it is accepted as a limitation that the sample size was of twenty single-sport multidirectional athletes. A replication of this study with a larger number of participants, and with players from different sports, would enhance the knowledge base beyond this study. A potential limitation of the current study is that the neuromuscular challenge tests examined were all pre-planned, with no indecision element. It may be argued that movement in response to a sudden stimulus may elicit different and more sport

Table 5 Significant inter-limb differences ($p < 0.05$) as identified in the analysis of characterising phases

Variable	Difference	Percentage of movement (%)	*p* value	Effect size
Drop landing				
Hip abductor moment (Nm/kg)	D > ND	12-16	0.02	0.62
Pelvis contralateral lift (deg)	D > ND	53-100	0.04	0.66
Hurdle Hop				
Pelvis contralateral drop (deg)	ND > D	1 - 100	0.02	0.88
Cut				
Ankle internal rotation moment (Nm/kg)	ND > D	23-38	0.04	0.52
Ankle dorsiflexion (deg)	ND > D	78 - 94	0.01	0.57

D: dominant; ND: non-dominant

specific movement patterns and thus may potentially provide a greater test of symmetry [47, 48]. Based on findings from a meta-analysis undertaken by Brown and colleagues [49], substantial increases in frontal plane knee abductor moments (approximately 63 %) and knee internal rotator moments (up to 127 %) may be expected when undertaking un-planned in comparison to pre-planned cuts. Knee angles in all three movement planes would also be expected to increase [49]. Increases such as this could facilitate the identification of asymmetries that may be masked in less challenging pre-planned cuts.

Conclusions

Elite, injury free, rugby union players tend to exhibit bilateral symmetry across a broad range of biomechanical variables in a single leg drop landing, a single leg hurdle hop and a cutting manoeuvre. This study provides useful normative values for inter-limb symmetry in these movement tests. In addition it is recommended to utilise data analysis techniques that allow an examination of continuous data as opposed to discrete points; a discrete point analysis was unable to detect two of the five asymmetries identified. Our findings highlighted that the use of an asymmetry index as a standard measure of symmetry in biomechanical variables is questionable due to its sensitivity to variable magnitude. Asymmetries identified in this study were limited to frontal plane pelvis angles and moments in the drop landing and hurdle hop, alongside ankle sagittal plane angles and internal rotation moment in the cut. Prospective studies are required to establish the relevance of these biomechanical asymmetries in the development of injuries.

Additional files

Additional file 1: Drop landing clip. Video clip of the drop landing movement test.

Additional file 2: Hurdle hop clip. Video clip of the hurdle hop movement test.

Additional file 3: Running cut clip. Video clip of the running cut movement test.

Additional file 4: Table S1. Hurdle hop discrete point findings—inter-limb differences in peak variable magnitudes during the concentric phase. Inter-limb differences in peak variable magnitudes during the concentric phase of the hurdle hop movement.

Additional file 5: Table S2. Running cut discrete point findings—inter-limb differences in peak variable magnitudes during the concentric phase. Inter-limb differences in peak variable magnitudes during the concentric phase of the running cut movement.

Additional file 6: Table S3. Intraclass correlation coefficient (test-retest reliability) of measures in the drop landing, hurdle hop and cut. Test-retest reliability scores of measures in the drop landing, hurdle hop and cut.

Abbreviations

ACP: Analysis of characterising phases; 3D: Three dimensional; AI: Asymmetry index.

Competing interests

The authors declare that they have no competing interests.

Authors' contributions

All authors have been involved in revising the manuscript for important intellectual content. BM contributed to study concept and design, collected data, assisted with data analysis, data interpretation and drafted the manuscript. AFM, EF and EK contributed to study concept, design and data interpretation. KM and SS contributed to study concept, data interpretation and assisted with drafting the manuscript. SG assisted with data collection, data analysis and manuscript drafting. CR undertook data analysis and contributed to data interpretation. All authors read and approved the final manuscript.

Acknowledgements

This study has emanated from research funding supported in part by a research grant from Science Foundation Ireland (SFI) under Grant Number SFI/12/RC/2289. The authors would like to thank David Breen for his help in collecting the data and Dr Carson Farmer for his help with figure generation. The authors have received consent from the individual seen in Additional file 1, 2 and 3 that these movie clips can be published.

Author details

[1]Sports Medicine Department, Sports Surgery Clinic, Santry Demesne, Dublin, Ireland. [2]School of Health and Human Performance, Dublin City University, Dublin, Ireland. [3]Department of Life Sciences, Roehampton University, London, UK. [4]Centre for Health, Exercise and Sports Medicine, University of Melbourne, Melbourne, Australia. [5]Insight Centre for Data Analytics, Dublin City University, Dublin, Ireland. [6]Department of Medicine, University College Cork, Cork, Ireland.

References

1. Kiesel K, Plisky PJ, Voight ML. Can serious injury in professional football be predicted by a preseason functional movement screen? North Am J Sports Phys Ther. 2007;2:147.
2. Lockie RG, Schultz AB, Callaghan SJ, Jordan CA, Luczo TM, Jeffriess MD. A preliminary investigation into the relationship between functional movement screen scores and athletic physical performance in female team sport athletes. Biol Sport. 2015;32:41–51.
3. Plisky PJ, Rauh MJ, Kaminski TW, Underwood FB. Star excursion balance test as a predictor of lower extremity injury in high school basketball players. J Orthop Sports Phys Ther. 2006;36:911–9.
4. Hodges SJ, Patrick RJ, Reiser RF. Effects of fatigue on bilateral ground reaction force asymmetries during the squat exercise. J Strength Cond Res. 2011;25:3107–17.
5. Hickey KC, Quatman CE, Myer GD, Ford KR, Brosky JA, Hewett TE. Methodological report: dynamic field tests used in an NFL combine setting to identify lower-extremity functional asymmetries. J Strength Cond Res. 2009;23:2500–6.
6. Zifchock RA, Davis I, Hamill J. Kinetic asymmetry in female runners with and without retrospective tibial stress fractures. J Biomech. 2006;39:2792–7.
7. Hewett TE, Myer GD, Ford KR, Heidt Jr RS, Colosimo AJ, McLean SG, et al. Biomechanical measures of neuromuscular control and valgus loading of the knee predict anterior cruciate ligament injury risk in female athletes: a prospective study. Am J Sports Med. 2005;33:492–501.
8. Paterno MV, Schmitt LC, Ford KR, Rauh MJ, Myer GD, Huang B, et al. Biomechanical measures during landing and postural stability predict second anterior cruciate ligament injury after anterior cruciate ligament reconstruction and return to sport. Am J Sports Med. 2010;38:1968–78.
9. Ford KR, Myer GD, Smith RL, Vianello RM, Seiwert SL, Hewett TE. A comparison of dynamic coronal plane excursion between matched male and female athletes when performing single leg landings. Clin Biomech. 2006;21:33–40.
10. Wilkerson GB, Pinerola JJ, Caturano RW. Invertor vs. evertor peak torque and power deficiencies associated with lateral ankle ligament injury. J Orthop Sports Phys Ther. 1997;26:78–86.

11. Cowan DN, Jones BH, Frykman PN, Polly DW, Harman EA, Rosenstein RM, et al. Lower limb morphology and risk of overuse injury among male infantry trainees. Med Sci Sports Exerc. 1996;28:945–52.
12. Zifchock RA, Davis I, Higginson J, McCaw S, Royer T. Side-to-side differences in overuse running injury susceptibility: a retrospective study. Hum Mov Sci. 2008;27:888–902.
13. Powers CM. The influence of abnormal hip mechanics on knee injury: a biomechanical perspective. J Orthop Sports Phys Ther. 2010;40:42–51.
14. Zazulak BT, Hewett TE, Reeves P, Goldberg B, Cholewicki J. Deficits in neuromuscular control of the trunk predict knee injury risk a prospective biomechanical-epidemiologic study. Am J Sports Med. 2007;35:1123–30.
15. Dayakidis MK, Boudolos K. Ground reaction force data in functional ankle instability during two cutting movements. Clin Biomech. 2006;21:405–11.
16. Willems T, Witvrouw E, Delbaere K, De Cock A, De Clercq D. Relationship between gait biomechanics and inversion sprains: a prospective study of risk factors. Gait Posture. 2005;21:379–87.
17. Cibulka MT, Threlkeld-Watkins J. Patellofemoral pain and asymmetrical hip rotation. Phys Ther. 2005;85:1201–7.
18. Zajac FE. Muscle coordination of movement: a perspective. J Biomech. 1993;26:109–24.
19. Karamanidis K, Arampatzis A, Bruggemann GP. Symmetry and reproducibility of kinematic parameters during various running techniques. Med Sci Sports Exerc. 2003;35:1009–16.
20. Edwards S, Steele JR, Cook JL, Purdam CR, McGhee DE. Lower limb movement symmetry cannot be assumed when investigating the stop-jump landing. Med Sci Sports Exerc. 2012;44:1123–30.
21. Kristianslund E, Faul O, Bahr R, Myklebust G, Krosshaug T. Sidestep cutting technique and knee abduction loading: implications for ACL prevention exercises. Br J Sports Med. 2013;48:779–83.
22. Kimura Y, Ishibashi Y, Tsuda E, Yamamoto Y, Hayashi Y, Sato S. Increased knee valgus alignment and moment during single-leg landing after overhead stroke as a potential risk factor of anterior cruciate ligament injury in badminton. Br J Sports Med. 2012;46:207–13.
23. Besier TF, Lloyd DG, Cochrane JL, Ackland TR. External loading of the knee joint during running and cutting maneuvers. Med Sci Sports Exerc. 2001;33:1168–75.
24. Herzog W, Nigg BM, Read LJ, Olsson E. Asymmetries in ground reaction force patterns in normal human gait. Med Sci Sports Exerc. 1989;21:110–4.
25. Pappas E, Carpes FP. Lower extremity kinematic asymmetry in male and female athletes performing jump-landing tasks. J Sci Med Sport. 2012;15:87–92.
26. Viitasalo JT, Salo A, Lahtinen J. Neuromuscular functioning of athletes and non-athletes in the drop jump. Eur J Appl Physiol Occup Physiol. 1998;78:432–40.
27. Richter C, O'Connor NE, Marshall B, Moran K. Analysis of Characterizing Phases on Waveforms - An Application to Vertical Jumps. J Appl Biomech. 2013;30(2):316–21.
28. Ramsay J, Silverman BW. Functional data analysis. 2nd ed. New York: Springer; 2005.
29. Laughlin WA, Weinhandl JT, Kernozek TW, Cobb SC, Keenan KG, O'Connor KM. The effects of single-leg landing technique on ACL loading. J Biomech. 2011;44:1845–51.
30. Zazulak BT, Ponce PL, Straub SJ, Medvecky MJ, Avedisian L, Hewett TE. Gender comparison of hip muscle activity during single-leg landing. J Orthop Sports Phys Ther. 2005;35:292–9.
31. Marshall BM, Franklyn-Miller AD, King EA, Moran KA, Strike SC, Falvey EC. Biomechanical factors associated with time to complete a change of direction cutting maneuver. J Strength Cond Res. 2014;28:2845–51.
32. Kristianslund E, Krosshaug T, van den Bogert AJ. Artefacts in measuring joint moments may lead to incorrect clinical conclusions: the nexus between science (biomechanics) and sports injury prevention! Br J Sports Med. 2013;47:470–3.
33. Kristianslund E, Krosshaug T. Comparison of drop jumps and sport-specific sidestep cutting: implications for anterior cruciate ligament injury risk screening. Am J Sports Med. 2013;41:684–8.
34. Winter DA. Biomechanics and motor control of human movement. 4th ed. New Jersey: J. Wiley; 2009.
35. Hammill J, Selbie WS, Kepple TM. Three-Dimensional Kinematics. In: Robertson DGE, Caldwell GE, Hamill J, Leeds KG, editors. Research Methods in Biomechanics. 2nd ed. United Kingdom: Human Kinetics; 2014. p. 35–60.
36. Hewett TE, Di Stasi SL, Myer GD. Current concepts for injury prevention in athletes after anterior cruciate ligament reconstruction. Am J Sports Med. 2013;41:216–24.
37. Richter C, NE OC, Marshall B, Moran K. Comparison of discrete-point vs. dimensionality-reduction techniques for describing performance-related aspects of maximal vertical jumping. J Biomech. 2014;47:3012–7.
38. Carpes FP, Mota CB, Faria IE. On the bilateral asymmetry during running and cycling - a review considering leg preference. Phys Ther Sport. 2010;11:136–42.
39. Ford KR, Myer GD, Hewett TE. Reliability of landing 3D motion analysis: implications for longitudinal analyses. Med Sci Sports Exerc. 2007;39:2021–8.
40. Zakas A. Bilateral isokinetic peak torque of quadriceps and hamstring muscles in professional soccer players with dominance on one or both two sides. J Sports Med Phys Fit. 2006;46:28–35.
41. Shorter KA, Polk JD, Rosengren KS, Hsiao-Wecksler ET. A new approach to detecting asymmetries in gait. Clin Biomech. 2008;23:459–67.
42. Theoharopoulos A, Tsitskaris G. Isokinetic evaluation of the ankle plantar and dorsiflexion strength to determine the dominant limb in basketball players. Isokinet Exerc Sci. 2000;8:181–6.
43. Griffin LY, Albohm MJ, Arendt EA, Bahr R, Beynnon BD, Demaio M, et al. Understanding and preventing noncontact anterior cruciate ligament injuries: a review of the Hunt Valley II meeting, January 2005. Am J Sports Med. 2006;34:1512–32.
44. Nakagawa TH, Moriya ET, Maciel CD, Serrao FV. Trunk, pelvis, hip, and knee kinematics, hip strength, and gluteal muscle activation during a single-leg squat in males and females with and without patellofemoral pain syndrome. J Orthop Sports Phys Ther. 2012;42:491–501.
45. Nakagawa TH, Moriya ET, Maciel CD, Serrao AF. Frontal plane biomechanics in males and females with and without patellofemoral pain. Med Sci Sports Exerc. 2012;44:1747–55.
46. Takacs J, Hunt MA. The effect of contralateral pelvic drop and trunk lean on frontal plane knee biomechanics during single limb standing. J Biomech. 2012;45:2791–6.
47. O'Connor KM, Monteiro SK, Hoelker IA. Comparison of selected lateral cutting activities used to assess ACL injury risk. J Appl Biomech. 2009;25:9–21.
48. Fedie R, Carlstedt K, Willson JD, Kernozek TW. Effect of attending to a ball during a side-cut maneuver on lower extremity biomechanics in male and female athletes. Sports Biomech. 2010;9:165–77.
49. Brown SR, Brughelli M, Hume PA. Knee mechanics during planned and unplanned sidestepping: a systematic review and meta-analysis. Sports Med. 2014;44:1573–88.

14

Metastability in plyometric training on unstable surfaces

Armin Kibele[1*], Claudia Classen[1†], Thomas Muehlbauer[2†], Urs Granacher[2†] and David G Behm[3†]

Abstract

Background: In the past, plyometric training (PT) has been predominantly performed on stable surfaces. The purpose of this pilot study was to examine effects of a 7-week lower body PT on stable vs. unstable surfaces. This type of exercise condition may be denoted as metastable equilibrium.

Methods: Thirty-three physically active male sport science students (age: 24.1 ± 3.8 years) were randomly assigned to a PT group (n = 13) exercising on stable (STAB) and a PT group (n = 20) on unstable surfaces (INST). Both groups trained countermovement jumps, drop jumps, and practiced a hurdle jump course. In addition, high bar squats were performed. Physical fitness tests on stable surfaces (hexagonal obstacle test, countermovement jump, hurdle drop jump, left-right hop, dynamic and static balance tests, and leg extension strength) were used to examine the training effects.

Results: Significant main effects of time (ANOVA) were found for the countermovement jump, hurdle drop jump, hexagonal test, dynamic balance, and leg extension strength. A significant interaction of time and training mode was detected for the countermovement jump in favor of the INST group. No significant improvements were evident for either group in the left-right hop and in the static balance test.

Conclusions: These results show that lower body PT on unstable surfaces is a safe and efficient way to improve physical performance on stable surfaces.

Keywords: Instability resistance training, Stretch-shortening cycle, Physical fitness test, Balance training

Background

In different sports, athletes must produce force and power in motor skills during stretch-shortening type of muscle contractions. In the past, plyometric exercises have been used to adapt the neuromuscular system for the corresponding type of force development [1]. However, in many instances, athletes, when executing plyometric skills, experience balance disturbances due to tackling opponents, cutting maneuvers, slippery turf, or strong winds. In these cases, plyometric skills incorporate balance demands during force development. While athletes are, for the most part, able to counterbalance the disturbances through muscular activity simplistic classifications referring to a stable or unstable state of equilibrium appear to be inappropriate. Instead, the above conditions of force and power production correspond to a metastable state of equilibrium. For metastable systems [2], slight disturbances do not change the present state of equilibrium. Only sufficiently strong disturbances will put the system out of the metastable state and the system will pass into another state of equilibrium. Examples of metastability [3] can be found in biology, climatology, economics, or physics. Accordingly, an athlete working out on a stability device to improve his balance skills would exercise in a state of metastable equilibrium. While small imbalances are being compensated by muscular activity to keep the athlete in the metastable equilibrium large disturbances will force him to drop from the device.

In the past, resistance training lacking stable support has been termed as instability training [4,5] incorporating muscular demands for balance and weight lifting at the same time. In contrast, plyometric training on unstable surfaces has not been investigated yet. To date, effects of instability training (IT) may be classified regarding

* Correspondence: akibele@uni-kassel.de
†Equal contributors
[1]Institute for Sports and Sport Science, University of Kassel, Damaschkestr. 25, Kassel 34121, Germany
Full list of author information is available at the end of the article

the limbs and muscles involved, the training contents and intensity, the length of the training, and subjects' expertise as independent variables [4,6]. For differences in the dependent variables, instability studies using exercises on unstable surfaces have conclusively shown improvements in strength and endurance measures [7-10]. In addition, studies have demonstrated significant improvements in power related skills as jump test and hopping tests [8,10,11]. Instability training was reported to strengthen the core [5,12], the upper extremities [11], the lower extremities [8,13], and to improve sports related skills [8,14]. However, researchers concluded that this type of training does not provide a sufficient stimulus to induce neuromuscular adaptations in the primary working muscles for the force development in the line of action [15-17]. Instead, instability exercises accounted for increased activity in the stabilizing muscles and, thus, provide essential stimuli for their neuromuscular adaptation [6].

For the lower extremities, studying IT effects showed that squat exercises on stable or unstable platforms provide similar improvements in strength and in sports related skills with only small amounts of instability as in the 20 m-sprint [8]. However, Kibele and Behm [8] detected superior effects of instability load training for sports related skills with larger amounts of instability (e.g., left-right hop). In contrast, Cressey on colleagues [14] could not detect any superior output of IT in jump tests or sprint tests as compared to stable training conditions. A possible reason for this discrepancy might be related to the instability devices used in both studies (inflatable rubber discs with a soft surface vs. inverted Bosu Balls and wooden rockers with a hard surface). In fact, Wahl and Behm [17] showed that moderately unstable training devices do not provide sufficient challenges to the neuromuscular system in experienced resistance trained individuals. Hence, IT effects might depend on the properties of the support devices. In addition, the expertise of the subjects could be a determinant of IT as well since the resistance training experience was different in the above studies (collegiate soccer players with considerable resistance training experience [14]; highly resistance-trained individuals [17], and sport students with no experience in resistance training [8]).

Aside from instability resistance training with loads, effects for the lower extremities have been investigated in numerous studies on balance training. For example, improvements in rate of force development under maximal isometric conditions were consistently observed [18,19] without any increases in maximal voluntary strength indicating that improvements in power related skills to be likely [20]. While these trainings effects were associated with neural adaptations on the spinal and the supraspinal level [21], the magnitude of the improvements remained small as compared to ballistic strength training [19,22]. While these results show that balance training alone has the potential to improve power related motor skills it is of interest to discover if plyometric exercises under metastable training conditions provides substantially greater improvements than a traditional stable resistance training program.

In regard to the plyometric training (PT), since the early work of Verhoshansky [23,24], numerous studies have been conducted. Although some conflicting results with no beneficial effects exist, meta-analyses indicated a positive effect of plyometric training on athletic performance [22,25]. In this regard, mean improvements in vertical jump performance were reported ranging between 5% for squat jumps and depth jumps and roughly 8% for countermovement type jumps [25]. In addition, de Villarreal and coworkers [26,27] showed that, although PT improvements in jump performance are observed independent of the physical condition of the subjects tested, experienced athletes obtained greater enhancements in the vertical jumps. However, among the various possibilities to perform PT, the surface stability (the resistance to disturbance of equilibrium) has been rarely evaluated. For instance, Impellizzeri and colleagues [28] found larger improvements in countermovement jumps but not in squat jumps when performed on grass as compared to sand surfaces. In addition, enhancements in the vertical jump in volleyball players were found following aquatic PT [29].

In summary, across the numerous studies conducted on the effects of IT, to the authors' knowledge, so far, no study has investigated the effects of metastability in PT on strength and power related skills. Thus, according to the principle of dynamic conformity by Verhoshansky [23], the means of specialized strength preparation should be chosen that it has maximum accordance with the force development during the real sport competition (For another version of the principle, see the concept of training specificity by Sale and MacDougall [30]). In other words, if instability is a major part of the plyometric force development in the real sport situation, it should be part of the PT routines as well. Therefore, the objective of the present study was to compare a PT performed on stable vs. unstable surfaces to evaluate their effectiveness in improving skills related to strength and power abilities. It was hypothesized that, according to an additive effect of PT and balance training, larger improvements are expected through PT under metastable equilibrium conditions on testing measures incorporating a stretch-shortening cycle and balance demands (e.g., 1 legged hopping) as compared to the stable PT. For a first approach to this issue, a pilot study with sport science students was conducted to explore the effects of metastability in PT on unstable surfaces. For simplicity reasons, stable and metastable states of equilibrium are further on referred to as stable and unstable exercise conditions. As care has to be taken to ensure that PT is safe for children and athletes [31,32] particular guidelines are built into the present intervention.

Methods

Experimental approach

To evaluate the effects of short-term PT on stable or unstable surfaces on athletic performance measures (i.e., tests for agility, jumping, hopping, balance, strength), physically active male sport science students who were inexperienced in resistance training were randomly divided into a lower-body stable and unstable PT group. Training was conducted twice per week for 7 weeks during summer months (see Figure 1).

Subjects

Fifty healthy and physically active male sport science students were randomly assigned to either a PT group on unstable (INST) or stable (STAB) surfaces. Course credit was given for their participation. Their average amount of everyday and sports-related physical activity ranged between 10 and 20 h per week including university courses in physical education and the practice of a favorite sport. However, none of the subjects had performed any systematic resistance training before the start of the study. Given that free-weight experienced subjects do not show the extent of muscle activation increases typically reported for untrained individuals when subjected to moderate levels of instability [17], inexperienced subjects were included in this investigation. Each training group comprised 25 participants. Due to a variety of reasons (i.e., schedules, muscle soreness, lack of motivation) other than injuries, a number of participants were unable to perform the entire 12 training sessions or to participate in the post-test measurements. These subjects were excluded from the data analysis, none of them suffering from any injury. In total, 13 subjects remained for statistical data evaluation in the stable group (age: 24.1 ± 4.6 y, body-mass: 75.8 ± 8.3 kg, height: 179 ± 5.3 cm) and 20 subjects in the unstable group (age: 24.1 ± 3.4 y, body-mass: 76.1 ± 8.9 kg, height: 182 ± 5.0 cm). There were no significant baseline differences in anthropometric data or age between the groups. All subjects were kindly asked not to make any significant changes to their diet during the testing or training program. Before the start of the study, all participants were thoroughly informed about potential risks and thereafter signed an informed consent document. The experiments were conducted according to the latest amendments of the declaration of Helsinki approved by the 59th World Medical Association in Seoul 2008. The institution's Human Research Ethics Board approved the study (File number 2013–0321).

Testing

All testing was performed indoors on a regular gym surface. Three consecutive trials were executed for each measure and the best performance was used for the statistical analysis. Prior to testing, subjects warmed up for approximately 10 minutes by light jogging and short bouts of dynamic muscle stretching. Pre- and post-testing (see Table 1, left side) consisted of the Hexagonal Obstacle Test (agility), the Countermovement Jump Test (bilateral power with moderate stretch-shortening type muscle action), a hurdle drop jump test (bilateral power with fast stretch-shortening type muscle action), the Left-Right-Hop-Test (unilateral power with stretch-shortening type muscle action), the Standing Stork-Test (static balance), a balance beam test (dynamic balance), and a isometric leg extension test (static leg strength).

The Hexagonal Obstacle Test (HOT) was administered according to Reiman and Manske [33]. The length of each hexagon side was 60 cm, and each angle was 120 degrees. The subjects started with both feet together in the middle of the hexagon facing the front line. On the "go" command, they jumped ahead across the line, then back over the same line into the middle of the hexagon. Then, continuing to face forward with feet together, jump over the next side and back into the hexagon. Subjects continued this pattern for three full revolutions and performed the test in a clockwise direction. The total testing

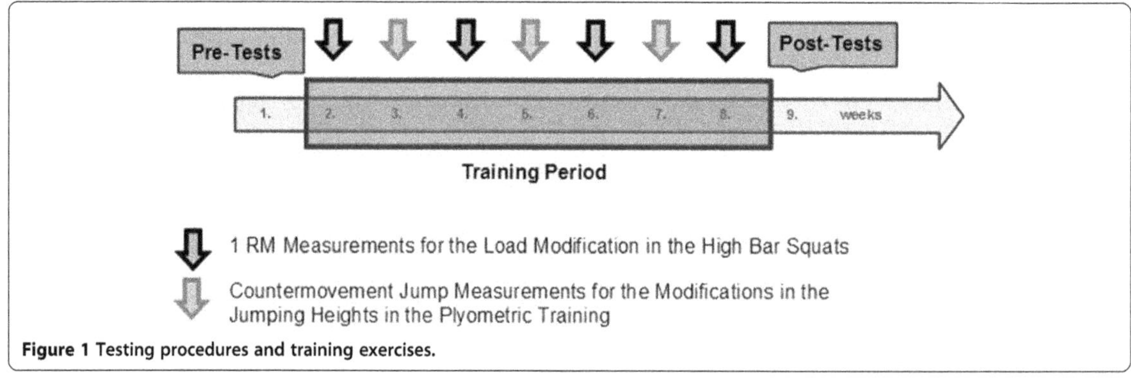

Figure 1 Testing procedures and training exercises.

Table 1 Testing procedures and training exercises

Testing	Training: STAB group	Training: INST group
• **Hexagonal Obstacle Test** (agility), • **Countermovement Jump Test** (bilateral power, moderate stretchshortening cycle)	exercises performed on stable surfaces	exercises performed on unstable surfaces (foam rocker boards, balance pads, inflatable discs, balance boards, wobble boards)
• **Hurdle Jump Test** (bilateral power, fast stretch-shortening cycle)	**Bilateral Countermovement Jumps,** 5 reps, 3 series, 5 min rest	**Bilateral Countermovement Jumps,** 5 reps, 3 series, 5 min rest
• **Left-Right-Hop-Test** (unilateral power, fast stretch-shortening cycle)	**Bilateral Drop Jumps,** 10 reps, 3 series, 5 min rest	**Bilateral Drop Jumps,** 10 reps, 3 series, 5 min rest
• **Standing Stork-Test** (static balance)	**Bilateral Hurdle Jumps,** 5 reps, 3 series, 5 min rest	**Bilateral Hurdle Jumps,** 5 reps, 3 series, 5 min rest
• **Balance Beam Test** (dynamic balance) • **Leg Extension Test** (isometric leg strength)	**High Bar Squats** (appr. 90° – 100°knee angle) 80% 1 RM, 5 reps, 3 series, 5 min rest	**High Bar Squats** (appr. 90° - 100°knee angle) 50% 1 RM, 5 reps, 3 series, 5 min rest

time was measured by a stop-watch to the nearest tenth of a second. According to Reiman and Manske [33] intra-class correlations (ICC) ranged between 0.86 and 0.95 for the HOT. In our study, an ICC value was calculated across the three trials during pre-test measurements and amounted to 0.98 (see Table 2).

The Countermovement Jump (CMJ) test was conducted to evaluate the bilateral plyometric power with a self-initiated stretch-shortening cycle and a moderate muscle stretch typical for many sport activities. Further, a hurdle drop jump test was conducted to evaluate the bilateral plyometric power during a fast stretch-shortening cycle in the course of a landing phase after a dropping movement. The CMJ test was performed according to the guidelines provided by Komi and Bosco [34]. The Optojump photo-cell system (Microgate, Bolzano, Italy) was used to estimate the individual jump performance. This system consists of two parallel bars (one receiver and one transmitter unit). Bars were placed approximately 1 m apart and parallel to each other. The transmitter contains 32 light emitting diodes, which are positioned 0.3 cm from ground level at 3.125-cm intervals. The Optojump system measures the flight time of CMJs with an accuracy of 1/1000 seconds (1 kHz). Optojump software (version 1.5.1.0) was used for quantification of jump height. Compared with a force plate, the Optojump system demonstrated strong validity (ICC = 0.99) and excellent test-retest reliability (ICC = 0.98) for the estimation of vertical jump height [15]. Our own data revealed an ICC of 0.99. To ensure that performance was predominantly dependent on the leg extensor muscles, subjects were asked to keep their hands on their hips throughout the movement task. After a brief verbal instruction prior to the jumps, subjects waited in an upright starting position for the final starting command of the experimenter ("go"). Briefly before the starting command, the computer based data acquisition was initialized by a keystroke. The subjects were instructed to jump as high as possible.

For the hurdle drop jump test, the Optojump system was used as well. Here, the subjects were instructed to jump over a knee high plastic bar prior to performing a bouncing drop jump to gain maximal height. The height in the latter drop jump was used as an estimate for the plyometric power associated with a short stretch shortening cycle. During the jumping task, the subjects kept their hands akimbo to ensure that the jumps were performed primarily by the leg extensor muscles. The ICC value for the hurdle drop jump test amounted to 0.99.

The 20-m Left-Right-Hop-Test (LRH) provided an indication of left and right leg power and possible right vs. left leg power imbalances [35]. Subjects were asked to perform single-leg hops with each leg for a distance of 20 m. A run-up distance of 15 m was provided prior to the hopping task. Two light barriers were used to examine the time taken for the hopping distance. The ICC value for the LRH amounted to 0.99 (as compared to ICC = 0.98 provided by Kibele and Behm [8]).

Dynamic balance testing was performed on a 3-m gymnastic beam slightly elevated above ground level [8]. Standing one step from the end of beam with one foot touching its surface and facing in the movement direction, subjects were asked to step forward (on a "go" signal) and walk on the beam until they touched its opposite end with one foot. At that time, subjects had to proceed with a backward movement to the starting line as fast as possible. The time for both directions was used as a testing criterion. Time measurements were performed with a stop watch while announcing the start with an acoustic signal. The ICC value for the dynamic balance test amounted to 0.98 (as compared to ICC = 0.90 reported by Kibele and Behm [8].

For the testing of static balance, the Stork-test was used according to Reiman and Manske [33]. In this task, subjects stood comfortably on both feet with their hands on their hips. They lifted their preferred leg and placed the sole of the corresponding foot against the side of the

Table 2 Pre- and post-test mean values, standard deviations, and relative differences in the left-right-hop (LRH), countermovement jump test (CMJT), hurdle drop jump test (HDJT), static balance stork test (ST), dynamic balance test (DBT), agility hexagonal obstacle test (HOT), and an isometric leg extension strength test (ILES) for the training groups exercising on stable (STAB) and unstable (INST) surfaces

		ICC	STAB (n = 13)	INST (n = 20)
Age (y)			24.1 ± 4.6	24.1 ± 3.4
Height (cm)			179 ± 5.3	182 ± 5.2
Mass (kg)			75.8 ± 8.3	76.0 ± 8.9
LRH (s)	Pre	0.99	3.8 ± 0.5	3.8 ± 0.4
Left-Right-Hop	Post		3.8 ± 0.5	3.8 ± 0.5
	% diff		−0.1%	+ 0.3%
CMJT (cm)	Pre	0.99	39.9 ± 4.3	35.3 ± 4.8
Countermovement jump test	Post		42.0 ± 6.0	40.1 ± 4.8
F^m = 28.1 (η^2 = 0.47) F^x = 4.4* (η^2 = 0.12)**	% diff		+5.1%	**+14.5%**°°**
HDJT (cm)	Pre	0.99	49.2 ± 6.7	44.2 ± 5.7
Hurdle drop jump test	Post		51.3 ± 6.8	48.4 ± 6.3
F^m = 17.7 (η^2 = 0.36)**	% diff		+4.6%	**+9.8%*°°**
ST (s)	Pre	0.82	17.3 ± 12.8	10.5 ± 8.0
Static balance stork-test	Post		15.2 ± 10.6	11.8 ± 6.6
	% diff		−1.0%	+39.7%
DBT (s)	Pre	0.98	3.9 ± 0.8	3.8 ± 0.7
Dynamic balance test	Post		3.2 ± 0.5	3.1 ± 0.5
F^m = 61.5 (η^2 = 0.67)**	% diff		**+15.9%*°°**	**+18.4%**°°**
HOT (s)	Pre	0.98	11.4 ± 1.2	10.9 ± 1.2
Agility hexagonal obstacle test	Post		10.3 ± 1.2	9.9 ± 1.0
F^m = 57.1 (η^2 = 0.65)**	% diff		**+9.7%*°°**	**+8.3%**°°**
ILES (kg)	Pre	0.98	162.9 ± 30	174.5 ± 36
Isometric leg extension strength	p ost		186.2 ± 42	194.9 ± 44
F^m = 12.3 (η^2 = 0.29)**	% diff		**+14.7%°**	**+13.4%°**

Single (*) and double (**) asterisks indicate α-error probabilities of 0.05 and 0.01 in the paired t-test for the pre-post differences for both groups separately and for the F-tests, single (°) and double (°°) circles indicate α-error probability of 0.05 and 0.01 in the non-parametric Wilcoxon-test.
In addition, F-values with effect size vales (partial η^2) are listed for significant pre-post main effects (F^m) and for the significant interactions of the pre-post factor and the group factor (F^x).
Reliability estimates (ICC) were calculated through Cronbach's α (internal consistency) across the three trials during pre-test measurements.

other leg's kneecap. On the "go" signal, a stopwatch was started and the subject raised the heel of the non-preferred foot to stand on the toes. The participant was asked to hold this position for as long as possible. The test was terminated when the heel of the supporting leg touched the ground or the foot moved away from the knee cap. Reiman and Manske [33] reported a reliability value of r = 0.87 for the Stork test. Our own data revealed an ICC = 0.82.

Isometric leg extension strength (ILES) was examined with a cable pull device (Takei A5002, Fitness Monitors, Wrexham, England) in an upright body posture. Individual cable lengths were chosen to provide a knee angle of approximately 160° [8]. Subjects were asked to start the pull initially with a moderate intensity and slowly increase the intensity to maximum exertion while keeping the trunk extended to prevent muscle injuries. Reliability scores (ICC) for the leg extension strength amounted to 0.98 (as compared to ICC = 0.93 provided by Kibele and Behm [8].

Training materials

The training lasted 7 weeks with 2 training sessions per week to achieve effective results for inexperienced strength training subjects [36]. Each training session lasted 40 minutes. Participants were monitored during training by one of the authors of this study to ensure that subjects exercised at maximal effort. Prior to every second training week, stable squats were used to test for 1 RM strength performance. The time course of the training sessions is sketched in Figure 1. The training was scheduled in the morning until noon time (8.30 a.m. to 1.30 p.m.) on regular work days. For both training groups, CMJs, drop jumps, and a series hurdle jumps were performed (see Table 1, right side and Figure 2). In addition, subjects executed high bar squats (described later on in greater detail) to additionally strengthen their leg extension muscles parallel to the plyometric exercises. While these exercises were conducted on a regular gym floor with a rigid surface for the STAB group, exercises for the INST group were executed on various unstable platforms (see below). Throughout the trainings sessions, subjects were advised to take particular care in performing the exercises on the unstable platforms and follow the given safety guidelines [32,33]. Aside from paying attention to safety considerations for the force development during metastable states of equilibrium, INST subjects were asked to focus on a stationary position in the unstable platform used for their exercises. In this regard, Makaruk and colleagues [37] showed that such an external focus of attention during PT may provide a greater stimulus to jump performance in slow stretch shortening cycle tasks by producing greater force than adopting the internal and no specific focus.

Prior to STAB training, subjects warmed up for approximately 10 minutes by doing light intensity jogging and short bouts of dynamic muscle stretching. After warm-up, subjects executed 3 sets with 15 repetitions for CMJs on stable surfaces with a 5 min rest between the sets.

The CMJs were performed onto an individually target height platform. In this respect, subjects jumped onto a judo mat platform with a height that corresponded to the nearest CMJ value during the pre-test by rounding up or down to the given judo mat levels. For example, a pre-test CMJ value of 31.5 cm was rounded up to a target height on level 3 = 34 cm. After every second week, the target height was increased by 2 cm. This increase was achieved by adding 2 cm layers underneath the judo mat piles. While level 0 indicated the lowest step at 16 cm, a difference between 6 cm was selected to the next step (level 1 = 22, level 2 = 28, ..., level 10 = 76 cm). For the DJs, subjects dropped from an individually determined platform level to a stable surface and executed a fast stretch-shortening cycle jump upon their given target height level. Three sets with 10 repetitions and a 5 min rest between the sets were required.

For the series of hurdle jumps, 3 sets with 5 jumps and a 5 min rest between the sets were performed. The adjustable hurdle heights were kept constant for the first four weeks of training at approximately 150% of the previously assessed CMJ best value during the pre-test. From the fifth week on, the hurdle heights were increased by 5 cm until the end of the training period. This set-up was chosen since subjects were expected to tuck up their legs while crossing the hurdle bars.

Finally, subjects performed high bar squats (from a starting point with a knee angle of approx. 90 to 100°) at 80% of their 1repetition maximum (RM) (stable) with 5 sets, 3 repetitions, and a 5 min rest between the sets. The training loads for the high bar squats were modified every second week according to the 1RM.

For the INST group, the same warm-up routine and the same amount of sets, repetitions, and rest period durations were used. However the high bar squats (with 50% of the 1RM stable) and the plyometric jumps were executed on unstable platforms. For the series of hurdle jumps, the hurdle heights were kept constant for the first four weeks during training at approximately 100% of the previously assessed CMJ best value during the pre-test. Landing and the take-off were performed on an Airex Pro SoftX foam rocker board and an Airex balance pad (Gaugler & Lutz, Aalen-Ebnat, Germany), inflatable

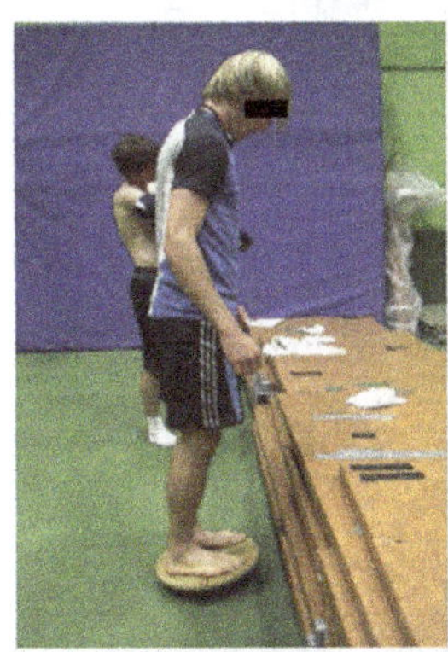
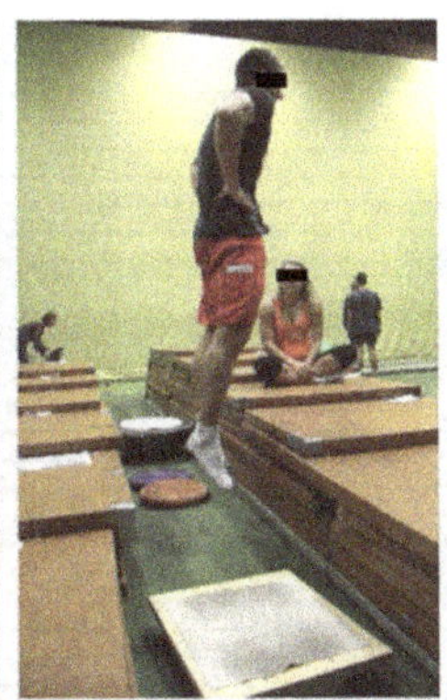
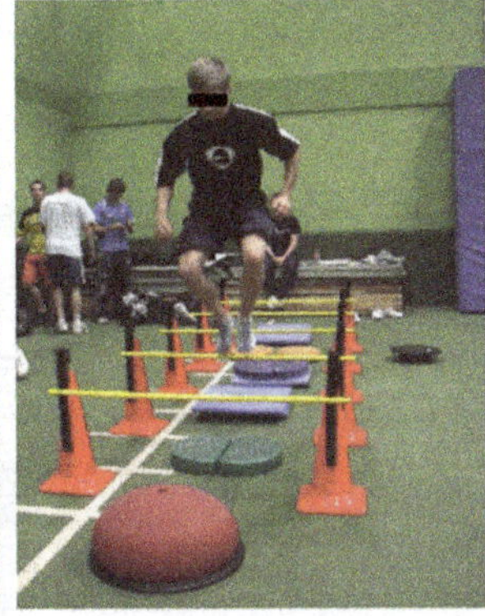

Figure 2 Left image: countermovement jump exercise on a wobble board, middle image: drop jump exercise on a wooden rocker board, right image: series of hurdle jumps (further details listed in the text).

discs and balance boards (DynAir Pro, AeroSteps XL, and Balance Board from Togu, Prien-Bachham, Germany), as well as a rigid wooden wobble/rocker board.

In terms of the individual load intensities during the PT routines, dropping heights and target heights for jumping were regulated by the following rationale. Throughout the training sessions, subjects with different training protocols practiced at the same time. Therefore, various dropping platforms and landing platforms for the individual target heights were required for the CMJ and drop jump exercises. For this purpose, two piles of judo mats with increasing heights were lined up parallel to provide the different platforms for the dropping levels and the target heights (see Figure 3). The distance between the two lines was approximately 90 cm. A total of 11 platform levels with 6 cm difference between the two levels were used.

While the target steps for the STAB group were matched with the CMJ performance during the pre-tests, two levels (i.e., 12 cm) were added to this platform height for the INST group due to the device heights of the unstable take-off surfaces. For the drop jumps, subjects were given an individual drop height and target jump height. Again, the best CMJ value during the pre-tests was used to establish this protocol. For the STAB group, subjects dropped from one step less than they jumped onto in the CMJ training. Their target height in the drop jump training was settled one level higher than for the CMJ training. This protocol was based on the results of a pilot study and served for convenience in the training organization.

For the INST group, this protocol was slightly modified depending on the surface height from which the subjects jumped during DJ training. For the DynAirX inflatable disc, subjects dropped from one step less than they jumped onto during CMJ training. Again, their target height was one step more than what they performed during CMJ training. For the Airex Pro SoftX™ foam rocker board, subjects dropped from one step more than they jumped onto during CMJ training and their target height was three steps beyond the CMJ training level. For the drop jumps on a BOSU™ Ball (hemispherical ball) (from Fitness Quest Inc., Canton, OH USA), larger add-on steps were required to settle the jumping height for drop jump performed from this device. Due to the larger construction height of this device and its elastic rebound behavior, subjects dropped from two steps more than they jumped onto during CMJ training and their target height was four steps beyond the CMJ training level.

Statistics

The Kolmogorov-Smirnov goodness-of-fit test was calculated separately for each training group. In addition, Levene's test for equality of error variances was computed for all variables. There were no significant differences detected with the Levene test and all data were normally distributed according to the Kolmogorov-Smirnov test. To analyze the training effects, a 2-way analysis of variance (ANOVA) with repeated measures (SPSS V19.0) was executed. The factors included training groups (unstable and stable training) and time (pre- and post-training). Eta^2 values were calculated to assess effect sizes. If significant interactions were detected, a Bonferroni-Dunn's procedure post hoc test was utilized. In addition to the ANOVA calculations, pre-post differences were analyzed by paired t-tests for both groups separately. In addition, a non-parametric Wilcoxon-test was calculated to confirm

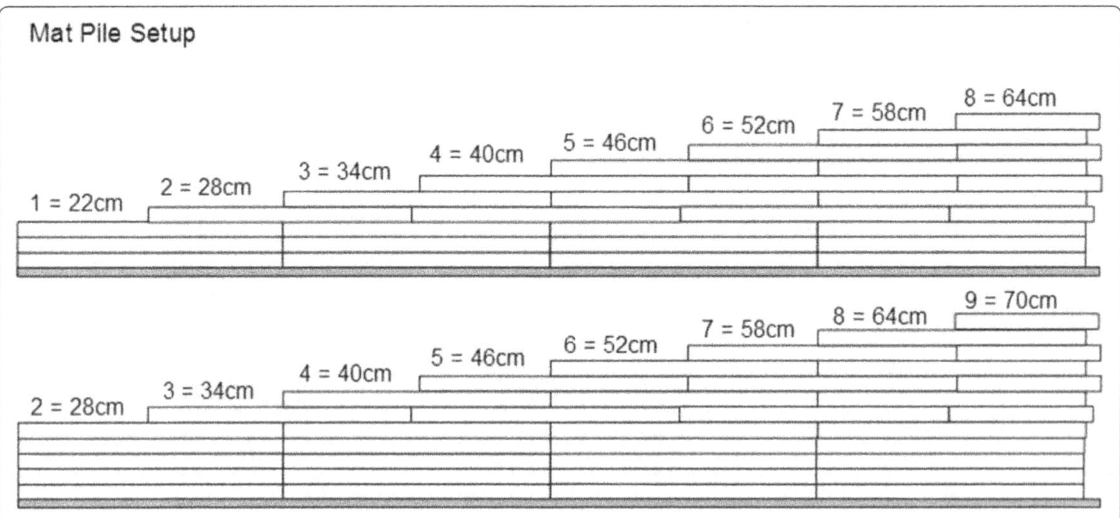

Figure 3 Two piles of judo mats to provide target heights for CMJs and dropping heights and target heights for the DJs. Both judo mat piles were lined up in parallel with a distance of approximately 90 cm.

the parametric results independent from any data distribution effect. Statistical significance was considered to be achieved at $p = 0.05$ for all tests administered. Intraclass correlations were calculated (according to Cronbach's alpha for internal consistency) to estimate the reliability of the tests applied [38]. For this purpose, the results of the three test repetitions during pre-tests of each subject were included in the reliability evaluations.

Results

Participants in both PT groups completed the training program according to the given schedule and none of them reported any training-related injury. However, five subjects from the INST group and 12 subjects from the STAB group were excluded from the study since they were unable to complete at least 75 percent of the training sessions in the course of the seven-week training program. For the remaining subjects (in both PT groups), a mean attendance rate of 98 (±4) percent was observed.

The means and standard deviations for all analyzed variables before and after training are displayed in Table 2. The ICCs ranged between 0.82 and 0.99. For the pre-post analysis, significant differences were found across both groups for the HOT (agility), dynamic balance, CMJ test, hurdle jumps, and ILES (leg extension strength) with η^2 effect sizes ranging between 0.29 and 0.67. There was one significant interaction observed for the CMJ test between the pre-post factor and the group factor ($\eta^2 = 0.12$) while the level of significance for this interaction was nearly achieved for the hurdle jump test. The specific training effect for the INST group was confirmed by the analysis of the paired t-tests in both groups. In this regards, a significant improvement was observed for the INST group only. To prevent for any specific effect of the baseline deviations in both groups, a t-test for independent samples was calculated for the pre-post differences in CMJ test [39] confirming the significant interaction effect in the repeated measures ANOVA ($t = 2.1$, $p < 0.05$). These results were substantiated by the paired t-tests and the non-parametric Wilcoxon-test for the STAB and the INST group separately. No significant improvements were found for either group in the LRH (Left-Right-Hop) and in the Stork test (static balance).

Discussion

The present results extend the findings of an earlier study that investigated the effects of traditional resistance training on sport related functional performance applying leg extension exercises on stable and unstable surfaces [8]. Overall, our results show that metastability in PT on unstable surfaces provided similar results as PT on stable surfaces. For the HOT (agility), dynamic balance, and ILES (leg strength), comparable improvements were found across both training groups. In contrast, no significant improvements could be detected in both groups in the LRH and the Stork test. Further, as a main result, the present study identified specific improvements for the INST group in the jumping tests (CMJ and hurdle jump tests) executed on stable surfaces. In fact, the CMJ test increases (+5.1%) for the STAB group corresponded in size to the trainings effects listed in the meta-analyses on PT [25]. However, these increases did not reach the level of statistical significance. In contrast, the INST improved their CMJ height significantly by approximately 15 percent. This result does not agree with the principle of dynamic conformity [1] as larger improvements on stable testing surfaces were expected for the STAB group as compared to the INST group. For the hurdle jump test, a significant interaction effect was missed ($p = 0.15$) although pre-post differences in the t-test and in the Wilcoxon-test indicated a tendency towards a specific improvement in the INST group.

The reported training effects for the jump tests (on stable platforms) appear to question the principle of dynamic conformity given that the STAB group's jump training exercises resembled the test jump conditions more specifically than those of the INST group. In this regard, the improvements reported in CMJ test for the INST group could be caused by a number of reasons including a higher neural adaptation stimulus for the primary leg extensors when exercising on unstable platforms, a more pronounced strengthening stimulus for the stabilizing leg extensor muscles (e.g., the adductor muscles), and/or an improvement in the overall intermuscular coordination pattern. Last not least, to some degree, the results could be attributed to the low training status of the sample as well. In contrast, due to the short intervention period and the chosen training volume, it seems unlikely that muscle mass increased to a greater degree in the INST group as compared to the STAB group.

To date, there is only limited evidence supporting the idea that IT has the potential to enhance the activation level of the primary leg extensors. While some exercise studies performed under unstable conditions with lower loads applied as compared to the stable condition showed higher limb muscle activations under unstable as compared to stable conditions [40,41]. In contrast, other studies were inconclusive or found similar activation levels [4,42]. Indirect evidence for a task-specific training effect in the instability group is also indicated by the study of Cressey and co-workers [14]. These authors examined the effects of lower leg extension tasks (e.g., squats, deadlifts, lunges) on unstable platforms and did not find any improvements in the countermovement jump and in the bouncing drop jump (on stable platforms). In addition, the cross-sectional study by Prieske and colleagues [43] showed that the primary leg extensors were less activated during drop jumps performed on unstable as compared to a stable surface. However, this study did not exclude that the neuromuscular activation of the primary leg extensors might increase in the course of a PT on unstable surfaces. In fact, increases in the muscle activation level were observed following a PT on stable surfaces [44]. Therefore, more longitudinal studies are needed to analyze the any potential change in the muscle activation pattern as a result of metastability in PT.

Earlier, Kibele and Behm [8] investigated the effects of unstable versus stable resistance training of the leg extensors (i.e., high bar squats on stable and unstable surfaces) and found similar strength gains for both training groups and conditions. In that study, the intervention groups performed high bar squats at intensities of 70% of the 1 RM (stable group) and 50% of the 1 RM (unstable group), indicating that an additional adaptive stimulus due to the unstable platform may have compensated through smaller load intensities and reduced muscle activation in the primary leg extensors. The presumed adaptive stimulus could relate both to the primary leg extensors and/or to the stabilizing muscles. More evidence for this line of argument comes from studies showing that balance training alone enhanced countermovement jump height [20]. Here, neural adaptive processes following balance training were shown to reduce postural sway (i.e., less centre of mass displacements in the horizontal plane) in terms of a stabilizing effect and additionally improve jumping height under stable conditions (i.e., larger centre of mass elevation in the vertical direction) in terms of a performance enhancing effect. In this regard, improving trunk stability by exercising on unstable surfaces could reduce the variations in the direction of the resultant force vector, and thus vertical force production, in the countermovement jump when compared to jump training under stable conditions. For this matter, the stabilizing effect might relate to the trunk stabilizers in concert with the leg stabilizer muscles [6]. In particular, for the leg stabilizers, the stabilizing and the motor functions of a muscle may change in a task-specific way [45,46].

Aside from a possible center of mass stabilizing effect, balance training improved performance in reactive drop-jumps by enhanced neuromuscular activity in the lower-leg muscles immediately after ground contact [18]. Therefore, a similar effect could have caused the superior CMJ performance of the INST group as postural sway and balance demands were more pronounced during a PT on unstable platforms. As a last possible argument, instability PT could have altered muscle activation strategies related to an improvement in the coordination between muscles. Such an effect was observed in the study by Chimera and co-workers [44]. On the other hand, reflex activity during the state of metastable equilibrium, prior to the jumps, could have evoked synchronization in the muscle activation of the stabilizing muscles to reduce the horizontal sway as was denoted by Horak and Nashner [47] as a hip strategy.

While improvements for the jump tests were detected following a PT on unstable surfaces, significant increases in the testing results were amiss for the STAB group. This somewhat surprising finding might be based on statistical as well as methodological reasons. For the latter, higher baseline values in the STAB group might have attenuated a significant increase in post-test jumping performance for both the CMJ test and the hurdle jump test due to a ceiling effect. Although subgroups were matched for all testing variables, significant group differences existed due to the drop-out incidence in the STAB group. In contrast, differences in the potential gains of the PT due to expertise seem implausible as de Villarreal and co-workers [26] have pointed out that training induced performance enhancements following plyometric exercises are independent of the fitness level. Nevertheless, it must be noted that existing meta-analyses identified, for the majority of the studies analyzed, longer training periods than in our study [25]. Therefore, the INST group, with a lower level of baseline plyometric performance, might have improved in CMJ test and the hurdle jump test earlier and with a smaller amount of training as compared to what might have been necessary for the subjects exercising on a stable surface. Aside from methodological reasons, for data evaluation, a statistical correction of baseline differences [39] did not alter the results given the ANOVA. However, a statistical significance of the improvements in CMJ test might have been missed due to a reduction in the number of subjects in the STAB group.

For another testing variable, it is interesting to note, that no improvements were found for the LRH as Kibele and Behm [8] were able to show specific improvements in this sports related task following 7 weeks of instability resistance training for the leg extensors. This finding appears to be related to differences in the applied training protocols. While both studies included high bar squats on unstable platforms, additional trunk muscle exercises to strengthen the core (according to Verstegen and Williams [48]) were only incorporated in Kibele and Behm [8]. It seems plausible, that the training protocol of the present study (only plyometrics, no trunk muscle exercises) was responsible for the lack of improvements in the LRH. In this regard, our results provide additional evidence showing that trunk muscle exercises appear to be a valuable tool to enhance athletic performance particularly under unstable conditions [49].

In terms of balance performance, this study, in line with Kibele and Behm [8], failed to show any sensitivity in static and dynamic balance following IT as compared to stable training surfaces. For resistance training and PT, on stable and on unstable surfaces roughly the same increases in the balance scores were observed. However, according to one side of the principle of dynamic conformity [1] more pronounced balance demands should have provided better balance scores after IT. A possible reason why plyometric/resistance IT did not induce improvements in balance performance could be related to the (different) primary muscles operating in specific balance tasks with little vertical displacement/lift in the center of mass as compared to powerful leg extension in the jumps or when lifting weights and elevating the center of mass in the high-bar squats. In this regard, balance demands prior to the leg extensions in vertical jumps and the squats were associated with smaller knee angles at approximately 90 degrees while the balance tasks were executed in more erect, less dynamic body postures. Therefore, the muscles responsible to keep the center of mass above the base of support might have been stressed to a similar extent in the stability and the instability groups. A similar lack of dynamic conformity was revealed with the Stork-test which did not show any systematic improvements for both PT groups following bilateral exercises. In this regard exercise related balance tasks would be needed as balance tests failed to show statistical correlations [50]. To further investigate this line of argument, 3D-force platforms should be incorporated when analyzing post-training high bar squats and any changes in the corresponding force vector in an instability and a stability group. Such a testing set-up would provide evidence whether a variation in the direction of the resultant force vector is reduced through IT with weights.

Conclusion

This study confirmed that PT is a useful tool to improve skill related performance. To our knowledge, no study has, to date, examined the effects of plyometric exercises performed on unstable surfaces. In this respect, our study indicated that metastability in PT can be safe and beneficial for improving jump performance on stable and unstable surfaces in healthy and physically active young men with no resistance training background. Further studies are needed to explore the trainings effects in other subgroups and for testing procedures on unstable surfaces concurring with the principle of dynamic conformity as related to the demands in various sports. Aside from a strengthening for the primary leg extensor muscles, it is assumed that metastability in PT and resistance training strengthens the stabilizing leg muscles. For both strengthening effects, a reduction in the variations for the direction of the resultant force during plyometric jumps might evolve.

Abbreviations

ANOVA: Analysis of variance; BOSU: Both sides up; CMJ: Countermovement jump; HOT: Hexagonal obstacle test; ICC: Intraclass correlation coefficient; ILES: Isometric leg extension strength; INSTAB: Unstable; IT: Instability training; LRH: 20 meter left right hop test; PT: Plyometric training; RM: Repetition maximum; STA: Stable.

Competing interests

There were no financial or non-financial competing interests.

Authors' contributions

AK was involved with data collection, analysis, interpretation and writing of the manuscript. CC was involved with organization of the training program and data acquisition. TM was involved with interpretation of results and writing of the manuscript. UG was involved with interpretation of results and writing of the manuscript. DGB was involved with interpretation of results and writing of the manuscript. All authors read and approved the final manuscript.

Author details

[1]Institute for Sports and Sport Science, University of Kassel, Damaschkestr. 25, Kassel 34121, Germany. [2]Division of Training and Movement Science, University of Potsdam, Potsdam, Germany. [3]School of Human Kinetics and Recreation, Memorial University of Newfoundland, St. John's, Newfoundland, Canada.

References

1. Chu DA, Meyer G: *Plyometrics*. Human Kinetics: Champaign; 2013.
2. Tschoegl NW: *Fundamentals of equilibrium and steady-state thermodynamics*. Amsterdam: Elsevier; 2000.
3. den Hollander F: **Three lectures on metastability under stochastic dynamics.** In *Methods of contemporary mathematical statistical physics*. Edited by Biskup M, Bovier A, den Hollander F, Ioffe D, Martinelli F, Netocný K, Toninelli C, Kotecký R. Berlin: Springer; 2009:1–24.
4. Behm DG, Anderson KG: **The role of instability with resistance training.** *J Strength Cond Res* 2006, **20**(3):716–722.
5. Behm DG, Drinkwater EJ, Willardson JM, Cowley PM: **Canadian society for exercise physiology position stand: the use of instability to train the core in athletic and non-athletic conditioning.** *J Appl Physiol Nutr Metab* 2010, **35**:109–112.
6. Anderson K, Behm D: **The impact of instability resistance training on balance and stability.** *Sports Med* 2005, **35**(1):43–53.
7. Stanforth D, Stanforth PR, Hahn SR, Phillips A: **A 10 week training study comparing resistaball and traditional trunk training.** *J Dance Med Sci* 1998, **2**:134–140.
8. Kibele A, Behm DG: **Seven weeks of instability and traditional resistance training effects on strength, balance and functional performance.** *J Strength Cond Res* 2009, **23**:2443–2450.
9. Sekendiz B, Cug M, Korkusuz F: **Effects of swiss-ball core strength training on strength, endurance, flexibility, and balance in sedentary women.** *J Strength Cond Res* 2010, **24**:3032–3040.
10. Sparkes R, Behm DG: **Training adaptations associated with an 8-week instability resistance training program with recreationally active individuals.** *J Strength Cond Res* 2010, **24**:1931–1941.
11. Cowley PM, Swensen T, Sforzo GA: **Efficacy of instability resistance training.** *Int J Sports Med* 2007, **28**:829–835.
12. Behm DG, Drinkwater EJ, Willardson JM, Cowley PM: **The use of instability to train the core musculature.** *Appl Physiol Nutr Metab* 2010, **35**:91–108.
13. Hamlyn N, Behm DG, Young WB: **Trunk muscle activation during dynamic weight-training exercises and isometric instability activities.** *J Strength Cond Res* 2007, **21**(4):1108–1112.
14. Cressey EM, West CA, Tiberio DP, Kraemer WJ, Maresh CM: **The effects of ten weeks of lower-body unstable surface training on markers of athletic performance.** *J Strength Cond Res* 2007, **21**:561–567.
15. Anderson K, Behm D: **Maintenance of emg activity and loss of force output with instability.** *J Strength Cond Res* 2004, **18**:637–640.
16. Drinkwater EJ, Pritchett EJ, Behm DG: **Effect of instability and resistance on unintentional squat-lifting kinetics.** *Int J Sports Physiol Perf* 2007, **2**:400–413.
17. Wahl MJ, Behm DG: **Not all instability training devices enhance muscle activation in highly resistance-trained individuals.** *J Strength Cond Res* 2008, **22**:1360–1370.
18. Bruhn S, Kullmann N, Gollhofer A: **The effects of a sensorimotor training and a strength training on postural stabilisation, maximum isometric contraction and jump performance.** *Int J Sports Med* 2004, **25**:56–60.

19. Gruber M, Gruber SB, Taube W, Schubert M, Beck SC, Gollhofer A: **Differential effects of ballistic versus sensorimotor training on rate of force development and neural activation in humans.** *J Strength Cond Res* 2007, **21**:274–282.
20. Granacher U, Gollhofer A, Kriemler S: **Effects of balance training on postural sway, leg extensor strength, and jumping height in adolescents.** *Res Quart Exer Sport* 2010, **81**(3):245–251.
21. Schubert M, Beck S, Taube W, Amtage F, Faist M, Gruber M: **Balance training and ballistic strength training are associated with task-specific corticospinal adaptations.** *Eur J Neurosci* 2008, **27**(8):2007–2018.
22. de Villarreal ESS, Requena B, Cronin JB: **The effects of plyometric training on sprint performance: a meta-analysis.** *J Strength Cond Res* 2012, **26**(2):575–584.
23. Verhoshanski Y: **Perspectives in the improvement of speed-strength preparation of jumpers.** *Track and Field* 1966, **9**:11–12.
24. Verhoshanski Y: **Are depth jumps useful?** *Track and Field* 1987, **12**(9):75–78.
25. Markovic G: **Does plyometric training improve vertical jump height? a meta-analytical review.** *British J Sports Med* 2007, **41**:349–355.
26. de Villarreal ESS, Kellis E, Kraemer WJ, Izquierdo M: **Determining variables of plyometric training for improving vertical jump height performance: a meta-analysis.** *J Strength Cond Res* 2009, **23**:495–506.
27. de Villarreal ESS, Requena B, Newton RU: **Does plyometric training improve strength performance? a meta-analysis.** *J Scie Med Sport* 2010, **13**:513–522.
28. Impellizzeri FM, Rampinini E, Castagna C, Martino F, Fiorini S, Wisloff U: **Effect of plyometric training on sand versus grass on muscle soreness and jumping and sprinting ability in soccer players.** *Br J Sports Med* 2008, **42**(1):42–46.
29. Martel GF, Harmer ML, Logan JM, Parker CB: **Aquatic plyometric training increases vertical jump in female volleyball players.** *Med Sci Sports Exerc* 2005, **37**(10):1814–1819.
30. Sale D, MacDougall JD: **Specificity in strength training: a review for the coach and athlete.** *Can J App Sports Sci* 1981, **6**:87–92.
31. Bobbert M: **Drop jump training as a training method for jumping ability.** *Sports Med* 1990, **9**(1):7–22.
32. Holcomb WR, Kleiner DM, Chu DA: **Plyometrics: considerations for safe and effective training.** *Strength Cond* 1998, **20**:36–39.
33. Reiman MP, Manske RC: *Functional testing in human performance.* Human Kinetics: Champaign, Ill; 2009.
34. Komi P, Bosco C: **Utilization of stored elastic energy in leg extensor muscles by men and women.** *Med Sci Sports* 1978, **10**:261–265.
35. Dintiman G, Ward B: *Sport Speed.* Windsor: Human Kinetics; 2003:45–78.
36. de Villarreal ESS, González-Badillo JJ, Izquierdo M: **Low and moderate plyometric training frequency produces greater jumping and sprinting gains compared with high frequency.** *J Strength Cond Res* 2008, **22**(3):715–725.
37. Makaruk H, Porter JM, Czaplicki A, Sadowski J, Sacewicz T: **The role of attentional focus in plyometric training.** *J Sports Med Phys Fitness* 2012, **52**(3):319–327.
38. Vincent WJ: *Statistics in kinesiology.* Human Kinetics: Champaign, Ill; 2012.
39. Overall JE, Ashby B: **Baseline corrections in experimental and quasi-experimental clinical trials.** *Neuropsychopharma* 1991, **4**(4):273–281.
40. Marshall PW, Murphy BA: **Changes in muscle activity and perceived exertion during exercises performed on a swiss ball.** *Appl Physiol Nutr Metab* 2006, **31**:376–383.
41. Marshall PW, Murphy BA: **Increased deltoid and abdominal muscle activity during Swiss ball bench press.** *J Strength Cond Res* 2006, **20**:745–750.
42. Goodman CA, Pearce AJ, Nicholes CJ, Gatt BM, Fairweather IH: **No difference in 1 RM strength and muscle activation during the barbell chest press on a stable and unstable surface.** *J Strength Cond Res* 2008, **22**:88–94.
43. Prieske O, Muehlbauer T, Mueller S, Krueger T, Kibele A, Behm DG, Granacher U: **Effects of surface instability on neuromuscular performance during drop jumps and landings.** *Eur J Appl Physiol* 2013, **113**:2943–2951.
44. Chimera NJ, Swanik KA, Swanik CB, Straub SJ: **Effects of plyometric training on muscle-activation strategies and performance in female athletes.** *J Athl Train* 2004, **39**(1):24–31.
45. Kornecki S, Zschorlich V: **The nature of the stabilizing functions of skeletal muscles.** *J Biom* 1994, **27**(2):215–225.
46. Wuebbenhorst K, Zschorlich V: **Effects of muscular activation patterns on the ankle joint stabilization: an investigation under different degrees of freedom.** *J Electromyogr Kinesiology* 2011, **21**(2):340–347.
47. Horak FB, Nashner LM: **Central programming of postural support-surface configurations movements: adaptation to altered.** *J Neurophysiol* 1986, **55**:1369–1381.
48. Verstegen M, Williams P: *The core performance: the revolutionary workout program to transform your body and your life.* Toronto, Canada: Benjamin Cummings Publisher; 2005:125–194.
49. Hibbs AE, Thompson KG, French D, Wrigley A, Spears I: **Optimizing performance by improving core stability and core strength.** *Sports Med* 2008, **38**(12):995–1008.
50. Sell TC: **An examination, correlation, and comparison of static and dynamic measures of postural stability in healthy, physically active adults.** *Phys Therapy Sport* 2012, **13**:80–86.

15

Reliability and validity of ten consumer activity trackers

Thea J. M. Kooiman[1*], Manon L. Dontje[2,3], Siska R. Sprenger[2], Wim P. Krijnen[1], Cees P. van der Schans[1] and Martijn de Groot[1,3]

Abstract

Background: Activity trackers can potentially stimulate users to increase their physical activity behavior. The aim of this study was to examine the reliability and validity of ten consumer activity trackers for measuring step count in both laboratory and free-living conditions.

Method: Healthy adult volunteers ($n = 33$) walked twice on a treadmill (4.8 km/h) for 30 min while wearing ten different activity trackers (i.e. Lumoback, Fitbit Flex, Jawbone Up, Nike+ Fuelband SE, Misfit Shine, Withings Pulse, Fitbit Zip, Omron HJ-203, Yamax Digiwalker SW-200 and Moves mobile application). In free-living conditions, 56 volunteers wore the same activity trackers for one working day. Test-retest reliability was analyzed with the Intraclass Correlation Coefficient (ICC). Validity was evaluated by comparing each tracker with the gold standard (Optogait system for laboratory and ActivPAL for free-living conditions), using paired samples t-tests, mean absolute percentage errors, correlations and Bland-Altman plots.

Results: Test-retest analysis revealed high reliability for most trackers except for the Omron (ICC .14), Moves app (ICC .37) and Nike+ Fuelband (ICC .53). The mean absolute percentage errors of the trackers in laboratory and free-living conditions respectively, were: Lumoback (−0.2, −0.4), Fibit Flex (−5.7, 3.7), Jawbone Up (−1.0, 1.4), Nike+ Fuelband (−18, −24), Misfit Shine (0.2, 1.1), Withings Pulse (−0.5, −7.9), Fitbit Zip (−0.3, 1.2), Omron (2.5, −0.4), Digiwalker (−1.2, −5.9), and Moves app (9.6, −37.6). Bland-Altman plots demonstrated that the limits of agreement varied from 46 steps (Fitbit Zip) to 2422 steps (Nike+ Fuelband) in the laboratory condition, and 866 steps (Fitbit Zip) to 5150 steps (Moves app) in the free-living condition.

Conclusion: The reliability and validity of most trackers for measuring step count is good. The Fitbit Zip is the most valid whereas the reliability and validity of the Nike+ Fuelband is low.

Keywords: Accelerometry, Activity trackers, Validation study, Reliability, Free-living

Background

Activity trackers are developed to increase an individual's awareness about physical activity behavior throughout the day. It is well known that regular physical activity decreases the risk of many chronic diseases and can improve quality of life [1–3]. A commonly used physical activity guideline is the 10,000 steps/day norm: healthy adults are recommended to take 10,000 steps per day to maintain physical fitness and health [4]. However, many people worldwide are not aware if they comply with this recommendation [1]. In addition, previous research has indicated that most people tend to overestimate their level of physical activity [5, 6]. Activity trackers may potentially overcome this issue.

Over the past five to ten years, an increasing number and variety of activity trackers have become available on the consumer market. Activity trackers are small and user friendly devices that measure the number of steps taken and/or the amount of time spent performing physical activities at different intensities. Most activity trackers also convert the number of steps with algorithms into measures such as the distance covered and the number of calories burned. Associated (mobile) applications provide users with insight into their individual

* Correspondence: t.j.m.kooiman@pl.hanze.nl
[1]Research group Healthy ageing, Allied health care and Nursing, Hanze University of Applied Sciences, Groningen, The Netherlands
Full list of author information is available at the end of the article

physical activity behavior over a certain period of time. This might work as a motivator to increase physical activity [7, 8]. Consumer activity trackers might also be beneficial for scientific research, due to their ease of usability and relatively low cost. Examples of popular devices are the Fitbit, Jawbone Up, and Withings Pulse.

For accurate measurement and interpretation of the data, these devices must be reliable and valid. A number of studies have examined consumer tracker accuracy [6, 9–18], however, six studies were based upon earlier versions of Fitbit devices, and the methodology for assessing reliability and validity varied considerably. For example, different types of activity were used (walking on a treadmill at different speeds, lab cycling, walking stairs, daily activities), and different gold standards were utilized (energy expenditure [EE] measured by breath-to-breath analysis, self-reported physical activity translated to EE [in METs], and real step count). Five studies were performed in a laboratory condition [9–11, 14, 16], and six studies examined the reliability or validity of activity trackers during (semi-structured) free-living conditions [6, 12, 13, 15, 17, 18]. The validity of activity trackers may differ in free-living conditions compared to standardized lab conditions because of the increased variety in walking speeds, directions, intensities, etc. in free-living. To date, no studies have assessed reliability and validity of consumer trackers in both laboratory and free-living conditions. The aim of this study was to determine the reliability and validity of ten consumer activity trackers, in both a standardized laboratory condition and in free-living conditions.

Methods

Study design

The following ten activity trackers were examined: the Lumoback, Fitbit Flex, Nike+ Fuelband SE, Jawbone Up, Misfit Shine, Withings Pulse, Fitbit Zip, Omron HJ-203, Yamax Digiwalker SW-200 and the Moves mobile application. The Optogait system *(OPTOGait, Microgate S.r.I, Italy, 2010)* was used as the gold standard on the treadmill in the laboratory condition. This system consists of two beams attached to the sides of the treadmill. The system uses an LED lighting system to precisely measure the number of steps which is a reliable and valid method for measuring step count (cadence) [19]. The ActivPAL *(PAL Technologies Ltd., Glasgow, UK)* was used as the gold standard in the free-living condition. The ActivPAL was worn on the thigh underneath the clothing. Previous research has demonstrated that the ActivPAL is a reliable and valid tool for measuring the number of steps taken both on a treadmill and in free-living conditions [20–22].

Study sample

Only healthy adult volunteers (age ≥18, <65 years) were included in the study. Participants were recruited through advertisements within the Hanze University and by using the individual networks of the researchers. Subscribers were excluded from participation if they experienced problems with standing or normal ambulation as well as if they performed daily activities which could possibly damage the activity trackers while being worn (when participating in the free-living study). All components of the study are described below in more detail. The study was in accordance with the principles as outlined in the Declaration of Helsinki and an exemption was obtained by the Medical Ethical Committee of the University Medical Center of Groningen for a comprehensive application. All participants were informed about the study procedures and provided informed consent prior to the initiation of this study.

Testing under laboratory conditions

In order to examine the test-retest reliability and the validity of the ten trackers in a standardized situation, the participants walked for 30 min on a treadmill at a walking speed of 4.8 km/h. This walking velocity was similar to velocities used in previous treadmill studies and is based on an average walking speed [14, 23]. During the treadmill test, the participants wore all ten activity trackers and the ActivPAL. The Optogait system on the treadmill was used as the gold standard. The primary outcome measure was the total number of steps measured within the duration of the 30 min treadmill test. All participants repeated this test one week later.

Testing under free-living conditions

In order to examine the validity of the ten trackers in free-living conditions during a working day, the activity behavior of the participants was measured during one working day between 9.00 am and 4:30 pm. The participants wore each ten different trackers and the ActivPAL simultaneously. During the specified day, participants performed their normal daily activities; however, they were requested to abstain from cycling or driving a vehicle during the test period. This was required in order to be able to make a realistic comparison between the trackers; because the different wearing positions of the trackers might influence step measurements during these activities. The primary outcome measure was the total number of steps measured between 9 am to 4:30 pm.

Activity trackers

All devices utilized in this study are able to track step count.

Lumoback

The Lumoback™ *(Lumo BodyTech, Inc. Palo Alto, California, USA)* was worn around the lower back and was calibrated to the user by utilizing the associated application.

Fitbit Flex

The Fitbit Flex™ *(Fitbit, Inc., San Francisco, CA, USA)* is a wrist-worn tri-axial accelerometer and was worn on the non dominant arm.

Jawbone UP

The Jawbone UP™ *(JAWBONE, San Francisco, CA, USA,* is a wrist-worn three-dimensional activity tracker and was worn on the non dominant arm.

Nike+ Fuelband

The Nike+ Fuelband SE ™ *(Nike Inc., Beaverton, OR, USA)* is a wrist-worn three-dimensional activity tracker and was worn on the non dominant arm.

Misfit Shine

The Misfit Shine™ *(Misfit Wearables, Burlingame, California, USA)* is a small tri-axial accelerometer which was carried in the front pocket of the trousers.

Pulse

The Withings Pulse™ *(Withings, Issy les Moulineaux, France)* is a small tri-axial accelerometer which was carried in the front pocket of the trousers.

Fitbit Zip

The Fitbit Zip™ *(Fitbit, Inc., San Francisco, CA, USA)* is a small tri-axial accelerometer which was carried in the front pocket of the trousers.

Omron

The Omron Walking Style III™ (type HJ-203) *(OMRON Healthcare Europe B.V., Hoofddorp, the Netherlands)* is a pedometer with a two-dimensional sensor which was carried in the front pocket of the trousers.

Digiwalker

The Yamax Digiwalker SW-200™ *(YAMAX Health & Sports, Inc. San Antonio, USA, $39.50)* is a two-dimensional pedometer that was attached to the participant's waistband.

Moves

The Moves^R is a smartphone application. It uses acceleration sensors from a smartphone and GPS to measure the number of steps taken. The mobile phone used in the laboratory study was an Iphone 4S *(Iphone 4S, Apple Inc., USA)*. During the free-living study the smartphone of the participant was used (IOS/Android) and carried in the front pocket of the trousers.

Statistical analysis

A sample size analysis was conducted to calculate the number of required participants. As previous data on relevant differences for sample size calculation does not exist, we reasoned that a difference of 10 % for the laboratory condition and 15 % for the free-living condition seemed appropriate. Using these relevant differences and expected mean number of steps in both conditions, it was calculated that at least 24 participants were necessary for participation in the laboratory condition and 58 participants for the free-living condition to enable substantiation of a relevant difference between the trackers and the gold standards with a power of 80 % and a significance level of 5 %. This number of participants is comparable to other validation studies [12, 14, 15]. This reassured our reasoned choice for using 10 % and 15 % as cut-off points for the mean difference.

Descriptive statistics were used to characterize the sample. Normality of the outcome measures was tested by Shapiro Wilk for all activity trackers in both parts of the study. Test-retest reliability of the trackers in the laboratory study was assessed by calculating the Intraclass Correlation Coefficient (ICC) (two-way random, absolute agreement, single measures with a 95 % confidence interval). Common cut-off points for reliability assessment were used; >.90 (excellent), .75-.90 (good), .60-.75 (moderate), and < .60 (low) [24].

The validity of the ten trackers was determined by several statistical tests. First, systematic differences between the activity trackers and the gold standards were assessed by the paired samples *t*-test. In the event of non-normally distributed data, the Wilcoxon Signed Rank test was used. Mean absolute percentage errors (c) compared to the gold standards were calculated with the following formula: mean difference activity tracker-gold standard x 100 / mean gold standard. Second, in order to examine the correlation between the trackers and the gold standards, the ICC was calculated (absolute agreement, two-way random, single measures, 95 % confidence interval). Third, to examine the level of agreement between the trackers and the gold standard, Bland-Altman plots were constructed with their associated limits of agreement. In addition, the ActivPAL scores from the laboratory study were compared with the corresponding Optogait scores by use of the three previously mentioned statistical tests, in order to assess the degree of consensus between the two gold standards used in this study.

Results

For the laboratory study, 33 participants were included (16 males, mean age (±SD) 39 (±13.1) years, mean BMI (±SD) 23.6 (±2.2) kg/m^2, and 17 females, mean age (±SD) 35 (±11.2), mean BMI 22.5 (±2.1) kg/m^2). Thirty of the 33 participants performed the test again one week later. Most individuals who participated in the laboratory study also participated in the free-living study ($N = 23$) wherein a total of 56 participants were included (18 males, mean age (±SD) 37.1 (±10.6), mean BMI (±SD) 24.1 (±2) kg/m^2, and 38 females, mean age (±SD) 30 (±9.5) years, mean BMI (±SD) 23.1 (±2.5) kg/m^2). Most of the participants were university employees, with an office job. Activities performed by the participants during the test day included sitting (e.g., at the computer), standing (e.g., teaching activities) and walking. A number of participants were highly active (e.g., took a long walk during lunch time) whereas others were mainly sedentary during the test day. The Nike+ Fuelband and Moves app were tested with a fewer number of participants in the free-living study ($N = 20$ and $N = 11$ respectively). The Nike+ Fuelband was not available at the beginning but was included during the study. The Moves app was unavailable at no cost for most participants in the free-living study. In all 11 cases, the Moves app was operating on an Android device.

Descriptive statistics

Figure 1 depicts the descriptive statistics (mean number of steps, 95 % CI) as measured by the gold standards and by the ten activity trackers in both the laboratory (A) and free-living condition (B). The mean number of steps (±SD) measured by the Optogait in the laboratory condition was 3314 (±162), and the mean number of steps (±SD) measured by the ten trackers ranged from 2716 (±672) [Nike+ Fuelband] to 3633 (±286) [Moves app]. The mean number of steps (±SD) measured by the ActivPAL in the free-living condition was 4070 (±2430), and the mean number of steps (±SD) measured by the ten trackers ranged from 3271 (±2136) [Nike+ Fuelband] to 4372 (±2562) [Fitbit Flex]. As shown in Fig. 1, the Nike+ Fuelband and Moves app provide a relatively large confidence interval for the mean number of steps in the free-living condition, which is partly due to a lower number of measurements of these devices. Therefore, additional power analyses were executed, which are shown below.

Agreement between the two gold standards

The ActivPAL was compared with the Optogait in the laboratory condition using the same statistical tests that were used for the ten activity trackers. The ActivPAL demonstrated a mean difference of 9 ± 6 steps [0.3 %] with the Optogait ($P < 0.001$, $N = 25$). The effect size of this significant difference was calculated using Cohens effect size [25] and indicated an effect size of 0.02, which is negligibly small. The ICC between the ActivPAL and the Optogait is 1. The Bland-Altman plot revealed a difference between the lower and upper limit of agreement of 24 steps. These results indicate excellent agreement of the two gold standards used in this study.

Test-retest reliability

The ICCs between the first test and the second test (one week later) in the laboratory condition varied between 0.14 and 0.96 (Table 1). The gold standards used in this study (Optogait and ActivPAL), demonstrated excellent test-retest reliability. Test-retest reliability of the Lumoback, Fitbit Zip, and Withings Pulse was excellent as well (i.e., ICC > .90). Test-retest reliability of the Jawbone Up, Fitbit Flex, and Misfit Shine was good (ICC .75 - .90); test-retest reliability of the Digiwalker was moderate (ICC .60 - .75); and test-retest reliability of the Nike + Fuelband, Omron, and Moves app was low (ICC < 0.60).

Systematic differences and mean absolute percentage error

In the laboratory condition, there was a significant difference between the number of steps measured by the Optogait (gold standard) and those measured by the Lumoback, Fitbit Flex, Nike+ Fuelband, Withings Pulse, Fitbit Zip, Omron, and the Moves app (Table 2). However, the size of the mean difference was less than 34 steps (MAPE = 1 %) or close to this MAPE for most of the trackers. There was a more substantial MAPE between the Optogait and Fitbit Flex; (188 steps [5.7 %]), the Moves app (319 steps [9.6 %]), and the Nike+ Fuelband (598 steps [18 %]). The Misfit Shine demonstrated the smallest MAPE compared with the Optogait [i.e., 0.18 %].

In the free-living condition, there was a significant difference in the number of steps between the ActivPAL (gold standard) and the Fitbit Flex, Nike+ Fuelband, Fitbit Zip, Withings Pulse, Digiwalker, and the Moves app (Table 2). Again, the MAPE values of the trackers were small (less than 10 %), except for the Nike+ Fuelband and the Moves app (24 % and 37.6 % respectively). The smallest MAPE values were between the ActivPAL and the Omron (0.4 %) and Lumoback (0.4 %). The power for the calculation of the Nike+ Fuelband and Moves app was 62 % and 39 %, respectively. The power for the remaining devices was high, i.e., greater than 99 %.

Correlations

Table 3 illustrates the Intraclass Correlation Coefficients between the ten activity trackers and the gold standard, for both the laboratory study and the free-living study.

In the laboratory study, the ICCs ranged from -.13 (Moves) to .99 (Lumoback, Withings Pulse, and Fitbit Zip). The ICCs in the free-living study ranged from 0.80 (Moves) to 1 (Fitbit Zip).

Level of agreement

Bland-Altman plots indicate the differences between the tracker and the gold standard (y-axis) against the average of the two methods (x-axis). Table 4 indicates the mean differences with the gold standard and the limits of agreement for all activity trackers. In the laboratory condition, the plots showed the narrowest limits for the Fitbit Zip (46 steps), Lumoback (78 steps), and Withings Pulse (92 steps). The broadest limits were for the Nike+ Fuelband (2422 steps), Moves app (1436 steps), and Fitbit Flex (855 steps). In the free-living condition, the plots showed the narrowest limits for the Fitbit Zip (866 steps), Misfit Shine (1400 steps), and the Lumoback (1590 steps). The broadest limits of agreement were determined for the Moves app (5150 steps), Nike+

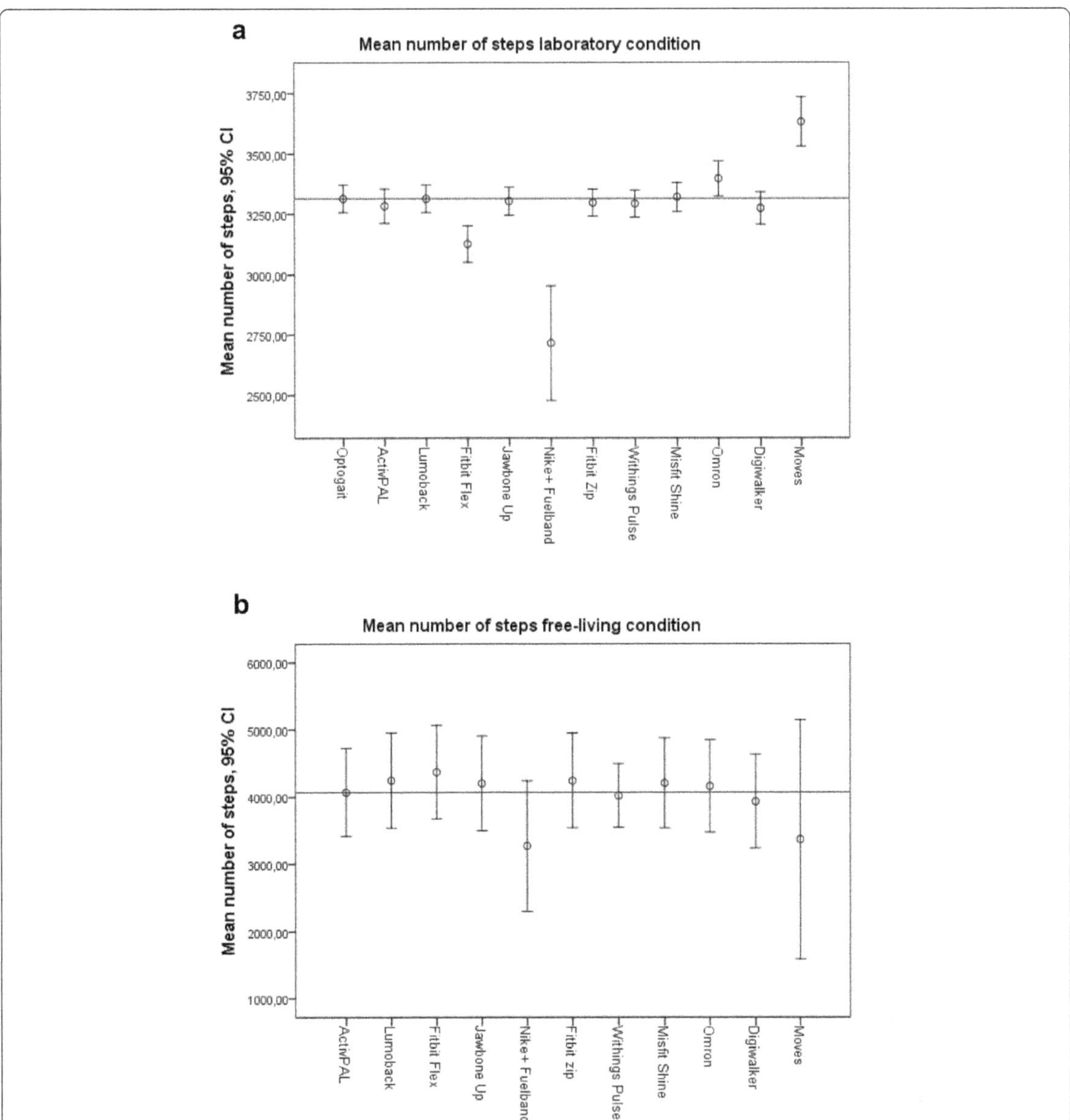

Fig. 1 Descriptive Statistics (mean number of steps, 95 % CI) as measured by the gold standards (horizontal lines) and the ten activity trackers in the laboratory and free-living condition

Table 1 Intraclass correlation coefficients between Test 1 and Test 2 of the treadmill walking test ($N = 30$)

Activity tracker	Intraclass Correlation Coefficient	95 % confidence Interval
Optogait	*0.92***	*0.85 –0.96*
ActivPAL	*0.96***	*0.90 –0.99*
Lumoback	0.90**	0.79 – 0.95
Fitbit Flex	0.81**	0.64 –0.91
Jawbone UP	0.83**	0.66 –0.91
Nike+ Fuelband	0.53**	0.22 –0.75
Misfit Shine	0.86**	0.73 –0.93
Withings Pulse	0.92**	0.83 –0.96
Fitbit Zip	0.90**	0.80 –0.95
Omron	0.14	−0.24 –0.47
Digiwalker	0.71**	0.47 –0.86
Moves app	0.37*	0.02 –0.64

*P<0.05
**P <0.01

Fuelband (4528 steps), and Jawbone Up (3350 steps). Figure 2 illustrates the Bland-Altman plots for the top three activity trackers (narrowest limits of agreement) for both the laboratory (Fitbit Zip, Lumoback, and Withings Pulse) and for the free-living condition (Fitbit Zip, Misfit Shine and Lumoback).

Discussion

Ten popular consumer activity trackers were tested for their reliability and validity for measuring step count. Seven out of ten trackers were reliable (Lumoback, Fitbit Flex, Jawbone UP, Misfit Shine, Withings Pulse, Fitbit Zip, and Digiwalker), and five of these trackers also demonstrated high validity in laboratory conditions (Lumoback, Jawbone Up, Misfit Shine, Withings Pulse, and Fitbit Zip). The Moves app and Nike+ Fuelband exhibited low reliability and a low validity in laboratory conditions. In free-living conditions, the Fitbit Zip showed the highest validity and the Nike+ Fuelband indicated a low validity.

The validity of the ten activity trackers in laboratory conditions was examined with three methods of which the first was to assess systematic differences. According to Tudor-Locke et al. [23], activity monitors should not exceed a 1 % error deviation (MAPE) from the gold standard during walking on a treadmill at a speed of 3 mph (4.8 km/h) in order to be considered accurate. In the controlled lab-condition, five trackers achieved this condition: the Lumoback, Jawbone Up, Misfit Shine, Withings Pulse, and Fitbit Zip. The Digiwalker and Omron had an error deviation slightly higher than the 1 % threshold, e.g., 1.2 % and 2.5 %, respectively, which still represents a very low MAPE. The Fitbit Flex (5.6 %), Moves app (9.6 %) and Nike+ Fuelband (18 %) exhibited greater deviation errors whereby the Fitbit Flex and Nike+ Fuelband underestimated the number of steps, and the Moves app overestimated the number of steps. Some trackers were examined in other studies as well for systematic differences using comparable conditions. Melanson et al. [26] found an accuracy of 97.8 % of the Digiwalker SW-200 during walking on the treadmill with speeds between 3.0 and 3.5 mph (4.8 – 5.6 km/h), which is in accordance with our finding of 1.2 % error. In the study of De Cocker et al. [27], the Omron differed on an average of 6.7 % compared to the gold standard. The slightly smaller difference of 2.5 % determined in our study could possibly be explained by the longer duration of the treadmill test in this study (30 min vs. 5 min) which decreases the relative size of measurement error. Case et al. [16] found an error of +6.2 % for the Moves app installed on an IOS device and an error of −6.7 % for the Moves app installed on an Android device. The MAPE found for the IOS device was a bit lower than the +9.6 % difference in our study. An explanation could be the different version of the Iphone that was utilized (Iphone 5S compared to the 4S in our study). For the Nike+ Fuelband, Case et al. found a mean underestimation of 22.7 %. This was in line with our finding of 18 % underestimation.

The second method to determine validity was to examine the ICCs between the trackers and the gold standard. In the laboratory study, all trackers demonstrated a good to excellent agreement with the gold standard, with the exception of the Moves app, Nike+ Fuelband, and Fitbit Flex. Two other studies also examined correlations between the activity trackers and the gold standard in laboratory conditions. For the Fitbit One, Tacacs et al. [14] ascertained concordance correlations between 0.97 and 1.0 for five different speeds on

Table 2 Mean difference scores (gold standard – activity tracker) and MAPE in the laboratory and free-living condition

Laboratory Condition [1]						Free-living condition [2]				
	N	Mean difference (SD) [a]	MAPE [b]	t-value/Z-value [c]	P-value	N	Mean difference [a]	MAPE [b]	Z-value [c]	P-Value
ActivPAL	*25*	*9 (6)*	*0.3*	*7.19*	*0.000 **	55				
Lumoback	32	8 (20)	0.2	2.24	0.033 *	51	17	0.4	−0.97	0.332
Fitbit Flex	33	188 (219)	5.7	4.93	0.000 *	54	−150	3.7	−2.23	0.026 *
Jawbone UP	32	34 (123)	1.0	1.60	0.119	53	−58	1.4	−0.24	0.851
Nike+ Fuelband	33	598 (618)	18.0	−4.36	0.000 *	20	977	24	−3.55	0.000 *
Misfit Shine	33	−6 (43)	0.2	−0.80	0.430	55	−43	1.1	−0.36	0.719
Withings Pulse	32	15 (23)	0.5	3.70	0.001 *	51	323	7.9	−5.24	0.000 *
Fitbit Zip	32	11 (12)	0.3	5.44	0.000 *	55	−49	1.2	−2.66	0.008 *
Omron	32	−82 (157)	2.5	−2.96	0.006 *	55	17	0.4	−0.71	0.479
Digiwalker	32	38 (145)	1.2	1.46	0.153	55	240	5.9	−2.04	0.041 *
Moves app	33	−319 (366)	9.6	−4.36	0.000 *	11	1529	37.6	−2.85	0.004 *

[1]Mean (±SD) Optogait = 3314 (±162) [2] Mean (±SD) ActivPAL = 4070(±2430) *significant p-value indicating a systematic difference of the activity tracker. [a]positive values indicate an underestimation of the activity tracker and negative values indicate an overestimation. [b] MAPE = mean absolute percentage error [c]In case of non-normality the Wilcoxon Signed Rank Test was used instead of the Paired Samples *T*-test

the treadmill with manual steps counting as the gold standard. This was in accordance with our finding for the Fitbit Zip (ICC .99). For the Digiwalker SW-200, Beets et al. determined an ICC of .99 compared to real step count for children walking on a treadmill at the same speed (4.8 km/h) [28]. This is somewhat higher than the ICC found in our study (ICC .65). However, if we removed the four outliers in our analyses our ICC increased to .94, which is more in line with the findings of Beets et al.

The third and last way to examine validity was to assess the level of agreement by visualizing the data with Bland-Altman plots [29]. The difference between the lower and upper limit of agreement (Mean difference ± 1.96SD of difference scores) ranged from 46 steps (Fitbit Zip) to 2422 steps (Nike+ Fuelband). The Lumoback, Jawbone Up, Misfit Shine, Withings Pulse, and Fitbit Zip indicated the narrowest limits of agreement (less than 300 steps) which equals less than 10 % and less than 3 min walking. This can be considered as a relatively small range. Taken together with the small systematic differences of these trackers (less than 1 %), it is suggested that the Lumoback, Jawbone Up, Misfit Shine, Withings Pulse, and Fitbit Zip can be used interchangeably with the gold standard when walking on a treadmill. The systematic differences and the range between the upper and lower limits of agreement of the Moves app (1436 steps) and the Nike+ Fuelband (2422 steps) are considered to be too large to be used interchangeably with the gold standard.

To summarize, the lab results show that most trackers are valid with the Lumoback, Jawbone Up, Misfit Shine, Withings Pulse, and Fitbit Zip demonstrating the highest validity. The Moves app and Nike+ Fuelband are clearly

Table 3 Intraclass Correlation Coefficients between the activity trackers and gold standards in the laboratory and free–living study

	Laboratory study (*N* = 33) (Optogait)	95 % confidence interval	Free–living study (*N* = 56) (ActivPAL)	95 % confidence interval
ActivPAL	*1*	*0.94 – 1*		
Lumoback	0.99 **	0.98 – 0.99	0.99 **	0.98 – 0.99
Fitbit Flex	0.22 *	−0.08 – 0.5	0.96 **	0.94 – 0.98
Jawbone UP	0.98 **	.095 – 0.99	0.94 **	0.90 – 0.97
Nike+ Fuelband	0.12	−0.1 – 0.37	0.83 **	0.37 – 0.94
Misfit Shine	0.97 **	0.93 – 0.98	0.99 **	0.98 – 0.99
Withings Pulse	0.99 **	0.95 – 0.97	0.96 **	0.91 – 0.98
Fitbit Zip	0.99 **	0.96 – 0.99	1 **	0.99 – 1
Omron	0.59 **	0.27 – 0.78	0.98 **	0.96 – 0.99
Digiwalker	0.65 **	0.39 – 0.81	0.96 **	0.93 – 0.98
Moves app	−0.13	−0.32 – 0.15	0.80 **	0.05 – 0.99

*P<0.05 **P<0.01

Table 4 Mean difference scores with the gold standards and limits of agreement of the activity trackers in the laboratory and free-living study

	Mean difference (Optogait – tracker, lab study)[a]	Limits of Agreement		Mean difference (ActivPAL- tracker, free-living study)[a]	Limits of Agreement	
		Lower	Upper		Lower	Upper
ActivPAL	*9*	*−3*	*21*			
Lumoback	8	−31	47	17	−778	812
Fitbit Flex	188	−240	615	−150	−1424	1124
Jawbone UP	34	−54	81	−58	−1732	1618
Nike+ Fuelband	598	−613	1809	977	−1288	3240
Misfit Shine	−6	−91	85	−43	−743	657
Withings Pulse	15	−31	61	323	−864	1510
Fitbit Zip	11	−12	34	−49	−482	384
Omron	−82	−390	226	17	−1006	1040
Digiwalker	38	−248	323	240	−1028	1508
Moves app	−319	−1037	399	1529	−1046	4104

[a] Positive values indicate an underestimation of the activity tracker and negative values indicate an overestimation

invalid. It should be noted that, in a controlled lab condition, there is no variation in walking speed, intensity, direction, etc. which is in contrast to real life. Therefore, validity was also tested in free-living conditions.

The first way to validate activity trackers in free-living conditions was to assess systematic differences. In free-living conditions, an acceptable mean deviation from the gold standard is 10 % [23]. Eight activity trackers achieved this criterion. The Nike+ Fuelband and Moves

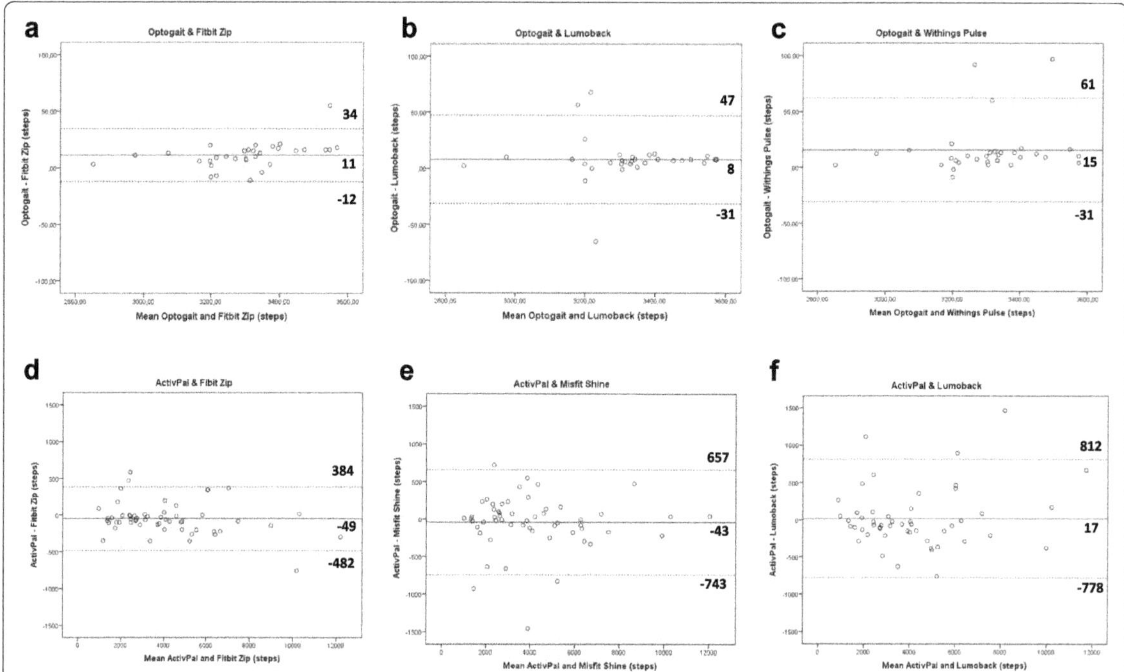

Fig. 2 Bland-Altman plots of the top three activity trackers in the laboratory condition (Optogait vs. Fitbit Zip, Lumoback, and Withings Pulse, figure **a-c**) and free-living condition (ActivPal vs. Fitbit Zip, Misfit Shine, and Lumoback, figure **d-f**). The middle line shows the mean difference between the tracker and the gold standard, and the dashed lines indicate the limits of agreement (±1.96 * SD of the difference scores)

app showed larger percentages of underestimation: 24.0 % and 37.6 %, respectively. Lee et al. [12] investigated various consumer trackers during different semi-structured activities (the participants followed a 69-min protocol), and compared total energy expenditure with the gold standard (breath-to-breath analysis). The Fitbit Zip, Jawbone Up, and Nike+ Fuelband differed 10.1 %, 12.2 %, and 13.0 %, respectively, from the gold standard. The differences are greater for the Fitbit Zip and Jawbone Up compared to the results of our study which could possibly be explained by the different outcome measure that was utilized in the study of Lee et al. (energy expenditure vs. step count). The difference between the Nike+ Fuelband and the gold standard is smaller compared to the present study (24 %). However, Lee et al. has already mentioned inconsistent results for the Nike+ Fuelband (a relatively small MAPE but also a low correlation with the gold standard) and, therefore, advised interpreting these results with caution. Ferguson et al. [17] investigated five similar devices (Jawbone UP, Nike+ Fuelband, Misfit Shine, Withings Pulse and Fitbit Zip) in free-living conditions for 48 h. They ascertained differences of 8.1 %, 25.6 %, 10.1 %, 6.3 % and 4.3 %, respectively. These values are in line with our findings in which the somewhat larger differences can be explained by the longer period of measurement. De Cocker et al., [27] investigated the Omron during free-living conditions and used the Digiwalker as a criterion measure. They reported a more substantial difference between the two devices compared to the findings of the present study (36.9 % vs. 0.4 %) which can be a result of non-walking activities, a longer period of measurement, and the different gold standard.

The second way to determine the validity of the activity trackers during free-living conditions was to calculate ICCs. All activity trackers were highly correlated to the gold standard (ActivPAL). The Nike + Fuelband and the Moves app showed ICCs which were a bit lower and had broad confidence intervals (.83 [CI .37; .94] and .80 [CI .05 – .99] respectively). The high ICCs in the free-living study can be partially attributed to the differences in activity patterns between the participants during the test day; more variation increases the chances of a high ICC. Lee et al. [12] indicated similar results for the Fitbit Zip, Jawbone Up, and the Nike+ Fuelband, i.e., high correlations for the Fitbit Zip and Jawbone Up and a lower correlation for the Nike+ Fuelband. Tully et al. investigated the validity of the Fitbit Zip in free-living conditions; the Fitbit Zip was worn for seven days along with the Actigraph accelerometer. They reported a high correlation (Spearman Rho = .91) between steps/day when measured by the Fitbit Zip and by the Actigraph [15]. In addition, Ferguson et al. reported similar correlations for the Jawbone UP, Nike+ Fuelband, Misfit Shine, Withings Pulse, and Fitbit Zip in their free-living study of 48 h [17].

Finally, the level of agreement of the activity trackers with the gold standard during free-living conditions was assessed by Bland-Altman plots. The difference between the lower and upper limit of agreement ranged from 861 steps (Fitbit Zip) to 5150 steps (Moves app). For the Fitbit Zip, the range of 861steps (less than 1000 steps, e.g., 10 min walking) appears to be sufficiently low enough to be a valid measure in scientific research. The Misfit Shine and Lumoback demonstrated slightly larger limits of agreement (1400 and 1590 steps, respectively) which still demonstrates a good validity. For the other trackers, the limits of agreement show that, despite the relatively small systematic error (below 400 steps [10 %] for eight of the ten trackers), larger individual differences are evident, resulting in a lower validity.

To summarize, the validity of eight of the ten trackers was good during free-living conditions whereby the Fitbit Zip showed the best validity. The validity of the Nike + Fuelband is low for measuring steps in free-living conditions.

Our study has some limitations. First, in the laboratory condition, only one type of activity was examined (walking), however, activity trackers can possibly perform differently during different activities or velocities (such as walking slow). The advantage of the 30-min measurement was that reliable data for average walking speed was obtained. Second, for examining free-living activity, we used a time span of 9:00–16:30 in which 'occupational activity' was mostly measured. The advantage of this method was that we were able to make a realistic comparison between the different trackers with different wearing positions because cycling was excluded. Cycling could have biased the results between centrally worn and wrist-worn trackers. However, the trackers might perform differently during a greater variety of activities such as more intensive exercise. These activities were not measured in this study. The third limitation was, that in the free-living condition, the Nike+ Fuelband and Moves app were tested with fewer number of participants. Because of a reasonable power (62 %), consistent results with the laboratory condition, and consistent results with other studies [12, 16, 17], the results of the Nike+ Fuelband are considered reliable. For the Moves app, only preliminary conclusions can be drawn on the validity in free-living conditions. This is due to the low N, consequently a lower power of 39 %, and because the Moves app was tested on different types of phones compared to the laboratory study (Android vs. IOS devices). Therefore, the results of the free-living condition cannot be compared with the lab condition because the different types of firmware may have influenced the results.

However, our results for the Moves app on the different types of phones are comparable with the study of Case et al. [16] who showed that Android devices are associated with a modest underestimation, and IOS devices show a modest overestimation of step counting, which is in line with our results.

By combining the results of both conditions, it can be concluded that the validity of most activity trackers is good (Fitbit Zip, followed by Misfit Shine and Lumoback) or acceptable (Fitbit Flex, Jawbone Up, Withings Pulse, Omron, and Digiwalker). Looking at the wearing position of the trackers (wrist-worn for the Fitbit Flex, Jawbone UP, and Nike+ Fuelband and centrally worn, e.g. close to the pelvis or trunk, for the remaining devices), our results indicate that activity trackers worn close to the body exhibit a better validity than the wrist-worn activity trackers, especially during free-living conditions. For wrist-worn activity trackers, more measurement error can occur due to more variation in the way the arms are used in free-living conditions. This finding is supported by the research of Atallah et al. [30].

For the choice of a device, different considerations can be taken into account. First, the goal of physical activity measurement should be considered. For individual users, it is most important that the change in physical activity is clearly displayed, therefore, devices should be reliable. For large-scale research, the validity of a tracker is important in order to be able to compare physical activity levels of different groups. In addition, the type of activity that will be measured should be considered so a choice for the wearing position can be made. For example, wrist-worn activity trackers are better able to measure higher limb activity, and ankle worn trackers are better able to measure lower limb activity (e.g. cycling) [31]. Furthermore, a consumer can choose between a more advanced -and mostly more expensive device-, or a more simple and affordable device. This study demonstrated that less expensive devices are not necessarily less valid.

Conclusions

In conclusion, the reliability of the Lumoback, Fitbit Flex, Jawbone UP, Misfit Shine, Withings Pulse, Fitbit Zip, and Digiwalker is good. These trackers are suitable for consumer usage and health enhancing programs. Of all ten trackers the Fitbit Zip shows the highest validity whereas the Nike+ Fuelband shows the lowest validity. The results of this study can assist consumers, researchers, and health care providers to make an evidence based choice for an activity tracker to measure step count.

Abbreviations

EE: Energy expenditure; MET: Metabolic equivalent; BMI: Body mass index; km/h: Kilometers per hour; MAPE: Mean absolute percentage error; ICC: Intraclass correlation coefficient; CI: Confidence interval.

Competing interests

The authors declare that they have no competing interests.

Authors' contributions

TJMK participated in the design of the study, undertook data collection for the laboratory study, undertook statistical analysis, and wrote the manuscript. MLD participated in the design of the study, undertook data collection for the free-living study, and contributed to writing the manuscript. SRS participated in the design of the study, contributed to data collection of the free-living study, contributed to statistical analysis of the free-living results, and contributed to writing the manuscript. WPK participated in the design of the study, advised for statistical analysis, and contributed to writing the manuscript. CPS participated in the design of the study and contributed to writing the manuscript. MG participated in the design of the study, gave supervision during the execution of this study and contributed to writing the manuscript. All authors have approved the final version.

Acknowledgements

This study was funded by the Hanze University and the Center for Physical Activity and Research (CBO Groningen). All trackers were purchased by Hanze University or by CBO Groningen.

Author details

[1]Research group Healthy ageing, Allied health care and Nursing, Hanze University of Applied Sciences, Groningen, The Netherlands. [2]CBO Groningen: Center for Physical Activity and Research, Groningen, The Netherlands. [3]Quantified Self Institute, Hanze University of Applied Sciences, Groningen, The Netherlands.

References

1. Lee IM, Shiroma EJ, Lobelo F, Puska P, Blair SN, Katzmarzyk PT, et al. Effect of physical inactivity on major non-communicable diseases worldwide: an analysis of burden of disease and life expectancy. Lancet. 2012;380(9838):219–29.
2. Warburton DE, Nicol CW, Bredin SS. Health benefits of physical activity: the evidence. CMAJ. 2006;174(6):801–9.
3. Haskell WL, Lee IM, Pate RR, Blair SN, Franklin BA, Macera CA, et al. Physical activity and public health: updated recommendation for adults from the American College of Sports Medicine and the American Heart Association. Med Sci Sports Exerc. 2007;39(8):1423–34.
4. Tudor-Locke C, Craig CL, Brown WJ, Clemes SA, De Cocker K, Giles-Corti B, et al. How many steps/day are enough? For adults. Int J Behav Nutr Phys Act. 2011;8:79-5868-8-79.
5. Godino JG, Watkinson C, Corder K, Sutton S, Griffin SJ, Van Sluijs EM. Awareness of physical activity in healthy middle-aged adults: a cross-sectional study of associations with sociodemographic, biological, behavioural, and psychological factors. BMC Public Health. 2014;14(1):421.
6. Vooijs M, Alpay LL, Snoeck-Stroband JB, Beerthuizen T, Siemonsma PC, Abbink JJ, et al. Validity and usability of low-cost accelerometers for internet-based self-monitoring of physical activity in patients with chronic obstructive pulmonary disease. Interact J Med Res. 2014;3(4):e14.
7. Bravata DM, Smith-Spangler C, Sundaram V, Gienger AL, Lin N, Lewis R, et al. Using pedometers to increase physical activity and improve health: a systematic review. JAMA. 2007;298(19):2296–304.
8. El-Gayar O, Timsina P, Nawar N, Eid W. A systematic review of IT for diabetes self-management: are we there yet? Int J Med Inform. 2013;82(8):637–52.
9. Adam Noah J, Spierer DK, Gu J, Bronner S. Comparison of steps and energy expenditure assessment in adults of Fitbit Tracker and Ultra to the Actical and indirect calorimetry. J Med Eng Technol. 2013;37(7):456–62.
10. Dannecker KL, Sazonova NA, Melanson EL, Sazonov ES, Browning RC. A comparison of energy expenditure estimation of several physical activity monitors. Med Sci Sports Exerc. 2013;45(11):2105–12.
11. Fortune E, Lugade V, Morrow M, Kaufman K. Validity of using tri-axial accelerometers to measure human movement - Part II: Step counts at a wide range of gait velocities. Med Eng Phys. 2014;36(6):659–69.
12. Lee JM, Kim Y, Welk GJ. Validity of consumer-based physical activity monitors. Med Sci Sports Exerc. 2014;46(9):1840–8.

13. Stahl ST, Insana SP. Caloric expenditure assessment among older adults: criterion validity of a novel accelerometry device. J Health Psychol. 2014;19(11):1382–7.
14. Takacs J, Pollock CL, Guenther JR, Bahar M, Napier C, Hunt MA. Validation of the Fitbit One activity monitor device during treadmill walking. Interact J Med Res. 2014;17(5):496–500.
15. Tully MA, McBride C, Heron L, Allen W, Hunter RF. The validation of Fibit ZipTM physical activity monitor as a measure of free-living physical activity. BMC Res Notes. 2014;7(1):952.
16. Case MA, Burwick HA, Volpp KG, Patel MS. Accuracy of smartphone applications and wearable devices for tracking physical activity data. JAMA. 2015;313(6):625–6.
17. Ferguson T, Rowlands AV, Olds T, Maher C. The validity of consumer-level, activity monitors in healthy adults worn in free-living conditions: a cross-sectional study. Int J Behav Nutr Phys Act. 2015;12:42-015-0201-9.
18. Dontje ML, de Groot M, Lengton RR, van der Schans CP, Krijnen WP. Measuring steps with the Fitbit activity tracker: an inter-device reliability study. J Med Eng Technol. 2015;39(5):286–90.
19. Lee M, Song C, Lee K, Shin D, Shin S. Agreement between the spatio-temporal gait parameters from treadmill-based photoelectric cell and the instrumented treadmill system in healthy young adults and stroke patients. Med Sci Monit. 2014;20:1210–9.
20. Dahlgren G, Carlsson D, Moorhead A, Hager-Ross C, McDonough SM. Test-retest reliability of step counts with the ActivPAL device in common daily activities. Gait Posture. 2010;32(3):386–90.
21. Dowd KP, Harrington DM, Donnelly AE. Criterion and concurrent validity of the activPAL professional physical activity monitor in adolescent females. PLoS One. 2012;7(10):e47633.
22. Ryan CG, Grant PM, Tigbe WW, Granat MH. The validity and reliability of a novel activity monitor as a measure of walking. Br J Sports Med. 2006;40(9):779–84.
23. Tudor-Locke C, Sisson SB, Lee SM, Craig CL, Plotnikoff RC, Bauman A. Evaluation of quality of commercial pedometers. Can J Public Health 2006;97:S10-S15.
24. Portney L, Watkins M. Foundations of clinical research: applications to practice. Upper Saddle River, NJ: Pearson/Prentice Hall; 2009.
25. Cohen J. A power primer. Psychol Bull. 1992;112(1):155.
26. Melanson EL, Knoll JR, Bell ML, Hill JO, Nysse LJ, Lanningham-Foster L, et al. Commercially available pedometers: considerations for accurate step counting. Prev Med. 2004;39(2):361–8.
27. De Cocker KA, De Meyer J, De Bourdeaudhuij IM, Cardon GM. Non-traditional wearing positions of pedometers: validity and reliability of the Omron HJ-203-ED pedometer under controlled and free-living conditions.
J Sci Med Sport. 2012;15(5):418–24.
28. Beets MW, Patton MM, Edwards S. The accuracy of pedometer steps and time during walking in children. Med Sci Sports Exerc. 2005;37(3):513–20.
29. Martin Bland J, Altman D. Statistical methods for assessing agreement between two methods of clinical measurement. Lancet. 1986;327(8476):307–10.
30. Atallah L, Lo B, King R, Yang G. Sensor positioning for activity recognition using wearable accelerometers. IEEE Trans Biomed Circuits Syst. 2011;5(4):320–9.
31. Mannini A, Intille SS, Rosenberger M, Sabatini AM, Haskell W. Activity recognition using a single accelerometer placed at the wrist or ankle. Med Sci Sports Exerc. 2013;45(11):2193–203.

16

The effect of external ankle support on the kinematics and kinetics of the lower limb during a side step cutting task in netballers

Andrew John Greene[1,2*], Max Christian Stuelcken[3], Richard Murray Smith[2] and Benedicte Vanwanseele[4,5]

Abstract

Background: Excessive knee valgus moments are considered to be a risk factor for non-contact injuries in female athletes. Knee injuries are highly prevalent in netballers and are significant in terms of cost and disability. The aim of the study was to identify if changes in external ankle support mechanisms effect the range of motion and loading patterns at the ankle and knee joint during a sidestep cutting manoeuvre in high performance netball players.

Methods: Netballers with no previously diagnosed ankle or knee injury (n = 10) were recruited from NSW Institute of Sport netball programme. Kinematic and kinetic data were collected simultaneously using a 3-D Motion Analysis System and a force platform to measure ground reaction forces. Players performed repeated side step cutting manoeuvres whilst wearing a standard netball shoe, the same shoe with a lace-up brace and a high-top shoe.

Results: The brace condition significantly reduced ankle joint ROM in the sagittal plane by 8.9° ± 2.4 when compared to the standard netball shoe ($p = 0.013$). No other significant changes were seen between conditions for either kinematic or kinetic data. All shoe conditions did however produce knee valgus moments throughout the cutting cycle that were greater than those considered excessive in the previous literature (0.59 Nm/kg-Bwt).

Conclusions: The results show that an external ankle support brace can be used to reduce the ROM at the ankle in the sagittal plane without affecting the loading of the joints of the lower limb. Internal varus moments generated at the knee during the task were however greater than values reported in the literature to classify excessive knee joint moments, regardless of the condition. All netballers exhibited lower extremity patterns and alignments previously associated with increased peak external valgus moments including; increasing hip abduction, peak hip flexion and internal rotation during early contact and high laterally directed ground reaction forces. Increased external valgus knee loads have been strongly linked to the development of non-contact injuries at the knee in female athletes and could highlight a potential mechanism for the development non-contact knee injuries in netballers performing side step cutting tasks.

Keywords: Netball, Sidestep cutting, Biomechanics, External ankle support, Knee joint loading, Internal valgus moment

Background

Netball is a sport played mainly in commonwealth countries and is one of the most popular team sports in Australia [1]. Netball is a predominantly female sport which places high physical demands upon players, requiring them to perform movements such as jumping, braking, lunging, leaping and hopping [2] often at high speed. As a result of this, injury to the joints of the lower limb, and specifically the ankle and knee joints are highly prevalent. Whilst ankle injuries are reported to be the most prominent site of injury in netballers [3-5], injuries to the knee have the potential to be more serious in terms of impairment and treatment costs [3,5,6]. In team sports, up to 70% of injuries to the knee joint, and specifically those injuries affecting the anterior cruciate ligament (ACL) have been shown to be non-contact in nature [7]. Non-contact injuries to the knee typically

* Correspondence: andrew.greene@anglia.ac.uk
[1]Postgraduate Medical Institute, Faculty of Medical Science, Anglia Ruskin University, Chelmsford, UK
[2]Discipline of Exercise and Sport Science, Faculty of Health Science, The University of Sydney, Sydney, Australia
Full list of author information is available at the end of the article

occur during the landing or stance phase of a high impact task that incorporates sudden deceleration and/or rapid changes in direction [8]. Excessive external knee valgus moments are thought to be a significant factor in placing the female knee at greater risk of ACL injury [9]. Added to this is the finding that female athletes are two to eight times more likely to sustain a non-contact ACL injury when compared to male athletes [7,10]. This may suggest that female netballers undertaking rapid landing and cutting movements such as the side step cutting manoeuvre could be highly susceptible to injuries at the knee.

The high risk of injury at the ankle in netball is one that has been given the most attention both by researchers and athletes. External ankle supports (prophylactic ankle brace; high top shoes) are commonly used in an attempt to protect the ankle joint or to prevent further injury [11] with their most important function being to ensure the necessary stability to avoid inversion injuries [12]. Ankle braces have been shown to be effective in restricting frontal plane motion at the ankle in a netball specific landing tasks [13] and have been shown to significantly reduce the occurrence of ankle sprains in athletes and particularly those with a history of ankle injury [14,15], although not specifically in netballers. However, some research has suggested that restricting the motion at the ankle may alter the loading at the knee joint. Restricting the ankle motion in the frontal plane using prophylactic ankle braces [16] and custom foot orthotics [17] has been linked to increased peak external rotation moments at the knee joint during vertical landing [16] and running tasks [17], which may have the potential to contribute to the development of knee injuries through altered knee loading [9,18]. Whilst ankle braces have been shown to restrict frontal plane ankle motion during a netball specific landing task without altering the mechanics at the knee [13], the effect of ankle bracing on side step cutting manoeuvres has not been examined. The literature examining the effect of high top shoes in preventing ankle sprains has been inconclusive as to whether high top shoes have a stabilising effect at the ankle and are able to restrict ankle inversion [19]. There have however been reports that high top shoes, whilst not restricting the ROM at the ankle, increased plantar flexion moments at the ankle, internal rotation moments at the knee and the ROM at the knee during a single leg netball landing whist receiving a pass [13]. Studies have also showed that wearing high top shoes in certain ankle strain situations brought about delayed muscular pre-activation timing, decreased amplitudes of muscle activity and changed proprioceptive feedback, which may have a detrimental effect on establishing and maintaining functional ankle joint stability [19].

A demanding and dynamic movement such as a side step-cut, which requires athletes to change their direction of motion after landing and has been implicated in the development of knee injuries [9], may produce changes in the interaction of the joints of the lower limb with different external ankle support mechanisms. Potential restriction of the ankle motion in the frontal plane from an external ankle support may alter the mechanics at the knee joint in female netballers undertaking this task. The primary objective therefore was to quantify and compare the effect of different ankle support conditions: a standard netball shoe, a standard netball shoe with a supportive ankle brace and a high-top shoe on the ankle joint movement and loading during a side step cutting task. We hypothesised that the external brace and the high-top shoes would restrict the peak ankle joint angles, range of motion (ROM) and position throughout the contact phase of the side step cut. The secondary aim was to examine ankle and knee joint moments during the side step cutting task in the different ankle support conditions. We hypothesised that the brace and the high-top shoes would increase knee joint moments compared to the standard shoes throughout the contact phase of the side step, as a result of restriction of the motion at the ankle.

Methods

Ten female netballers (mean age, 18.3 ± 1.9 years; height, 178.1 ± 4.0 cm; mass, 69.9 ± 8.5 kg) elected to participate in this part of the study. Each player provided written consent prior to commencement. For those players under the age of 18, parental consent was also obtained. Initially, 44 players from the New South Wales Institute of Sport (NSWIS) netball program completed a self-administered questionnaire which sought information about their experiences with knee and ankle problems. Nineteen players were excluded from the study because they satisfied one or more of the exclusion criteria: (1) a history of knee or ankle surgery; (2) knee or ankle pain in the previous six months that required consultation with a medical practitioner and/or caused a formal netball training session or game to be missed; or (3) current knee or ankle pain or instability that would have prevented performance of the side step cutting task at the required intensity. Of the 25 players that met the inclusion criteria, many were unavailable to participate in the study due to; travel distance, representative netball, other commitments or injuries sustained between completing the screening questionnaire and the time of testing. Players were assessed in an indoor biomechanics laboratory using a protocol that was approved by the Human Research Ethics Committee at the University of Sydney.

A three-dimensional kinematic analysis was performed to track the position of all segments of the right lower limb (pelvis, thigh, shank, rear foot and fore foot, respectively) in space. The data were collected at 200Hz using 14-camera 3-D motion analysis system (Cortex, Motion Analysis Corporation, Santa Rosa, CA, USA). Additionally, one Kistler force plate (Kistler Instruments AG, Winterhur, Switzerland) sampling at 1000 Hz was used to simultaneously measure ground reaction forces. Each subject had twenty-one reflective surface markers attached to specific anatomical landmarks on the pelvis, thigh, shank, calcaneous and shoe to calculate three dimensional kinematic data [13].

Motion at the ankle joint was calculated using a previously described model [20], in which the ankle joint has three degrees of freedom. The multi-segment foot model is based on one used previously in the literature with moderate to high inter session reliability [21,22]. For all shoe conditions, motion of the rear foot segment was defined by a detachable wand triad marker which was attached directly to the calcaneous. This has been shown to be a valid and reliable method of obtaining in-shoe motion [23]. Wand-based markers are commonly used to measure three-dimensional rear foot kinematics [24]. The wand triad markers extended through a 16 mm diameter hole in the heel counter of the shoe. The use of the detachable rear foot wand cluster ensured marker placement was not altered between conditions, as the base for the markers remained in place during the data collection process. Forefoot motion was tracked by placing reflective markers on the outer of the shoe's upper [25,26]. For the ankle brace condition, markers to track the medial and lateral malleolus were palpated and attached to the surface of the ankle brace, so as not to alter the integrity of the ankle brace.

The movement pattern assessed was a side step cutting task during which each player was instructed to use a 5 m straight line approach to the landing area at a self-selected, match appropriate speed. This was calculated using the horizontal velocity of the sacrum marker in the five frames prior to heel contact. All players were required to land on the ground embedded and level force platform and sidestep cut off the right leg at a cutting angle of approximately 45° towards a designated marked location [27]. Players were allowed as many practice trials as necessary to become familiar with the procedures and testing environment and all players identified as right handed/footed. Once data collection commenced players were required to complete 8–10 successful trials. A trial was considered successful if it satisfied the requirements of the task and the right foot landed within the border of the force plate. Players performed this movement with a standard netball shoe (Ignite3, ASICS) (standard condition), the same netball shoe with a lace-up brace (E-Professional) (brace condition) and a high-top shoe (Jordan, Nike) (high-top condition). The order of the conditions was randomized.

Kinematic and kinetic data were processed using Visual3D software (C-motion, Rockville, MD, USA). The lower extremity segments were modeled as a frustra of right cones while the pelvis was modeled as a cylinder. Anthropometric data was used based on [28]. Internal moments were calculated at the proximal end of the distal segment of each joint. The local coordinate systems of the pelvis, thigh, leg, rear-foot and fore-foot were derived from the standing reference position in which participants stood in a relaxed stance with both feet aligned with the laboratory X axis. Players adopted this reference position prior to undertaking the side step cut for each condition. Coordinate data were low-pass filtered using a fourth-order Butterworth filter with a 6–15 Hz cutoff frequency. Ground reaction force data were low-pass filtered using a fourth-order Butterworth filter with a 20 Hz cut-off frequency. Six degrees-of-freedom for each segment were determined from the segment's set of reflective markers. Subsequently, lower extremity 3-D joint angles were calculated using a XYZ Cardan rotation sequence.

All data were time-normalized to 100% of the cut cycle and all players contacted the ground with their right (dominant) foot. The cut cycle was defined as the period from initial contact of the right foot (0%) to the toe off of the right foot, as determined by the vertical ground reaction forces with a threshold of 20 N. Four trials per subject per condition were analysed. Discrete variables (peak joint angles, joint range of motion, peak joint moments, peak ground reaction forces) were extracted from each individual trial and averaged for each player. All trials were time normalized across stance and averaged for each player. The individual mean curves were then averaged across conditions to produce ensemble curves.

Statistical analyses were undertaken in SPSS 21.0 (IBM SPSS Statistics for Windows, Armonk, NY, USA). For the primary discrete variables of the footwear conditions: Standard shoe vs Brace condition vs High Top Shoe, a repeated measures analysis of variance was undertaken for the ankle and knee joint range of motion, peak joint moments and peak ground reaction forces. A Bonferroni adjustment was applied to each condition to test significant differences between footwear conditions. All p values of less than 0.05 were considered statistically significant. Data were expressed as mean and standard deviation.

Results

No significant differences existed between the approach velocities in each of the three conditions (Standard: 3.2 $m.s^{-1} \pm 0.4$; Brace: 3.3 $m.s^{-1} \pm 0.4$; High Top: 3.3 $m.s^{-1} \pm 0.4$). No significant difference existed for foot progression angle at flat foot between conditions, with all conditions landing within 1° of the zero alignment, as defined by the standing reference trial (Standard: 0.1° ± 1.6; Brace: 0.8° ± 1.5; High Top: 0.1° ± 1.9). The brace condition was shown to significantly reduce the range of motion (ROM) at the ankle in the sagittal plane when compared to the standard shoe condition (39.7° ± 8.4° vs. 48.6° ± 10.6°, $p = 0.013$) (Table 1). There was no significant effect of the brace or high top condition at the ankle or knee in any of the other planes of motion (Table 1). No significant differences existed at either the ankle or the knee joint for the peak joint moments (Table 2) or for the peak ground reaction forces (Table 3) between the different conditions.

Figure 1 shows the ensemble curves for the sagittal plane kinematics at the ankle and the knee for all conditions. At initial contact, the ankle is slightly plantar flexed and undergoes a slight increase in plantar flexion through the initial loading phase. This occurs with a relatively static knee angle through the first 10% of the phase. The ankle and knee joints simultaneously undergo increases in dorsi flexion and flexion respectively through the next 30% of the phase. The knee reaches peak flexion at approximately 40% of landing after which it undergoes extension through to approximately 80% of ground contact. Ankle dorsi flexion continues to increase until approximately 50%, after which the ankle plantar flexes through to toe off at 100%. The knee once again flexes from approximately 80% of the phase through to toe off.

Figure 2 shows the kinematics of the hip joint throughout the landing phase of the side step cut. The hip is relatively flexed at initial ground contact and undergoes continual extension throughout the entire phase. Hip extension plateaus at approximately 85% of the landing through to toe off at 100%. In the fontal plane, the hip is abducted at ground contact which continues to rise through to approximately 65-70% of the landing phase, after which the hip adducts through to toe off. The hip is internally rotated at initial contact and this increases slightly through the initial contact phase, up to approximately 15% of the phase. The hip then externally rotates through the remainder of the landing, rapidly from 15-35% of the phase, and then more gradually though to toe off.

Table 1 Range of motion at the ankle and knee joint for all ankle support conditions

	Standard	Brace	High Top
Ankle Sagittal ROM	48.6 ± 10.6	**39.7 ± 8.4***	45.8 ± 6.5
Ankle Frontal ROM	13.5 ± 4.6	13.5 ± 4.4	14.7 ± 6.4
Ankle Transverse ROM	16.1 ± 9.1	14.1 ± 7.4	17.9 ± 5.1
Knee Sagittal ROM	41.1 ± 6.5	38.9 ± 9.1	39.2 ± 7.2
Knee Frontal ROM	8.6 ± 2.8	8.5 ± 3.6	8.4 ± 2.1
Knee Transverse ROM	17.5 ± 4.2	17.6 ± 5.4	17.9 ± 3.3

Values are presented in degrees (°) as mean ± SD. *Significant difference between the Standard shoe condition and the Standard shoe with ankle brace condition ($p \leq 0.05$).

Table 2 Peak joint moments at the ankle and knee joint for all ankle support conditions

	Standard	Brace	High Top
Ankle Flexor Moment	0.04 ± 0.01	0.04 ± 0.02	0.04 ± 0.01
Ankle Extensor Moment	0.07 ± 0.02	0.06 ± 0.02	0.07 ± 0.02
Ankle Inversion Moment	0.01 ± 0.01	0.01 ± 0.01	0.01 ± 0.01
Ankle Eversion Moment	0.01 ± 0.01	0.01 ± 0.01	0.01 ± 0.01
Ankle Adduction Moment	0.03 ± 0.01	0.02 ± 0.01	0.02 ± 0.01
Ankle Abduction Moment	0.03 ± 0.02	0.02 ± 0.02	0.01 ± 0.01
Knee Flexion Moment	3.81 ± 0.42	3.77 ± 0.57	3.91 ± 0.38
Knee Extensor Moment	1.66 ± 0.39	1.58 ± 0.46	1.70 ± 0.32
Knee Varus Moment	0.78 ± 0.29	0.80 ± 0.40	0.87 ± 0.34
Knee Valgus Moment	0.44 ± 0.27	0.36 ± 0.25	0.48 ± 0.29
Knee Internal Rotation Moment	0.34 ± 0.17	0.32 ± 0.13	0.36 ± 0.14
Knee External Rotation Moment	0.37 ± 0.17	0.40 ± 0.18	0.42 ± 0.16

Values are presented in Nm / kg.Bwt as mean ± SD. Positive moments are determined at the ankle as: dorsiflexion, inversion and adduction; and at the knee as: flexion, adduction (varus) and internal rotation.

Discussion

The brace condition significantly reduced ankle joint range of motion in the sagittal plane by 8.9° ± 2.4° throughout ground contact of the side step cut, when compared to the standard netball shoe. These results differ from previous research that has investigated the effect of ankle bracing in a netball specific landing task [13] in that no restriction of motion in the frontal plane at the ankle was observed in the current study. Restriction of ankle ROM in the current study came without any changes in the ROM at the knee joint, or any increases in the loading at the ankle or knee joint. This is not entirely surprising however, as previous studies [16] have linked frontal plane ROM restriction at the ankle using an external ankle support with increased external rotation moments at the knee, which were not demonstrated in this study. As such, it can be suggested that an external ankle support brace can be used successfully to

Table 3 Peak ground reaction forces for all ankle support conditions

	Standard	Brace	High Top
Vertical GRF	23.1 ± 0.8	23.3 ± 2.7	22.9 ± 2.2
Medial GRF	9.9 ± 0.7	10.1 ± 1.6	9.7 ± 1.4
Breaking GRF	−7.0 ± 2.8	−6.9 ± 2.6	−6.8 ± 2.3
Propulsive GRF	1.6 ± 0.6	1.8 ± 0.3	1.7 ± 0.5

Values are presented in degrees N / kg.Bwt as mean ± SD. Breaking (posterior) GRF is presented at negative as it acts in the opposite to that of the direction of motion.

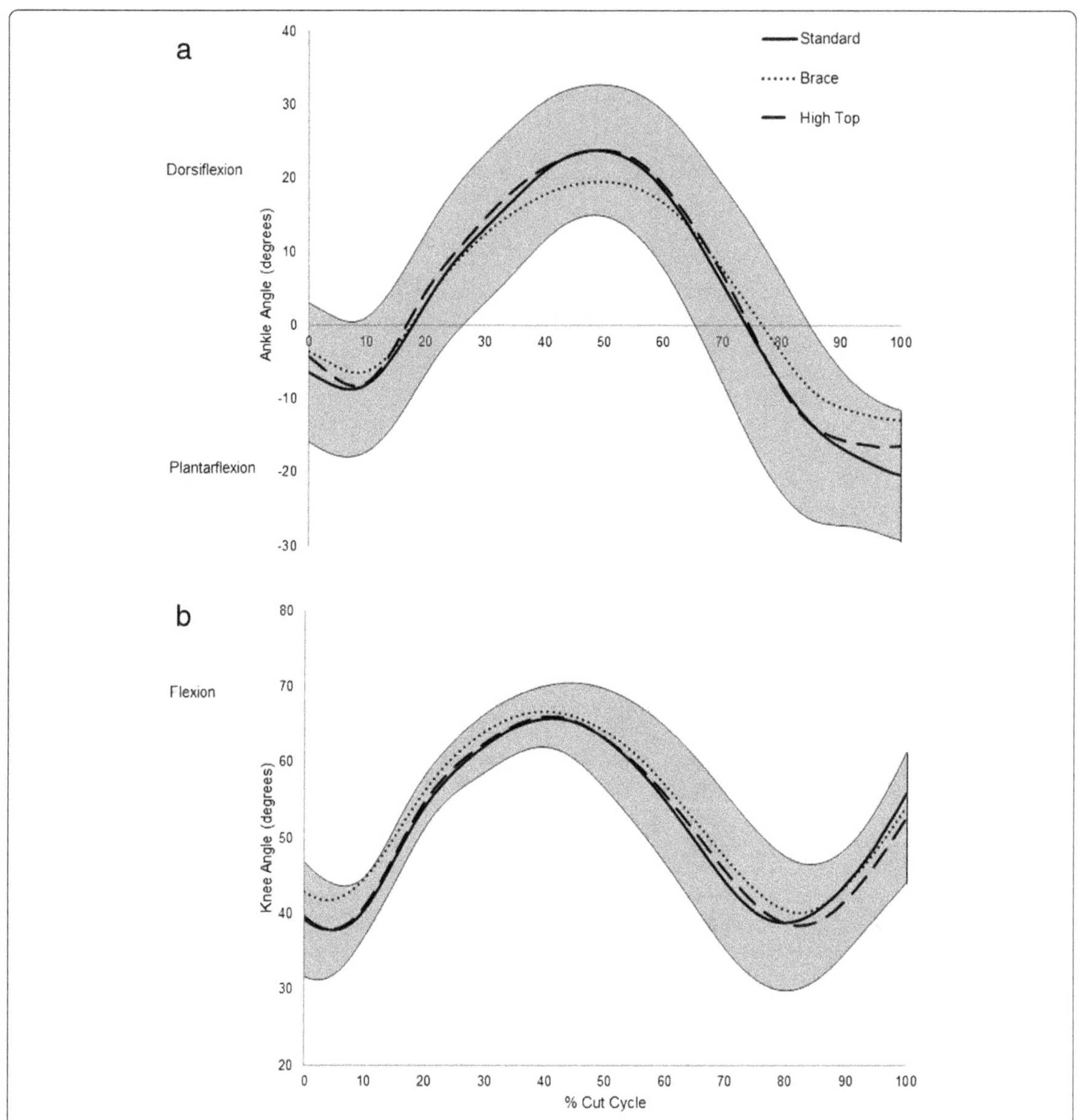

Figure 1 Sagittal plane angular displacement at the ankle and knee joint. Mean ensemble curves for **(a)** the sagittal plane ankle angular displacement and **(b)** the sagittal plane knee angular displacement during the cut cycle. The shaded area shows the 95% confidence interval of the mean curve for the standard shoe condition. Dorsiflexion and Flexion are depicted at positive in the figure.

stabilise the ankle joint and limit range on motion in the sagittal plane during a side step cutting task without increasing the potential for knee injury due to altered mechanics and loading of the knee joint. No significant restrictions were seen for the ankle ROM in the high top shoe condition. It can therefore be suggested that despite observing some minor restriction in the sagittal plane range of motion at the ankle (Table 1), the use of a high top shoe in an attempt to stabilise and restrict the ankle ROM during a side step cutting task is not as effective as an external ankle brace. Unlike in previous studies that examined the effect of external ankle support during a netball specific landing task [13], no alterations to the plantar flexion moments at the ankle, internal rotation moments at the knee or the ROM at the knee were seen in the high top condition. As previously mentioned, it might have been expected that the ankle brace condition would have brought about

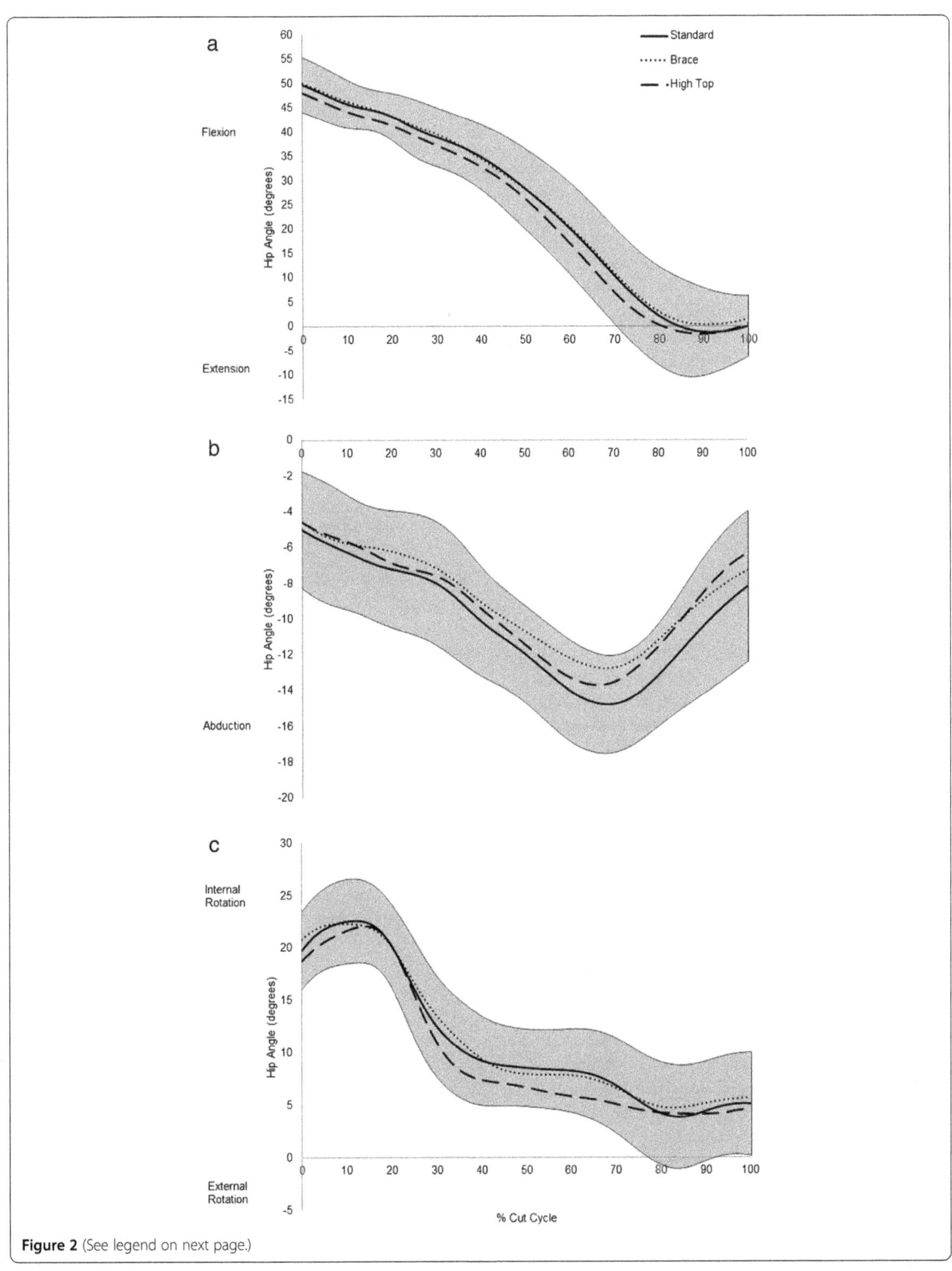

Figure 2 (See legend on next page.)

(See figure on previous page.)
Figure 2 Sagittal, Frontal and Transverse place angular displacement at the hip joint. Mean ensemble curves for **(a)** the sagittal plane hip angular displacement **(b)** the frontal plane hip angular displacement and **(c)** the frontal plane hip angular displacement the during the cut cycle. The shaded area shows the 95% confidence interval of the mean curve for the standard shoe condition. Flexion, Adduction and Internal Rotation are depicted as positive in the figure.

restrictions in the frontal plane ROM at the ankle throughout the task, and in the ankle inversion eversion angle at initial contact, however this did not occur (data for inversion eversion angle at initial contact not shown). It has been reported in the literature that the most important function of ankle braces is to ensure the necessary stability immediately prior to landing to avoid lateral ankle injuries, however this was assessed in vertical landing tasks where the ankle was loaded on a 30° tilting platform [12]. Previous studies that have found restrictions in the frontal plane ROM in external brace conditions have done so in tasks where the ankle was passively forced into internal or external rotation [29,30] or where a task involved the stabilisation of the ankle during the active slowing of a forward landing [13]. In the side step cutting task performed in the current study, the athlete is not trying to actively slow down her landing at contact in preparation for a rapid stop as in a catch and land task [13] and is maintaining forward movement which will then be transferred and used to facilitate an effective cutting movement. Otago [1] reported that run-on landing conditions (similar to the side step cut), as opposed to landing conditions that required a rapid deceleration or stop, were the least stressful on the body. As there is less demand on the ankle joint to actively brake and slow down the movement throughout landing during the side step cutting task as opposed to a land and stop task [13], it may therefore be the case that in the side step cutting task, the ankle joint is not subjected to frontal plane loads which require the ankle brace to provide stability and ROM restriction in the frontal plane. It is not entirely evident from the results of this study whether the restriction of the ankle ROM in the sagittal plane in the brace condition is beneficial to the athlete, especially as no significant differences were seen in the joint moments or ground reaction forces experienced by the athletes. These results may however be of benefit to those athletes suffering from chronic ankle instability or recurrent ankle sprains, who may require joint range of motion limitation to provide a greater feeling of stability at the ankle joint, whilst not altering the action of the other joints of the lower limb.

No significant differences existed between conditions for the motion and loading at the knee joint throughout the task. However, all shoe conditions produced internal knee varus moments throughout ground contact (Table 2) that were larger than the external valgus moments considered to be excessive during a side step cutting task in previous literature [9]. The data reported in the current study depicts the internal varus moment at the knee, whereas the previously presented literature [9] shows the external valgus moment at the knee. Due to the different conventions used, these two variables depict comparable loading in the frontal plane on the medial side of the knee. Irrespective of the adopted convention (internal or external joint moment), studies in general report consistent joint moment profiles for the sagittal and frontal planes during able-bodied adult gait [31]. Nine of the ten netballers tested produced internal knee varus moments for at least one of the shoe conditions of a magnitude greater than 0.59 Nm/kg-Bwt, the value used in the study by Sigward and Powers [9] to group athletes that were identified as exhibiting excessive external valgus moment at the knee joint during a side step cut. Whilst the values in the current paper (Standard: 0.78 ± 0.3 Nm/kg-Bwt; Brace: 0.80 ± 0.4 Nm/kg-Bwt; High Top: 0.87 ± 0.34 Nm/kg-Bwt) are not as large as those reported by Sigward and Powers [9] (1.2 ± 0.4 Nm/kg-Bwt), they are still much larger than the 0.59 Nm/kg-Bwt used to define excessive external knee valgus moments, and the external knee valgus values of 0.62 ± 0.2 Nm/kg-Bwt reported by McLean et al. [32] in females during side stepping tasks. The reason for the reduced knee valgus moments in the current study can more than likely be attributed to the reduced approach velocity of the athletes (3.3 ± 0.07 m.s^{-1}) as compared to the increased approach velocity (5.1 ± 0.4 m.s^{-1}) used previously in other studies [9]. In the context of a netball population however, this would more than likely be an accurate representation of the speeds at which players would carry out such tasks, due to the restrictive court conditions and the relatively short duration of sprint activities that occur in netball games [33].

External knee valgus loading has been reported to be the predominant mechanism of non-contact injury to the ACL during the side step cutting task, and this has been shown to be elevated in female athletes [9,27,34]. It is thought that poor or altered neuromuscular control of the knee during sidestep cutting could potentially expose the knee to dangerous combinations of knee joint loading [8,34,35]. Increased peak external valgus moments have also been correlated with a number of kinematic actions at the hip which appear to act to increase the valgus load on the knee joint [32]. Athletes exhibiting excessive external valgus knee moments [9] demonstrated increased internal rotation and abduction at the hip and greater laterally directed GRF's during the side step. Kipp et al. [36] reported that less overall hip flexion throughout the side step cut task had an important role with respect to controlling the frontal and transverse plane loading of the knee, and specifically that reduced hip flexion acted to increase the peak internal knee rotation moments, which are considered to be important dynamic loading mechanisms of the knee [8]. It can be seen from Figure 2 that the netballers assessed in the current study demonstrate a number of these lower extremity patterns and alignments, with continual hip extension and hip abduction throughout the task, initial internal rotation with a rapid shift into external rotation of the hip, as well as high laterally directed GRF's (Table 3). This may therefore indicate that the netballers tested in the current study are demonstrating kinematic actions at the hip joint which may contribute to the elevated internal valgus moments at the knee joint. A possible mechanism for these actions at the hip would be to facilitate the change in direction during the cutting task, which requires the rotation of the body towards the direction of the cut and the lateral translation of the centre of mass to this direction [9]. Hip internal rotation at initial contact would act to rotate the landing limb towards the direction of motion of the cut. The rapid hip external rotation after landing would suggest that the body is being rotated to the direction of the cut whilst the foot is still planted on the ground. The continual hip extension through the contact phase suggests a more upright body position through the landing, which is similar to previous findings [36] and may therefore increase the demands on the knee joint throughout ground contact. Large laterally directed ground reaction forces as the athlete executes the cutting aspect of the manoeuvre, coupled with the orientation of the body towards the direction of the movement and the increase in hip abduction could act to increase the loading on the medial aspect of the knee.

Given the relatively high incidence and potential severity of knee injuries in netballers, it is important to identify the underlying mechanisms that increase the internal varus/external valgus knee loading, and subsequently the potential risks of injury. The identification of risk factors and the development of prevention strategies may have widespread health and economic implications [34]. It has been suggested that increased hip internal rotation and/or flexion at initial contact may compromise the ability of the medial muscle groups to adequately support the resultant knee valgus loading, and that increased neuromuscular control during sidestepping may reduce the likelihood of ACL injury via valgus load in females [32]. Poor and/or altered neuromuscular control during side step cutting tasks has been suggested as a major contributor to the production of potentially hazardous knee joint loading combinations that place the ACL at risk [8,34]. Sigward and Powers [9] reported that athletes that displayed normal frontal plane moments during the side step cutting task maintained a more neutral alignment with the centre of pressure of the ground reaction forces closer to the centre of mass throughout the movement. They suggested that instructions of body alignments with the goal of maintaining a more vertical tibia and reduced medio-lateral forces through landing should be included in injury prevention training. This idea for providing postural alignment training to prevent injury may be particularly valid in a netball population, who in previous studies [37] have been shown to have difficulty in consistently aligning the knee and foot during single leg landing tasks. An investigation of netballers that demonstrate both normal and excessive ranges of internal varus or external valgus knee loading is necessary to determine if the side step cutting techniques undertaken by the groups significantly differed, and to see whether the actions at the hip, which have been previously linked to increased external valgus knee loading were present or active in netballers exhibiting reduced internal varus knee moments. Since these actions at the hip throughout the landing have been linked to potential neuromuscular weaknesses in the athletes with elevated valgus knee loads, it would also be advantageous to undertake further work to see whether neuromuscular training interventions to target improvements in the strength of the hip musculature may be beneficial for netballers.

There were a number of limitations of the current study. The sample size of netballers tested was small, which may impact upon the power of our findings and the extent to which the findings can be generalised. Whilst netballers were recruited from the same source to maintain a homogenous sample, access to and the availability of high performance netballers was limited. The current study calculated the internal joint moments at the joints to describe the loads being applied to joints throughout the side step cut. Previous studies [9,32,35] have however reported external joint moments acting throughout the side step cutting manoeuvre. Whilst it is suggested that regardless of the convention, internal and external moments are comparable in able bodied gait [31], differences in the methods used to calculate the moments including marker sets, reference frames and joint expression could not be standardised and so should be considered when comparing and reviewing the results. This being said, all moments have been displayed with the same units of Nm/kg-Bwt with the purpose of the results being used to provide some context to suggest possible mechanisms of knee injury in female netballers during a side step task. The velocity of the side step cut in the current study was much slower than those studies that reported external valgus knee loads side step cutting tasks [9,32] which could potentially have limited the findings of the current study. The approach velocity demonstrated by the netballers in the current study is however close to the 4 m.s^{-1} that has been recommended as the standardised value of approach speed to be used when examining side step cutting tasks in female athletes [38]. All netballers were asked to perform the task at a self-selected game related speed, and as mentioned previously, the velocity of the task in the current study does not seem unreasonable for a sample of netballers given the demands of the game. The side step cutting tasks in the current study was also anticipated by the players, and so they had the opportunity to prepare for the task prior to carrying it out. Studies [36,39,40] have suggested that loads are increased when the task is unanticipated in nature, so this needs to be taken into account when evaluating the findings of the current study. Whilst it would be beneficial and interesting to look at unanticipated side step tasks in the netball cohort, in a netball game, athletes would undertake a number of side step cuts where they were anticipating making the move in order to run into space to receive a pass.

Conclusions

The result show that an external ankle support brace can be used to successfully reduce the sagittal plane ROM at the ankle during a side step cutting task without having any effects upon the loading of the joints of the lower limb. There were no changes in the frontal plane ROM at the ankle between the brace and the other shoe conditions. The data does however show that netballers demonstrated high internal varus moments of the knee joint during the side step cutting task regardless of the external ankle support mechanism. The internal varus loading of the knee in the current study was greater than the external valgus loading values reported by previous studies [9] to highlight athletes that produced valgus knee loads that were classed as excessive. These findings may suggest that the side step cut places greater loads on the knee joint throughout the task with a reduced need to stabilise the ankle joint laterally. Increased external valgus knee loads have been strongly linked to the development of non-contact injuries at the knee in female athletes, and so the results of the current study may highlight a potential mechanism for the development of non-contact injuries at the knee joint in netballers performing side step cutting tasks.

Abbreviations

ACL: Anterior Cruciate Ligament; ROM: Range of Motion.

Competing interests

The authors declare that they have no competing interests.

Authors' contributions

AG participated in the acquisition of the data, undertook analysis and interpretation of the data and drafted the manuscript. MS participated in the design of the study, coordinated the study, undertook the acquisition of the data and helped to revise the manuscript. RS participated in the design of the study and helped to revise the manuscript. BV conceived of the study, participated in its design and coordination, undertook the analysis of the data and helped to revise the manuscript. All authors read and approved the final manuscript.

Acknowledgements

We would like to acknowledge all netball players who were willing to volunteer for this study and took time out of their busy training schedules to participate. We would like to thank Caleb Wegener and Angus Chard for their assistance in the data collection. This research project was funded by the Research and Injury Prevention Scheme of the NSW Sporting Injury Committee.

Author details

[1]Postgraduate Medical Institute, Faculty of Medical Science, Anglia Ruskin University, Chelmsford, UK. [2]Discipline of Exercise and Sport Science, Faculty of Health Science, The University of Sydney, Sydney, Australia. [3]School of Health and Sport Sciences, Faculty of Science, Health, Education and Engineering, University of the Sunshine Coast, Queensland, Australia. [4]Department of Kinesiology, KU Leuven, Leuven, Belgium. [5]Chair of Health Innovation and Technology, Fontys University of Applied Sciences, Eindhoven, Netherlands.

References

1. Otago L: **Kinetic analysis of landings in netball: is a footwork rule change required to decrease ACL injuries?** *J Sci Med Sport* 2004, **7**:85–95.
2. Williams R, O'Donoghue PG: **Lower limb injury risk in netball: a time-motion analysis investigation.** *J Hum Mov Stud* 2005, **49**:315–331.
3. McManus A, Stevenson MR, Finch CF: **Incidence and risk factors for injury in non-elite netball.** *J Sci Med Sport* 2006, **9**(1–2):119–124.
4. Hume PA, Steele JR: **A preliminary investigation of injury prevention strategies in Netball: are players heeding the advice?** *J Sci Med Sport* 2000, **3**(4):406–413.
5. Hopper D, Elliott B, Lalor J: **A descriptive epidemiology of netball injuries during competition: a five year study.** *Br J Sports Med* 1995, **29**(4):223–228.
6. Flood L, Harrison JE: **Epidemiology of basketball and netball injuries that resulted in hospital admission in Australia, 2000–2004.** *Med J Aust* 2009, **190**:87–90.
7. Boden BP, Dean GS, Feagin JA, Garrett WE: **Mechanisms of anterior cruciate ligament injury.** *Orthopedics* 2000, **23**:573–578.
8. Griffin LY, Albohm MJ, Arendt EA, Bahr R, Beynnon BD, Demaio M, Dick RW, Engebretsen L, Garrett WE Jr, Hannafin JA, Hewett TE, Huston LJ, Ireland ML, Johnson RJ, Lephart S, Mandelbaum BR, Mann BJ, Marks PH, Marshall SW, Myklebust G, Noyes FR, Powers C, Shields C Jr, Shultz SJ, Silvers H, Slauterbeck J, Taylor DC, Teitz CC, Wojtys EM, Yu B: **Understanding and preventing noncontact anterior cruciate ligament injuries: a review of the Hunt Valley II meeting, January 2005.** *Am J Sports Med* 2006, **34**(9):1512–1532.
9. Sigward SM, Powers CM: **Loading characteristics of females exhibiting excessive valgus moments during cutting.** *Clin Biomech (Bristol, Avon)* 2007, **22**:827–833.
10. Hootman JM, Dick R, Agel J: **Epidemiology of collegiate injuries for 15 sports: summary and recommendations for injury prevention initiatives.** *J Athl Train* 2007, **42**:311–319.
11. Hume PA, Stacoff A, Steele JR: **Your body: your choice. Have you checked your shoes?** In *Are You Ready for Netball Pamphlet Series, LINZ Activity and Health and Research Unit, University of Auckland, New Zealand 1995.* Edited by Wilson N. Netball New Zealand: 1995.
12. Eils E, Rosenbaum D: **The main function of ankle braces is to control the joint position before landing.** *Foot Ankle Int* 2003, **24**(3):263–268.
13. Vanwanseele B, Stuelcken M, Greene A, Smith R: **The effect of external ankle support on knee and ankle joint movement and loading in netball players.** *J Sci Med Sport* 2013, **17**(5):511–515.
14. Sitler M, Ryan J, Wheeler B, McBride J, Arciero R, Anderson J, Horodyski M: **The efficacy of a semirigid ankle stabilizer toreduce acute ankle injuries**

in basketball—a randomized clinical-study at west-point—reply. *Am J Sports Med* 1994, **22**(4):454–461.
15. Surve I, Schwellnus MP, Noakes T, Lombard C: **A fivefold reduction in the incidence of recurrent ankle sprains in soccer players using the sport-stirrup orthosis.** *Am J Sports Med* 1994, **22**(5):601–606.
16. Venesky K, Docherty CL, Dapena J, Schrader J: **Prophylactic ankle braces and knee varus-valgus and internal-external rotation torque.** *J Athl Train* 2006, **41**(3):239–244.
17. Mundermann A, Nigg BM, Humble RN, Stefanyshyn DJ: **Foot orthotics affect lower extremity kinematics and kinetics during running.** *Clin Biomech (Bristol, Avon)* 2003, **18**(3):254–262.
18. Oh YK, Lipps DB, Ashton-Miller JA, Wojtys EM: **What strains the anterior cruciate ligament during a pivot landing?** *Am J Sports Med* 2012, **40**(3):574–583.
19. Fu W, Fang Y, Liu Y, Hou J: **The effect of high-top and low-top shoes on ankle inversion kinematics and muscle activation in landing on a tilted surface.** *J Foot Ankle Res* 2014, **7**:14–24.
20. Chard A, Greene A, Hunt A, Vanwanseele B, Smith R: **Effect of thong style flip-flops on children's barefoot walking and jogging kinematics.** *J Foot Ankle Res* 2013, **6**(1):8.
21. Hunt AE, Smith RM, Torode M, Keenan AM: **Inter-segment foot motion and ground reaction forces over the stance phase of walking.** *Clin Biomech* 2001, **16**(7):592–600.
22. Rattanaprasert U, Smith R, Sullivan M, Gilleard W: **Three-dimensional kinematics of the forefoot, rearfoot, and leg without the function of tibialis posterior in comparison with normals during stance phase of walking.** *Clin Biomech* 1999, **14**(1):14–23.
23. O'Meara D, Smith RM, Hunt AE, Vanwanseele BM: **In shoe motion of the child's foot when walking.** In *Proceedings of the 8th Footwear Biomechanics Symposium*. Taipei, Taiwan: Footwear Biomechanics Group; 2007.
24. Shultz R, Jenkyn T: **Determining the maximum diameter for holes in the shoe without compromising shoe integrity when using a multi-segment foot model.** *Med Eng Phys* 2012, **34**(1):118–122.
25. Stacoff A, Reinschmidt C, Nigg BM, Van den Bogert AJ, Lundberg A, Denoth J, Stüssi E: **Effects of shoe sole construction on skeletal motion during running.** *Med Sci Sports Exerc* 2001, **33**(2):311–319.
26. De Wit B, De Clerq D, Aerts P: **Biomechanical analysis of the stance phase during barefoot and shod running.** *J Biomech* 2000, **33**:269–278.
27. McLean SG, Huang XM, Su A, van den Bogert AJ: **Sagittal plane biomechanics cannot injure the ACL during sidestep cutting.** *Clin Biomech (Bristol, Avon)* 2004, **19**:828–838.
28. Dempster WT, Gabel WC, Felts WJ: **The anthropometry of the manual work space for the seated subject.** *Am J Phys Anthropol* 1959, **17**:289–317.
29. Greene TA, Hillman SK: **Comparison of support provided by a semi rigid orthosis and adhesive ankle taping before, during, and after exercise.** *Am J Sports Med* 1990, **18**(5):498–506.
30. Gross MT, Bradshaw MK, Ventry LC, Weller KH: **Comparison of support provided by ankle taping and semi rigid orthosis.** *J Orthop Sports Phys Ther* 1987, **9**(1):33–39.
31. Schache AG, Baker R, Vaughan CL: **Differences in lower limb transverse plane joint moments during gait when expressed in two alternative reference frames.** *J Biomech* 2007, **40**:9–19.
32. McLean SG, Huang X, van den Bogert AJ: **Association between lower extremity posture at contact and peak knee valgus moment during sidestepping: implications for ACL injury.** *Clin Biomech (Bristol, Avon)* 2005, **20**:863–870.
33. Fox A, Spittle M, Otago L, Sunders N: **Activity profiles of the Australian female netball team players during international competition: implications for training practice.** *J Sports Sci* 2013, **31**(14):1588–1595.
34. Weinhandl JT, Earl-Boehm JE, Ebersole KT, Huddleston WE, Armstrong BSR, O'Connor KM: **Anticipatory effects on anterior cruciate ligament loading during sidestep cutting.** *Clin Biomech (Bristol, Avon)* 2013, **28**:655–663.
35. McLean SG, Neal RJ, Myers PT, Walters MR: **Knee joint kinematics during the sidestep cutting maneuver: potential for injury in women.** *Med Sci Sports Exerc* 1999, **31**:959–968.
36. Kipp K, McLean SG, Palmieri-Smith RM: **Patterns of hip flexion motion predict frontal and transverse plane knee torques during a single-leg land-and-cut maneuver.** *Clin Biomech (Bristol, Avon)* 2011, **26**:504–508.
37. Stuelcken M, Greene A, Smith R, Vanwanseele B: **Knee loading patterns in a simulated netball landing task.** *Eur J Sport Sci* 2013, **13**(5):475–482.
38. Vanrenterghem J, Venables E, Pataky T, Robinson MA: **The effect of running speed on knee mechanical loading in females during side cutting.** *J Biomech* 2012, **45**:2444–2449.
39. Brown SR, Brughelli M, Hume P: **Knee mechanics during planned and unplanned sidestepping: a systematic review and meta-analysis.** *Sports Med* 2014, **44**:1573–1588.
40. Besier TF, Lloyd DG, Ackland TR, Cochrane JL: **Anticipatory effects on knee joint loading during running and cutting maneuvers.** *Med Sci Sports Exerc* 2001, **33**:1176–1181.

17

Age profiles of sport participants

Rochelle M. Eime[1,2*], Jack T. Harvey[1,2], Melanie J. Charity[1,2], Meghan M. Casey[2], Hans Westerbeek[1] and Warren R. Payne[1]

Abstract

Background: Participation in sport has many health benefits, and is popular amongst children. However participation decreases with age. While the membership records of peak sports organisations have improved markedly in recent years, there has been little research into sport participation trends across the lifespan. This study investigates age profiles of participation in sport and compares these trends between genders and residential locations.

Methods: De-identified 2011 participant registration data for seven popular Australian sports (Australian Football, Basketball, Cricket, Hockey, Lawn Bowls, Netball and Tennis) were obtained and analysed according to age, gender and geographical location (metropolitan v non-metropolitan) within the state of Victoria, Australia. All data were integrated and sports were analysed collectively to produce broadly based participation profiles while maintaining confidentiality of membership data for individual sports.

Results: The total number of registered participants included in the data set for 2011 was 520,102. Most participants (64.1 %) were aged less than 20 years. Nearly one third (27.6 %) of all participants were aged 10–14 years, followed by the 5–9 year age group (19.9 %). Participation declined rapidly during adolescence. A higher proportion of males than female participants were young children (4–7 years) or young adults 18–29 years; this pattern was reversed among 8–17 year-olds. A higher proportion of metropolitan participants were engaged between the ages of 4–13 and 19–29, whereas a higher proportion of non-metropolitan participants played during adolescence (14–18 years) and throughout mature adulthood (30+ years).

Conclusions: Increasing participation in sport is an objective for both government and sporting organisations. In order to have both mass population-based participation, from a health policy and elite performance perspective, we need to further explore the findings arising from the analysis of this extensive data set. Such an examination will lead to better understand of the reasons for attrition during adolescence to inform program and policy developments to retain people participating in sport, for a healthy and sport performing nation.

Keywords: Sport, Participation, Age patterns

Background

Sport is a common form of Leisure Time Physical Activity (LTPA) [1, 2] which has been shown to result in many health benefits. Recent systematic reviews found that there are many psychological and social health benefits specifically associated with participation in sport for children, adolescents and adults [3, 4]. There is consistent evidence that those who participate in club-based and/or team-based sport participation can have better psychological and social health outcomes than those that only engage in individual types of physical activity (PA) [3, 4]. The social nature of club- and team-based sport is suggested to mediate these health outcomes, although the psychological and social health benefits of sport participation differ between children, adolescents and adults. For children and adolescents social health benefits are more prominent, such as development of social skills through opportunities for social interaction and improved self-esteem, whereas sport participation among adults is more likely to lead to better psychological health, including reduced stress and distress [3, 4]. In addition to the mental and social health benefits, club sport has been shown to be associated with greater physical health benefits at low

* Correspondence: rochelle.eime@vu.edu.au
[1]Institute of Sport, Exercise and Active Living, Victoria University, PO Box 14428, Melbourne, Victoria 8001, Australia
[2]School of Health Sciences and Psychology, Federation University, Ballarat, Australia

and moderate levels of participation, than participation in individual-based physical activities such as walking [5]. From a public health perspective, sport during adolescence is a strong predictor of PA later in life [6, 7].

Understanding participation patterns in sport is also important for a range of key stakeholders including government, sport and recreation, and health organisations, and in particular sport governing bodies [2]. Population-level sport participation patterns can inform evidence-based strategic and policy planning and development [8, 9] and facilitate the achievement of desirable outcomes. For instance, in Australia the National Sport Policy Framework provides a guide outlining the importance of sport policies and coordinated strategies at both the community and elite levels for increased participation and a healthy nation, as well as for international success of elite athletes [10].

Sport participation patterns are typically explored according to age and gender. There is evidence that sport participation is a young persons' activity [11], with reports that participation levels peak at ages 12–13 years [12]. However, others have found that for Belgian boys aged 13–18 years, there was a linear increase in sport participation until age 16.8 years, before participation declined [13]. Another study of sport and PA participation by girls found that overall PA levels did not significantly change throughout adolescence, but that the context of participation changed [14]. Older adolescent females (16–18 years) shifted their participation away from organised, competitive modes and settings towards non-organised and non-competitive modes and settings and were more likely to then participate in individual types of PA [14].

For adults, the relationship between sport participation, age and gender has been found to differ amongst European countries [15]. In France, Latvia, Slovakia and the UK, males reported significantly more sport participation than women in the young adult age group (18–34 years). In Belgium and Greece, males were more likely to participate than females in both the young adult (18–34 years) and older adult (55 years and older) categories [15]. In contrast, Swedish women were more active than males in the young adult category (18–34 years); whilst in Finland this was only true for the middle-age group (35–54 years) and in Denmark for the older adults (55 years and older) [15]. In Australia, sport participation in an organised context was dominated by those aged 15–34 years compared to all older age groups, for both males and females [2]. Similarly in Spain, the prevalence of participation in sport decreased as age increased [16]. Amongst older adults aged 58–67, sport participation has also been found to decrease with age [17].

There are significant gender differences in sports participation in European countries, where males were more likely to participate in sport more regularly than females in Belgium, France, Greece, Latvia, Lithuania, Slovakia, Spain and the UK, whilst the opposite was true for Denmark, Finland, Sweden and the Netherlands [15]. The authors point out that historically male participation in sport has dominated over female participation, however some policy developments targeted at increasing participation in sport for females may have contributed to higher participation rates for females in some countries [15]. For instance in Belgium, available data show a greater level of male than female participation, females have closed the gap considerably since the 1970s [18]. However, with regard to the club based, organised context of sport participation, there were no gender differences detected in the Belgian study [18]. Amongst older Dutch adults, males and females were equally likely to participate in sport, or to be a sports club member, however participation in competition was more likely to occur amongst males rather than females [17].

In general, the above research provides evidence that as age increases participation in sport decreases. However, these studies are often limited to self-report sample surveys and/or to specific age ranges. Furthermore, most studies do not compare different residential locations. It is important to better understand participation in sport and how it relates to age, gender and geographical location, in order to inform evidence-based, well targeted program and policy development. The aim of this study was to use a unique, very large set of comprehensive membership registration data, effectively a census of participation, to provide age profiles of participation across seven major sports [14, 19], across the lifespan, and to compare these trends between genders and residential locations.

Methods

We investigated profiles of sport participation according to age, gender and geographical region in the Australian state of Victoria. As part of the Sport and Recreation Spatial project (www.sportandrecreationspatial.com.au) the authors of this study have initiated a large repository of sport registration data to inform evidence-based decision making across the sport sector. The seven sports incorporated in the study (Australian Football, Basketball, Cricket, Hockey, Lawn Bowls, Netball and Tennis) include six of the 10 most popular adult club-based physical activities in Australia, and five of the 10 most popular organised physical activities for children [20]. De-identified data on participant registrations were obtained from the respective state sporting associations (SSAs), the sports' state governing bodies. In this way the study was able to overcome the limitations of many studies in this area, such as the use of self-reported data, narrowly defined player population segments and failure to examine geographical variation.

Of the seven SSAs engaged in the study, five register participants for a calendar year with age determined at 1 January, and two register participants for a financial year, with age being calculated as at 1 July. The scope of this study was nominally the calendar year 2011; we included 2011 registrations for five sports and 2011–12 registrations for two sports. Ethics approval was granted by the Federation University Australia Human Research Ethics Committee.

All data were integrated and sports were analysed collectively in order to produce broadly based participation profiles while maintaining confidentiality of membership data for individual sports. An individual could engage in more than one sport and was counted separately in each sport, with the result that counts of participants are to some extent weighted by individuals' levels of participation. Because of anonymity provisions, it was not possible to identify participation of a particular individual in more than one sport, but based on an analysis of demographic characteristics and residential postcodes, the proportion of individuals who were registered in more than one sport was estimated to be around 12 % across Victoria. The methods of data integration and analysis have been reported previously [21].

Regional breakdowns were based on residential postcodes. Although postcode areas are not precisely geographically specified, the Australian Bureau of Statistics (ABS) precisely defines approximations to postcode areas entitled postal areas [22]. ABS also produces a correspondence table for assigning population-weighted proportions of postal areas to local government areas (LGAs) [23], which enabled estimated numbers of participant registrations in each LGA to be calculated. The 79 Victorian LGAs are classified as metropolitan (31 LGAs) or non-metropolitan (48 LGAs) by the Victorian state government [24].

It is important to emphasise that the age profiles reported throughout this paper are based on proportions of all participants, not on age-specific participation rates. The outcome variable, the proportion of participants in an age category, was defined as the number of registered members in that age category, expressed as a percentage of the total number of participants of all ages. This resulted in standardised profiles that could be directly compared between genders and regions. The alternative approach of expressing each number of participants as a proportion of the population in the same age category (i.e. a participation rate) would result in profiles with different scales due to different overall participation rates for the different genders and regions. Furthermore, ABS inter-censal population estimates are only published for 5-year age cohorts, whereas there is no such limitation for participant age profiles because the birthdate, and hence the exact age, of each participant is known.

Two sets of age profiles were tabulated and graphed. The first covers the whole life span, tabulated in 5-year age ranges and graphed in single-year age ranges, and the second provides a more detailed single-year picture of the 4–29 year age range. In each case, overall age profiles and separate profiles for each gender and region are presented.

Because data were collected from the whole population of members of each sport, i.e. a census rather than a sample, statistical inference was not applicable. Analyses were conducted using Excel and SPSS Version 21.

Results

The seven sports have been de-identified in all results presented. While a small proportion of participants registered in Victoria resided in other states, only those residing in Victoria were included. After consultation with SSAs, the valid age range was considered to be 4–100 years. Those for whom no birthdate were recorded ($n = 34{,}341$; 6.2 %) were excluded from the analysis, as were those whose calculated ages at the appropriate registration date were outside the valid age range ($n = 974$; 0.2 %). The remaining number of registered participants in the seven sports ranged from 13,275 to 171,304, with the total number of registered participants for 2011 being 520,102.

Overall trends

Table 1 provides age profiles of registered sport participants, and breakdowns by gender and region, within standard ABS 5-year age cohorts (plus a separate 4-year-old cohort). Most participants (64 %) were aged less than 20 years. Nearly one third of all participants were aged between 10–14 years (27.6 %), followed by the 5–9 year age group (19.9 %) and the 15–19 year age group (15.3 %). Fewer than 10 % of participants were over the age of 50 years. Given that the great majority of participants (79.1 %) in the seven sports were aged from 4–29 years more detailed age profiles are presented in Table 2.

Gender

Tables 1 and 2 and Figs. 1 and 2 show that, in terms of sport participation by gender, a higher proportion of male participants were very young (4–7 years) (13.8 %) compared to females (7.3 %); this pattern was repeated in young adulthood (18–29 years; 20.4 % and 17.5 % for males and females, respectively). A higher proportion of female participants were aged 8–17 (53.9 %) than males (45.0 %). The proportion of female participants aged

Table 1 Age profiles of registered sport participants: percentage of total sport participants

Age (years)	Participants (%)	Male (%)	Female (%)	Metropolitan (%)	Non-Metropolitan (%)
4	1.3	0.5	1.7	1.5	0.9
5–9	19.9	17.1	21.5	21.5	17.0
10–14	27.6	32.1	25.6	28.1	26.7
15–19	15.3	15.8	15.1	14.7	16.5
20–24	8.8	7.8	9.1	9.0	8.5
25–29	6.1	5.4	6.3	6.3	5.8
30–34	4.1	3.8	4.2	4.0	4.2
35–39	3.0	3.5	2.8	2.9	3.4
40–49	5.0	6.0	4.6	4.9	5.2
50–59	2.5	2.5	2.6	2.3	3.0
60–69	2.6	2.6	2.6	2.0	3.8
70+	3.6	3.0	3.9	2.8	5.1

Table 2 Age profiles of registered sport participants aged 4–29 years: percentage of total sport participants

Age (years)	Participants (%)	Male (%)	Female (%)	Metropolitan (%)	Non-Metropolitan (%)
4	1.3	1.7	0.5	1.5	0.9
5	3.0	3.8	1.4	3.3	2.5
6	3.5	4.1	2.2	3.8	2.8
7	3.8	4.2	3.2	4.2	3.2
8	4.5	4.5	4.6	4.8	4.0
9	5.0	4.8	5.6	5.3	4.5
10	5.9	5.4	6.9	6.2	5.4
11	5.9	5.4	6.9	6.1	5.5
12	5.7	5.3	6.4	5.7	5.6
13	5.3	4.9	6.2	5.3	5.3
14	4.9	4.6	5.6	4.8	5.0
15	4.2	3.9	4.8	4.0	4.5
16	3.6	3.4	4.0	3.3	4.0
17	2.8	2.8	2.9	2.6	3.2
18	2.5	2.6	2.2	2.4	2.5
19	2.3	2.4	2.0	2.3	2.2
20	2.1	2.1	1.9	2.1	2.0
21	1.9	2.0	1.7	1.9	1.9
22	1.7	1.8	1.5	1.8	1.7
23	1.6	1.7	1.4	1.7	1.5
24	1.5	1.5	1.3	1.5	1.4
25	1.4	1.5	1.3	1.5	1.3
26	1.3	1.3	1.2	1.3	1.2
27	1.2	1.2	1.1	1.2	1.1
28	1.1	1.2	1.0	1.2	1.1
29	1.0	1.1	0.9	1.1	1.0
Total % in 4–29 year age range	79.1	79.3	78.6	81.2	75.4

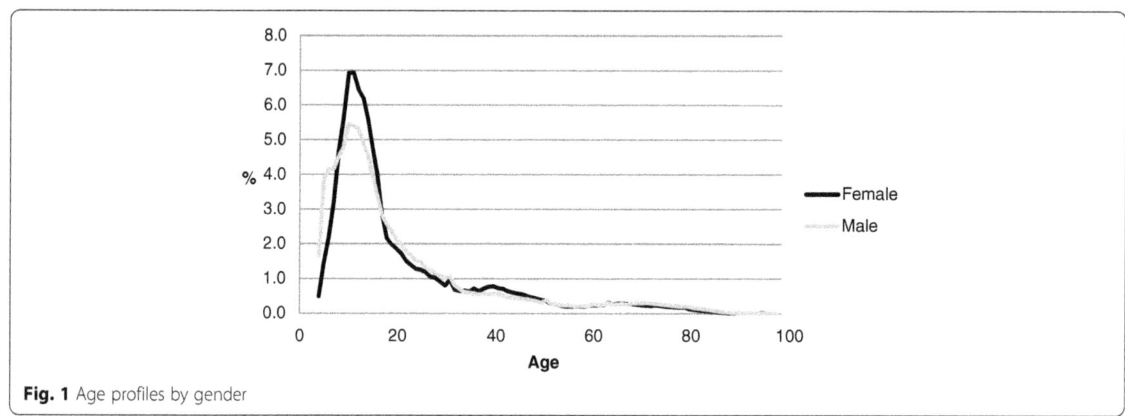

Fig. 1 Age profiles by gender

30–49 was again slightly higher compared to males. Beyond age 50, gender differences were negligible.

A deeper examination of the data revealed that the highest proportion of participants for both males and females was in the 10–11 age group (5.4 % and 6.9 % for males and females, respectively). For all age groups with a proportion of participants of 4 % or more, the males were younger (aged 6–14) than the females (aged 8–16). This represented a 9-year span for both genders. A much higher proportion of male participants were aged 4–5 (5.5 %) than was the case for females (1.9 %).

Region

Tables 1 and 2 and Figs. 3 and 4 provide details of the age profiles by geographical region. Higher proportions of metropolitan than non-metropolitan registered sport participants were engaged in the seven sports between the ages of 4–12 and ages 19–29; whereas higher proportions of non-metropolitan registered participants were engaged during adolescence (14 – 18 years) and throughout most of adulthood (30+ years).

A closer analysis of the 4–29 year age group, where around 80 % of the participation occurs, showed some key differences in age between metropolitan and non-metropolitan registered sport participants. The ages of 4–12 years represented a higher proportion of all metropolitan registered sport participants than for non-metropolitan. This difference was reversed from ages 14–18 years onward.

Discussion

This study is unique in providing population-derived age profiles of club sport participation within popular organised sports in Australia. A strength of this study is in the number of total participants (n = 520,102 member records), representing the whole population of registered participants for seven popular sports in the state of Victoria, Australia in 2011. However, it must be noted

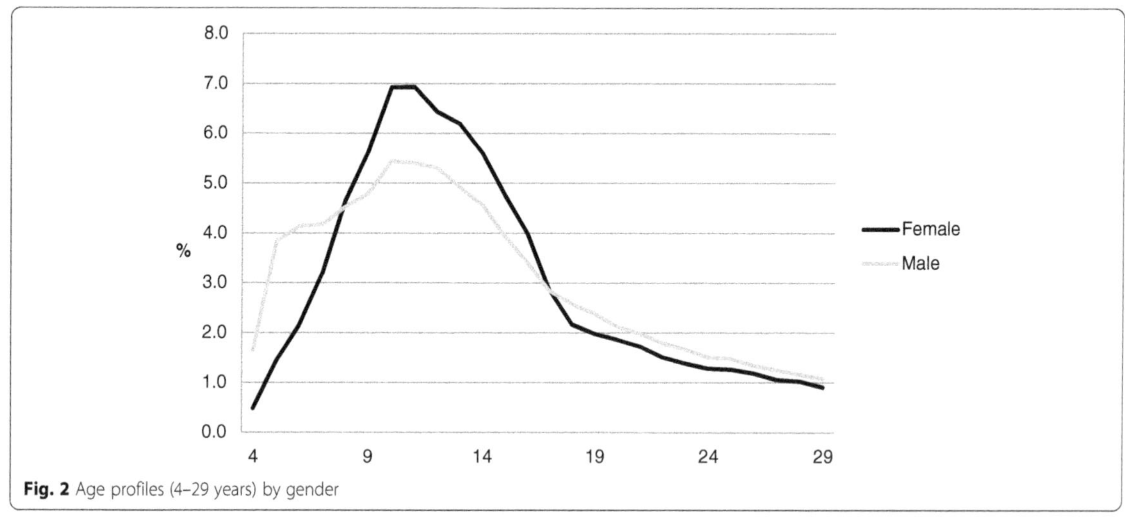

Fig. 2 Age profiles (4–29 years) by gender

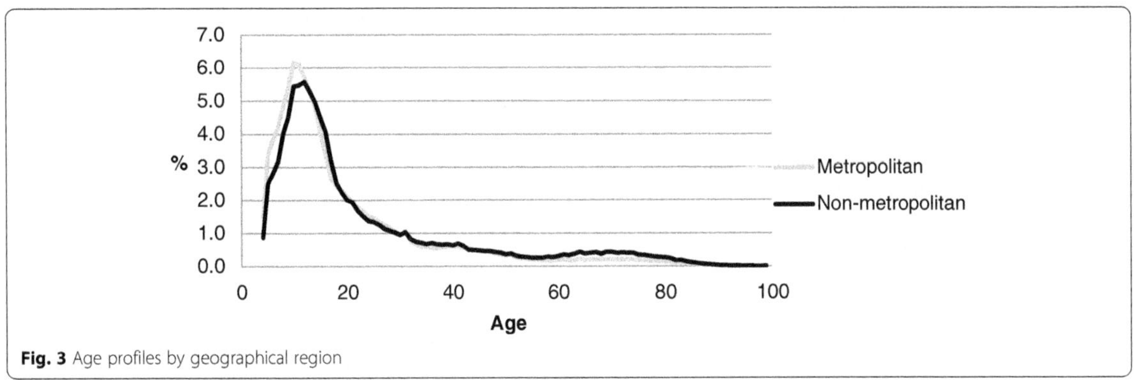

Fig. 3 Age profiles by geographical region

that this does not include all participants in these sports, such as those participating in school based programs or 'involved' participants for example those engaged in a non-physical manner such as coaches and officials [11].

Participation in club sport is clearly an activity dominated by young people. The peak representation for both males and females was 10–11 years. However, the 9-year age range across childhood for which the representation for each year of age was greater than 4 % was younger for males (6–14 years) than for females (8–16 years). Furthermore, there were considerably more males participating aged 4–5 years (6 %) than females at these ages (2 %).

Very few studies have provided age profiles of all registered participants in a sport; rather, the proportion of a study sample in sport at a given time has been reported [16, 25]. Nevertheless, other studies in Australia have reported that sports participation peaked at 12–13 years for boys and girls and fell by 50 % by age 16 [12]. In a national Australian population survey, it was reported that in the 12 months prior to the survey 60 % of all children aged 5 to 14-years participated in at least one organised sport activity outside of school hours [19]. The participation rates were 56 % for 5–8 year olds, 66 % for 9–11 and 60 % for 12–14 year olds [19]. While the present study focuses on the age profile rather than participation rates, our results are consistent with the 2012 study; both report a lower peak participation age than the 2009 study. This may be the result of a growing trend to get children engaged in organised sport at a younger age via the increasing availability of modified sports programs. However the apparent increase in younger participants in sport and especially rising numbers in 4–5 year olds raises another issue. Younger children tend to sample sports, that is they typically play several different sports, and only when older, around 13 years, do they tend to specialise and focus their attention on one sport [26]. This is also the age when they are most likely either become involved in organised competitive sport or drop out of sport altogether [27]. However, the apparent tendency towards earlier participation in modified programs, and the consequent longer period between commencement and preparedness for specialisation and competition, may lead to a greater risk

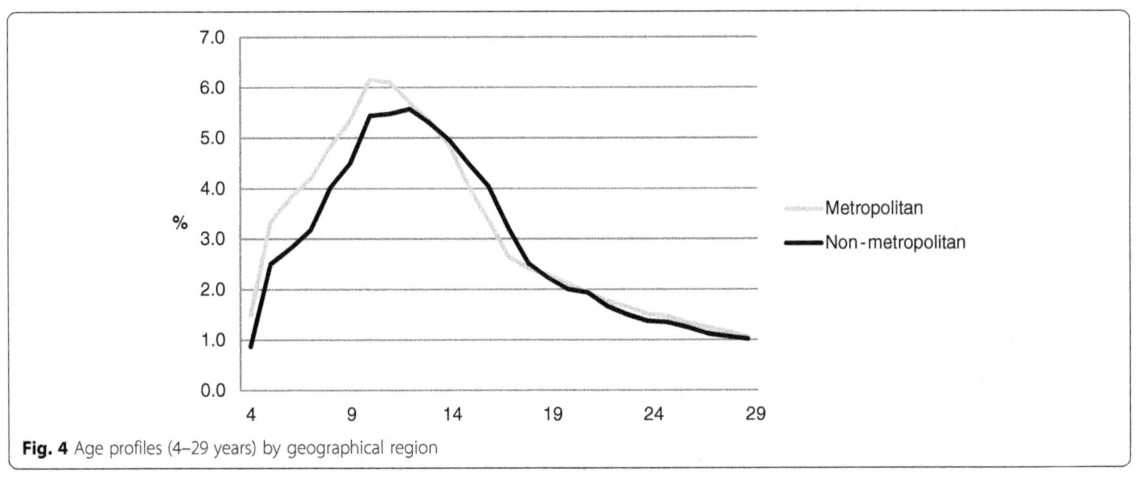

Fig. 4 Age profiles (4–29 years) by geographical region

of dropout, either through boredom with an extended period in modified programs, or because of the temptation and/or pressure to transition prematurely into standard competitive forms of sport before their capacities are adequately developed [21]. Is there a risk that the specific targeting of very young children could have a negative effect on long term sport participation and potentially on social, mental and physical health outcomes? Further research is required to investigate whether the participation of very young children leads to higher or lower uptake of (organised) competitive sport later in childhood, and any affect that this may have on their health.

The reason that a greater proportion of males participate at a younger age than females is not known, however it may relate to boys being encouraged more to participate in sport at a young age than girls. There is some evidence to suggest that in families with male and female children, fathers tend to be more involved with their sons' sport than their daughters' [28]. Furthermore, parents influence children's sport participation [29] and this is shaped by the parents' own sporting backgrounds [28]. Since adult males are more likely to participate in sport than females [2], this may be a factor in encouraging the participation of young boys more than young girls.

While the development of modified sports programs for young children provide sporting opportunities to a new, wider, consumer segment, there are fewer opportunities for adolescents or adults to participate in sport outside standard club competition. Generally, sporting opportunities for children in the 10–14 age group in Australia and other nations such as the UK and Germany are focused on standard club competitions. Our study showed that the participation peaked for both males and females at age 11, and nearly a third of participants were aged between 10–14 years. This raises the question as to whether the available sport programs/opportunities are meeting the needs of adolescents and adults. Research has shown that whilst for those aged 15 years and older participation in leisure-time physical activity significantly increased over a 10 year period, participation in organised and/or club sport remained relatively stable [2]. It is evident that there are many individuals who wish to be active in their leisure-time, and health is often a major driver, but their interest in being physically active shifts away from traditional (organised, competitive) sport [2, 30]. Participation in organised leisure-time activities (such as sport) is not as popular as non-organised activities among those aged 15 years and over, with roughly 27 % participating in organised activities compared to 53 % participating in non-organised activities at least once within a 12-month period [19]. It seems that the drop-off in sport participation during adolescence towards non-organised activities occurs at the same time when people would enter the elite sport pathway. Indeed, it has been suggested that as young people progress through early- to mid-adolescence, there are fewer and fewer opportunities to play sport for all but the most able and mature [31].

From an elite sport policy perspective, fewer individuals participating after the age of around 12 years would make the pool available for talent identification and elite pathway progression smaller. Researchers suggest that "talent identification models are likely to exclude many, especially late maturing, 'promising' children from development programmes due to the dynamic and multidimensional nature of sport talent" [32]. From a health policy perspective, fewer people active through sport may contribute to a range of negative health outcomes [33].

Fewer than ten per cent of the registered sport participants were adults aged 50 years and over. Exercise, fitness and team sports make up a greater proportion of the moderate and vigorous physical activity of young adults (16–24 years) compared to older adults (65+) [34]. A recent study found that, across both genders, there was no significant difference in the proportion of club sport participants across the ages from 15 to 75+ [2]. However for younger females aged 15–34 participation was significantly higher than all other age groups (35–54, 55–74, and 75+ age groups), which did not differ significantly from each other [2]. As an ageing society, we should consider strategies to increase participation in sport for adults and older adults. In doing so, modifications may be required in sport products and equipment. There are many health benefits of sport participation for older adults, and many participate for social reasons, and enjoy playing with family members across generations [35].

In addition to age-related differences there were some notable geographic differences. A higher proportion of metropolitan children aged 4–13 participated in sport compared to non-metropolitan. The peak metropolitan participation age was younger, at age 10–11 years, compared to non-metropolitan, which peaked at 11–12 years. This may be related to the earlier provision (and a broader range of choice) of modified sports programs in metropolitan regions. However, adults and older adults represented a higher proportion of non-metropolitan than metropolitan participants. This may relate to the central role of community sport in Australian regional communities, where sport can be considered the 'social cement' [36], contributing to local identity [37], being 'held up as gauges of the health of country communities' [38], and crucial for increasing social connections and community cohesion [39]. It has been reported that in rural and regional areas, participation in sport for adolescent girls is a socially and culturally privileged activity, whereby involvement or lack of participation in club sport positions girls on one side of the physically active/inactive binary categorisation [40]. This is sometimes related to perceived level of competency and lack of choices of activities in rural and regional areas.

Sports governing organisations generally have a strategic goal of increasing the level of participation within their sport. However, operationally their focus is often on development of the player/athlete segment of the population rather than recreational participants. Similarly, sport policy and funding in Australia, and other countries such as the UK and Canada, have been entrenched and focused on the elite level, often prioritising high performance over mass participation [41]. For example, an international analysis of government sport policies revealed that despite the existence of 'sport for all' policies emerging in a number of countries, these policies do not enjoy significant infrastructure or human resources support from governments to operationalise the policies, and in particular, do not enjoy the existence and stability of national institutes for elite sport [41]. The development of recreational pathways for sport participants therefore, requires a system-wide approach with cross-sectoral engagement of government and the sport and recreation industry if policy and organisational goals such as increasing sport participation are to be achieved. Ireland is one country that has proposed a hybrid model for participant/player development which not only maps out player/athlete development but also maps recreational pathways to ensure lifelong involvement in sport and physical activity [42]. Finland and the Netherlands also have a political and funding bias towards mass participation, and as a consequence have reported high participation rates compared to Australia, England, Canada and a number of European countries [41]. However, the definition and measurement of what constitutes sport participation varies between nations, which makes it difficult to make comparisons [41].

Redirecting sport policy and funding towards mass participation and the development of recreational pathways is one strategy to increase population levels of sport participation, and promote the health of individuals and communities. In this approach sporting organisations would need to be supported by government to monitor sport participation levels and the impact of sports programs. In another approach, the interests and needs of various population groups require consideration by governments and sporting organisations. However, it is much easier to argue changes to pathways and policies based on theory than it is to determine what are the critical process levers, community interests and stakeholders that will drive those changes. Researchers have suggested that socio-ecological models taken from physical activity research, and sport development concepts taken from sport management theory, be integrated to enhance efforts to increase sport participation [8, 9]. This is particularly important as the determinants of sport participation are often examined within the broader context of leisure-time physical activity [43]. Most studies have examined sport participation focusing on adolescents [44–46]. For instance, a Canadian study of adolescent sport participation identified the need to fit sport into the "time-challenged, gender-stereotyped, highly technologized, cyber-filled lives of today's youth" [44]. Others have found that different sports have diverse participation determinants, particularly in regard to demographic and economic variables [47]. For instance, in a German study, swimming participation was positively influenced by being young or old (U-form relationship), female, well-educated and a native of the country; whilst football (soccer) participation was positively influenced by being young, male, less-educated and having a foreign nationality [47]. Individual and unorganised physical activities such as running, fitness/gymnasium and going for a walk or hiking were associated with middle age [47]. In Australia, market segmentation studies were recently conducted to better understand the Australian community's participation in sport and physical activities for both adults (aged 14–65) and children (aged 5–13 years) [48]. Consumer segments amongst the population were characterised to identify challenges and opportunities to engage and/or re-engage individuals in sport. For example, among children segments considered as potential sport participants included 'thrifty enthusiasts' who are positive about physical activity, but may not participate in activities organised in a community club; and 'ponderers' who would like to do more sport but are unsure how to get involved [48]. The underlying motivation for many sports participants, and especially young people is to have fun and socialise [39, 49]. Key factors that affect participation in sport include: 1) sport delivery that focuses on competition rather than fun and enjoyment; 2) a lack of flexibility around traditional sport club scheduling; 3) teams organised on the basis of talent rather than friendship groups; 4) limited opportunities for those with less sports competency; and 5) self-consciousness amongst adolescents, embarrassed by their lack of sporting ability [48].

This research on the determinants of sport participation and market segmentation raises some important questions regarding the delivery of sport and recreation. For instance, we contemplate whether organised sport can be modified in ways to cater for the needs of adolescent and adults, such as smaller fields, reduced time commitment, or flexibility in player rotations. In doing so, appropriate marketing would be required, as this has been a strength of modified sports programs for children [11]. The voluntary nature of the delivery of sport also needs to be considered in planning and implementing such programs. Others have suggested that alliances with more powerful organisations, particularly in the area of health, are required before sufficient resources can be allocated to promote mass participation [41] and that further collaboration between public health and sport management is required [2, 8].

Conclusion

In conclusion, this study is the first to examine the age profile of all registered participants in a major sub-national geographical region within seven popular organised sports, across the lifespan. The majority of organised sport participation within these sports was by children aged 10–14 years, peaking at ages 10–11. The proportion of individuals engaged in these sports declined rapidly during adolescence, which may have health implications. Furthermore males and metropolitan participants were more likely to be represented in younger age categories compared to non-metropolitan participants.

Governments and sporting organisations alike have strategic and policy objectives to increase sport participation/mass participation; although these objectives are not sufficiently supported through the provision of infrastructure or resources that measure and analyse participation. A twin track approach to mass participation and elite performance may be required to achieve increases in sport participation as suggested by others [50], such as exemplified in Ireland [42]. In order to implement a twin track approach, further research is required to investigate reasons for attrition more closely especially relating to the very young participant cohorts, to inform program design and to test the efficacy of such programs for promoting an active and healthy nation.

Abbreviations

ABS: Australian Bureau of Statistics; LGA: local government areas; LTPA: leisure time physical activity; PA: physical activity; SSA: state sporting associations.

Competing interests

The authors declare that they have no competing interests.

Authors' contributions

RME, MMC contributed to the study design, interpretation of results, manuscript conceptualisation and preparation. JTH and MJC contributed to the study design, data management, statistical analysis and interpretation, manuscript conceptualisation and preparation. HW and WRP contributed to the interpretation of results and manuscript preparation. All authors have read and approved the final manuscript.

Acknowledgements

We thank the Victorian State Sporting Associations (Australian Football League, Tennis, Netball, Basketball, Cricket, Hockey and Lawn Bowls) for providing the data on which this research was based. Rochelle Eime was supported by a VicHealth Research Practice Fellowship- Physical Activity

References

1. Kumar A, Rossiter P, Olczyk A. Children's participation in organised sporting activity. In: Research Paper Cat No 1351055028. Canberra: Australian Bureau of Statistics; 2009.
2. Eime R, Sawyer N, Harvey J, Casey M, Westerbeek H, Payne W. Integrating public health and sport management: sport participation trends 2001–2010. Sport Manage Rev. 2015;18(2):207–17.
3. Eime R, Young J, Harvey J, Charity M, Payne W. A systematic review of the psychological and social benefits of participation in sport for children and adolescents: informing development of a conceptual model of health through sport. Int J Behav Nutr Phys Act. 2013;10:98.
4. Eime R, Young J, Harvey J, Charity M, Payne W. A systematic review of the psychological and social benefits of participation in sport for adults: informing development of a conceptual model of health through sport. Int J Behav Nutr Phys Act. 2013;10:135.
5. Eime R, Harvey J, Payne W. Dose–response of women's Health-Related Quality of Life (HRQoL) and life satisfaction to physical activity. J Phys Act Health. 2014;11:330–8.
6. Dohle S, Wansink B. Fit in 50 years: participation in high school sports best predicts one's physical activity after Age 70. BMC Public Health. 2013;13(1):1100.
7. Scheerder J, Thomis M, Vanreusel B, Lefevre J, Renson R, Enynde B, et al. Sports participation among females from adolescence to adulthood: a longitudinal study. Int Rev Sociol Sport. 2006;41(3):413–30.
8. Rowe K, Shilbury D, Ferkins L, Hinckson E. Sport development and physical activity promotion: an integrated model to enhance collaboration and understanding. Sport Manag Rev. 2013;16(3):364–77.
9. Henderson KA. A paradox of sport management and physical activity interventions. Sport Manag Rev. 2009;12(2):57–65.
10. Commonwealth of Australia. National sport and active recreation policy framework. In. Canberra: Commonwealth of Australia; 2011.
11. Eime R, Payne W, Harvey J. Trends in organised sport membership: Impact on sustainability. J Sci Med Sport. 2009;12(1):123–9.
12. Olds T, Dollman J, Maher C. Adolescent sport in Australia: Who, when, where and what? ACHPER Healthy Lifestyles Journal. 2009;56(1):11–6.
13. Maia JAR, Lefevre J, Claessens AL, Thomis MA, Peeters MW, Beunen GP. A growth curve to model changes in sport participation in adolescent boys. Scand J Med Sci Sports. 2010;20(4):679–85.
14. Eime R, Harvey J, Sawyer N, Craike M, Symons C, Polman R, et al. Understanding the contexts of adolescent female participation in sport and physical activity. Res Q Exerc Sport. 2013;84(2):157–66.
15. Van Tuyckom C, Scheerder J, Bracke P. Gender and age inequalities in regular sports participation: a cross-national study of 25 European countries. J Sports Sci. 2010;28(10):1077–84.
16. Palacios-Ceña D, Fernandez-de-Las-Peñas C, Hernández-Barrera V, Jiménez-Garcia R, Alonso-Blanco C, Carrasco-Garrido P. Sports participation increased in Spain: a population-based time trend study of 21 381 adults in the years 2000, 2005 and 2010. Br J Sports Med. 2012;46(16):1137–9.
17. Cozijnsen R, Stevens N, Van Tilburg TG. The trend in sport participation among Dutch retirees, 1983–2007. Ageing Soc. 2013;33(04):698–719.
18. Scheerder J, Vanreusel B, Taks M. Stratification patterns of active sport involvement among adults: social change and persistence. Int Rev Sociol Sport. 2005;40(2):139–62.
19. Sports and physical recreation: A statistical overview, Australia 2012 [http://www.abs.gov.au/ausstats/abs@.nsf/Latestproducts/4156.0Main%20Features12012?opendocument&tabname=Summary&prodno=4156.0&issue=2012&num=&view=].
20. Standing Committee on Recreation and Sport: Participation in exercise, recreation and sport. In. Canberra: Australian Sports Commission; 2010.
21. Eime R, Casey M, Harvey J, Charity M, Young J, Payne W. Participation in modified sports programs: a longitudinal study of children's transition to club sport competition. BMC Public Health. 2015;15:649.
22. Australian Bureau of Statistics. Australian Statistical Geography Standard (ASGS): Volume 3- Non ABS Structures, Cat.No.1270.0.55.003. In. vol. Catalogue number 1270.0.55.003. Canberra: Australian Bureau of Statistics; 2011.
23. Australian Bureau of Statistics. ABS Postal Area Concordances, Cat.No.1270.0.55.006. In., vol. Catalogue number 1270.0.55.006. Canberra: Australian Bureau of Statistics; 2011.
24. Local Government Areas in Metropolitan Melbourne [http://www.liveinvictoria.vic.gov.au/living-in-victoria/melbourne-and-regional-victoria/melbourne#.VNBGp00cTiw].

25. Stamatakis E, Chaudhury M. Temporal trends in adults' sports participation patterns in England between 1997 and 2006: the Health Survey for England. Br J Sports Med. 2008;42(11):901–8.
26. Cote J, Vierimaa M. The developmental model of sport particiation: 15 years after its first conceptualization. Rev Sci Sports. 2014;29:S63–9.
27. Côté J, Hay J. Children's involvement in sport: A developmental perspective. In: Silva JM, Stevens DE, editors. Psychological foundations of sport. 2nd ed. Boston, MA: Allyn & Bacon; 2002. p. 503–19.
28. Wheeler S. The significance of family culture for sports participation. Int Rev Sociol Sport. 2012;47(2):235–52.
29. Eime R, Harvey J, Craike M, Symons C, Payne W. Family support and ease of access link socio-economic status and sports club membership in adolescent girls: a mediation study. Int J Behav Nutr Phys Act. 2013;10:50.
30. Hajkowicz S, Cook H, Wilhelmseder L, Boughen N. The future of Australian sport: Megatrends shaping the sports sector over coming decades. In.: CSIRO; 2013.
31. Kirk D. Physical education, youth sport and lifelong participation: the importance of early learning experiences. Eur Phys Educ Rev. 2005;11(3):239–55.
32. Vaeyens R, Lenoir M, Williams AM, Philippaerts RM. Talent identification and development programmes in sport: current models and future directions. Sports Med. 2008;38(9):703.
33. Eime R, Harvey J, Charity M, Casey M. Physical activity, sport and health in the City of Brimbank: A report to Mitchell Institute for Health and Education Policy. In.: Federation University, Victoria University; 2014.
34. Bélanger M, Townsend N, Foster C. Age-related differences in physical activity profiles of English adults. Prev Med. 2011;52(3–4):247–9.
35. van Uffelen J, Jenkin CW, HW, Biddle S, Eime R. Active and healthy ageing through sport. Report prepared for the Australian Sports Commission. Melbourne: Victoria University; 2015.
36. Mugford S. The status of sport in rural and regional Australia: Literature, research and policy options. In.: Qualitative and Quantitative Social Research, Adelaide, Australia; 2001.
37. Tonts M. Competitive sport and social capital in rural Australia. J Rural Stud. 2005;21:137–49.
38. Gard M. Sport, physical education and country towns: diverse enough? Educ Rural Aust. 2001;11:19–26.
39. Eime R, Payne W, Casey M, Harvey J. Transition in participation in sport and unstructured physical activity for rural living adolescent girls. Health Educ Res. 2010;25(2):282–93.
40. Mooney A, Casey M, Smyth J. "You're no-one if you're not a netball girl": rural and regional living adolescent girls' negotiation of physically active identities. Ann Leis Res. 2012;15:19–37.
41. Nicholson M, Hoye R, Houlihan B. Participation in Sport: International Policy Perspective. London: Routledge; 2010.
42. Macphail A, Kirk D. Young people's socialisation into sport: experiencing the specialising phase. Leis Stud. 2006;25(1):57–74.
43. Craggs C, Corder K, van Sluijs EMF, Griffin SJ. Determinants of change in physical activity in children and adolescents: a systematic review. Am J Prev Med. 2011;40(6):645–58.
44. Berger IE, O'Reilly N, Parent MM, Séguin B, Hernandez T. Determinants of sport participation among Canadian adolescents. Sport Manag Rev. 2008;11(3):277–307.
45. Cox L, Coleman L, Roker D. Determinants of sports and physical activity participation amongst 15–19 year-old young women in England - Final report on research commissioned by Sport England. In.: Trust for the Study of Adolescence (TSA); 2005.
46. Taggart A, Sharp S. Adolescents and sport: determinants of current and future participation In. Perth: Sport and Physical Activity Research Centre, Edith Cowan University; 1997.
47. Breuer C, Hallmann K, Wicker P. Determinants of sport participation in different sports. Manag Leis. 2011;16(4):269–86.
48. Australian Sports Commission. Market segmentation for sport participation-adults. In., vol. March. Canberra: Australian Sports Commission; 2013.
49. Casey M, Eime R, Payne W, Harvey J. Using a socioecological approach to examine participation in sport and physical activity among rural adolescent girls. Qual Health Res. 2009;19(7):881–93.
50. Collins D, Bailey R, Ford PA, MacNamara Á, Toms M, Pearce G. Three worlds: new directions in participant development in sport and physical activity. Sport Educ Soc. 2011;17(2):225–43.

18

Pre-pubertal males practising Taekwondo exhibit favourable postural and neuromuscular performance

Mohamed Chedly Jlid[1], Nicola Maffulli[2,3*], Nisar Souissi[4], Mohamed Souheil Chelly[1] and Thierry Paillard[5]

Abstract

Background: The postural and neuromuscular performances in healthy children taekwondo (TKD) practitioners in comparison with control children were examined.

Methods: Seventeen healthy pre-pubertal males undertaking only physical education at school (age: 11.88 ± 0.33 years) and 12 pre-pubertal male TKD practitioners (>3 years, 4 sessions a week) (age 11.66 ± 0.49 years) were recruited. Performances in the dynamic postural control (Star Excursion Balance Test -SEBT), vertical jump [squat jump (SJ) and countermovement jump (CMJ)] and sprint running (distances: 5, 10, 20 and 30 m) tests were compared between the two groups.

Results: The performances of the TKD practitioners were better than those of the non-TKD active for the SEBT (for 14 of 16 conditions, $p < 0.05$), SJ ($p < 0.01$), CMJ ($p < 0.03$) sprint running (5 m, $p < 0.01$; 10 m, $p < 0.04$; the performances for the 20 and 30 m sprints were not significant, $p > 0.05$).

Conclusions: TKD practice would stimulate sensory input and motor output of the postural system that would enhance its efficiency. In addition, the dynamic nature of TKD would develop the muscle power of the lower limbs. In our sample of healthy pre-pubertal males, TKD appears to improve postural and neuromuscular functions, but further research is required.

Keywords: Taekwondo, Postural control, Sprint running, Vertical jump, Pre-pubertal male

Background

Motor experiences facilitate the maturation of the central nervous system in children, refining their postural and motor skills [1]. Moreover, certain physical and/or sport activities stimulate the postural and motor functions more than others. To improve these functions in an optimal way, physical and/or sport activity requires be completed by trying to react very quickly to a signal, to develop a muscle power or strength, to perform fast and well-coordinated motors skill and/or to perform technique movements in difficult postural conditions e.g. on monopodal dynamic stance.

Taekwondo (TKD) stimulates these motor abilities [2]. TKD focuses on kicking techniques. Rotation of the body and pivoting on one leg is an essential component in all of these kicking skills [3]. Elite TKD athletes turn and kick at high speeds (5.2 m/s to 16.26 m/s), and produce high striking forces (390.7 to 661.9 N) without losing balance [4]. The ability to perform fast and well-coordinated attack and defense actions are determining factors in TKD performance. To complete fast and powerful kicks, TKD practitioners require high muscle power and speed for kicking, and great dynamic postural control on the supporting leg. Therefore, the neuromuscular and postural abilities are determining factors for the athletes' performance in competitions.

TKD training can improve knee and calf muscle strength in athletes at different levels of training [5–7]. Heller et al. [6] reported that the leg muscle powers are above normal in elite TKD athletes. Elite semiprofessional

* Correspondence: n.maffulli@qmul.ac.uk
[2]Department of Musculoskeletal Disorders, Faculty of Medicine and Surgery, University of Salerno, 84081 Baronissi, Salerno, Italy
[3]Centre for Sports and Exercise Medicine, Mile End Hospital, Barts and The London School of Medicine and Dentistry, London, UK
Full list of author information is available at the end of the article

TKD athletes also demonstrate greater knee muscle strength than TKD novices. Recreational athletes may also benefit from TKD training in terms of neuromuscular qualities [8].

Few studies have addressed the effect of TKD training on postural control performance [9–13]. Noorul et al. [8] showed that, even with low-level TKD training (less than 4 h per week), recreational TKD practitioners had better balance performance than their sedentary counterparts when standing with their eyes closed after dropping from a height. TKD practitioners might even develop sport-specific balance ability [9, 14]. Seventeen weeks of TKD training could improve the balance time in single leg stance in elderly subjects [12]. Similarly, TKD training produced positive effects on balance and mobility in older adults, as indicated by the improvement in functional reach distance, Timed Up-and-Go test, walking velocity, and gait stability [11].

These two studies consistently showed that older adults could benefit from TKD training in terms of various balance components. To date, few studies have investigated the effects of TKD training in young healthy adolescents [9, 10, 14]. A study has shown that adolescents undertaking TKD training may have better balance performance than untrained subjects [9].

However, the effects of TKD training on the postural and neuromuscular functions were separately studied in healthy adults and adolescents, which does not allow the establishing of global effects of their functional abilities relative to posture and movement. In addition, these effects were not studied in healthy pre-pubertal children. Yet, with the increasing popularity of this sport and as many practitioners start training at a very young age [15], there is a need to examine the effect of TKD to ascertain whether TKD induces improvements in postural and neuromuscular functions in pre-pubertal healthy children. Hence, the aim of this study is to examine the postural and neuromuscular performances in healthy pre-pubertal male TKD practitioners in comparison to control males. It was hypothesized that the postural and neuromuscular performances of healthy pre-pubertal male TKD practitioners would perform significantly better in these tests than their non-TKD practicing counterpart.

Methods

All the procedures described in the present investigations were approved by the Ethics Committee of the University of Manouba, Tunisia.

Signed written consent to publish was obtained from the children's parent or legal guardian.

Participants

Our population consisted of 17 pre-pubertal healthy males (age: 11.88 ± 0.33 years) taking only part in physical education lessons at school, for at least 3 years (non sport children), and 12 pre-pubertal healthy male TKD practitioners (age 11.66 ± 0.49 years) who had practiced TKD for 3.33 ± 0.49 years for four sessions a week (1 h30 per session). All the subjects were at Tanner's stage 1 of puberty [16], with no differences in anthropometric characteristics between the 2 groups (Table 1). None of the subjects reported a history of hip, knee or ankle injury, or reported known pathological condition of the lower limb. All practitioners were right leg dominant, as ascertained by asking them which leg they preferred to kick a football with. All procedures were approved by Manouba University Institutional Review Committee. Written informed consent was obtained from all participants and their guiardian/parent after they had received both verbal and a written explanations of the experimental protocol and its potential risks and benefits. All participants and their parents were assured that they could withdraw from the trial without penalty at any time.

Procedures

The experiment consisted in examining the anthropometric characteristics and the postural and neuromuscular (vertical jumps and sprint running) abilities for the two groups of subjects. Postural tests, vertical jump, sprint run tests, were administered over three different days, with one day of recovery between each day (i.e. between the postural control test, the vertical jump tests, and the sprint test) to avoid possible fatigue effects. All the tests were completed between 3 and 6 pm.

Measures

Height and body mass

Subject's height was measured (in cm) using a graduated and non-deformable measuring rod and their weight [body mass (BM) in kg] was evaluated using the EKS apparatus (Focus 9800, Sweden), without clothes and barefoot.

Leg length

Leg length of both legs were measured (in cm) with the subjects lying supine on an examination couch using a standard tape measurer from the anterior superior iliac spine to the distal end of the medial malleolus [17].

Table 1 Comparison of anthropometric measures (means ± standard deviations) between the non-athletic children and the taekwondo practitioners children. The significance level was set at *P* <0.05 (NS = non significant)

	Non sport children	TKD practitioners children	*P*
Height (cm)	148.31 ± 3.93	145.42 ± 3.75	NS
Leg length (cm)	79.83 ± 3.54	82.29 ± 3.180	NS
Body mass (kg)	42.52 ± 11.10	36.93 ± 5.11	NS

Dynamic Postural Control (DPC) test

The Star Excursion Balance Test (SEBT) measured DPC. This functional, unilateral balance test integrates a single-leg stance with maximum reach of the opposite leg [18] The SEBT was performed with the subjects standing in the middle of a grid placed on the floor with 8 lines extending at 45° increments from the center of the grid. The 8 lines on the grid were named in relation to the direction of reach with regard to the stance leg: Anterolateral (AL), Anterior (A), Anteromedial (AM), Medial (M), posteromedial (PM), Posterior (P), Posterolateral (PL), and Lateral (L) (Fig. 1).

The protocol by Hertel et al. [18] was followed and the reach distances were normalized by dividing each excursion distance (in cm) by the subject's leg length (in cm) and then multiplying the value obtained by 100.

Vertical jump tests

After a 10 min warm up (including progressive running exercises and stretching exercises), jumping height was assessed using an infrared photocell mat connected to a digital computer (Optojump System, Microgate SARL, Bolzano, Italy) by the same investigator. The optical acquisition system allowed the measurement of the contact time (t_c) and the flight time (t_f) during a jump, and calculated the height of the jump (h) to a precision of 1/1000s [19]. The height is measured using the equation as follows: h(cm) = g (t_f) 2/8 (g : gravity).

For the squat jump (SJ) tests, the subjects started in the semi squat position with a knee flexion angle of nearly 90° and without moving, and the subjects had their hands placed on their hips. At the signal, the subject pushed off.

Countermovement jump (CMJ) tests started from an upright standing position with the subjects' hands on their hips. At the signal, the subjects made a downward movement until reaching an approximate knee angle of 90°, and subsequently began to push-off. All subjects performed familiarization trials before undertaking three consecutive experimental trials for the two tests (SJ and CMJ). The highest value for each jump (test) was retained. Every subject was given a 15-s interval between attempts.

Sprint run (30 m)

After a 15 min warm-up, the subject ran at his maximum speed a distance of 30 m from a standing start. Photoelectric cells (radio system, Microgate, Bolzano, Italy) were placed at 5, 10, 20 and 30 m. Each subject took the test three times with an interval of 5 min of recovery after each test. The best value (in s) for each distance was used for statistical analyses.

Analysis

Statistical analyses were performed using SPSS for Windows software (version 17.0). The descriptive values are presented as mean and standard deviation. The reproducibility of measurements of DPC, SJ, CMJ and 30 m sprint were determined by calculating the interclass coefficient of correlation (ICC). The estimation of this coefficient was based on a process of analysis of variance (ANOVA): an ICC from 0.80 to 1.00 is considered very reproducible, 0.60 to 0.79 moderately reproducible, and less than 0.60 representing a questionable reproducibility. Before using parametric statistics, it was checked the normality of the test variables Shapiro-Wilk W. The independent *t* Test was used to detect any differences between two groups. Cohen's effect sizes were also calculated using GPOWER software (Bonn FRG, Bonn University, Department of Psychology) [20]. The results were interpreted using the following criteria: 0.20 [small]; 0.50 [medium]; 0.80 [large] [21]. Significance level was set at $p < 0.05$.

Results

The interclass correlation coefficients on the reproducibility (ICCs) showed an excellent reliability for the DPC test concerning the right and the left supporting legs and for the SJ, CMJ and sprint tests (Table 2).

Most of the results on postural data were significantly different between the non-athletic practitioners and the

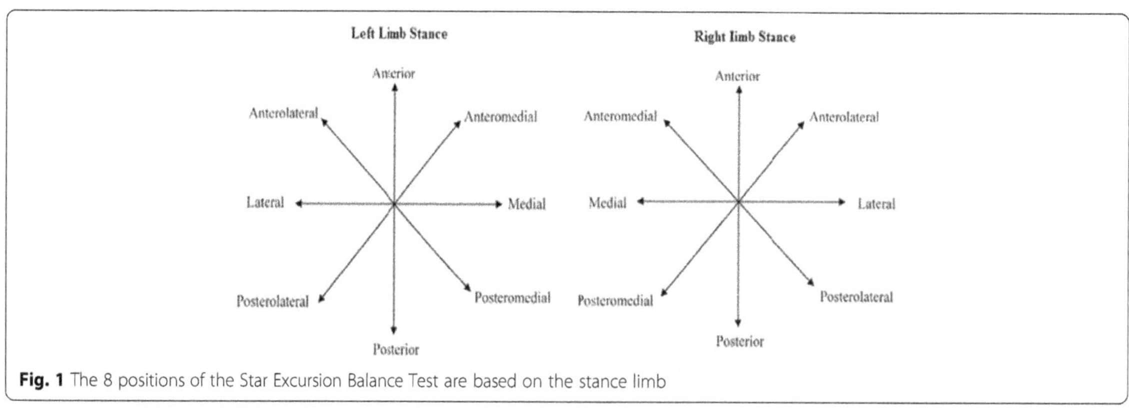

Fig. 1 The 8 positions of the Star Excursion Balance Test are based on the stance limb

Table 2 The coefficient of intraclass correlation on the reproducibility of vertical jumps, speed run and dynamic postural control tests

			ICC	95 % IC
Vertical jumps (cm)	SJ		0.952	0.981–0.983
	CMJ		0.961	0.911–0.985
Speed run (s)	5 m		0.883	0.624–0.934
	10 m		0.929	0.841–0.972
	20 m		0.964	0.919–0.986
	30 m		0.967	0.926–0.987
Dynamic postural control (cm)	Anterolateral	Right	0.994	0.988–0.997
		Left	0.997	0.994–0.998
	Anterior	Right	0.996	0.993–0.998
		Left	0.990	0.982–0.995
	Anteromedial	Right	0.993	0.988–0.997
		Left	0.995	0.991–0.997
	Medial	Right	0.997	0.995–0.999
		Left	0.998	0.996–0.999
	Posteromedial	Right	0.995	0.991–0.998
		Left	0.997	0.994–0.998
	Posterior	Right	0.997	0.994–0.998
		Left	0.996	0.992–0.998
	Posterolateral	Right	0.997	0.994–0.998
		Left	0.997	0.995–0.999
	Lateral	Right	0.997	0.994–0.998
		Left	0.993	0.987–0.996

ICC interclass correlation coefficients, *CI* Confidence interval

TKD practitioners. Fourteen of 16 measures were significantly different between the two groups (Table 3).

The performances in vertical jumps (SJ and CMJ) were significantly different between the non-athletic practitioners and the TKD practitioners (Table 3).

The sprint performances differed between the two groups only for the very short distances (5 and 10 m). The performances for the other distances (20 and 30 m) did not differ between the non-sport and TKD practitioners (Table 3).

All the raw data are available in Additional files 1, 2, 3, and 4 enclosed.

Discussion

The present investigation showed that the performances in dynamic postural control, vertical jumps (SJ and CMJ) and very short sprint (5 and 10 m) were significantly better for the TKD practitioners than for the non-athletic males.

The fact that the performance in the DPC test was better for the TKD practitioners than for the non-athletic children is not surprising. First, in general, regular sport practice improves the postural system output [22] by refining its sensory and motor functions as well as its central integration of sensory information [23–26]. Moreover, in children, motor experience facilitates the building of a repertoire of postural strategies and enables the child to select the most appropriate postural strategy, depending on the ability to anticipate the consequence of the movement to maintain balance control and optimal efficiency of the motor task [1]. The DPC test aims to reach the maximal distance with the opposite leg while on monopodal stance. The movements involved by this test are destabilizing, and require anticipation of the consequence of movement. This could mean that TKD practice can favorably influence the ability to anticipate the consequence of the movement in children.

Previous studies have shown that TKD practice improves postural control in adolescents, adults, older subjects [9, 10, 27] and in children with a variety of pathologies [5]. However, no study has shown that TKD can enhance postural abilities in healthy children. Obviously, TKD requires dynamic stability on the supporting leg (e.g. rotation of the body and pivoting on one leg) to perform fast, ballistic movements by the kicking leg aimed to hit the opponent [14]. To maintain balance in this context, the TKD practitioner children strongly stimulate their different sensory receptors, particularly proprioceptive, vestibular, visual and cutaneous receptors. Repetitive and regular stimulations of these receptors related to TKD practice would refine their sensitivity. This would explain why young TKD practitioners exhibited more efficient somatosensory and vestibular inputs than untrained children [9, 10, 27]. In addition, learning of technique movements during the practice of combat sports can influence postural adaptation by motor program acquisitions that include specific postural adaptations [28]. As the postural task of DPC (i.e. moving one leg by supporting the body on the other leg) is relatively close to that observed for kicking techniques in TKD (i.e. performing a kicking technique while supporting on one leg ony), one could hypothesize that specific postural adaptations could occur in healthy children. The motor function of the postural system involving movement control and command could benefit specific postural adaptations. Fong et al.' study [29] reinforces this hypothesis, since it reported that TKD practitioners seem to exhibit sport-specific balance ability. These authors demonstrated that adolescent TKD practitioners required less time to complete a 180°-turn and swayed less during turning than non-practitioners. This hypothesis can be also corroborated through neurophysiological considerations since Chung and Ng [30] showed that professional TKD practitioners have better neuromotor ability than non-athletes in both large and small muscles, with faster reactions to sport-specific stimuli, suggesting a generalized motor experience effect across various muscles.

Table 3 Comparison of values (means ± standard deviations) and effect size of vertical jumps, speed run and dynamic postural control between the non sport children and the TKD practitioners children. The significance level was set at $P < 0.05$ (NS = non significant)

			Non sport children	TKD practitioners children	Effect size	P
Vertical jumps (cm)	SJ		18.85 ± 4.00	24.30 ± 4.85	1.22 [large]	0.003
	CMJ		19.54 ± 4.23	23.53 ± 5.44	0.81 [large]	0.035
Speed run (s)	5 m		1.30 ± 0.10	1.54 ± 0.33	0.98 [large]	0.008
	10 m		2.23 ± 0.16	2.43 ± 0.30	0.83 [large]	0.038
	20 m		3.98 ± 0.30	4.06 ± 0.31	0.26 [medium]	NS
	30 m		5.72 ± 0.41	5.74 ± 0.38	0.05 [small]	NS
Dynamic postural control (cm)	Anterolateral	Right	78.4 ± 10.8	83.5 ± 6.6	0.56 [large]	NS
		Left	77.2 ± 10.6	93.8 ± 7.5	1.80 [large]	0.000
	Anterior	Right	79.4 ± 9.4	83.9 ± 1.01	0.67 [large]	NS
		Left	79.6 ± 8.7	86.1 ± 5.4	0.59 [large]	0.031
	Anteromedial	Right	83.5 ± 1.08	91.5 ± 8.4	1.33 [large]	0.042
		Left	82.8 ± 8.9	94.0 ± 7.6	1.35 [large]	0.002
	Medial	Right	80.7 ± 11.4	93.1 ± 9.8	1.16 [large]	0.005
		Left	80.04 ± 10.0	96,3 ± 9,5	1.67 [large]	0.000
	Posteromedial	Right	85.1 ± 1.48	95.9 ± 9.2	1.63 [large]	0.034
		Left	81.7 ± 9.2	92.1 ± 6.9	1.27 [large]	0.003
	Posterior	Right	73.2 ± 14.7	94.4 ± 9.01	1.73 [large]	0.000
		Left	74.9 ± 12.8	94.1 ± 7.6	1.82 [large]	0.000
	Posterolateral	Right	69.1 ± 1.04	87.1 ± 1.1	1.68 [large]	0.000
		Left	71.9 ± 1.1	94.2 ± 7.8	4.00 [large]	0.000
	Lateral	Right	61.2 ± 12.3	79.4 ± 9.9	1.63 [large]	0.000
		Left	65.66 ± 10.3	93.5 ± 7.4	3.10 [large]	0.000

In addition, better neuromotor ability could explain why the postural performances for both dominant and non-dominant supporting legs were better for the TKD practitioners than for the non-sporting children. However, two of 16 postural conditions were non significant for the dominant supporting leg while all the conditions were significant for the non-dominant leg. The specific postural adaptations would be thus more marked for the non-dominant supporting leg than for the dominant supporting leg. This phenomenon would be linked to the fact that kicking techniques are more frequently performed on the non-dominant supporting leg than on the dominant supporting leg in TKD practitioners. Hence, the solicitation time was longer on the non-supporting leg than on the dominant leg and thus would induce further postural adaptations.

TKD practitioners exhibited better performance in vertical jump with or without downward movement (SJ and CMJ). This may mean that the muscle power and myotendineous elasticity were greater for the young TKD practitioners than for the age matched non-athletic children [31]. Power is the product of force by velocity: our results represent either a greater force or a greater speed, or both, in favour of the TKD practitioners. Thus, TKD practice could induce either an improvement of muscle strength through better spatial and temporal recruitment of motor units, or an improvement in the speed of muscle action through better synchronisation of motor units firing during the vertical jump test [32]. As the anthropometric characteristics of the young TKD practitioners did not differ from those of the non-athletic children, they were unlikely to influence the performance in vertical jump. Hence, the best performance in vertical jump for the practitioners TKD children would be related to better intrinsic qualities of the neuromuscular function. Indeed, improvements in neuromuscular performance can be observed with or without increase in muscle mass [33]. Moreover, multiple and repetitive skipping and jumps during TKD practice would stimulate the myotendineous structures of the lower limb, and would thus enhance the myotendineous elasticity in healthy children.

The fact that TKD children had greater muscle power than the non-athletic children could explain why they were better in short sprint run (5 and 10 m) i.e. for distances whose power abilities are determining in terms of performance [34]. The children practicing TKD were not faster than the non-athletic children over 20 and 30 m. This is not surprising, as specificity of sport would suggest that, as TKD is based on extremely fast accelerations over very short distances, the experience effect in TKD would manifest itself only over the shorter sprint distances [34]. To analyze more precisely the locomotor effects induced by the TKD practice, future studies could use gait analysis to investigate the biomechanics of sprint running in relation to stride length and stride rate over the different distances considered.

This study presents limitations: for example, it did not evaluate the effects of TKD training but only compared the postural and neuromuscular performances between healthy pre-pubertal males TKD practitioners and healthy non-athletic males of the same age. The study did show that young male TKD practitioners were more performant than the non-practitioner children, but only a longitudinal study would determine whether TKD training improves performance in these performance variables.

Conclusions

The performances in postural control, vertical jumps and very short sprint running were significantly better in healthy pre-pubertal males TKD practitioners than for non-athletic males of the same age. TKD practice would stimulate sensory input and motor output of the postural system, which would improve its efficiency particularly in specific postural conditions, i.e. on one leg support. In addition, the dynamic nature of TKD could develop the power of the muscles of the lower limb. TKD training is likely to facilitate postural and neuromuscular functions in healthy children.

Additional files

Additional file 1: Vertical Jump NO SPORTS. (DOC 46 kb)
Additional file 2: Dynamic Postural Control NO SPORTS. (DOC 116 kb)
Additional file 3: Dynamic Postural Control (TKD). (DOC 87 kb)
Additional file 4: SPEED NO SPORTS. (DOC 47 kb)

Abbreviations

A: anterior; AL: anterolateral; AM: anteromedial; BM: body mass; CMJ: countermovement jump; DPC: dynamic postural control; L: lateral; M: medial; P: posterior; PL: posterolateral; PM: posteromedial; SEBT: Star Excursion Balance Test; SJ: squat jump; TKD: Taekwondo

Acknowledgements

The authors would like to thank the "Ministère de l'enseignement supérieur et de la Recherche Scientifique, Tunisia" for financial support.

Funding

The present investigation was partially funded by the Ministère de l'enseignement supérieur et de la Recherche Scientifique, Tunisia.

Authors' contribution

MCJ, NS and MSC conceived the study and performed the measurements. They analysed the results. MCJ wrote the first draft of the manuscript. NM and TP supervised the work, and helped in the interpretation of the results. They supervised the writing of the manuscript. All the authors read and approved the final version of the manuscript.

Authors' information

Mohamed Chedly Jlid, PhD; Assistant Professor of Sport Science, University of Manouba.
Nicola Maffulli, PhD, MD; Professor, Department of Musculoskeletal Disorders, Faculty of Medicine and Surgery, University of Salerno, 84081 Baronissi, Salerno, Italy.
Centre for Sports and Exercise Medicine, Mile End Hospital, Barts and The London School of Medicine and Dentistry, London, UK.
Nisar Souissi, PhD; Professor of sports science, University of Manouba.
Mohamed Souheil Chelly, PhD, Associate Professor of sports science, University of Manouba.
Thierry Paillard, PhD; Professor of Sport Science, Movement, Balance, Performance and Health Laboratory, University of Pau and Pays de l'Adour.

Competing interests

The authors declare that they have no competing interests.

Author details

[1]Research Unit of Sport Performance and Health, Higher Institute of Sport and Physical Education of Ksar Said, Tunis, Tunisia. [2]Department of Musculoskeletal Disorders, Faculty of Medicine and Surgery, University of Salerno, 84081 Baronissi, Salerno, Italy. [3]Centre for Sports and Exercise Medicine, Mile End Hospital, Barts and The London School of Medicine and Dentistry, London, UK. [4]Unité de Recherche Evaluation, Sport, Santé, Centre National de Médecine et Science en Sport, Tunis, Tunisie. [5]Laboratoire Activité Physique, Performance et Santé (EA 4445), Université de Pau et des Pays de l'Adour, Département STAPS, ZA Bastillac Sud, 65000 Tarbes, France.

References

1. Assaiante C. Development of locomotor balance control in healthy children. Neurosci Biobehav Rev. 1998;22:527–32.
2. Bridge CA, Ferreira da Silva Santos J, Chaabène H, Pieter W, Franchini E. Physical and physiological profiles of taekwondo athletes. Sports Med. 2014;44:713–33.
3. Toskovic NN, Blessing D, Williford HN. Physiologic profile of recreational male and female novice and experienced Tae Kwon Do practitioners. J Sports Med Phys Fitness. 2004;44:164–72.
4. Pieter F, Pieter W. Speed and force in selected Taekwondo techniques. Biol Sport. 1995;12:257–66.
5. Fong SM, Tsang WW, Ng GY. Taekwondo training improves sensory organization and balancecontrol in children with developmental coordination disorder: a randomized controlled trial. Res Dev Disabil. 2012;33:85–955.
6. Heller J, Peric T, Dlouha R, Kohlikova E, Melichna J, Novakova H. Physiological profiles of male and female taekwon-do (ITF) black belts. J Sports Sci. 1998;16:243–9.
7. Pieter W, Taaffe D, Troxel R, Heijmans J. Isokinetic peak torque of the quadriceps and hamstrings of college age Taekwondo athletes. J Hum Mov Stud. 1989;16:17–25.
8. Noorul HR, Pieter W, Erie ZZ. Physical fitness of recreational adolescent Taekwondo athletes. Brazil J Biomotricity. 2008;2:230–40.
9. Fong SM, Ng GY. Sensory integration and standing balance in adolescent taekwondo practitioners. Pediatr Exerc Sci. 2012;24:142–51.
10. Leong HT, Fu SN, Ng GY, Tsang WW. Low-level Taekwondo practitioners have better somatosensory organisation in standing balance than sedentary people. Eur J Appl Physiol. 2011;111:1787–93.
11. Cromwell RL, Meyers PM, Meyers PE, Newton RA. Taekwondo: an effective exercise for improving balance and walking ability in older adults. J Gerontol A Biol Sci Med Sci. 2007;62:641–6.
12. Brudnak MA, Dundero D, Van Hecke FM. Are the 'hard' martial arts, such as the Korean martial art, Taekwon-Do, of benefit to senior citizens? Med Hypotheses. 2002;59:485–91.
13. Fong SS, Ng SS. Can Taekwondo footwear affect postural stability in young adults? J Am Podiatr Med Assoc. 2013;103:291–6.
14. Negahban H, Aryan N, Mazaheri M, Norasteh AA, Sanjari MA. Effect of expertise in shooting and Taekwondo on bipedal and unipedal postural

control isolated or concurrent with a reaction-time task. Gait Posture. 2012, Epub ahead of print (doi:10.1016)
15. Kordi R, Maffulli N, Wroble RR, Wallace WA. Combat sports medicine. London, IL: Springer Science; 2009. p. 1–359.
16. Tanner JM. Growth at adolescence, 2nd Edition. Oxford: Blackwell Scientific Publications, IL; 1962. p. 1–236.
17. Alyson F, Robyn B, Mark VP, Gregory DM, Timothy EH. Neuromuscular training improves performance on the star excursion balance test in young female athletes. J Orthop Sports Phys Ther. 2010;9:551–7.
18. Hertel J, Miller JS, Denegar CR. Intratester and intertester reliability during the Star Excursion Balance Tests. J Sport Rehabil. 2000;9:104–16.
19. Lehance C, Croisier JL, Bury T. Optojump system efficiency in the assessment of lower limbs explosive strength. Sci Sport. 2005;20:131–5.
20. Faul F, Erdfelder E. GPOWER. A Priori, Post-Hoc, and Compromise Power Analyses for MS-DOS (Computer Program). Bonn, FRG: Bonn University, Department of Psychology; 2004.
21. Jacob Cohen. Statistical Power Analysis for the Behavioral Sciences (second ed.). New Jersey, USA: Lawrence Erlbaum Associates; 1988.
22. Hrysomallis C. Balance ability and athletic performance. Sports Med. 2011;41:221–32.
23. Paillard T, Margnes E, Portet M, Breucq A. Postural ability reflects the athletic skill level of surfers. Eur J Appl Physiol. 2011;111:1619–23.
24. Paillard T, Bizid R, Dupui P. Do sensorial manipulations affect subjects differently depending on their postural abilities? Br J Sports Med. 2007;41: 435–8.
25. Paillard T, Noé F, Rivière T, et al. Postural performance and strategy in the unipedal stance of soccer players at different levels of competition. J Athl Train. 2006;41:172–6.
26. Taube W, Gruber M, Gollhofer A. Spinal and supraspinal adaptations associated with balance training and their functional relevance. Acta Physiol (Oxf). 2008;193:101–16.
27. Fong SM, Fu SN, Ng GY. Taekwondo training speeds up the development of balance and sensory functions in young adolescents. J Sci Med Sport. 2012;15:64–8.
28. Paillard T, Montoya R, Dupui P. Specific postural adaptations according to the throwing techniques practiced in competition-level judoists. J Electromyogr Kinesiol. 2007;17:241–4.
29. Fong SM, Cheung CKY, Ip JY, Chiu JHN, Lam KLH, Tsang WWN. Sport-specific balance ability in Taekwondo practitioners. J Hum Sport Exerc. 2012;7:520–6.
30. Chung P, Ng GY. Taekwondo training improves the neuromotor excitability and reaction of large and small muscles. Phys Ther Sport. 2012;13:163–9.
31. Bosco C, Luhtanen P, Komi PV. A simple method for measurement of mechanical power in jumping. Eur J Appl Physiol. 1983;50:273–82.
32. Paillard T, Noe F, Bernard N, Dupui P, Hazard C. Effects of two types of neuromuscular electrical stimulation training on vertical jump performance. J Strength Cond Res. 2008;22:1273–8.
33. Sale DG. Neural adaptation to resistance training. Med Sci Sports Exerc. 1988;20 Suppl 5:135–45.
34. Mero A, Komi PV, Gregor RJ. Biomechanics of sprint running. A review. Sports Med. 1992;13:376–92.

19

Joint torque variability and repeatability during cyclic flexion-extension of the elbow

Laurent Ballaz[1,3], Maxime Raison[2,3,5*], Christine Detrembleur[4], Guillaume Gaudet[2,3] and Martin Lemay[1,3]

Abstract

Background: Joint torques are generally of primary importance for clinicians to analyze the effect of a surgery and to obtain an indicator of functional capability to perform a motion. Given the current need to standardize the functional evaluation of the upper limb, the aim of this paper is to assess (1) the variability of the calculated maximal elbow joint torque during cyclic elbow flexion-extension movements and (2) participant test-retest repeatability in healthy young adults. Calculations were based on an existing non-invasive method including kinematic identification and inverse dynamics processes.

Methods: Twelve healthy young adults (male $n = 6$) performed 10 elbow flexion-extension movement carrying five different dumbbells (0, 1, 2, 3 and 4 kg) with several flexion-extension frequencies (½, $^1/_3$, ¼ Hz) to evaluate peak elbow joint torques.

Results: Whatever the condition, the variability coefficient of trial peak torques remained under 4 %. Bland and Altman plot also showed good test-retest, whatever the frequency conditions for the 0, 1, 2, and 3 kg conditions.

Conclusion: The good repeatability of the flexion-extension peak torques represents a key step to standardize the functional evaluation of the upper limb.

Keywords: Modeling, Inverse dynamics, Kinematic solidification, Elbow joint torques, Variability, Repeatability

Background

In many musculoskeletal diseases muscular weakness leads to functional disability and decreased quality of life. For therapists, it is important to assess and quantify muscle strength in order to choose the most appropriate treatment or to evaluate therapy effects [1, 2]. Joint torques are generally of primary importance for clinicians to analyze the effect of a surgery on symmetry and comfort, and to obtain an indicator of functional capability to perform a motion. Joint torques are very often analyzed in patients with osteoarthritis (e.g.: [3, 4]) or scoliosis (e.g.: [5, 6]). Especially at the elbow, the change in elbow torque is an indicator of incremental release of the brachioradialis insertion footprint, for surgeons performing open reduction or internal fixation of distal radius fractures [7]. For physio/ergo-therapists, the elbow torque is an indicator of functional capability to perform a motion, e.g. in stroke patients, and a control variable for assistive devices developed for these patients [8]. In the rehabilitation field, strength is assessed though the measurement of the maximal joint torque [9–11], which represents the resultant action of all muscles crossing the joint, but do not provide each muscle force contribution. Studies have shown the potential of musculoskeletal simulation tools to determine the contribution of each muscle crossing a joint during movement which was otherwise impractical or impossible to obtain experimentally [12]. According to the clinical relevance and accuracy of the used method, such quantification would help clinicians to target the best therapeutic solution. Indeed, computational model could give the opportunity to predict the effect of the muscle property modifications on joint torque production [13]. For example, the effect of antagonist muscle release (e.g.: spasticity treatment) on joint torque production could be anticipated.

* Correspondence: maxime.raison@polymtl.ca
[2]Department of mechanical engineering, École Polytechnique de Montréal, Montreal, Qc, Canada
[3]Research & Engineering Chair Applied to Pediatrics (RECAP), Marie Enfant Rehabilitation Centre (CRME) – Research Center – Sainte-Justine UHC, and École Polytechnique de Montréal, Montreal, Qc, Canada
Full list of author information is available at the end of the article

The upper limb function is of utmost importance in improving the quality of life and enhancing functional independence. Especially, elbow flexion movement has been related to motor impairment and performance [14]. Thus, accurate modeling of elbow muscle involvement could provide an interesting tool to better understand the movement limitation. Within this process of calculating the muscle forces, joint torque is an essential intermediate variable [15–17]. Moreover, precise and repeatable quantification of the upper limb joint torque is of major importance for numerous applications (e.g. [18–20]) including exoskeletons and interactive rehabilitation devices development (e.g. [18, 21]), the understanding of the mechanisms resulting in joint rigidity (e.g. [22, 23]), or the impact of joint co-contraction on joint constraint (e.g. [17, 24]).

However, it is not always obvious to obtain accurate joint torque results that could be usefully exploited in model [25–27]. Applied to human motion analysis, several parameters can be a source of error. The major problems are linked to the inverse dynamic solution repeatability, which is affected by both the data processing and the experimental procedure. More specifically, in a top down approach, inaccuracy in movement coordinate data, joint centre of rotation location, and kinematic data processing can impact on inverse dynamics solution [25]. Indeed, using marker-based optical motion capture systems, marker misallocation and skin movement greatly influence joint centre localisation [28, 29]. The inertia parameters of the body segments can also influence inverse dynamic solution [30]. Lastly, the estimate of internal efforts, i.e. joint torques and muscle forces, is particularly sensitive to accelerations [31–33]. As a result, kinematic data analysis is also of greatest importance and mainly impact inverse dynamic results. Riemer et al. found that these various inaccuracies can result in uncertainties of estimated joint torques ranging from 6 % to 232 % of the peak torque during gait. As suggested in the literature however, more accurate results can be obtained with corrected kinematics based on a kinematic identification process, named solidification procedure [34], compared to inverse dynamics using either raw kinematic data, smoothing or low-pass filtering [35–37].

Additionally, in order to use inverse dynamics to follow patient progress, the experimental procedure should (1) allow the spontaneous adaptation of the participant to perform the task (e.g.: minimally constraint movement) and (2) result in within-subject test-retest task repeatability, according to the kinematic and dynamic movement parameters used in the model.

In light of this information, we have developed a model which quantifies the contribution of muscles crossing the elbow joint during flexion and extension movements [17] in order to use it as a clinical tool. The model-based process includes two consecutive steps: a kinematic identification based on procedure of solidification [34], combined with inverse kinematics and an inverse dynamics process that provides the elbow joint net torque (for more details, see [17]). As a first step to test the accuracy of the model, the aim of the present study is (1) to assess the maximal elbow joint torque variability during cyclic elbow flexion extension movements and (2) to assess participant test-retest repeatability in healthy young adults.

Methods

Participants

Twelve healthy young adults (age = 23 ± 2; male $n = 6$) were included in the present study. Exclusion criteria were known musculoskeletal or orthopaedic pathology, on the basis of a questionnaire in participants. The study was approved by the Research Ethics Board of Ste-Justine Hospital, Montreal, Canada (Ethics case #3362). A written informed consent was obtained from participants. The research was in compliance with the Helsinki Declaration.

Procedure

Experimental set-up

The experiments were conducted on cyclic elbow flexion-extension movement with the upper arm maintained vertical. As illustrated in Fig. 1, an experimental chair was designed to enable standardized motion of elbow flexion-extension in the sagittal plane. The person depicted in Fig. 1c gave a special consent to publish this one. Particularly, our incentive was to minimize the elbow joint motion during the task, but without mechanically blocking it, to highlight the behaviour of only one joint, i.e. the elbow. Consequently, right elbow optokinetic sensors were inserted in specific holes created on the side of the chair rest (Fig. 1a). Further, to limit the range of the flexion-extension motion (approximately 50°), 'sensitive' stops were placed to keep the movement between 70 and 120 degrees of flexion (Fig. 1a). This arc (70–120) was chosen because it corresponds to range of movement involve in many functional tasks [38]. The chair was adapted in height and depth in order to seat the participant with their hips and knees flexed at 90 degrees, and the right arm placed vertically downward. The participants were equipped with optokinetic sensors, placed on the following anatomical landmarks: the acromion, the middle of the arm (technical marker), the lateral epicondyle, the middle of the forearm (technical marker), the radial styloid, and both extremities of the dumbbells. This placement was set to enable the three-dimensional kinematic reconstruction of the upper limb and the

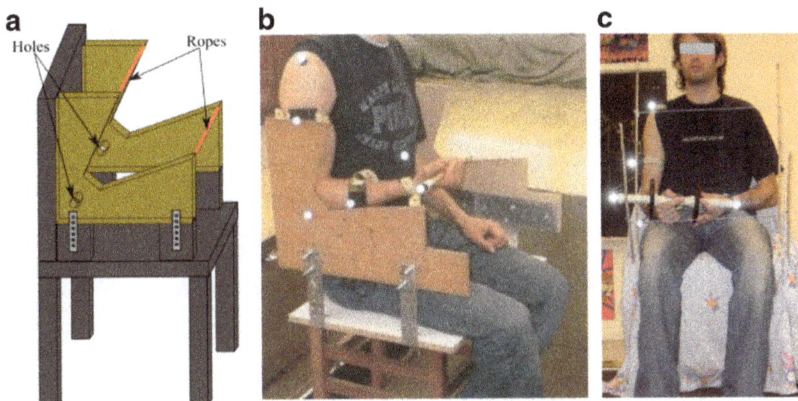

Fig 1 Experimental chair designed to perform elbow flexion/extension in the sagittal plane. Legend: **a** Design plan of the chair, featuring the ropes that limit the motion amplitude and the holes into which the elbow optokinetic sensor is inserted to avoid the elbow motion; **b** Side view of the chair, pointing out the elbow optokinetic sensor is inserted to avoid the elbow motion; **c** Front view of the chair, pointing out the ropes that limit the motion amplitude

dumbbell. The displacement of the markers was filmed by six infrared cameras (Elite-BTS, Milano, Italy) cadenced at 100 Hz.

Participant instructions

During experimentation, the participant sat on the chair. The participants were asked to perform 10 cycles of flexion-extension, following the rhythm of a given metronome, with and without dumbbells. Participants had to keep the shoulder and elbow joint as motionless as possible and the dumbbell axis horizontal. Participants were involved a few minutes with the dumbbells, before beginning the experiments.

The participants had to perform ten elbow flexion-extension movements with five different masses: 0, 1, 2, 3 and 4 kg, and at three motion frequencies, 0.5 Hz (i.e. a cycle in 2 seconds), 0.33 Hz (1 cycle in 3 seconds) and 0.25 Hz (1 cycle in 4 seconds). The order of the masses and frequencies was drawn randomly by the operator. Each male participant performed the whole experimental protocol twice in order to assess test and retest reproducibility of the joint torques. The retests were performed approximately 20 min after the tests, without removing the kinematic sensor.

Joint torque quantification process

Using the measurements of kinematic sensors, a 3D multibody model of the human body [17] provides the elbow joint torques via these three consecutive steps:

1. The full model joint kinematics: the system is modeled as a constrained multibody system, using kinematic loops.
2. The joint kinematic identification: the joint coordinates q, velocities q and accelerations q are numerically determined by an optimization process that estimates the joint coordinates of the multibody model that best fit the experimental joint positions.
3. The inverse dynamics: using recursive Newton-Euler formalism, a 3D multibody model [17] provides the vector Q_{inv} of joint forces and torques during movement as follows:

$$Q_{inv} = f(q, \dot{q}, \ddot{q}, F_{ext}, M_{ext}, g) \quad (1)$$

where f is a function of the kinematics q, $\dot{q}$, q and represents the inverse dynamical model of the human body, on the basis of the external forces F_{ext} and torques M_{ext} applied to the system, and also gravity g. The inertia parameters of the body segments have been defined using the Table from de Leva [39].

These equations were symbolically generated by the ROBOTRAN software [40], UCL, which allows us to straightforwardly interface these equations with any numerical process, such as the optimization process presented above and the time simulation of the trials.

Statistical analysis

Data was reported as mean (standard deviation) (SD). Normality of the distributions was determined using the Kolmogorov–Smirnov test. For each frequency (0.5, 0.3, and 0.25 Hz) and mass (0, 1, 2, 3, 4 kg), the peak torque variability within each trial was assessed by computing the coefficient of variation (%CV). The aim of this intra-test variability analysis was to enable to average the peak torques of each trial for the repeatability analysis. Paired t-tests were performed to detect possible systematic bias between test and retest trial. The possibility of heteroscedasticity was examined on the basis of the Pearson product-moment correlation (r) between the mean and the absolute differences. If the correlation coefficient was significant the data were considered as heteroscedastic [41]. Bland and Altman plots and limits of agreement analyses were also calculated to determine whether peak torque is in agreement between tests and retest trial [42]. This method (Bland & Altman, 1986) was extensively used in different research fields in test-retest studies [43–46] and is suitable in the case of the present study [41]. A corrected standard deviation of differences for repeated measurements, $SD_{corrected} = \sqrt{(2 \bullet SD^2)}$, was used based on Bland and Altman (1986) [42]. Statistical analysis was performed using SPSS 17.0 (IBM, Chicago, USA).

Results

In each condition, the peak torque values were normally distributed (Kolmogorov–Smirnov test, $p > 0.05$).

Intra-test variability

Whatever the test conditions, the variation coefficient of the peak torque ranged between 0.8 and 4 % (see Table 1).

Table 1 Peak torque coefficients of variation within trial

	Peak torque CV ($n = 12$)	
Test conditions mass (Kg)/Frequency (Hz)	Mean (SD)	95 % confidence interval
0/0.25	1.3 (1.1)	0.6-2.0
0/0.33	0.8 (0.4)	0.5-1.0
0/0.5	0.9 (0.5)	0.6-1.2
1/0.25	3.9 (3.9)	1.4-6.4
1/0.33	4.0 (3.1)	2.1-6.1
1/0.5	3.0 (2.9)	1.2-4.9
2/0.25	1.2 (1.1)	0.5-2.0
2/0.33	1.3 (1.5)	0.3-2.3
2/0.5	1.1 (0.6)	0.7-1.5
3/0.25	0.8 (0.4)	0.6-1.1
3/0.33	1.0 (1.0)	0.4-1.7
3/0.5	1.3 (0.9)	0.7-1.9
4/0.25	1.3 (0.5)	1.0-1.8
4/0.33	1.1 (0.9)	0.5-1.7
4/0.5	0.9 (0.3)	0.7-1.2
Mean	1.6	
SD	1.1	

Legend: *CV* coefficient of variation, *SD* standard deviation

Test-retest repeatability

Test-retest repeatability was performed with the male participants ($n = 6$). Whatever the condition, test and retest values were not significantly different ($p > 0.05$). Considering that the assumption of homoscedasticity was not met when the 4 kg conditions were included in the analysis, the conditions involving 4 kg were no longer considered in the present study. Whatever the other test conditions, the limits of agreement were -0.52 Nm to 0.62 Nm, which represent a variation of 8.5 % of the averaged peak torques (6.7 Nm) around the mean test-retest difference (See Bland and Altman plots, Fig. 2, right panel).

Whatever the mass condition, with a frequency of 0.25, 0.33, and 0.5 Hz, the limits of agreement values were -0.64 Nm to 0.86 Nm, -0.75 Nm to 0.92 Nm, and -0.49 Nm to 0.72 Nm, which represent a variation of 9.1, 9.9, and 7.2 % of the averaged peak torques (8.3 Nm, 8.4 Nm, and 8.3 Nm) around the mean test-retest differences, respectively (see Fig. 3).

Whatever the frequency condition, with a mass of 0, 1, 2, and 3 kg, the limits of agreement values were -0.16 Nm to 0.24 Nm, -0.64 Nm to 0.60 Nm, -0.34 Nm to 0.44 Nm, -0.74 Nm to 0.99 Nm, which represent a variation of 9.3, 12, 4.6, and 7.6 % of the averaged peak torques torques (2.2 Nm, 5.2 Nm, 8.5 Nm, and 11.4 Nm) around the mean test-retest differences, respectively (see Fig. 4).

Discussion

This study showed that the data processing and the experimental procedure implemented in the present study resulted in a low within-trial variability, i.e. a low variability inside each trial, and a good within-participant test-retest repeatability, i.e. a good repeatability between tests of the same participant, of the elbow peak torque in typically developing young adults. As shown by the limit of agreements, expressed as a percentage of the averaged peak torque, the result repeatability was equivalent whatever the frequency, amongst 0.25, 0.33, and 0.5 Hz, or the load, amongst 0 1, 2, and 3 kg, imposed during the movement.

This study highlighted that the 4 kg resulted in a more important variability compared to the lower masses. Based on this observation, it can be assumed that increasing the mass higher than 4 kg would result in a more important variability that would not be appropriated to evaluate the joint torques. On the contrary, using lower masses, such as 0 kg, are recommended for the good repeatability, and certainly do not imply fatigue, especially in female participants.

In summary, to evaluate muscle efforts in the rehabilitation field, the repeatability of the model at low frequencies and with light loads was a key result. In

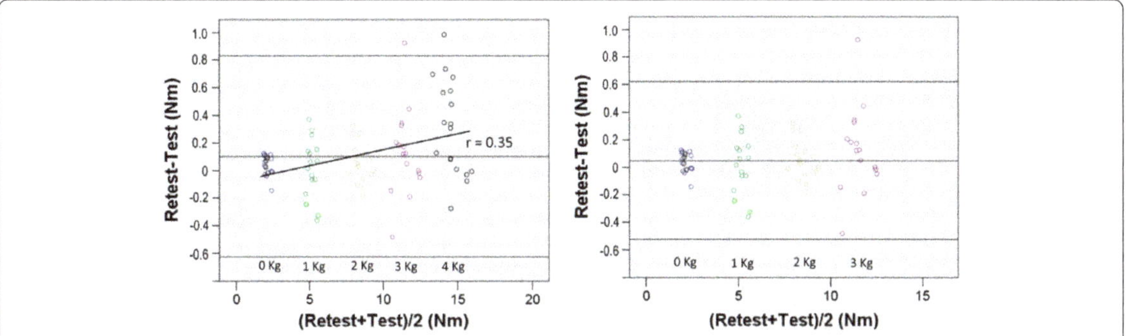

Fig 2 Bland and Altman plot for peak torque repeatability. Legend: Bland and Altman plot of the difference between test and retest peak torque values. The left panel illustrates that the homoscedasticity assumption would be violated if the 4 kg condition were included in the analysis (a correlation exists, $p < 0.05$). The right panel illustrates that the homoscedasticity assumption is met (no correlation exists, $p > 0.05$) if the 4 kg condition is dropped

patients with neurological disorder, muscular strength and movement velocity is potentially very low depending on their functional capacity. As supported by the Bland and Altman analysis (Fig. 3), at low frequency (0.25Hz) the limit of agreement represented 9.1 % of the averaged peak torque, and considering the condition without dumbbells, the limit of agreement represented 9.3 % of the averaged peak torque. Even if the literature still has no consensus on the clinically important difference in elbow torque for humans, because this torque relates to each joint and each motion, Laitenberger et al. (2015) [47] reported an elbow torque variability up to 24 % in healthy subjects, which confirms that the obtained repeatability of 8.5 % when all test conditions are viewed together (Fig. 2) is relevant compared to the magnitude of this measurement. As described earlier, kinematic

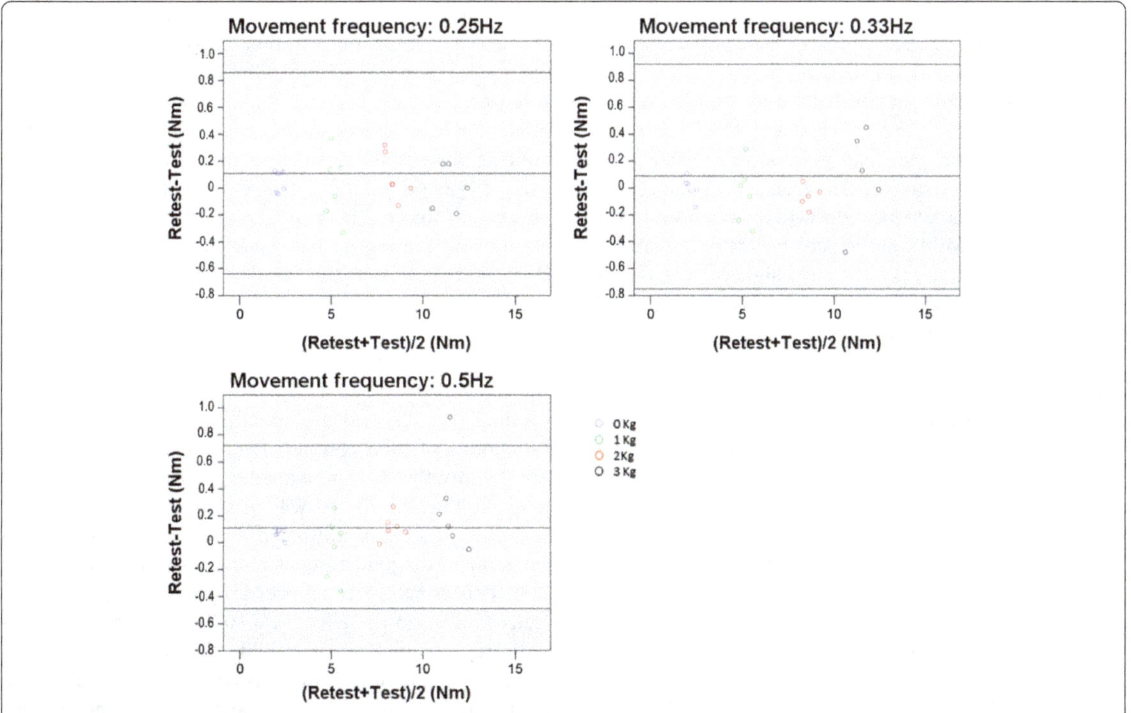

Fig 3 Bland and Altman plots for peak torque repeatability at each frequency condition. Legend: Bland and Altman plots of the difference between test and retest peak torque values for each frequency condition

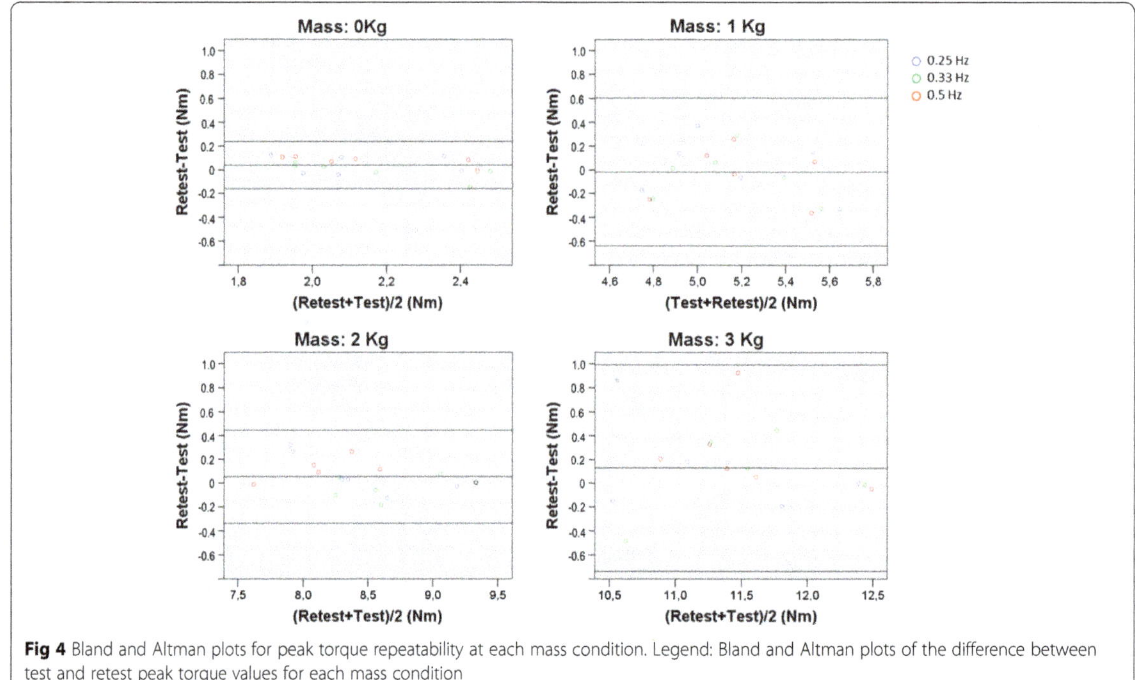

Fig 4 Bland and Altman plots for peak torque repeatability at each mass condition. Legend: Bland and Altman plots of the difference between test and retest peak torque values for each mass condition

data processing, marker misallocation and skin movement could greatly influence joint centre localisation [28, 29] and in turn greatly impact inverse dynamic solution repeatability [25]. Riemer et al. found that these various inaccuracies can result in uncertainties of estimated joint torques ranging from 6 % to 232 % of the peak torque during gait. The methodology used in the present study in terms of kinematic data processing, based on solidification procedure [34], was adequate to result in a good within-participant test-retest repeatability. At the same time, these results showed that the device used (Fig. 4) was adequate to obtain a repeatable elbow flexion-extension maximal torque.

Several limits were inherent with this study. First the repeatability of the data processing and the experimental procedure was tested with a limited number of participants. Nevertheless, many conditions were tested (frequency*mass), resulting in a test-retest repeatability analysis based on 90 trials. The test-retest repeatability analysis was performed only in male because fatigue could be more present in female compared to male participants. Secondly, the present study included healthy participants, the repeatability of the data processing and the experimental procedure implemented in the present study should be tested for each targeted disease. Thirdly, the repeatability of the model has been tested without removing the maker. A Further study is required to test the reproducibility with markers replacement because markers location could impact the inverse dynamic solution. Fourthly, the gender effect on repeatability was not studied and could be a further perspective. Fifthly, the trials were randomised and a 3 min. rest period was allocated between the trials, as recommended by Kollmitzer et al. (1999) [48] to avoid the muscle fatigue effect in the context of a sub-maximal effort of the upper limb. However, it is never excluded that either a fatigue or a time effect may have influenced the CV results. Especially concerning the higher CV reported for the 1 kg condition, we believe that this results from the method variation that might also be seen in other conditions. Nevertheless, the CV reported for the 1 kg condition remains low, even if it represents twice the CV reported in the other conditions. Sixthly, a method with a good reproducibility does not necessarily guarantee an accurate estimation of joint torques. Reproducibility is a necessary feature that is complementary to the accuracy, guaranteeing that the results will be similar for any trial. Let us remind that it is still not possible today to check the accuracy of the joint torques in a non-invasive way, even if this information is of primary importance for clinicians to analyze the effect of a surgery and to obtain an indicator of functional capability. Being aware of these limitations, the incentive of this paper was to analyse the quality of our joint torque quantification. The present inverse dynamical model of the human body, necessarily preceded by a kinematic identification of the model configurations, is proposed as a satisfying method to estimate the joint efforts in dynamical context. This problem being deterministic, Q_{inv} becomes a sufficiently accurate result that can be exploited as a reference for the optimization process that attempts to solve the muscle force redundancy. These results represent the first step leading to the development of an accurate assessment of elbow muscle strength in clinical environment. The ability of giving accurate elbow joint net torques during motion, without requiring an important computational cost, is the main benefit of this method. Based on these results, multibody model refinement and clinical analysis will be implemented in further studies.

Conclusion

The aim of this study was to assess the peak torque elbow variability and repeatability. Whatever the flexion-extension movement conditions imposed, within-trial peak torque variability was low and within-participant test-retest repeatability of the elbow joint torques resulted in good agreement. This method is promising for potential clinical applications and can be used as a basis for further comparison between efforts quantification methods or refined multibody models in the human body during motion.

Competing interests

The authors declare that they have no competing interests.

Authors' contributions

LB has made substantial contributions to the analysis and interpretation of data, and has been involved in drafting the manuscript. MR has made substantial contributions to the study design, the acquisition of data, the analysis and interpretation of data, and has given final approval of the version to be published. CD has made substantial contributions to the study design, and has made substantial contributions to the analysis and interpretation of data. GG has made substantial contributions to the acquisition of data, the analysis and interpretation of data. ML has made substantial contributions to the analysis and interpretation of data, and revising the manuscript critically for important intellectual content. All authors read and approved the final manuscript.

Acknowledgments

The authors wish to thank MÉDITIS program supported by FONCER-CSNG for financial support.

Author details

[1]Department of kinanthropology, Université du Québec à Montréal, Montreal, Qc, Canada. [2]Department of mechanical engineering, École Polytechnique de Montréal, Montreal, Qc, Canada. [3]Research & Engineering Chair Applied to Pediatrics (RECAP), Marie Enfant Rehabilitation Centre (CRME) – Research Center – Sainte-Justine UHC, and École Polytechnique de Montréal, Montreal, Qc, Canada. [4]Institute of NeuroSciences (IoNS), Université catholique de Louvain, Bruxelles, Belgium. [5]CRME – Research Center, Office GR-123, 5200, East Bélanger Street, H1T 1C9 Montréal, QC, Canada.

References

1. Damiano DL, Abel MF, Pannunzio M, Romano JP. Interrelationships of strength and gait before and after hamstrings lengthening. J Pediatr Orthop. 1999;19:352–8.
2. Hinderer KA, Hinderer SR. Muscle strength development and assessment in children and adolescents, in: H.-R. K. (Ed.), Muscle strength. Edinburgh: Churchill Livingstone 1993;p.93-140
3. Schache AG, Fregly BJ, Crossley KM, Hinman RS, Pandy MG. The effect of gait modification on the external knee adduction moment is reference frame dependent. Clin Biomech (Bristol, Avon). 2008;23(5):601–8.
4. Schwachmeyer V, Damm P, Bender A, Dymke J, Graichen F, Bergmann G. In vivo hip joint loading during post-operative physiotherapeutic exercises. PLoS One. 2013;8(10), e77807.
5. D'Amico M, D'Amico G, Paniccia M, Roncoletta P, Vallasciani M. An integrated procedure for spine and full skeleton multi-sensor biomechanical analysis & averaging in posture gait and cyclic movement tasks. Stud Health Technol Inform. 2010;158:118–26.
6. Raison M, Ballaz L, Detrembleur C, Mahaudens P, Lebleu J, Fisette P, Mousny M. Lombo-sacral joint efforts during gait: comparison between healthy and scoliotic subjects. Stud Health Technol Inform. 2012;176:113–6.
7. Tirrell TF, Franko OI, Bhola S, Hentzen ER, Abrams RA, Lieber RL. Functional consequence of distal brachioradialis tendon release: a biomechanical study. J Hand Surg Am. 2013;38(5):920–6.
8. Cheng HS, Ju MS, Lin CC. Improving elbow torque output of stroke patients with assistive torque controlled by EMG signals. J Biomech Eng. 2003;125(6):881–6.
9. Florence JM, Pandya S, King WM, Robison JD, Baty J, Miller JP, Schierbecker J, Signore LC. Intrarater reliability of manual muscle test (Medical Research Council scale) grades in Duchenne's muscular dystrophy. Phys Ther. 1992;72:115–22.
10. Cuthbert SC, Goodheart Jr GJ. On the reliability and validity of manual muscle testing: a literature review. Chiropr Osteopat. 2007;15:4.
11. Stark T, Walker B, Phillips JK, Fejer R, Beck R. Hand-held dynamometry correlation with the gold standard isokinetic dynamometry: a systematic review. PM R. 2011;3:472–9.
12. Bessonet G, Sardain P, Chéssé S. Optimal motion synthesis – dynamic modeling and numerical solving aspects. Multibody System Dynamics. 2002;8:257–78.
13. Hoy MG, Zajac FE, Gordon ME. A musculoskeletal model of the human lower extremity: the effect of muscle, tendon, and moment arm on the moment-angle relationship of musculotendon actuators at the hip, knee, and ankle. J Biomech. 1990;23(2):157–69.
14. Massie CL, Fritz S, Malcolm MP. Elbow extension predicts motor impairment and performance after stroke. Rehabil Res Pract. 2011;381978.
15. Amarantini D, Martin L. A method to combine numerical optimization and EMG data for the estimation of joint moments under dynamic conditions. J Biomech. 2004;37:1393–404.
16. De Groote F, Pipeleers G, Jonkers I, Demeulenaere B, Patten C, Swevers J, De Schutter J. A physiology based inverse dynamic analysis of human gait: potential and perspectives. Comput Methods Biomech Biomed Engin. 2009;12:563–74.
17. Raison M, Detrembleur C, Fisette P, Samin JC. Assessment of antagonistic muscle forces during forearm flexion/extension. Comput Methods Appl Sci. 2011;23:215–38.
18. Gilliaux M, Lejeune T, Detrembleur C, Sapin J, Dehez B, Stoquart G. A robotic device as a sensitive quantitative tool to assess upper limb impairments in stroke patients: a preliminary prospective cohort study. J Rehabil Med. 2012;44(3):210–7.
19. Zampagni ML, Casino D, Zaffagnini S, Visani A, Marcacci M. Trend of the carrying angle during flexion-extension of the elbow joint: a pilot study. Orthopedics. 2008;31(1):76.
20. Lin JH, McGorry RW, Banks JJ. Exposures and physiological responses in power tool operations: fastening vs. unfastening threaded hardware. J Occup Environ Hyg. 2010;7(5):290–7.
21. Malosio M, Pedrocchi N, Vincenti F. Tosatti LM. Rehabilitation Robotics. 2011;5975393.

22. Endo T, Okuno R, Yokoe M, Akazawa K, Sakoda S. A novel method for systematic analysis of rigidity in Parkinson's disease. Mov Disord. 2009;24:2218–24.
23. Park BK, Kwon Y, Kim JW, Lee JH, Eom GM, Koh SB, Jun JH, Hong J. Analysis of viscoelastic properties of wrist joint for quantification of parkinsonian rigidity. IEEE Trans Neural Syst Rehabil Eng. 2011;19(2):167–76.
24. Gross R, Leboeuf F, Rémy-Néris O, Perrouin-Verbe B. Unstable gait due to spasticity of the rectus femoris: gait analysis and motor nerve block. Ann Phys Rehabil Med. 2012;55(9-10):609–22.
25. Riemer R, Hsiao-Wecksler ET, Zhang X. Uncertainties in inverse dynamics solutions: a comprehensive analysis and an application to gait. Gait Posture. 2008;27:578–88.
26. Vaughan CL, Davis BL, O'Connor JC. Dynamics of Human Gait. 2nd ed. Cape Town, South Africa: Kiboho; 1992. p. 137.
27. Winter DA. Biomechanics and motor control of human movement. Thirdth ed. Hoboken, New-Jersey: John Wiley & Sons, Inc; 2005. p. 720.
28. Kuo YL, Tully EA, Galea MP. Skin movement errors in measurement of sagittal lumbar and hip angles in young and elderly subjects. Gait Posture. 2008;27:264–70.
29. Stagni R, Leardini A, Cappozzo A, Grazia Benedetti M, Cappello A. Effects of hip joint centre mislocation on gait analysis results. J Biomech. 2000;33:1479–87.
30. Rao G, Amarantini D, Berton E, Favier D. Influence of body segments' parameters estimation models on inverse dynamics solutions during gait. J Biomech. 2006;39:1531–6.
31. Cahouet V, Luc M, David A. Static optimal estimation of joint accelerations for inverse dynamics problem solution. J Biomech. 2002;35:1507–13.
32. Cappozzo A, Leo T, Pedotti A. A general computing method for the analysis of human locomotion. J Biomech. 1975;8:307–20.
33. Challis JH, Kerwin DG. Quantification of the uncertainties in resultant joint moments computed in a dynamic activity. J Sports Sci. 1996;14:219–31.
34. Cheze L, Fregly BJ, Dimnet J. A solidification procedure to facilitate kinematic analyses based on video system data. J Biomech. 1995;28:879–84.
35. Cappozzo A, Catani F, Leardini A, Benedetti MG, Croce UD. Position and orientation in space of bones during movement: experimental artefacts. Clin Biomech (Bristol, Avon). 1996;11:90–100.
36. Chiari L, Della Croce U, Leardini A, Cappozzo A. Human movement analysis using stereophotogrammetry. Part 2: instrumental errors. Gait Posture. 2005;21:197–211.
37. Lu TW, O'Connor JJ. Bone position estimation from skin marker co-ordinates using global optimisation with joint constraints. J Biomech. 1999;32:129–34.
38. Kim K, Song WK, Lee J, Lee HY, Park DS, Ko BW, Kim J. Kinematic analysis of upper extremity movement during drinking in hemiplegic subjects. Clin Biomech (Bristol, Avon). 2014;29(3):248–56.
39. de Leva P. Adjustments to Zatsiorsky-Seluyanov's segment inertia parameters. J Biomech. 1996;29(9):1223–30.
40. Samin JC, Fisette P. Symbolic modeling of multibody systems. Netherlands: Kluwer Academic Publishers; 2003. p. 479.
41. Atkinson G, Nevill AM. Statistical methods for assessing measurement error (reliability) in variables relevant to sports medicine. Sports Med. 1998;26(4):217–38.
42. Bland JM, Altman DG. Statistical methods for assessing agreement between two methods of clinical measurement. Lancet. 1986;1:307–10.
43. Høyer E, Opheim A, Strand LI, Moe-Nilssen R. Temporal and spatial gait parameters in patients dependent on walking assistance after stroke: reliability and agreement between simple and advanced methods of assessment. Gait Posture. 2014;40(1):101–6.
44. Thompson P, Beath T, Bell J, Jacobson G, Phair T, Salbach NM, Wright FV. Test-retest reliability of the 10-metre fast walk test and 6-minute walk test in ambulatory school-aged children withcerebral palsy. Dev Med Child Neurol. 2008;50(5):370–6.
45. Birmingham TB, Hunt MA, Jones IC, Jenkyn TR, Giffin JR. Test-retest reliability of the peak knee adduction moment during walking in patients with medial compartment knee osteoarthritis. Arthritis Rheum. 2007;57(6):1012–7.
46. de Zwart BC, Frings-Dresen MH, van Duivenbooden JC. Test-retest reliability of the Work Ability Index questionnaire. Occup Med (Lond). 2002;52(4):177–81.
47. Laitenberger M, Raison M, Périé D, Begon M. Refinement of the upper limb joint kinematics and dynamics using a subject-specific closed-loop forearm model. Multibody System Dynamics. 2015;33(4):413–38.
48. Kollmitzer J, Ebenbichler GR, Kopf A. Reliability of surface electromyographic measurements. Clin Neurophysiol. 1999;110(4):725–34.

20

Cancer patients participating in a lifestyle intervention during chemotherapy greatly over-report their physical activity level: a validation study

Karianne Vassbakk-Brovold[1,2*], Christian Kersten[1], Liv Fegran[1,3], Odd Mjåland[4], Svein Mjåland[1], Stephen Seiler[2] and Sveinung Berntsen[2]

Abstract

Background: The short form of the International Physical Activity Questionnaire (IPAQ-sf) is a validated questionnaire used to assess physical activity (PA) in healthy adults and commonly used in both apparently healthy adults and cancer patients. However, the IPAQ-sf has not been previously validated in cancer patients undergoing oncologic treatment. The objective of the present study was to compare IPAQ-sf with objective measures of physical activity (PA) in cancer patients undergoing chemotherapy.

Methods: The present study was part of a 12-month prospective individualized lifestyle intervention focusing on diet, PA, stress management and smoking cessation in 100 cancer patients undergoing chemotherapy. During the first two months of the lifestyle intervention, participants were wearing an activity monitor (SenseWear™ Armband (SWA)) for five consecutive days while receiving chemotherapy before completing the IPAQ-sf. From SWA, Moderate-to-Vigorous intensity PA (MVPA) in bouts ≥10 min was compared with self-reported MVPA from the IPAQ-sf. Analyses both included and excluded walking in MVPA from the IPAQ-sf. Results were extrapolated to a wearing time of seven days.

Results: Sixty-six patients completed IPAQ-sf and wore the SWA over five days. Mean difference and limit of agreement between the IPAQ-sf and SWA including walking was 662 (±1719) min·wk^{-1}. When analyzing time spent in the different intensity levels separately, IPAQ-sf reported significantly higher levels of moderate (602 min·wk^{-1}, $p = 0.001$) and vigorous (60 min·wk^{-1}, $p = 0.001$) PA compared to SWA.

Conclusions: Cancer patients participating in a lifestyle intervention during chemotherapy reported 366 % higher MVPA level from the past seven days using IPAQ-sf compared to objective measures. The IPAQ-sf appears insufficient when assessing PA level in cancer patients undergoing oncologic treatment. Activity monitors or other objective tools should alternatively be considered, when assessing PA in this population.

Keywords: Validation, Physical activity, Accelerometer, IPAQ, Cancer patient, Oncology

* Correspondence: karianne.vassbakk.brovold@sshf.no
[1]Oncologic Department, Southern Hospital Trust, Postbox 416, 4604 Kristiansand, Norway
[2]Department of Health and Sport Science, University of Agder, Postbox 422, 4604 Kristiansand, Norway
Full list of author information is available at the end of the article

Background

The number of new cancer cases is continuously rising and is estimated to grow from 12.7 million new cases in 2008 to more than 22 million new cases worldwide in 2030 [1, 2]. Parallel to this increase, the possibilities for surviving cancer has never been better with 32.6 million cancer survivors worldwide in 2012 [3]. Many cancer survivors are expected to return to normal and productive lives following their diagnosis. However, cancer and its treatments are often associated with long-term impairment of physical, mental and psychosocial health and survivors are at risk of developing co-morbidities [4, 5].

Physical activity (PA) is recommended as a strategy both during and after chemotherapy to manage treatment-related symptoms, prevent early and late co-morbidities, improve quality of life, increase the rate of chemotherapy completion and possibly extend overall and disease-specific survival in cancer patients [6–8]. Consequently, the American Cancer Society has provided a set of general PA recommendations for cancer patients and survivors. Accordingly, cancer patients should avoid inactivity, try to return to normal daily activities as soon as possible following diagnosis, and follow the general PA guidelines for aerobic and strength exercise. This recommendation is >150 min of moderate PA per week combined with strength training two days per week. Further, the importance of individualizing these PA recommendations to the patient's condition and preferences is pointed out, and it is emphasized that cancer patients may need to exercise at a lower intensity and/or for a shorter duration during their treatment [6]. These global PA recommendations are largely based on self-reports of cancer patients' PA levels [6].

The International Physical Activity Questionnaire (IPAQ) is a validated questionnaire developed to monitor self-reported PA levels in healthy adults [9], and the most commonly used self-report tool of PA worldwide [10, 11]. However, limitations of the IPAQ include its length, low compliance and difficulties in completing the questionnaire [12]. These difficulties may be of even greater magnitude for cancer patients experiencing disease and treatment-related side-effects like fatigue, loss of interest, and cognitive difficulties [13, 14] when undergoing chemotherapy. A short form of the IPAQ (IPAQ-sf) is therefore preferred and previously used in cancer patients [15], but has not been validated in cancer patients. Cancer is primarily a disease of the elderly [16], which can make the use of the IPAQ-sf challenging since the questionnaire is developed for adults aged 18–65 years [9]. Secondly, the IPAQ-sf defines moderate PA as activities that make you breathe somewhat harder than normal [17]. In this regard it is of major importance to be aware of the fact that cancer patients undergoing chemotherapy usually are fatigued, which may impair the patients' perceived level and intensity of PA. A validation study of IPAQ-sf across 12 countries revealed large variations with respect to correlation between IPAQ and objective measures of PA by activity monitors [9]. Thus, it is likely that the accuracy of the IPAQ varies when different populations are assessed, dependent on the populations' demographics, cultural backgrounds, physical fitness, level of physical functioning and disease status [12, 18]. The objective of the present study was therefore to compare time in Moderate-to-Vigorous intensity PA (MVPA) recorded with the short form of the IPAQ with activity directly quantified using SenseWear™ Armband (SWA) in cancer patients receiving chemotherapy with curative or palliative intent.

Methods

The present validation study is part of the I CAN-study [19]; a 12-month prospective feasibility intervention with the aim to increase population based adherence to healthy lifestyle behaviors including diet, PA, mental stress management and smoking cessation. The intervention was delivered to 100 cancer patients undergoing chemotherapy with curative or palliative intent through: 1) a grouped start-up course with patients and nearest relatives, 2) an information binder with recommendations, recipes and tips on how to manage possible disease and treatment-related symptoms themselves, and 3) monthly counseling with a lifestyle supervisor with recommendations individualized to the patients' abilities, barriers and preferences. The study is described in detail elsewhere [19].

Participants

All cancer patients receiving chemotherapy for all cancer types, with either curative or palliative intent, at one oncology center in Kristiansand, Norway were considered for study participation against the following inclusion criteria: 1) age ≥ 18 years; 2) life expectancy ≥ 6 months; 3) Eastern Cooperative Oncology Group performance status (ECOG) ≤ 2; and 4) able to speak and read Norwegian. The only exclusion criterion was suspected anorexia cachexia syndrome. The study was conducted according to the guidelines of the Helsinki Declaration. The Regional Committee for Medical and Health Research Ethics, South-East approved the study (ref.no. 2012/1717/REK). Written informed consent was obtained from all patients before inclusion.

Procedures

Medical and demographic characteristics were collected via self-report and medical records. These included date of birth, height (collected by the physicians before start-up of chemotherapy), tumor type (later categorized into 1 = breast cancer; 2 = colorectal cancer; 3 = prostate cancer; 4 = other cancer types), tumor stage (I-IV), ECOG

(0–2), treatment intention (curative or palliative), marital status, cigarette smoking status and education level. Weight was measured to the nearest 0.5 kg (Mechanical scale, Seca 761, Birmingham, United Kingdom) and body mass index (BMI) was calculated by dividing weight (kg) by height (m) squared. Self-reported PA was assessed using the IPAQ-sf. Objective quantification of PA was acquired via the SWA, either in conjunction with the participants' first or the second appointed visit in the I CAN-study. The participants had undergone chemotherapy from five to twelve weeks at this time point. Participants were instructed to wear the SWA for five consecutive days; both including work week and weekend days. Since the present study was part of a comprehensive lifestyle study, participants' diet, mental stress, cigarette smoking and quality of life were assessed in addition to their PA level; a total of 59 questions.

Short form of the International Physical Activity Questionnaire (IPAQ-sf)

The IPAQ-sf questionnaire assesses PA in bouts of ≥ 10 min as part of leisure time, domestic and gardening activities, and work and transportation activities the past seven days. PA is classified as either Vigorous PA (VPA), Moderate PA (MPA) or as walking [17]. All walking was included to MPA, as proposed by Craig et al. [9]. Additionally, MPA minus time spent on walking is presented. Total PA was defined as the sum of time in MVPA.

SenseWear Armband

SenseWear™ Armband Pro3 and Mini (BodyMedia Inc. Pittsburgh, PA) has been shown valid compared to indirect calorimetry in cancer patients (underestimation of daily energy expenditure by 9%, $r = 0.68$; $p < 0.01$) [20] and doubly labeled water in healthy adults (underestimation of daily energy expenditure by 5%, $r = 0.81$; $p < 0.01$) [21]. The sensor array includes an accelerometer, heat flux-sensor, galvanic skin response sensor, skin temperature sensor and a near-body ambient temperature sensor [21]. The SWA was worn on the triceps muscle halfway between the acromion and olecranon processes of the upper arm, as recommended by the manufacturer. Participants were instructed to remove the SWA during water-based activities, such as swimming or bathing, as the monitor is not waterproof. Data were downloaded with software developed by the manufacturer (SenseWear Professional Research Software V.6.1 for Pro3 and V7.0 for Mini, algorithm V.2.2.4) after entering necessary demographic characteristics (sex, age, height, weight, smoking status).

The SWA was programmed to record PA in 1-min epochs. The cut-points defined MPA as 3–6 METs and VPA >6 METs in bouts ≥10 min. Total PA was defined as the sum of MVPA in bouts of ≥10 min. Min·wk^{-1} from the SWA for each participant was calculated by multiplication of mean MVPA min·day^{-1} by seven. Complete measurements required SWA wearing-time ≥19.2 h·day^{-1} on at least one day.

Data analysis

Descriptive characteristics are presented as mean and standard deviation (SD). The PA data are presented as min·wk^{-1} in the present study. The mean difference (IPAQ-sf minus SWA) ± 1.96 SD was calculated according to Bland and Altman [22]. To test if the IPAQ-sf overestimated PA compared to SWA, we applied a Wilcoxon signed-rank test for the absolute values for each activity monitor. Differences are presented as means with 95 % Confidence Intervals (CI). Additionally, the percentage discrepancy between IPAQ-sf and the SWA was calculated for each individual within different intensity categories. A linear regression with MVPA from SWA as the independent variable and the difference between IPAQ-sf and SWA for MVPA as the dependent variable was applied to test for systematic over-reporting. Level of significance was set to 0.05. Statistical analysis was performed with SPSS statistical software version 22 (SPSS Inc., Chicago, IL, USA). A post hoc power analysis using G*Power [23] yielded a power of 0.99 to detect differences between means, based on an effect size of 0.5.

Results

From the 100 I CAN participants, 16 participants dropped out before enrolment in the present validation study. The remaining 84 participants received a SWA and completed the IPAQ-sf. Of these, 18 were eliminated due to 1) SWA malfunction ($n = 14$) or 2) not sufficient wearing-time of the SWA ($n = 4$). In total 66 participants had valid registrations on the SWA and were included to the present validation study. There were no significant differences in self-reported MVPA between participants vs. non-participants at baseline ($p = 0.414$). Participants wore the SWA for an average of 3.6 days and 23.7 h·day^{-1} of all valid days. Demographic, medical and physical characteristics of the participants ($n = 66$) and non-participants ($n = 34$) are presented in Table 1.

Time in MPA, VPA and MVPA, including and excluding walking

The mean differences and limits of agreements between the IPAQ-sf and SWA from the Bland-Altman plots for time in MVPA were 662 (1719) min·wk^{-1} and 203 (1070) min·wk^{-1} with walking included and excluded in the analyses, respectively (Fig. 1a and b). Figure 1c and d depicts the mean differences and limits of agreements

Table 1 Characteristics of participants ($n = 66$) and non-participants ($n = 34$). Presented as frequencies and percentages in parenthesis unless otherwise stated*

	Participants		Non-participants		*P*-value
	n = 66	(%)	*n* = 34	(%)	
Age, mean (SD)*	59 (11)		62 (12)		.254
Height, mean (SD)*	169 (9)		172 (8)		.111
Weight, mean (SD)*	72 (14)		78 (16)		.085
BMI, mean (SD)*	25.2 (4.3)		26.1 (4.4)		.335
Waist circumference, mean (SD)*	91 (12)		96 (13)		.097
Sex					
- Men	18	(28)	12	(35)	.407
- Women	48	(72)	22	(65)	
Marital status					
- Married/living together	57	(86)	23	(68)	.027
- Single/divorced/widowed	9	(14)	11	(32)	
Education level[a]					
- High school or less	34	(52)	13	(41)	.279
- College/university	31	(48)	19	(59)	
Cigarette smoking					
- Smoker	8	(12)	5	(15)	.716
- Non-smoker	58	(88)	29	(85)	
ECOG					
- 0	49	(74)	29	(85)	.312
- 1	16	(24)	4	(12)	
- 2	1	(2)	1	(3)	
Treatment intention					
- Curative	44	(67)	17	(50)	.106
- Palliative	22	(33)	17	(50)	
Tumor stage					
- I	12	(18)	4	(12)	.564
- II	14	(21)	7	(20)	
- III	16	(24)	6	(18)	
- IV	24	(37)	17	(50)	
Diagnosis					
- Breast cancer	35	(53)	11	(32)	.036
- Colorectal cancer	22	(33)	10	(30)	
- Prostate cancer	2	(3)	2	(6)	
- Other	7	(11)	11	(32)	
Self-reported moderate-to-Vigorous PA, mean (SD)* (min·wk^{-1})	833 (989)		675 (694)		.414

[a]Missing value
*standard deviation

between the IPAQ-sf and the SWA from the Bland-Altman plots for time in MPA with walking included and excluded from the analyses; 602 (1694) min·wk^{-1} and 143 (1009) min·wk^{-1}, respectively. Furthermore, Fig. 1 shows that several of the participants also under-reported their PA compared to the SWA (plots under the solid line). From the IPAQ-sf, 23 participants reported VPA during the last week. The SWA only identified three participants conducting VPA during the same seven-day period, and VPA is thus not depicted in a Bland-Altman plot. Linear regression revealed no significant systematic over-reporting; indicating those who had

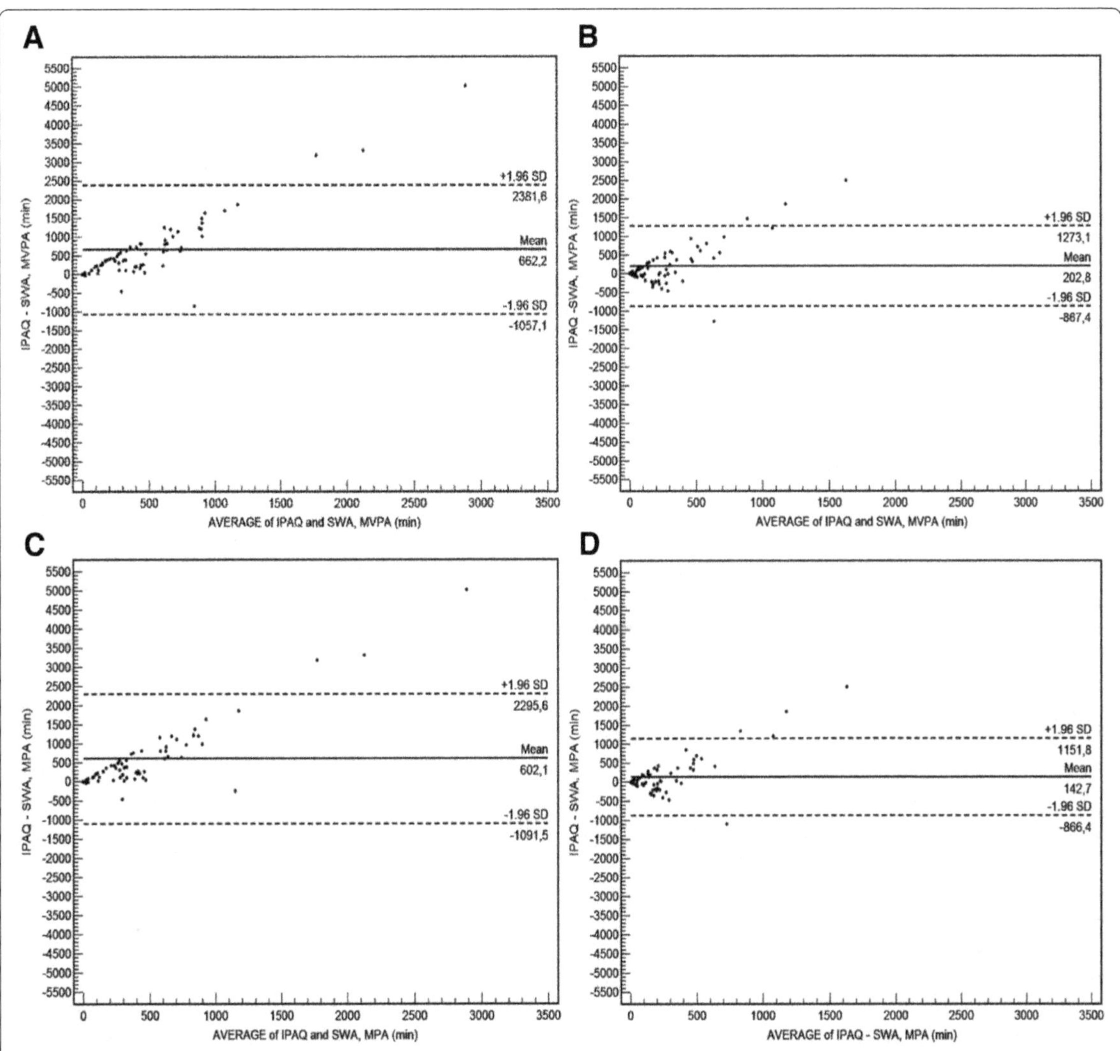

Fig. 1 Bland-Altman plots depicting the mean differences (IPAQ-sf minus SenseWear Armband) for minutes spent in **a** Moderate-to-Vigorous intensity Physical Activity (MVPA) including walking, **b** MVPA excluding walking, **c** Moderate intensity PA (MPA) including walking and **d** MPA excluding walking. The solid line represents the mean, and the dashed lines represent the 1.96 SDs of the observations

the highest levels of PA did not significantly over-report their PA levels the most. When comparing the min·wk^{-1} differences between IPAQ-sf and the MVPA recorded with SWA, analyses revealed a 366 % higher MVPA level reported on the IPAQ-sf compared to SWA ($p = 0.001$) (Table 2). After excluding walking from the analysis, the IPAQ-sf still reported statistically significant higher levels of MVPA; 112 % higher compared to the SWA ($p = 0.007$). When time in the different intensity categories were analyzed separately, IPAQ-sf reported significantly more time spent in MPA (602 min·wk^{-1}, $p = 0.001$) and VPA (60 min·wk^{-1}, $p = 0.001$) compared to SWA; 342 % and 1200 % more, respectively. Stratified analyses on mean differences between patients undergoing curative vs. palliative chemotherapy revealed no significant difference between the groups in over-report of MVPA (733 (443, 1023) vs. 521 (211, 832) min·wk^{-1}, respectively, $p = 0.395$).

Accommodation of PA guidelines

Participants were categorized into fulfilling the American Cancer Society PA guidelines of ≥150 min·wk^{-1} or not when comparing MVPA obtained from the IPAQ-sf vs. the SWA. Analyses revealed significant differences between the IPAQ-sf and the SWA when walking was included to the MVPA; IPAQ-sf identified 58 of the participants as meeting the PA guidelines vs. 32 by SWA ($p = 0.001$). After excluding walking from the analyses, 35 of the participants self-reported accommodating the PA guidelines ($p = 0.532$).

Table 2 Mean difference and 95 % Confidence Intervals (95 % CI) for PA obtained by the IPAQ-sf and SenseWear Armband data ($n = 66$)

	IPAQ-sf – SWA		P-value
	Mean difference (min·wk^{-1})	(95 % CI)	
Moderate PA			
- Walking included	602	(390, 815)	.001
- Walking excluded	143	(16, 269)	.107
- Walking vs. Moderate (IPAQ-sf vs. SWA)	283	(145, 421)	.001
Vigorous PA[a]	60	(28, 94)	.001
Moderate-to-Vigorous PA			
- Walking included	662	(447, 878)	.001
- Walking excluded	203	(69, 337)	.007

[a]Missing values

Discussion

In the present study, cancer patients participating in a comprehensive lifestyle intervention while undergoing chemotherapy over-reported time in MVPA compared to SWA, when completing the IPAQ-sf. Specifically, these cancer patients over-reported their moderate-to-vigorous PA by nearly 100 min·day^{-1}. No differences in over-reporting were observed between patients undergoing chemotherapy with curative or palliative intent.

Almost 90 % of the participants in the present study perceived themselves as meeting the PA guidelines of 150 min·wk^{-1} of MPA while less than 50 % actually met the PA guidelines according to the objective measures. Our findings are supported by previous studies, where more than half of healthy adults included perceived themselves as accommodating the PA guidelines [24, 25]. Objective measures in the same population revealed that only 15 % were reaching the guidelines [26]. The higher percentage of participants self-reporting accommodating the PA recommendations observed in the present study compared to previous studies [26] may be a result from drawing our participants from a lifestyle intervention focusing on the participants' diet, mental stress and smoking cessation in addition to their PA. In addition to measuring the participants' lifestyle behaviors, participants also received recommendations on how to maintain or adhere to a healthy lifestyle during their cancer treatment. It is a well-known phenomenon that individuals participating in a study often improve aspects of their behavior as a response to being studied or they believe they have improved more than what they actually have (the Hawthorne effect) [27–29]. In the present study, the IPAQ-sf identified significantly more participants as accommodating the PA guidelines of 150 min·wk^{-1} of MVPA vs. the SWA. Six of the participants reported from 420 to 840 min·wk^{-1} of MVPA, while less than 60 min·wk^{-1}was registered on their SWA. These findings are not only statistical significant, but also of great clinical importance. Health care professionals should take these findings into consideration when delivering PA recommendations in this population and if using IPAQ-sf as an assessment tool in the clinic. In terms of this knowledge, individualized PA recommendations can be delivered with barriers such as fatigue, feeling sick, loss of interest and nausea, in mind [13, 30], so that cancer patients undergoing oncologic treatment can harvest the known health benefits from adhering to the developed PA guidelines [6].

Participants in the present validation study self-reported being in MVPA 662 min·wk^{-1} more than what was objectively registered by the SWA; an over-reporting that is supported in the literature [9, 31–33]. Of the 844 min·wk^{-1} MVPA reported on the IPAQ-sf in the present study, participants reported 459 min·wk^{-1} as walking activities. As reported previously, IPAQ-sf may over-report MPA because it includes walking at any intensity [33]. In the present study, IPAQ-sf over-reported time spent on walking by 283 min·wk^{-1} or 1.6 times compared to MPA obtained by the SWA. When including MPA from the IPAQ-sf in the analysis, IPAQ-sf over-reported walking by 602 min·wk^{-1} or 3.4 times compared to MPA data on the SWA. To include time spent on walking in the MVPA but not differentiate the intensity of the walking may be a potential source of over-reporting in cancer patients undergoing chemotherapy, and time spent on walking was thus both included and excluded to MVPA in the present study. A significant amount of the walking performed by these patients may be objectively registered as light intensity [34], while being experienced and self-reported as moderate [35]. The IPAQ-sf defines MPA as activities that make you breathe somewhat harder than normal [17]. Importantly, cancer patients dealing with disease- and treatment-related side-effects such as reduced physical capacity, fatigue, pain, depression and anxiety [36–39] may feel short of breath at a much lighter intensity than they have previously or compared to the population which the questionnaire is developed for. Consequently, the experienced side-effects are a great source of over-reporting since the patients might experience and report the PA as moderate, while the SWA assesses the PA as light intensity. This is important to have in mind when using self-reports in cancer patients; many PA self-reports, like the IPAQ-sf, are developed for use in a healthy population. Gil-Rey et al. [39] thus suggest cancer-specific PA guidelines to maximize the health benefits in this population.

The participants did not systematically over-report their PA levels when completing the IPAQ-sf; in other words, higher physical activity levels from the SWA was not associated with more over-reporting of MVPA reported from the IPAQ-sf. Our findings are in contrast to the findings of Johnson-Kozlow et al. [31], who revealed larger over-reporting in the breast cancer survivors who reported the highest PA levels on the long form of the IPAQ. Reasons for our conflicting findings may be the use of different accelerometer in the two studies and the use of the long versus the short form of the IPAQ in the study of Johnson-Kozlow and colleagues [31] and the present study, respectively. The long form of the IPAQ gives a total of 35 examples of PA across different activity domains, i.e. recreational sports, leisure time and housework PA. This provides many opportunities for "forward telescoping"; a recall bias occurring if the activities were recalled as taking place during the same seven-day period which is monitored, but actually took place previously [40]. Secondly, while the participants were undergoing chemotherapy in the present study and may not have been able to perform much vigorous PA, the participants in the study of Johnson-Kozlow et al. [31] were cancer survivors two years post diagnosis. Recall of vigorous PA is more likely to be subject to "forward telescoping" on PA self-reports, since these activities are often easier to remember due to strong, distinct physiological signals [40].

Importantly, IPAQ has been criticized for being complicated to complete [41] due to difficulties in remembering which activities they performed the past seven days, to distinguish the intensity of the different activities and last but not least trying to identify whether or not the activities lasted ≥ 10 min [42]. These aspects may be even harder to recognize for cancer patients experiencing disease- and treatment-related side effects such as pain, mental stress, cognitive difficulties and fatigue [13, 14, 37]. When comparing the IPAQ-sf to the SWA, activities lasting ≥ 10 min from the SWA was applied in the analyses, which may lead to great over-reporting if the activity lasted < 10 min. Thus, post hoc PA comparisons assessed by the IPAQ-sf and minute-by-minute SWA data were conducted in the present study (data not shown). Analyses revealed that IPAQ-sf still significantly over-reported VPA but IPAQ-sf now significantly under-reported MPA by 44 % compared to the SWA. The difficulties in completing the IPAQ-sf are reasonably clear. Importantly, there are currently no gold-standard for quantifying PA [43]; however, accelerometers are a precise and valid tool and thus commonly used in validating self-reports of PA [32]. Consequently, it is of concern that both the evidence regarding PA in cancer patients and the PA recommendations in this population is developed on the basis of self-reported PA data, which in turn has impact on the validity of those recommendations [6]. Another question that arises in this context is why self-reports only addresses PA in bouts >10 min, when there is rapidly growing evidence on health benefits in shorter bouts of PA [44, 45]. This is; however, an unexplored field in cancer patients, which needs further investigation, especially since activities of longer duration may be hard to complete for cancer patients with impaired physical capacity due to the oncologic treatment.

There are strengths and limitations of the present study. To our knowledge, this is the first time the IPAQ-sf has been compared to an objective PA monitor in cancer patients undergoing chemotherapy with either curative or palliative intent. One key aspect when designing the present study was to make the objective registrations feasible to the patients. Many different guidelines regarding days wearing the activity monitors are previously provided, with a minimum wearing time of four days recommended [46, 47]. One weakness of the present study is that only 66 % of the eligible patients were included, despite wearing the SWA for only five days, due to voluntary dropout, SWA malfunction or insufficient wearing time, leading to a higher inclusion of breast cancer patients who were either married or living together with someone compared to the total sample. These observations may indicate that a shorter wearing time is preferred in this population with regard to feasibility. Secondly, the participants were instructed to remove the SWA during water-based activities and activities such as swimming were thus not recorded. However, cancer patients at our clinic were advised to refrain from activities such as swimming in public pools due to reduced immune function and increased infection risk during chemotherapy. Further, the present study, as previous lifestyle interventions, is limited by including the healthier and fitter participants compared to the population from which they are drawn [19, 30]. Unfortunately, no Bland-Altman plot was calculated for VPA since only three of the participants had bouts of ≥10 min of VPA recorded on the SWA. Further, the present study is limited by the amount of questions asked. The present validation study was part of a comprehensive lifestyle intervention, which focused on the participants' diet, mental stress, smoking cessation and quality of life in addition to their PA level. The large amount of questions asked, perhaps in combination with side effects from the disease and its treatment, may have affected the accuracy of the participants' answers.

Conclusion

Based on our findings, cancer patients participating in a lifestyle intervention while undergoing chemotherapy grossly over-report their PA level from the past seven days when using the IPAQ-sf. Thus, the IPAQ-sf seems to be insufficient when assessing PA level in cancer patients undergoing oncologic treatment. Activity monitors or other objective tools should be considered in this population as an attempt to bridge the gap between how physical active the cancer patients perceive themselves and how physical active they actually are, in order to provide each patient with correct and individualized PA recommendations.

Ethics approval and consent to participate

The Regional Committee for Medical and Health Research Ethics, South-East approved the study (ref.no. 2012/1717/REK). Written informed consent was obtained from all patients before inclusion.

Consent for publication

Not applicable.

Additional file

Additional file 1: Availability of data and materials. (XLSX 47 kb)

Abbreviations

ECOG: Eastern Cooperative Oncology Group performance status; IPAQ-sf: international physical activity questionnaire, short form; METs: metabolic equivalent tasks; Min: minutes; Min·wk^{-1}: minute per week; MPA: moderate physical activity; MVPA: moderate-to-vigorous physical activity; PA: physical activity; SWA: SenseWear Armband; VPA: vigorous physical activity.

Competing interests

The authors declare that they have no competing interests.

Authors' contributions

KVB drafted the manuscript, contributed in the statistical analysis and carried out the data collection. CK, LF and SB supervised the first author throughout the study and helped draft the manuscript. SB helped coordinate the data collection and performed the statistical analysis. All authors have contributed in the study design and in poof-reading and revising the final manuscript. All authors read and approved the final manuscript.

Acknowledgements

We would first like to acknowledge and thank the Oddrun Mjåland Foundation for Cancer Research, who funded this study. The authors humbly thank the participants of the present study for providing their valuable time and effort. We also thank the outpatient clinic at the Oncologic Department at the Southern Hospital Trust for their collaboration. Special thanks to the oncologic nurses Brit Hausken Haddeland and Marit Kristin Bjelland Lund who greatly contributed in the study by collecting data and supervising the I CAN participants.

Funding

The present study was funded by the Oddrun Mjåland Foundation for Cancer Research.

Author details

[1]Oncologic Department, Southern Hospital Trust, Postbox 416, 4604 Kristiansand, Norway. [2]Department of Health and Sport Science, University of Agder, Postbox 422, 4604 Kristiansand, Norway. [3]Department of Health and Nursing Science, University of Agder, Postbox 4224604 Kristiansand, Norway. [4]Surgical Department, Southern Hospital Trust, Postbox 4164604 Kristiansand, Norway.

References

1. Torre L, Bray F, Siegel R, Ferlay J, Lortet-Tieulent J, Jemal A. Global cancer statistics, 2012. CA Cancer J Clin. 2015;65(2):87–108.
2. Vineis P, Wild C. Global cancer patterns: causes and prevention. Lancet. 2014;383(9916):549–57.
3. Ferlay J, Soerjomataram I, Ervik M, Dikshit R, Eser S, Mathers C, et al. GLOBOCAN 2012 v1.0, Cancer Incidence and Mortality Worldwide: IARC CancerBase No. 11 International Agency for Research on Cancer, Lyon, France. 2013. http://globocan.iarc.fr. Accessed 17 Mar 2015.
4. Courneya KS. Exercise in cancer survivors: an overview of research. Med Sci Sports Exerc. 2003;35(11):1846–52.
5. Aziz N. Cancer survivorship research: state of knowledge, challenges and opportunities. Acta Oncologica. 2007;46(4):417–32.
6. Rock C, Doyle C, Demark-Wahnefried W, Meyerhardt J, Courneya K, Schwartz A, et al. Nutrition and physical activity guidelines for cancer survivors. CA Cancer J Clin. 2012;62(4):243–74.
7. Schmitz K, Courneya K, Matthews C, Demark-Wahnefried W, Galvão D, Pinto B, et al. American college of sports medicine roundtable on exercise for cancer survivors. Med Sci Sports Exerc. 2010;42(7):1409–26.
8. van Waart H, Stuiver M, van Harten W, Geleijn E, Kieffer J, Buffart L, et al. Effect of Low-Intensity Physical Activity and Moderate- to High-Intensity Physical Exercise During Adjuvant Chemotherapy on Physical Fitness, Fatigue, and Chemotherapy Completion Rates: Results of the PACES Randomized Clinical Trial. J Clin Oncol. 2015;33(17):1918–27.
9. Craig C, Marshall A, Sjöström M, Bauman A, Booth M, Ainsworth B, et al. International physical activity questionnaire: 12-country reliability and validity. Med Sci Sports Exerc. 2003;35(8):1381–95.
10. Bauman A, Ainsworth B, Bull F, Craig C, Hagströmer M, Sallis J, et al. Progress and pitfalls in the use of the International Physical Activity Questionnaire (IPAQ) for adult physical activity surveillance. J Phys Act Health. 2009;6:5–8.
11. van Poppel M, Chinapaw M, Mokkink L, van Mechelen W, Terwee C. Physical activity questionnaires for adults: a systematic review of measurement properties. Sports Med. 2010;40(7):565–600.
12. Bertheussen G, Oldervoll L, Kaasa S, Sandmæl J-A, Helbostad J. Measurement of physical activity in cancer survivors - a comparison of the HUNT 1 Physical Activity Questionnaire (HUNT 1 PA-Q) with the International Physical Activity Questionnaire (IPAQ) and aerobic capacity. Support Care Cancer. 2013;21(2):449–58.
13. Courneya K, McKenzie D, Reid R, Mackey J, Gelmon K, Friedenreich C, et al. Barriers to supervised exercise training in a randomized controlled trial of breast cancer patients receiving chemotherapy. Ann Behav Med. 2008;35(1):116–22.
14. Ganz P. Doctor, will the treatment you are recommending cause chemobrain? J Clin Oncol. 2011;30(3):229–31.
15. Kang S. The association of physical activity and colorectal and breast cancer: The Fifth Korea National Health and Nutrition Examination Survey (2008–2011). J Exerc Rehabil. 2015;11(3):155–60.
16. WHO (World Health Organization). Cancer. Fact sheet No. 297. 2015. http://www.who.int/mediacentre/factsheets/fs297/en/. Accessed February 2015.
17. IPAQ-group. Guidelines for Data Processing and Analysis of the International Physical Activity Questionnaire (IPAQ) - Short Form. 2004. http://www.institutferran.org/documentos/Scoring_short_ipaq_april04.pdf. Accessed April 2004 2004.
18. Shook R, Gribben N, Hand G, Paluch A, Welk G, Jakicic J et al. Subjective Estimation of Physical Activity Using the IPAQ Varies by Fitness Level. J Phys Act Health. 2015. [Epub ahead of print].
19. Vassbakk-Brovold K, Berntsen S, Fegran L, Lian H, Mjåland O, Mjåland S, et al. Individualized Comprehensive Lifestyle Intervention in Patients Undergoing Chemotherapy with Curative or Palliative Intent: Who Participates? PLoS One. 2015;10(7). doi:10.1371/journal.pone.0131355.
20. Cereda E, Turrini M, Ciapanna D, Marbello L, Pietrobelli A, Corradi E. Assessing energy expenditure in cancer patients: a pilot validation of a new wearable device. JPEN J Parenter Enteral Nutr. 2007;31(6):502–7.
21. St-Onge M, Mignault D, Allison D, Rabasa-Lhoret R. Evaluation of a portable device to measure daily energy expenditure in free-living adults. Am J Clin Nutr. 2007;85(3):742–9.
22. Bland J, Altman D. Statistical methods for assessing agreement between two methods of clinical measurement. Lancet. 1986;1:307–10.
23. Faul F, Erdfelder E, Buchner A, Lang A-G. Statistical power analyses using G*Power 3.1: Tests for correlation and regression analyses. Behavior Research Methods. 2009;41:1149–60.

24. Bryan S, Katzmarzyk P. Are Canadians meeting the guidelines for moderate and vigorous leisure-time physical activity? Appl Physiol Nutr Metab. 2009;34(4):707–15.
25. Ready A, Butcher J, Dear J, Fieldhouse P, Harlos S, Katz A, et al. Canada's physical activity guide recommendations are a low benchmark for Manitoba adults. Appl Physiol Nutr Metab. 2009;34(2):172–81.
26. Colley R, Garriguet D, Janssen I, Craig C, Clarke J, Tremblay M. Physical activity of Canadian adults: accelerometer results from the 2007 to 2009 Canadian Health Measures Survey. Health Rep. 2011;22(1):7–14.
27. Rosén M. On randomized controlled trials and lifestyle interventions. Int J Epidemiol. 1989;18(4):993–4.
28. Forbes G. Diet and exercise in obese subjects: self-report versus controlled measurements. Nutr Rev. 1993;51(10):296–300.
29. Lichtman S, Pisarska K, Berman E, Pestone M, Dowling H, Offenbacher E, et al. Discrepancy between self-reported and actual caloric intake and exercise in obese subjects. N Engl J Med. 1992;327(27):1893–8.
30. Courneya K, Segal R, Gelmon K, Mackey J, Friedenreich C, Yasui Y, et al. Predictors of adherence to different types and doses of supervised exercise during breast cancer chemotherapy. Int J Behav Nutr Phys Act. 2014;11(85). doi:10.1186/s12966-014-0085-0.
31. Johnson-Kozlow M, Sallis J, Gilpin E, Rock C, Pierce J. Comparative validation of the IPAQ and the 7-day PAR among women diagnosed with breast cancer. Int J Behav Nutr Phys Act. 2006;3(7). doi:10.1186/1479-5868-3-7.
32. Lee P, Macfarlane D, Lam T, Stewart S. Validity of the International Physical Activity Questionnaire Short Form (IPAQ-SF): a systematic review. Int J Behav Nutr Phys Act. 2011;8(115). doi: 10.1186/1479-5868-8-115.
33. Rzewnicki R, Vanden Auweele Y, De Bourdeaudhuij I. Adressing over-reporting on the International Physical Activity Questionnaire (IPAQ) telephone survey with a population sample. Public Health Nutr. 2003;6(3):299–305.
34. Rogers L, Markwell S, Courneya KS, McAuley E, Verhulst S. Physical activity type and intensity among rural breast cancer survivors: patterns and associations with fatigue and depressive symptoms. J Cancer Surviv. 2011;5(1):54–61.
35. Ainsworth B, Haskell W, Herrmann S, Meckes N, Bassett DJ, Tudor-Locke C, et al. 2011 Compendium of Physical Activities: a second update of codes and MET values. Med Sci Sports Exerc. 2011;43(8):1575–81.
36. Bränström R, Petersson L, Saboonchi F, Wennman-Larsen A, Alexanderson K. Physical activity following a breast cancer diagnosis: Implications for self-rated health and cancer-related symptoms. Eur J Oncol Nurs. 2015. Epub ahead of print.
37. Pinto B, Eakin E, Maruyama N. Health behavior changes after a cancer diagnosis: what do we know and where do we go from here? Ann Behav Med. 2000;22(1):38–52.
38. Vardar-Yagli N, Sener G, Saglam M, Calik-Kutukcu E, Arikan H, Inal-Ince D, et al. Associations among physical activity, comorbidity, functional capacity, peripheral muscle strength and depression in breast cancer survivors. Asian Pac J Cancer Prev. 2015;16(2):585–9.
39. Gil-Rey E, Quevedo-Jerez K, Maldonado-Martin S, Herrero-Román F. Exercise Intensity Guidelines for Cancer Survivors: a Comparison with Reference Values. Int J Sports Med. 2014. [Epub ahead of print]. doi:10.1055/s-0034-1389972.
40. Durante R, Ainsworth B. The recall of physical activity: using a cognitive model of the question-answering process. Med Sci Sports Exerc. 1996;28(10):1282–91.
41. Hallal P, Gomez L, Parra D, Lobelo F, Mosquera J, Florindo A, et al. Lessons learned after 10 years of IPAQ use in Brazil and Colombia. J Phys Act Health. 2010;7:S259–64.
42. Prokop N, Hrubeniuk T, Sénéchal M, Bouchard D. People who perceive themselves as active cannot identify the intensity recommended by the international physical activity guidelines. J Sports Med. 2015;17(5):234–41.
43. Terwee C, Mokkink L, van Poppel M, Chinapaw M, van Mechelen W, de Vet H. Qualitative attributes and measurement properties of physical activity questionnaires: a checklist. Sports Med. 2010;1(40):525–37.
44. White D, Gabriel K, Kim Y, Lewis C, Sternfeld B. Do Short Spurts of Physical Activity Benefit Cardiovascular Health? The CARDIA Study. Med Sci Sports Exerc. 2015;47(11):2353–8.
45. Clarke J, Janssen I. Sporadic and bouted physical activity and the metabolic syndrome in adults. Med Sci Sports Exerc. 2014;46(1):76–83.
46. Maddocks M, Byrne A, Johnson C, Wilson R, Fearon K, Wilcock A. Physical activity level as an outcome measure for use in cancer cachexia trials: a feasibility study. Support Care Cancer. 2010;18(12):1539–44.
47. Scheers T, Philippaerts R, Lefevre J. Variability in physical activity patterns as measured by the SenseWear Armband: how many days are needed? Eur J Appl Physiol. 2012;112(5):1653–62.

21

Effect of fatigue caused by a simulated handball game on ball throwing velocity, shoulder muscle strength and balance ratio: a prospective study

Marília Santos Andrade[1], Fabiana de Carvalho Koffes[1], Ana Amélia Benedito-Silva[2], Antonio Carlos da Silva[1] and Claudio Andre Barbosa de Lira[3*]

Abstract

Background: Arm throwing represents a deciding element in handball. Ball velocity, aim accuracy, and dynamic stability of the shoulder are factors that influence throwing effectiveness. The purpose of this study was to examine the influence of muscle fatigue caused by simulated game activities (SGA) on shoulder rotational isokinetic muscle strength, muscle balance and throwing performance, and to examine the relationship between muscle strength and throwing performance.

Methods: Ten national elite adult handball athletes were evaluated. Isokinetic internal (IR), external (ER) rotators peak torque, and balance ratio were measured before and after SGA. Ball throwing velocity was assessed by radar gun.

Results: Both internal (IR) and external (ER) rotators peak torque were significantly lower after SGA ($p = 0.0003$ and $p = 0.02$, respectively). However, the deleterious effect was more evident for IR than ER muscles (effect size $r = 0.39$ and $r = 0.18$, respectively). Balance ratio before and after SGA did not differ ($p = 0.06$). Ball throwing velocity was not impaired by SGA. Moreover, isokinetic variables correlated positively with ball velocity ($r \geq 0.67$).

Conclusions: SGA affected the muscle strength of IR more than ER, predisposing the shoulder joint to muscular imbalance. The muscular impairment after SGA was insufficient to impair ball throwing velocity.

Keywords: Isokinetic dynamometer, Handball, Shoulder strength, Ball throwing velocity

Background

Throwing velocity in overarm throwing is crucial in sports such as baseball, handball, javelin, volleyball, and water polo [1]. Glenohumeral stabilization and muscle strength are among the most important factors for developing ball velocity [2, 3], and several authors have studied the association of this factor [4–6]. Joint stabilization and muscular strength are also of fundamental importance to prevent joint injury [7–9]. With regard to this strength component, recent findings have shown that some overhead athletes have a strength imbalance between internal and external rotator shoulder muscles [4, 10–12] and consequently exhibit poor joint stabilization. In order to reduce this strength imbalance, core stability exercises have been suggested [13].

Another interesting finding drawn from the literature is that there is a higher incidence of injuries late in the game *vs* early in the game [14]. Thus, the muscular fatigue caused by repetitive movement during a game may be more evident in the agonist throwing muscles than in the antagonist muscles. This selective fatigue can affect muscular strength balance and consequently shoulder joint stabilization, which may be a factor contributing to the higher injury incidence late in the game. A greater involvement of elastic tissues in the presence of muscular fatigue, reducing the need for muscle activation, may

* Correspondence: andre.claudio@gmail.com
[3]Setor de Fisiologia Humana e do Exercício, Faculdade de Educação Física e Dança, Universidade Federal de Goiás (UFG), Avenida Esperança s/n, Campus Samambaia, Goiânia, GO CEP: 74690-900, Brazil
Full list of author information is available at the end of the article

also be associated with joint injury [15]. In addition, this fatigue may represent a factor impairing ball throwing performance, as previously demonstrated for basketball players [16].

Traditionally, muscle performance is assessed by isokinetic dynamometer, however adequate patient stabilization and clear instructions during the test are fundamental for good quality and reproducible data [4, 17]. This device provides coaches, clinicians, and physical therapists an objective evaluation of muscle strength and strength balance ratio between shoulder external (ER) and internal rotators (IR) muscles [4, 11, 12].

Although many authors agree on the importance of muscle strength for arm throwing, only limited conclusions can be drawn about the relationship between upper limb strength and throwing performance because results available are conflicting [18–21].

Therefore, we hypothesized that muscular strength, muscular balance between internal and external rotator muscles and ball throwing velocity are affected by the muscular fatigue caused by a game, or in the present case by a simulated game involving several muscle actions present in a real game. Moreover, we also hypothesized that there is a significant relationship between isokinetic muscle strength and ball throwing velocity.

Therefore, the purpose of this study was: i) to examine the influence of muscular fatigue caused by simulated game activities (SGA) on isokinetic muscle strength, balance ratio and ball throwing velocity; and ii) to examine the relationship between shoulder rotational strength and ball velocity in handball athletes.

Methods

Participants

Participants in this study comprised a convenience sample of 10 highly trained, competitive, professional male handball players from Brazil. The players had a mean age of 23.1 ± 2.8 years (range: 20–29 years), mean height of 185.0 ± 7.7 cm (range: 172–193 cm), and mean body mass of 87.1 ± 11.3 kg (range: 66–105 kg). All participants were recruited from an elite team that participates in national and international championships and had engaged in handball training for a mean of 10.2 ± 4.0 years (range: 5–18 years). Exclusion criteria were shoulder pain or injury within the year leading up to the study. Four athletes had shoulder injuries predating this time period.

Participants were informed of the potential risks and benefits of the study and signed an informed consent form to take part. All experimental procedures were approved by the Federal University of São Paulo Human Research Ethics Committee and conformed to the principles outlined in the Declaration of Helsinki.

Study design

Upon arrival at the laboratory, participants underwent isokinetic evaluation of their dominant upper limb. Tests began at 2 pm for all the athletes in order to avoid the influence of the circadian rhythm on muscle strength [22]. Limb dominance was determined by identifying the upper limb that the participant prefers to use to throw a ball [23]. Ten minutes after isokinetic evaluation, the participants performed eight standing and eight jumping arm throws on the handball court to measure ball velocity.

Immediately after completion of the throwing activities, athletes performed a program of simulated game activities (SGA) to simulate the upper limb muscular stress of a real handball game. Five minutes after the end of the SGA, arm throwing action was repeated to measure ball velocity . Finally, the athletes were submitted to another isokinetic strength test. All the evaluation tests were done in this sequence and on the same day.

Isokinetic assessment

Before isokinetic testing, a 5-min warm-up was performed on an arm-cycle ergometer (Cybex Inc., Ronkonkoma, NY, USA) at a resistance level of 25 W, and standardized static stretching exercises were performed, since it has been demonstrated that these static exercises in association with warm-up exercises performed prior to isokinetic strength tests have no influence on strength results [24, 25]. To stretch the glenohumeral joint muscles, the following exercises were performed in this order: arm abduction at 90 deg with horizontal flexion targeting the posterior deltoid fibers; shoulder abduction with the upper limb behind the head targeting the triceps muscle; upper limb abduction to 135 deg with horizontal extension targeting the pectoralis major muscle; upper limb abduction at 90 deg with horizontal extension targeting the pectoralis minor muscle; and shoulder internal rotation with the hand behind the body targeting the external rotator muscles. All the static stretching exercises were performed in two unassisted successive repetitions for 15-s up to a threshold of mild discomfort, with no pain acknowledged by the athletes. Between each stretching repetition, during stretching exercises and at each muscle group change, the upper limb was rested for a 15-s period in a neutral position. Following the stretching period, participants were placed in the isokinetic dynamometer (Biodex Medical Systems Inc., Shirley, NY, USA) to evaluate maximal strength during positive (concentric) and negative (eccentric) exercises for the dominant limb [26].

The IR and ER muscles were assessed in the seated position, with the upper limb abducted at 90 deg on the frontal plane and the elbow flexed at 90 deg. The range of motion reached 50 deg for internal rotation and 70 deg for external rotation. The isokinetic velocities selected were 60 deg·s^{-1}

and 300 deg·s^{-1} in the concentric mode (positive exercise) and 90 deg·s^{-1} and 300 deg·s^{-1} in the eccentric mode (negative exercise). Participants performed three submaximal trials to familiarize themselves with the range of motion and the accommodating resistance of the dynamometer. Participants then performed a maximum of five repetitions to test each velocity used. Positive exercise tests were done first; lower test velocities were performed before faster velocities. Peak torque, total work, and conventional strength ratio (calculated as positive external rotation-to-positive internal rotation ratio) was assessed at 60 deg·s^{-1}, peak torque and average power was assessed at 300 deg·s^{-1}, and functional strength ratio was calculated as negative external rotator peak torque at 90 deg·s^{-1} to positive internal rotator peak torque at 300 deg·s^{-1}. Successive velocity testing was separated by one-minute rest intervals.

Before testing, the dynamometer was calibrated according to the manufacturer's specifications and checked prior to testing each participant. Standardized verbal encouragement was given during all testing. Visual feedback from the computer screen was not allowed.

Throwing performance

Ball velocity was measured by a radar gun (Stalker Sport, Stalker Radar, Texas, USA) according to Cools et al. [27]. To this end, participants performed two types of throw: one was in a standing position seven meters from the goal; the second (from the nine meter line) was a jumping throw preceded by two steps. All participants threw the ball in this order, and performed eight arm throws in a standing position and eight in a jumping position, two into each corner of the goal. Ball velocity was measured for all arm throws, where the velocity used was the mean of the eight throws. This test was performed on an official handball court.

To establish test-retest reliability, subjects were invited to participate in a second measurement session at 3–4 days after the initial assessment, during which ball velocity on both tests was assessed in the same way as in the first session. A time interval of 3–4 days was chosen to avoid the training effect.

Simulated game activities (SGA)

Simulated game activities were designed to simulate the upper limb muscular stress of a real handball game. The SGA were based on the mean number of steps and throws toward goal registered for each team player position in the last three games. Therefore, the exercise protocol devised included 100 steps and 20 arm throws at goal.

During the SGA, the heart rate (HR) of all participants was monitored using a heart rate monitor (Suunto Team Pod, Suunto Oy, Vantaa, Finland) with the purpose of monitoring exercise intensity. The mean HR during SGA was 153 ± 13 bpm, which represents approximately 77 % of the maximal predicted HR (220-age) [28] for the group of handball players.

Statistical analysis

All variables presented normal distributions according to the Shapiro-Wilk test. In the pre-SGA condition, the association between ball velocity and isokinetic muscular performance was evaluated by calculating Pearson's correlation coefficients (r) and classifying according to the following rule: no correlation for $r < 0.50$; moderate for $0.50 \le r < 0.75$; and good-to-strong for $r \ge 0.75$ [29].

Paired *t*-tests were used to compare the effect of SGA on isokinetic muscular strength and ball velocity. The significance level (α) was set at 0.05 for all statistical procedures. The results were also assessed for clinical significance by using effect size (ES) of changes. ES was calculated and classified as follows: large for ES ≥ 0.8, moderate for 0.5 ≤ ES < 0.8, small for 0.2 ≤ ES < 0.5 and trivial for ES < 0.2 [30]. Confidence intervals (90 %) were also calculated. All statistical analyses were performed with Statistica version 7.0 software (Statsoft Inc., Oklahoma, USA).

An intraclass correlation coefficient (ICC) was used to assess test-retest reliability of both ball velocity tests (jumping or in standing position). ICC values of less than 0.40 were considered poor, 0.40–0.59 fair, 0.60–0.74 good, and .075–1.0 excellent [31].

Results

Analysis of the ICC for the ball velocity test in a standing position, the value was classified as good (0.71) while in the jumping throw preceded by two steps, ICC was classified as excellent (0.99).

Table 1 depicts the mean and standard deviations of shoulder ER and IR positive peak torque and total work (at 60 deg·s^{-1}), positive peak torque and mean power (at 300 deg·s^{-1}), and negative peak torque (at 90 deg·s^{-1} and 300 deg·s^{-1}), as well as balance ratio (conventional and functional strength ratios). Values shown represent before and after SGA.

Student's *t*-test for dependent samples showed significantly lower values of peak torque and total work (at 60 deg·s^{-1}) for ER and IR muscles after SGA. Effect size of SGA on IR muscles was higher for IR muscles than for ER muscles across all isokinetic variables.

Conventional strength ratios ranged from 0.61 ± 0.10 to 0.67 ± 0.10 at 60 deg.s^{-1} ($p = 0.06$) and functional strength ratios from 0.68 ± 0.10 to 0.67 ± 0.20 at 300 deg·s^{-1} ($p = 0.81$). Changes in conventional ratio after SGA had moderate ES.

In a subset analysis, the four athletes reporting history of injury predating the year before the study had a functional strength ratio of 0.62 ± 0.10, whereas the

Table 1 Effects of simulated game activities on isokinetic parameters for dominant limbs of handball athletes

	Before	After	*P* value	ES	IC
External rotator					
Positive peak torque at 60 deg.s^{-1} (Nm)	43.3 ± 7.7*	40.6 ± 6.4	0.02	0.38	−0.13 to −0.63
Positive total work at 60 deg.s^{-1} (J)	51.7 ± 9.8*	46.7 ± 8.5	0.01	0.54	−0.24 to-0.84
Positive peak torque at 300 deg.s^{-1} (Nm)	35.2 ± 5.0	34.5 ± 2.5	0.41	0.17	0.19 to −0.53
Average power at 300 deg.s^{-1} (W)	65.3 ± 14.4	59.2 ± 10.3	0.12	0.48	0.032 to −0.99
Negative peak torque at 90 deg.s^{-1} (Nm)	45.2 ± 9.8	38.9 ± 9.5	0.06	0.65	−0.096 to −1.2
Negative peak torque at 300 deg.s^{-1} (Nm)	44.7 ± 6.2*	40.4 ± 4.5	0.04	0.79	
Internal rotator					
Positive peak torque at 60 deg.s^{-1} (Nm)	71.3 ± 13.7*	60.9 ± 10.2	0.01	0.86	−0.37 to −1.3
Positive total work at 60 deg.s^{-1} (J)	90.9 ± 16.9*	77.8 ± 13.1	0.00	0.86	−0.86 to −0.86
Positive peak torque at 300 deg.s^{-1} (Nm)	66.5 ± 12.3*	61.3 ± 12.3	0.00	0.42	−0.42 to −0.42
Average power at 300 deg.s^{-1} (W)	113.3 ± 29.4*	94.8 ± 29.1	0.02	0.63	−0.22 to −1
Negative peak torque at 90 deg.s^{-1} (Nm)	79.8 ± 13.6	68.9 ± 17.2	0.06	0.70	−0.1 to −1.3
Negative peak torque at 300 deg.s^{-1} (Nm)	69.9 ± 14.6	62.9 ± 12.9	0.16	0.51	0.051 to −1.1
Balance ratios					
Conventional ratio	0.61 ± 0.1	0.67 ± 0.1	0.063	0.60	−0.081 to −1.1
Functional ratio	0.68 ± 0.1	0.67 ± 0.2	0.806	0.06	0.37 to −0.49

Data are expressed as mean ± standard deviation. *ES* effect size, *IC* interval confidence
*$p < 0.05$, differs from after, Student *t* test

remaining 6 players had a functional ratio of 0.75 ± 0.10. The conventional strength ratio for the four previously injured athletes was 0.58 ± 0.12 and for the remaining six athletes was 0.63 ± 0.14. There was no significant difference between the injured and uninjured groups.

Table 2 shows Pearson's correlation coefficients for isokinetic and throwing performance (*r*-values ranged from 0.67 to 0.82). Concerning ER muscles, a negative, moderate and significant correlation with ball velocity on the standing arm throw was found for functional ratio ($r = -0.65$, $p = 0.043$).

Table 2 Correlation coefficients between isokinetic parameters and ball velocity during standing or jumping arm throwing in male handball players

		Standing arm throwing		Jumping arm throwing	
		R value	*P* value	*R* value	*P* value
Positive peak torque at 60 deg.s^{-1}	External rotator	0.61	0.060	0.77	0.009
	Internal rotator	0.82	0.004	0.89	0.001
Positive total work at 60 deg.s^{-1}	External rotator	0.62	0.058	0.71	0.020
	Internal rotator	0.79	0.006	0.82	0.004
Positive peak torque at 300 deg.s^{-1}	External rotator	0.68	0.029	0.75	0.012
	Internal rotator	0.83	0.003	0.86	0.001
Average power at 300 deg.s^{-1}	External rotator	0.63	0.052	0.60	0.065
	Internal rotator	0.62	0.058	0.62	0.054
Negative peak torque at 90 deg.s-1	External rotator	0.53	0.118	0.67	0.036
	Internal rotator	0.67	0.022	0.73	0.031
Negative peak torque at 300 deg.s^{-1}	External rotator	0.29	0.424	0.40	0.258
	Internal rotator	0.71	0.022	0.68	0.031
	Conventional ratio	−0.23	0.525	0.12	0.732
	Functional ratio	−0.65	0.043	0.57	0.081

Variability of ball velocity among handball players was high at almost 30 %. Student's *t*-test for dependent samples showed no significant differences in ball velocity for throwing in jumping or standing positions before and after SGA ($p > 0.05$) (Table 3). The statistical power for these analyses ranged from 5.6 to 14.4 %.

Discussion

The primary purpose of this study was to ascertain whether SGA could affect muscular strength and balance as well as ball velocity in male handball players. The study also sought to determine whether isokinetic muscle variables were associated with ball throwing velocity in male handball players. To our knowledge, this is the first paper to demonstrate the effect of SGA on a functional task (ball velocity) and on isokinetic parameters in male handball players. The findings reported lead us to conclude that SGA causes a decrease in muscle strength and probably induces muscular imbalance, without significant changes in ball throwing velocity. Moreover, the data also showed a significant correlation between isokinetic muscle strength and ball throwing velocity. Statistical significance and ES were employed to interpret the data because it allows researchers to move away from the simple identification of statistical significance toward a more generally interpretable, quantitative description of an effect, independent of the potentially misleading influence of sample size.

Isokinetic variables of the positive IR test were reduced after SGA for all variables evaluated but this strength reduction was greater in IR than in ER. The muscle strength balance ratio tended to be affected by SGA ($p = 0.06$) and the ES was moderate. In this context, the higher incidence of injuries late in the game *vs* early in the game, suggested by Hawkins and Fuller [14], may be related to a loss of muscular balance due to the greater muscular fatigue in IR than in ER muscles caused by SGA. Therefore, it is likely that rehabilitation or injury prevention programs aimed at improving IR muscles endurance may be helpful to avoid muscular strength loss and consequently muscular joint imbalance at end of games.

Zapartidis et al. [32] examined the influence of SGA on throwing effectiveness and rotational strength of the shoulder. They found that SGA did not impair rotational strength of the shoulder except in the case of ER at 180 deg·s^{-1}. One possible explanation for the discrepancy between the present study results and those of Zapartidis et al. [32] is that our volunteers were men whereas the cited authors' were women. Fatigue caused by the game might produce different levels of impairment in muscle performance in men and women. Future studies, including muscle endurance evaluation, are necessary to elucidate this question.

Table 3 Throwing performance before and after simulated game activities

	Simulated game activities		
	Before	After	*P* value
Ball velocity - standing throwing (m.s^{-1})	23.6 ± 3.1	23.2 ± 3.2	0.09
Ball velocity - jumping throwing (m.s^{-1})	22.8 ± 2.5	22.5 ± 3.2	0.23

Data are expressed as mean ± standard deviation

The mean throwing velocity achieved by athletes in the present study before SGA was 23.6 m·s^{-1} (18.1–27.1 m·s^{-1}). These results were higher than values reported by Jöris et al. [2] and Zapartidis et al. [32], a difference likely explained by the fact that the subjects in the previous studies were female handball players, where higher ball velocities are to be expected among male athletes.

A plethora of studies have investigated muscle strength and balance of the shoulder muscles in an attempt to identify a relationship with throwing arm velocity [18, 20, 33]. It is reasonable to presume a relationship between ball velocity and strength developed by the throwing arm, but a review of other sports activities described in the literature has shown that the relationship between isokinetic results and field performance varies widely [18, 20, 33].

Our results showed a strong relationship between ER and IR peak torque at 60 and 300 deg·s^{-1}, total work at 60 deg·s^{-1}, and ball velocity in both jumping and standing throws. One finding is that IR shoulder strength almost always correlates more strongly with ball velocity than ER shoulder strength. This is expected because IR muscles are responsible for accelerating the limb during the throwing action.

It is important to emphasize that related findings do not necessarily prove cause and effect between muscle strength and ball velocity. Since throwing is a multi-joint action, a variety of factors may contribute to this movement. Indeed, Atwater [34] showed throwing to be a complex motion involving all body parts. It has been suggested that approximately 50 % of ball throwing velocity is the result of body rotation, while the remainder is the result of upper-extremity action. Further, Pappas et al. [35] have described the anatomical sequence of throwing as proceeding from the fixed foot, up through the pelvis and trunk, to the upper extremity and therefore the importance of the lower extremity movement and trunk rotation should not be underestimated when examining throwing movements. Thus, high ball velocity is not produced solely by greater shoulder muscle strength, but athletes who have strong shoulder muscles may also have greater strength in their lower limbs, pelvis and trunk musculature. This implies that their ball velocity test would be higher as a consequence of the greater strength in their entire body. The findings presented in this study lead us to postulate that improvement of IR and ER strength, whether at low or high velocities, may increase ball velocity during throwing. However, for the reasons given above this conclusion should be interpreted with caution.

Interestingly, ball velocity showed a significant negative relationship with functional strength ratio at 300 deg·s^{-1}. Forthomme et al. [19] also showed a significant negative relationship between the functional strength ratio at 400 deg·s^{-1} and spike velocity in volleyball players. These findings may suggest that lower strength ratios are beneficial for high arm throwing velocity. However, it is well known that shoulder stability is largely maintained by the ligaments and musculotendinous units [36] and sports such as handball that involve repetitive overarm motion require shoulder stability with well-coordinated and synchronized actions of shoulder muscles to prevent injury in this joint [9, 18, 19]. Several authors agree that in an overhead throwing athlete, an adequate ratio of negative antagonist muscle strength to positive agonist muscle strength is critical for dynamic stability and optimal function [9, 36]. In the present study, the four players reporting a history of shoulder tendinosis or superior labrum from anterior to posterior lesion, showed a tendency towards lower functional strength ratios. There was no significant difference between the groups but since the sample size for this analysis was very small, statistical analysis of this data should be analyzed cautiously. The four players who had previous injuries exhibited a mean functional strength ratio of 0.62 ± 0.10 whereas the remaining six uninjured players presented a mean functional ratio of 0.75 ± 0.10. The conventional strength ratio also showed a tendency to be lower among athletes who had a history of shoulder lesion than for those who presented no lesion (0.58 ± 0.12 and 0.63 ± 0.14, respectively). Therefore, although IR strengthening and low functional strength ratio seems to be beneficial for enhanced ball throwing velocity, we advise against shoulder strength imbalance because of the increased risk of injuries [10, 37].

To our knowledge, this paper is the first which demonstrate the effect of SGA on ball velocity and isokinetic strength parameters in male handball players. Another strength is the use of statistical significance and ES in data analysis, allow researchers to move away from the simple identification of statistical significance toward a more generally interpretable, quantitative description of an effect, independent of the possible misleading influence of sample size. However, data after a real handball game was not analyzed where SGA data was used instead, representing a possible limitation of the study. Further studies verifying the effects of a real handball game on shoulder muscular strength balance should be carried out. Studies investigating whether there is a causal effect between shoulder muscular balance and ball velocity should also be conducted.

Conclusion

SGA had a greater effect on IR than ER muscle strength, likely creating a muscle imbalance in the shoulder joint, which may predispose this to a higher injury risk. These findings may be helpful to exercise and sports science professionals since improving IR muscles endurance may prevent muscular imbalance at end of games. Despite this muscle strength reduction, ball velocity was not affected. Functional strength ratio had a negative correlation with ball velocity. However, muscular imbalance should be discouraged because of the increased risk of injury.

Ethics approval

Participants were informed of the potential risks and benefits of the study and signed an informed consent form to take part. All experimental procedures were approved by the Federal University of São Paulo Human Research Ethics Committee and conformed to the principles outlined in the Declaration of Helsinki.

Additional file

Additional file 1: Availability of raw data. (XLS 25 kb)

Abbreviations

ER: External rotators; ES: Effect size; HR: Heart rate; IR: Internal rotators; r: Pearson's correlation coefficient; SGA: Simulated game activities.

Competing interests

The authors declare that they have no competing interests.

Authors' contributions

MSA and FCK participated in the study design, conducted the experiment, analyzed the data and drafted the manuscript, AAB-S and ACS participated in the study design and provided critical comments on the manuscript, CABL participated in the study design, analyzed the data, participated in data collection and provided critical comments on the manuscript. All authors read and approved the final manuscript.

Acknowledgements

We would like to thank all the athletes who volunteered their time to participate in this study.

Funding

MSA had a fellowship from the Fundação de Amparo à Pesquisa do Estado de São Paulo-FAPESP/Brazil (grant no. 07/59686-8). This paper was partially supported by Financiadora de Estudos e Projetos-Brazilian Science and Technology Ministry (FINEP-MCT-Brazil) and the Brazilian Sports Ministry.

Author details

[1]Departamento de Fisiologia, Universidade Federal de São Paulo (UNIFESP), Rua Botucatu, 862, 5º andar, Vila Clementino, São Paulo, SP CEP: 04023-062, Brazil. [2]Escola de Artes, Ciências e Humanidades, Universidade de São Paulo (USP), Av. Arlindo Béttio, 1000, Ermelino Matarazzo, São Paulo, SP CEP: 03828-000, Brazil. [3]Setor de Fisiologia Humana e do Exercício, Faculdade de Educação Física e Dança, Universidade Federal de Goiás (UFG), Avenida Esperança s/n, Campus Samambaia, Goiânia, GO CEP: 74690-900, Brazil.

References

1. van den Tillaar R, Ettema G. Influence of instruction on velocity and accuracy of overarm throwing. Percept Mot Skills. 2003;96:423–34.
2. Jöris HJ, van Muyen AJ, van Ingen Schenau GJ, Kemper HC. Force, velocity and energy flow during the overarm throw in female handball players. J Biomech. 1985;18:409–14.
3. Noffal GJ. Isokinetic eccentric-to-concentric strength ratios of the shoulder rotator muscles in throwers and nonthrowers. Am J Sports Med. 2003;31:537–41.
4. Andrade Mdos S, Fleury AM, de Lira CA, Dubas JP, da Silva AC. Profile of isokinetic eccentric-to-concentric strength ratios of shoulder rotator muscles in elite female team handball players. J Sports Sci. 2010;28:743–9. doi:10.1080/02640411003645687.
5. Ellenbecker TS, Mattalino AJ. Concentric isokinetic shoulder internal and external rotation strength in professional baseball pitchers. J Orthop Sports Phys Ther. 1997;25:323–8.
6. Wilk KE, Meister K, Andrews JR. Current concepts in the rehabilitation of the overhead throwing athlete. Am J Sports Med. 2002;30:136–51.
7. Codine P, Bernard PL, Pocholle M, Herisson C. Isokinetic strength measurement and training of the shoulder: methodology and results. Ann Readapt Med Phys. 2005;48:80–92.
8. Stickley CD, Hetzler RK, Freemyer BG, Kimura IF. Isokinetic peak torque ratios and shoulder injury history in adolescent female volleyball athletes. J Athl Train. 2008;43:571–7. doi:10.4085/1062-6050-43.6.571.
9. Wang HK, Cochrane T. Mobility impairment, muscle imbalance, muscle weakness, scapular asymmetry and shoulder injury in elite volleyball athletes. J Sports Med Phys Fitness. 2001;41:403–10.
10. Edouard P, Degache F, Oullion R, Plessis JY, Gleizes-Cervera S, Calmels P. Shoulder strength imbalances as injury risk in handball. Int J Sports Med. 2013;34:654–60. doi:10.1055/s-0032-1312587.
11. Andrade Mdos S, de Lira CA, Vancini RL, de Almeida AA, Benedito-Silva AA, da Silva AC. Profiling the isokinetic shoulder rotator muscle strength in 13-to-36-year-old male and female handball players. Phys Ther Sport. 2013;14: 246–52. doi:10.1016/j.ptsp.2012.12.002.
12. Andrade MS, Vancini RL, de Lira CA, Mascarin NC, Fachina RJ, da Silva AC. Shoulder isokinetic profile of male handball players of the Brazilian National Team. Braz J Phys Ther. 2013;17:572–8. doi:10.1590/S1413-35552012005000125.
13. Dello Iacono A, Padulo J, Ayalon M. Core stability training on lower limb balance strength. J Sports Sci. 2016;34:671–8. doi:10.1080/02640414.2015.1068437.
14. Hawkins RD, Fuller CW. A prospective epidemiological study of injuries in four English professional football clubs. Br J Sports Med. 1999;33:196–203.
15. Padulo J, Tiloca A, Powell D, Granatelli G, Bianco A, Paoli A. EMG amplitude of the biceps femoris during jumping compared to landing movements. Springerplus. 2013;2:520. doi:10.1186/2193-1801-2-520.
16. Padulo J, Attene G, Migliaccio GM, Cuzzolin F, Vando S, Ardigò LP. Metabolic optimisation of the basketball free throw. J Sports Sci. 2015;33:1454–8. doi:10.1080/02640414.2014.990494.
17. di Vico R, Ardigò LP, Salernitano G, Chamari K, Padulo J. The acute effect of the tongue position in the mouth on knee isokinetic test performance: a highly surprising pilot study. Muscles Ligaments Tendons J. 2014;3:318–23.
18. Bayios IA, Anastasopoulou EM, Sioudris DS, Boudolos KD. Relationship between isokinetic strength of the internal and external shoulder rotators and ball velocity in team handball. J Sports Med Phys Fitness. 2001;41:229–35.
19. Forthomme B, Croisier JL, Ciccarone G, Crielaard JM, Cloes M. Factors correlated with volleyball spike velocity. Am J Sports Med. 2005;33:1513–9.
20. Bartlett LR, Storey MD, Simons BD. Measurement of upper extremity torque production and its relationship to throwing speed in the competitive athlete. Am J Sports Med. 1989;17:89–91.
21. De Siati F, Laffaye G, Gatta G, Dello Iacono A, Ardigò LP, Padulo J. Neuromuscular and technical abilities related to age in water-polo players. J Sports Sci. 2015;8:1–7 [Epub ahead of print].
22. Squarcini CF, Pires ML, Lopes C, Benedito-Silva AA, Esteves AM, Cornelissen-Guillaume G, Matarazzo C, Garcia D, da Silva MS, Tufik S, de Mello MT. Free-running circadian rhythms of muscle strength, reaction time, and body temperature in totally blind people. Eur J Appl Physiol. 2013;113:157–65. doi:10.1007/s00421-012-2415-8.
23. Dover G, Powers ME. Reliability of joint position sense and force-reproduction measures during internal and external rotation of the shoulder. J Athl Train. 2003;38:304–10.
24. Chaouachi A, Padulo J, Kasmi S, Othmen AB, Chatra M, Behm DG. Unilateral static and dynamic hamstrings stretching increases contralateral hip flexion range of motion. Clin Physiol Funct Imaging. 2015. doi: 10.1111/cpf.12263. [Epub ahead of print].
25. Mascarin NC, Vancini RL, Lira CA, Andrade MS. Stretch-induced reductions in throwing performance are attenuated by warm-up before exercise. J Strength Cond Res. 2015;29:1393–8. doi:10.1519/JSC.0000000000000752.
26. Padulo J, Chamari K, Concu A, Dal Pupo J, Laffaye G, Zagatto AM, Ardigò LP. Concentric and eccentric: muscle contraction or exercise? New perspective. Muscles Ligaments Tendons J. 2014;4(2):158.
27. Cools AM, Geerooms E, Van den Berghe DF, Cambier DC, Witvrouw EE. Isokinetic scapular muscle performance in young elite gymnasts. J Athl Train. 2007;42:458–63.
28. Fox 3rd SM, Naughton JP, Haskell WL. Physical activity and the prevention of coronary heart disease. Ann Clin Res. 1971;3:404–32.
29. Dancey C, Reidy J. Statistics without Maths for Psychology: using SPSS for Windows. 5th ed. London: Prentice Hall; 2011.
30. Cohen J. Statistical power analysis for the behavioral sciences. 2nd ed. Oxford: Lawrence Erlbaum Associates; 1988.
31. Fleiss JL. Balanced incomplete block designs for inter-Rater reliability studies. Appl Psych Meas. 1981;5:105–12. doi:10.1177/014662168100500115.
32. Zapartidis I, Gouvali M, Bayios I, Boudolos K. Throwing effectiveness and rotational strength of the shoulder in team handball. J Sports Med Phys Fitness. 2007;47(2):169–78.
33. Marques MC, van den Tilaar R, Vescovi JD, Gonzalez-Badillo JJ. Relationship between throwing velocity, muscle power, and bar velocity during bench press in elite handball players. Int J Sports Physiol Perform. 2007;2(4):414–22.
34. Atwater AE. Biomechanics of overarm throwing movements and of throwing injuries. Exerc Sport Sci Rev. 1979;7:43–85.
35. Pappas AM, Zawacki RM, Sullivan TJ. Biomechanics of baseball pitching. A preliminary report. Am J Sports Med. 1985;13(4):216–22.
36. Yildiz Y, Aydin T, Sekir U, Kiralp MZ, Hazneci B, Kalyon TA. Shoulder terminal range eccentric antagonist/concentric agonist strength ratios in overhead athletes. Scand J Med Sci Sports. 2006;16:174–80.
37. Niederbracht Y, Shim AL, Sloniger MA, Paternostro-Bayles M, Short TH. Effects of a shoulder injury prevention strength training program on eccentric external rotator muscle strength and glenohumeral joint imbalance in female overhead activity athletes. J Strength Cond Res. 2008;22:140–5. doi:10.1519/JSC.0b013e31815f5634.

22

Maximal strength training as physical rehabilitation for patients with substance use disorder; a randomized controlled trial

Runar Unhjem[1*], Grete Flemmen[1,2], Jan Hoff[1,3] and Eivind Wang[1,4,5]

Abstract

Background: Patients with substance use disorder (SUD) suffer from multiple health and psychosocial problems. Because poor physical capacities following an inactive lifestyle may indeed contribute to these problems, physical training is often suggested as an attractive supplement to conventional SUD treatment. Strength training is shown to increase muscle strength and effectively improve health and longevity. Therefore we investigated the feasibility and effect of a maximal strength training intervention for SUD patients in clinical treatment.

Methods: 16 males and 8 females were randomized into a training group (TG) and a control group (CG). The TG performed lower extremities maximal strength training (85-90 % of 1 repetition maximum (1RM)) 3 times a week for 8 weeks, while the CG participated in conventional clinical activities.

Results: The TG increased hack squat 1RM (88 ± 54 %), plantar flexion 1RM (26 ± 20 %), hack squat rate of force development (82 ± 29 %) and peak force (11 ± 5 %). Additionally, the TG improved neural function, expressed as voluntary V-wave (88 ± 83 %). The CG displayed no change in any physical parameters. The TG also reduced anxiety and insomnia, while the CG reduced anxiety.

Conclusion: Maximal strength training was feasible for SUD patients in treatment, and improved multiple risk factors for falls, fractures and lifestyle related diseases. As conventional treatment appears to have no effect on muscle strength, systematic strength training should be implemented as part of clinical practice.

Trial registration: ClinicalTrials.gov Identifier: NCT02218970 (August 14, 2014).

Keywords: Muscle strength, One repetition maximum, Rate of force development, V-wave, Physical health, Mental health

Background

In addition to their drug abuse, patients with substance use disorder (SUD) suffer from multiple health and psychosocial comorbidities, resulting in a life expectancy 20–30 years less than the general population [1, 2]. Compared to the average population these patients are more frequently represented in medical care, with an elevated incidence of cardiovascular disease [1, 2], diabetes [1, 2], cancer [1, 2], suicide [1, 2], as well as traumas, falls and fractures [3–5]. Recent findings in our laboratory show that muscle strength and aerobic fitness are markedly reduced in SUD patients compared to healthy age-matched individuals [6]. Low muscle strength is associated with increased incidence of falls and fractures [7, 8], poor mechanical efficiency [9], elevated risk of cancer [10] and cardiovascular disease [11], and is even shown to be an independent predictor of all-cause mortality in both patient populations and healthy [12–14].

Strength training has become an increasingly common measure to improve muscle strength in different patient populations, and effectively reduce the risk of medical conditions and mortality. Maximal strength training, with heavy loads (>85 % of 1 repetition maximum (1RM)) and emphasis on intended concentric velocity has been successfully applied in multiple patient

* Correspondence: Runar.Unhjem@gmail.com
[1]Department of Circulation and Medical imaging, Faculty of Medicine, the Norwegian University of Science and Technology, Prinsesse Kristinas gt. 3, 7006 Trondheim, Norway
Full list of author information is available at the end of the article

populations in our labs, and is shown to induce particularly large improvements in rate of force development (RFD) and muscle strength [15–19]. The improvements in maximal strength and RFD are suggested to predominantly rely on neural factors, with little or no change in body mass [9, 18, 20], which results in the training being even more suitable in populations where gains in weight are not sought after. Importantly, no injuries have been reported following these interventions, indicating that the training is not only effective, but also safe. Perhaps even more than the maximal strength, rapid force development is shown to be important for functional status, mechanical efficiency, balance adjustments and the prevention of falls and fractures [21–23]. Because the RFD relies mainly on neuromuscular properties [24], strength training applied to induce functional gain in patient populations should target neural adaptations. Assessed by the use of evoked reflex recordings, our research group has previously documented neural adaptations in both patient and healthy populations following maximal strength training [17, 25].

Although SUD patients are reported to have low muscle strength and aerobic capacity [6], there are few studies of systematic physical training as a part of clinical SUD treatment [26]. While physical activity is commonly used in conventional treatment [27], it appears not to apply a sufficient overload for taxing the muscular strength. Thus, maximal strength training would likely offer additional health benefits, and effectively reduce the risk of medical conditions. In addition to physical benefits, strength training is shown to have a positive effect on mental health, reducing anxiety and depression levels [28–30]. A low muscle strength has even been shown to independently be associated with an elevated rate of suicide [31]. In general, adherence to an exercise regime is also suggested to improve treatment outcomes and possibly reduce relapse rates in patients suffering from alcohol and substance abuse [26, 32].

Since physical activity in clinical treatment often appear random and unstructured [33], without the sufficient overload to produce gains in muscular strength, the aim of this study was to assess if a maximal strength training intervention was feasible for SUD patients, and would yield the previously documented beneficial physical and mental effects of such a training regime. We hypothesized that (1) SUD patients would be able to carry out the 8 week maximal strength training intervention, and (2) that the training group would improve maximal strength, RFD, efferent neural drive, depression, anxiety and insomnia more than the control group that participated in conventional treatment.

Methods

Subjects

24 patients diagnosed with SUD, classified within ICD-10: F10-F19 (mental and behavioral disorders due to psychoactive substance use), were included in the study from February to March 2013. All subjects participated in a ~3 month residential long term treatment at a substance abuse clinic at the University hospital, and had amphetamine as their primary drug. After providing their informed consents subjects were randomized to either a maximal strength training group (TG) or a control group (CG) participating in conventional activities (Fig. 1). Subjects were assigned a number between 1 and 24, and randomization was performed using a publicly accessible official website designed for research randomization (https://www.randomizer.org). Subjects were excluded if they had been abstinent and/or systematically participated in strength training for the last six months. Other exclusion criteria were cardiovascular or respiratory disease, not being able to carry out the testing procedure or failure to participate in at least 20/24 training sessions. Patient characteristics and medical use are shown in Table 1. The study was approved by the regional ethical committee (REK-nord) and conducted in accordance with the declaration of Helsinki.

Extent of drug use

To get an overview of the extent of drug use the first page of EuropASI was applied [34]. The index quantifies which substances the subject has used, age at first time drug use and years of use. Further the clinic provided information of prescribed medicine for the overall participating group of patients. Patient characteristics and medical use are given in Table 1.

Testing procedure

All subjects conducted the testing procedure before and after the 8 week training intervention. On the day of testing, neuromuscular measurements (V-wave) were carried out first, followed by 1RM hack squat, 1RM plantar flexion and hack squat RFD. After the strength measurements, psychological questionnaires were filled out to assess levels of insomnia, anxiety and depression. Subjects were asked to not engage in any physical training on the day of testing or the day before.

Strength measurements

One repetition maximum (1RM) was measured in hack squat and plantar flexion. Hack squat 1RM was obtained in a hack squat machine (Impulse Fitness IT7006, Shandong, China) angled 45° to vertical. For the plantar flexion test, the participants were seated in a calf rise machine (Impulse Health Tech IT7005, Shandong, China),

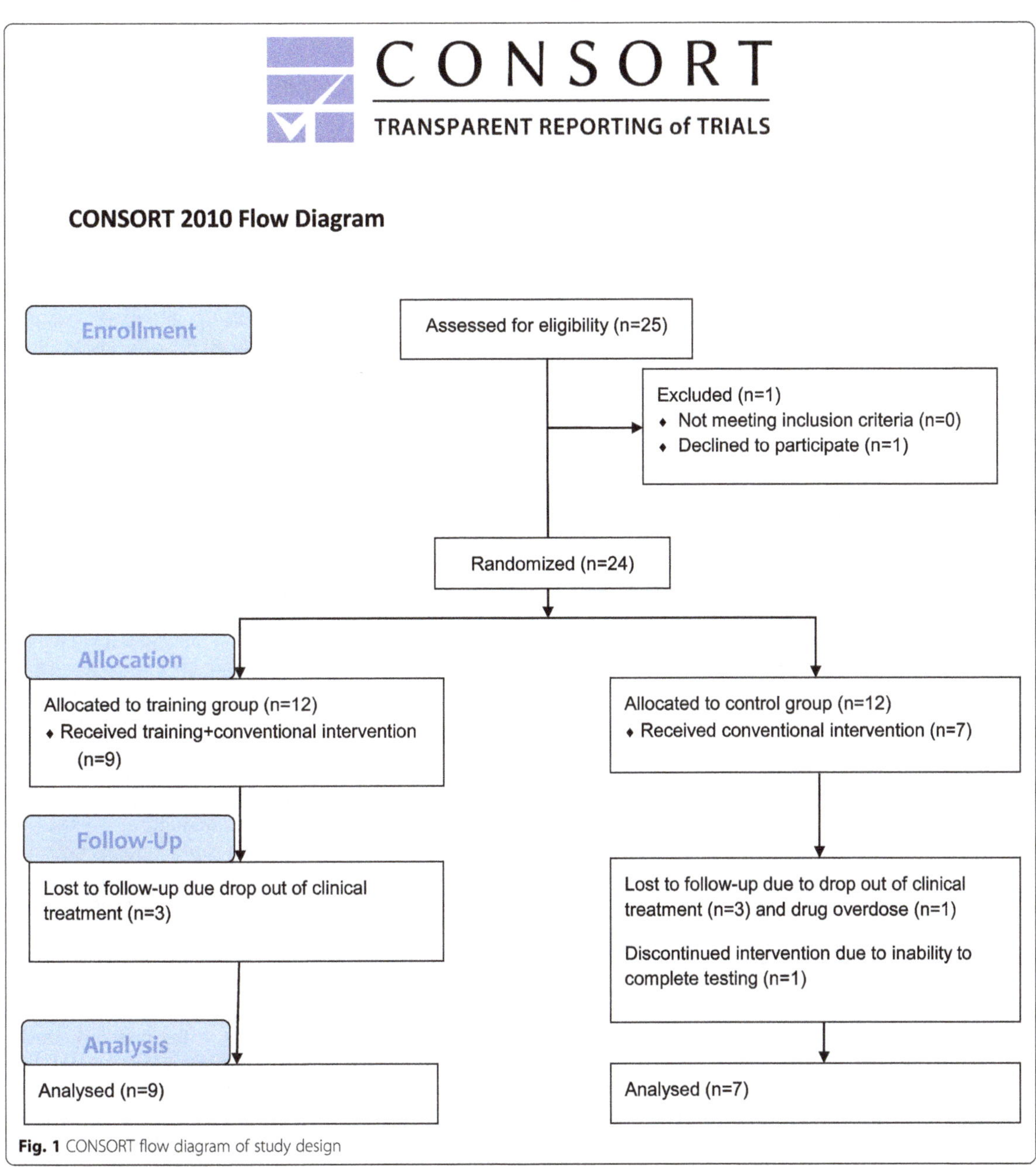

Fig. 1 CONSORT flow diagram of study design

with a knee joint angle of ~90°, and performed their lifts from an ankle joint angle of ~20° dorsiflexion in the lower position, up to ~30° plantar flexion in the upper position. Before testing the subjects were familiarized with the testing apparatus during an extensive warm up procedure, however no additional familiarization session was arranged. For both hack squat and plantar flexion, 1RM was achieved by increasing the load by 5-10 kg until the subject was not able to complete the lift. A three minutes rest was given between each trial, and correct joint angles were ensured. 1RM was achieved within 6–9 trials, and the highest load completed was recorded as 1RM.

RFD was recorded in the hack squat machine with a force platform at 2000Hz (9286AA, Kistler, Switzerland) attached to the foot plate. Each subject was given three attempts with a load corresponding to 80 % of pretest 1RM. Only the best trial was used for analyzes. The subjects were instructed to move slowly down to a knee

Table 1 Patient characteristics and medical use

	TG (n = 9)	CG (n = 7)	Combined (n = 16)
Men/Women (n)	6/3	7/0	13/3
Age (yr)	33 ± 9	29 ± 5	32 ± 8
Weight (kg)	80.2 ± 18.2	81.8 ± 9.6	80.9 ± 14.3
Height (cm)	173 ± 10	181 ± 5	177 ± 9
First time drug use (age)	14 ± 2	15 ± 2	14 ± 2
Duration of abuse (yr)	13 ± 10	11 ± 4	12 ± 8
Current Smoker	7	6	13
Primary drug:			
Amphetamine	9	7	16
Secondary drug:			
Alcohol	4	1	5
Cocaine		1	1
Cannabis	5	5	10
Symptoms for medicine prescription:			
ADHD	1	1	2
Allergies	3	4	7
Anxiety		3	3
Arthiritis	2		2
Asthma/COPD	3	1	4
Depression	3	1	4
Epilepsy		1	1
Hypertension	5		5
Schizofenia/Bipolar	4	1	5
Migrene	3		3
Substitutional treatment		1	1
Other	5	1	6

Data are presented as mean ± SD, *TG*; training group, *CG*; control group. Type of medication is reported on indication of symptoms according to common directory. The prescribed medicine in substitutional treatment is subuxone. Others: atherothrombosis, diabetes, infections

joint angle of 90°, have a short stop to avoid eccentric action involvement, and then mobilize maximally in the concentric phase of the movement. Three minutes rest was given between each trial. The highest concentric force was recorded as peak force and RFD was calculated as Δforce between 10 % and 90 % of peak force [9].

Neuromuscular measurements

Neuromuscular measurements were assessed by voluntary V-waves, with the subjects seated in a fixed version of the plantar flexion apparatus used for dynamic strength measurements. The V-wave method involves electrical stimulation of the tibial nerve, applied to evoke reflex potentials and motor potentials in afferent and efferent nerves. During supramaximal electrical stimulations all afferent and efferent nerve fibers are recruited simultaneously, and the reflex volley traveling the muscle spindle reflex circuit will collide with electrically evoked action potentials traveling antidromically in the efferent axons. Because of these collisions the reflex volley will be completely abolished during rest and not reach the muscle. In contrast, during maximal voluntary contraction (MVC) the efferent drive to the muscle will collide with the antidromic potentials, leaving some efferent axons open for transmission of the reflex. A higher efferent drive will clear more axons for reflex transmission, and will thus allow more of the reflex volley to pass through to the muscle, where it is recorded as a V-wave. Based on this, the amplitude of V-wave is used to express the efferent neural drive during MVC.

Reflex potentials were evoked by a current stimulator (DS7AH, Digitimer, Welwyn Garden City, UK), in the tibial nerve, in the popliteal fossa. The electrical current was delivered by gel-coated (Lectron 2 conductive gel, Pharmaceutical innovations INC, Newark, NJ, USA) bipolar felt pad electrodes, 25 mm between tips, 8 mm diameter (Digitimer, Welwyn Garden City, UK). The electrodes were held by hand throughout the testing procedure, and positioned at the site evoking the largest reflex amplitude. Evoked potentials were recorded through self-adhesive AG/AgCI electrodes (Ambu, M-00-S/50, Ballerup, Denmark) placed as recommended by SENIAM [35] on m. soleus. Before electrode attachment the skin was carefully preparated to minimize the inter-electrode impedance; impedance level <5 kΩ were required. To provide equal conditions from pre- to post-test, pictures were taken of the electrode placement at pretest, and used for identical positioning at posttest.

Searching for the maximal direct motor potential (M_{max}) the current intensity was gradually increased by 2–5 mA until the M-wave reached a plateau. Between 70 and 180 mA was needed to evoke M_{max}. To validate the M_{max} three supramaximal stimuli at 150 % of the current intensity needed to reach the plateau were given. Eight V-waves were evoked during MVC by delivering a supramaximal (150 %) stimulus at the point where the subject reached ~90 % of MVC force. Each MVC was separated by 1 min rest. Only V-wave recordings, in which the M-wave was > 90 % of $M_{max,}$ were used for analyzes. The maximal V-wave amplitude (V_{max}) was expressed relative to M_{max} (V/M-ratio), to allow between subjects comparisons. Changes in V/M-ratio are used to express changes in efferent drive following training.

Psychological questionnaires

In addition to the physical testing two questionnaires were implemented; Insomnia Severity Index (ISI) to measure level of insomnia, and Hospital Anxiety & Depression Scale (HAD), used to estimate symptoms of anxiety and depression. These self-report questionnaires were answered in conjunction with the pre- and posttest of muscular strength, as measures of psychological changes during the period of the study. The ISI has been evaluated to be a clinically useful tool for screening and quantifying perceived insomnia severity [36]. It is composed of 7 items targeting different categories of sleep disturbance severity. The items are rated at a five-point Likert scale (0–4) summed up to provide a total score ranging from 0–28, where a higher score indicates more severe insomnia. The score categories are 0–7 (no clinically significant insomnia), 8–14 (subthreshold insomnia), 15–21 (clinical insomnia, moderate severity) and 22–28 (clinical insomnia, severe). The HAD self-assessment scale consists of a fourteen item scale, seven items relate to anxiety and seven relate to depression. On the seven item HADS subscales a score of 0–7 for either subscale is estimated within the normal range, a score of 11 or higher implies a probable presence of a mood disorder. A score of 8–10 is considered signs of a mood disorder [37].

Training intervention

Both the TG and the CG attended the regular treatment program at the substance abuse clinic during the intervention period. The treatment program activities included: Ballgames (indoor-soccer, bandy and volleyball), yoga, stretching, outdoor walking, low resistance strength training (estimated <50 % of 1RM), ceramics, TV games and card games. Together this resulted in a total of ~3 h of physical activity per week. In addition, the TG received maximal strength training 3 times a week for a period of 8 weeks. The training intervention consisted of two exercises; hack squat and plantar flexion. Both exercises consisted of 4 sets of 4–5 repetitions, corresponding to 85-90 % of 1RM. The training load was increased with 5 kg if 5 repetitions were accomplished in the last set. Both exercises were conducted with a slow controlled movement in the eccentric phase, a short stop, and then maximal mobilization of force in the concentric movement. Hack squat was performed with 90° knee joint angle, while the plantar flexion exercise was performed from an ankle joint angle of ~20° dorsiflexion up to ~30° plantar flexion. Every training session was supervised to ensure proper technique and progression throughout the training period. While the TG participated in the supervised strength training, the CG chose to participate in self-elected supervised activities among the offered sports or games in the clinical treatment program.

Statistical analyzes

Statistical analyzes were done using IBM SPSS Statistics 21 (Chicago, IL, USA), while figures were created using GraphPad Prism 5 (San Diego, USA). Independent and paired t tests were used to examine differences between groups at baseline and within groups following training, respectively. Between group differences following training were determined by use of two-way repeated ANOVAS. The Pearson test for linear regression was applied to assess correlations. Statistical significance level was set to $p < 0.05$. All variables exhibited normal distribution, as confirmed by quantile-quantile plots. Data are presented as mean ± SD unless otherwise noted.

Results

Completion

Of the 24 patients that were included in the study, 16 subjects completed the study period. 3 patients in the TG dropped out of the clinical treatment, and hence also dropped out of the study. In the CG 5 subjects dropped out; 3 patients dropped out of clinical treatment, 1 patient were not able to complete the testing procedure and 1 patient died from drug overdose. The withdrawal in the two groups resulted in an uneven distribution of genders, leaving no females in the CG at posttest. The participants in the TG adhered to 23 ± 1 of the 24 scheduled training sessions during the training period. The patients completed all commenced training sessions and the targeted intensity (85–90 % of 1RM) was reached in all sessions.

Muscle strength measurements

For the 16 subjects that completed the study, there was no significant difference between the TG and the CG in any of the measured strength parameters at pretest. After 8 weeks of maximal strength training the TG increased 1RM hack squat by 88 ± 54 % ($p < 0.01$) (Fig. 2), whereas plantar flexion 1RM increased from 98 ± 23 kg to 121 ± 17 kg (26 ± 20 %, $p < 0.01$). The TG also increased RFD by 82 ± 28 % ($p < 0.01$) (Fig. 3), whereas peak force increased from 1846 ± 357 N to 2045 ± 415 N (11 ± 5 %, $p < 0.01$). No significant changes were observed in the CG for any of the strength parameters.

Neuromuscular measurements

Maximal strength training led to an enhanced efferent neural drive in the TG. Following the 8 week training intervention the TG increased m. soleus V_{max} from 1583 ± 1596μv to 2189 ± 1375μv (92 ± 95 % ($p < 0.01$)). As there was no observed change in m. soleus M_{max} (6379 ± 2188μv vs. 6332 ± 2244μv), this resulted in an 88 ± 83 % ($p < 0.01$) increase in m. soleus V/M-ratio (Fig. 4). No significant changes were observed for the CG. Finally, ΔV/M-ratio correlated with Δhack squat 1RM ($r = 0.44$, $p < 0.05$) and Δplantar flexion 1RM ($r = 0.57$, $p < 0.05$).

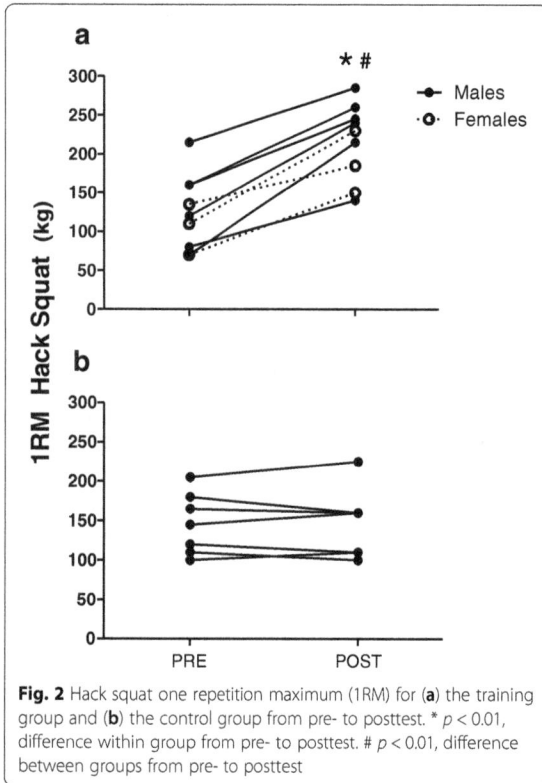

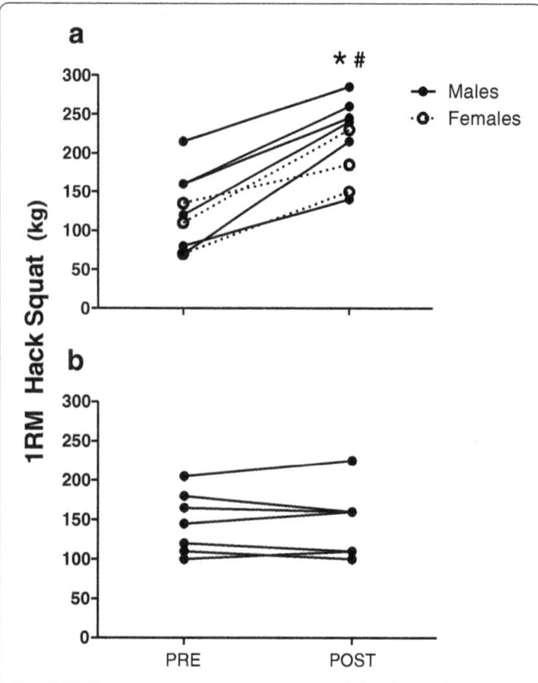

Fig. 2 Hack squat one repetition maximum (1RM) for (**a**) the training group and (**b**) the control group from pre- to posttest. * $p < 0.01$, difference within group from pre- to posttest. # $p < 0.01$, difference between groups from pre- to posttest

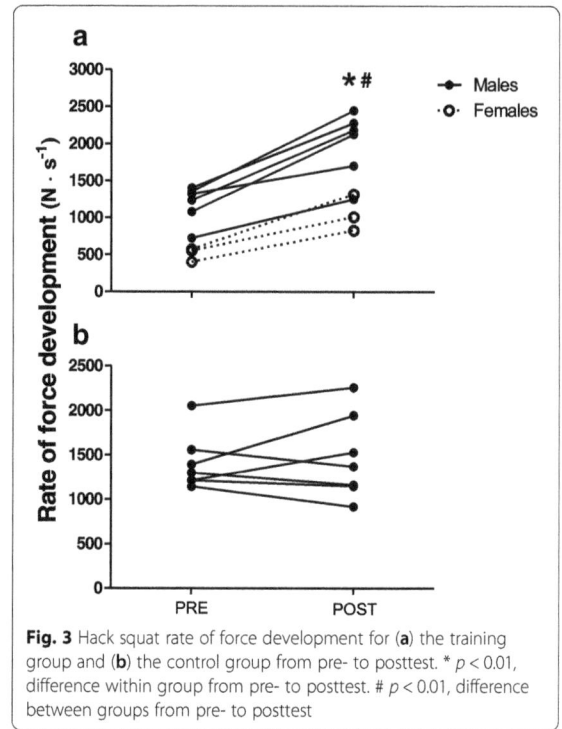

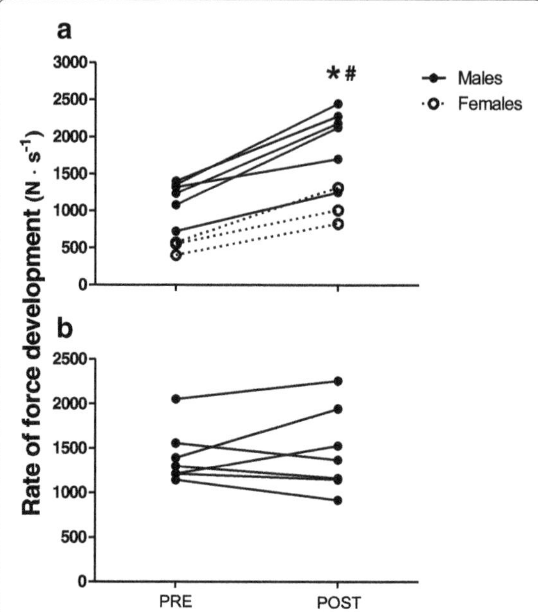

Fig. 3 Hack squat rate of force development for (**a**) the training group and (**b**) the control group from pre- to posttest. * $p < 0.01$, difference within group from pre- to posttest. # $p < 0.01$, difference between groups from pre- to posttest

Psychosocial variables

Both the TG and the CG scored within "probable presence of mood disorder" at inclusion, with elevated scores of anxiety and insomnia. Following the study period both the TG and the CG displayed significant within group reductions in anxiety level ($p < 0.05$), while the level of insomnia significantly decreased only in the TG ($p < 0.05$) (Table 2). Also the level of depression tended to decrease in both groups ($p = 0.11$ for the TG and $p = 0.10$ for the CG). Neither of the within group differences were apparent as between-group differences.

Discussion

Main findings

SUD patients suffer from physical and psychological deconditioning as a consequence of their detrimental lifestyle. Since strength training is documented to improve both physical and mental health, we sought to investigate the feasibility and efficiency of a maximal strength training regime for a group of SUD patients in residential treatment. The main findings were that 1) A maximal strength training intervention was feasible for SUD patients in treatment, 2) Maximal strength training effectively improved maximal strength and muscle force development characteristics, likely caused by alterations in the central nervous system, 3) Anxiety and insomnia were improved following the clinical treatment period.

Improved maximal strength and muscle force development characteristics

As expected the SUD patients that completed the strength training intervention displayed large improvements in all the measured strength parameters. The 88 % increase in hack squat 1 RM after 8 weeks of

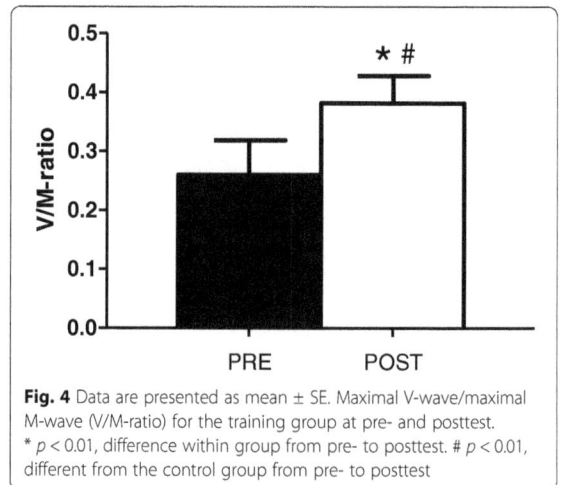

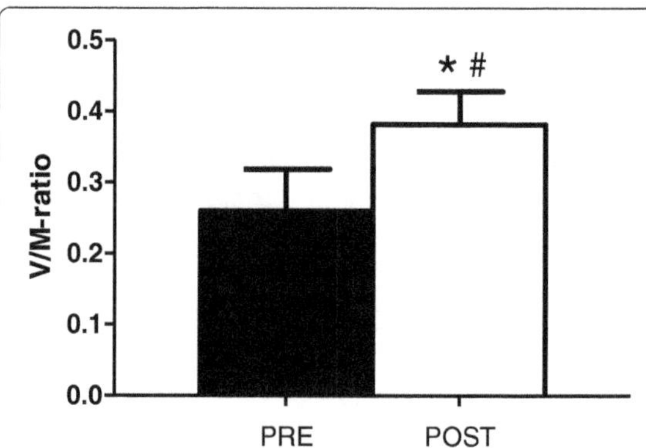

Fig. 4 Data are presented as mean ± SE. Maximal V-wave/maximal M-wave (V/M-ratio) for the training group at pre- and posttest. * $p < 0.01$, difference within group from pre- to posttest. # $p < 0.01$, different from the control group from pre- to posttest

Table 2 Psychological measurements, changes from pre- to posttest (scores from insomnia severity index and hospital anxiety and depression scale questionnaires)

	TG ($n = 9$)		CG ($n = 7$)	
	Pre	Post	Pre	Post
Anxiety (0–21)	12.3 ± 5.8	6.3 ± 3.9 *	11.1 ± 4.5	8.0 ± 4.8 *
Depression (0–21)	5.2 ± 2.1	3.0 ± 1.6	7.4 ± 4.7	4.9 ± 3.8
Insomnia (0–28)	9.2 ± 6.5	3.0 ± 2.0 *	13.3 ± 6.2	10.1 ± 5.3

Data are presented as mean ± SD, *TG*; Training group, *CG*; Control group. Score categories anxiety and depression: Normal (0–7); signs of mood disorder (8–10); probable presence of mood disorder (11–21). Score categories insomnia: No clinically significant insomnia (0–7); subthreshold insomnia (8–14); clinical insomnia, moderate severity (15–21); clinical insomnia, severe (22–28). * $p < 0.05$, difference within group pre- to posttest

training is even somewhat higher than most previous maximal strength training studies, typically ranging between 25–45 % [9, 18, 19, 38, 39]. Since familiarization was included as a part of the training intervention in this study, this likely contributed to the large strength gain. Additionally, the very low baseline of the weakest subject, which allowed for a very large percentage improvement of ~200 %, also contributed to the high percentage improvement of the TG. Nevertheless, our findings demonstrate the large strength gain achievable when heavy loads and maximal intended concentric velocity are emphasized in strength training. Recognizing that the low physical baseline of the patients in the current study allows large training adaptations, both physiologically and mathematically, the large increase in hack squat 1RM highlights the clinical benefit of a high intensity training intervention in effective physical rehabilitation. The health benefits from an 88 % improvement in leg muscle strength are unquestionable. Ortega et al. [31] reported that Swedish men with high muscular strength had 35 % lower risk of developing cardiovascular disease, 15–65 % lower risk of having any psychiatric diagnosis and 20 % lower risk of all cause mortality when compared to men with low muscle strength. Also Ruiz et al. [10, 12] found the risk of mortality from cancer, cardiovascular disease and other causes to be inversely correlated with muscle strength. Both the Ortega et al. (2012) study and the Ruiz et al. [10, 12] studies emphasize that subjects with low and very low muscle strength particularly suffer an increased risk of medical complications. Considering this, increasing the strength of the weakest individuals would provide the largest health benefit. Although we did not compare our subjects with a reference group some of the patients in the current study stood out as particularly weak. Interestingly it was these patients who apparently seemed to benefit the most from the training. This visual observation was also reflected in the psychosocial questionnaires, where the three weakest subjects exhibited substantial improvements in the psychosocial variables following the training period.

High muscle strength is also associated with lower risk of falls and fractures [7, 8]. Moreland et al. [40] reported that subjects with low and very low muscle strength exhibited elevated risk of single and recurrent falling (Odds ratio: 1.31–5.06). Considering the high incidence of non-drug related hospitalizations among SUD-patients, typically including traumas, falls and fractures [3–5], it is likely that the improved muscle strength would have a preventive effect on these high injury- and hospitalization rates. Balance adjustments and fall prevention do not only require maximal strength; the ability of rapid muscle contractions is often just as important, since the time frame to avoid a fall is short [21, 22, 41]. Because strength training with heavy loads and maximal concentric mobilization is associated with large gain in explosive strength, maximal strength training is argued to be particularly beneficial to induce gain in motor function. The 82 % increase in RFD in the current study adds evidence of the large improvements in explosive strength following maximal strength training regimes, and is similar to previous reports from our research group [18, 38, 39].

Neuromuscular alterations and maximal strength training

The ~ twofold increase in V/M-ratio highlights that neuromuscular changes largely contributed to the gain in muscle strength. Although there is agreement that training-induced changes in muscle strength relies on a combination of neuromuscular and anabolic adaptations [42], studies involving maximal strength training have often claimed that the improvements were mainly of neuromuscular origin, due to large improvements in 1RM and RFD, with no change in body weight [9, 18, 20]. Based on the comparable large improvements in V/M-ratio and maximal strength, as well as the lack of change in body weight, our findings are in line with this notion. It is unlikely that the low number of repetitions, and thus low anabolic effect, was sufficient to induce any significant muscle growth, while the heavy loads and maximal mobilization seems to be optimal for neural adaptations [20, 43]. The 88 % increase in V/M-ratio is slightly higher compared to other strength training studies, typically displaying improvements of 50–80 % [44, 45]. However, these interventions have been conducted with a lower training intensity than the current, consequently also resulting in smaller improvements maximal strength. Therefore, in combination, our findings and previous studies, exhibits corresponding improvements in neuromuscular adaptations and muscular strength. Specifically, the changes in V-wave amplitude in the current study likely reflects an enhanced efferent neural drive to the muscle, probably due to increased motor unit firing frequency and/or increased motoneuron recruitment [44, 46]. This is because a higher efferent drive would allow more of the electrically evoked reflex volley to pass through to the muscle, hence resulting in the increased amplitude of the V-wave.

Feasibility of maximal strength training in substance use clinical treatment

The 75 % completion rate of the TG in the current study exemplifies that although maximal strength training may be considered strenuous, SUD patients are in general capable of engaging in physically demanding training regimes. To date there have been few studies examining intensive physical training in SUD patients, but we have recently shown that also intensive endurance training is feasible for this patient group [33]. In agreement with our findings from the endurance training study, the SUD patients reported no difficulties carrying out the strength training, and the targeted intensity (85–90 % of 1 RM) was reached in all commenced training sessions, without any reports of pain or discomfort. Importantly, most of the subjects that participated reported that they found the simple and robust training motivating, and that they enjoyed observing their own steady and impressing large progression throughout the study. Although SUD is commonly associated with high rates of nonattendance and relapse [47, 48], we experienced no issues regarding subject compliance and attendance to the scheduled training sessions. None of the participating subjects in clinical treatment dropped out solely from the training intervention. Despite being simple and time-efficient to carry out, the training intervention likely benefits from supervision from a trained professional to provide commitment to, and understanding of, the training regime. This notion is also in agreement with previous studies employing training interventions in SUD-patients [33, 49]. Notably, our experience involves only patients participating in residential treatment. It should therefore be considered that the same feasibility and completion rates may not apply for outpatients.

Maximal strength training and psychosocial health

The SUD patients in the current study revealed significant signs of mood disorder at inclusion, reflected in elevated scores of anxiety and insomnia. The TG showed a reduction in both anxiety and insomnia scores, as well as a trend towards less depression. However, a reduction in depression following endurance training has previously been reported [33]. In combination, this is evidence that effective, intensive exercise training is not mentally harmful but, again, feasible. Since these improvements in this study are not significantly different from the CG it is difficult to conclude whether the mental health improvements were related to the clinical treatment itself or if they were a result of the improvements in muscle strength. Physical activity is in general shown to positively affect mental health [29], and it may therefore be that the mental health improvements are more related to physical activity performed by both groups, rather than the improvements in muscle strength. However, given the large beneficial effect of an improved physical capacity, and the substantial risk-reduction for diseases and thus likely improvement in quality of life, a clinical treatment including effective physical training should be advocated. Indeed, a close association between physical training and mental health has previously been reported [50–52]. Furthermore, it should be questioned whether self-reporting questionnaires that are not able to detect large training-induced decreases in risk of lifestyle-related diseases are good enough.

Clinical considerations for effective physical training in clinical treatment

Recognizing the close relationship between physical capacities, life style related diseases and mortality [10, 53], it is likely that implementation of effective physical training as standard part of the treatment for SUD patients would decrease the high rates of non-drug related hospitalizations. This study shows that maximal strength training not only is feasible as a part of the treatment, it also has a large effect size and is time efficient. Previously we have shown similar findings for endurance training [33]. Adding to the arguments for implementation of effective physical training in the clinic is also the poor rehabilitation results observed in the CG participating in conventional physical activity. The current study observed that the muscular strength and force characteristics in the CG remained unchanged following the 8 week period. In a previous study similar observations were also reported for endurance capacity [33]. Although SUD patients suffer from many challenges, it is important to recognize that their physical health constitutes an important part of the overall health. Since muscle strength and aerobic capacity are known to be important contributors to the physical health, we would argue that strength- and endurance training should be carried out concurrently in clinical SUD treatment. Not only are these physical characteristics shown to be very low in SUD patients [6], today's treatment also appears to have very limited, if any endurance and strength effects. Importantly, this study, as well as a recent endurance training study [33] suggests that effective strength- and endurance training regimes are feasible and safe to carry out within this patient group.

Interestingly, the dropout rate in the TG (3 subjects) in the current study was lower than in the CG (5 subjects). Again, a similar finding was documented following endurance training (3 subjects) vs. conventional treatment (5 subjects) [33]. It is also of importance that the three subjects that dropped out of this study dropped out of the general clinical treatment, and not solely the adherence to the maximal strength training intervention. In support of this notion, it has previously been suggested that participation and adherence to an exercise program may have a positive effect on the relapse rates during alcohol recovery [32]. In combination, these findings suggest that implementation of effective physical training will improve the patients' physical health more than conventional treatment, and it is likely that it may also lead to gains in psychosocial health.

Study limitations

The training-induced changes of the main physiological variables were statistical significant in this study. However, a larger sample size may have been beneficial for the psychosocial variables, or perhaps a replacement by more detailed psychosocial questionnaires. While this study exemplifies that high intensity strength training is effective and feasible in SUD treatment, it should be noted that all patients in the current study had amphetamine as their primary drug, and that they were all recruited from the same clinic. While the conventional treatment in this clinic did not have any effect on the physical variables, it cannot be excluded that other clinics may have more effective treatment programs. Similarly, it can also be questioned whether our results would have been different if we had included patients with other primary drugs than amphetamine. As both patient characteristics and clinical treatment programs may vary between clinics, future studies should aim to investigate the effect of effective physical training in multiple clinics, and also aim for larger sample sizes to target psychosocial variables and include patients with different primary drugs.

Conclusion

This study shows that maximal strength training is a feasible, safe and effective method to improve muscle strength and function during SUD treatment. The large improvements in maximal strength and RFD that were observed following two months of training seemed to rely largely on neuromuscular adaptations. The improvements in physical health implies that the SUD patients have reduced their risk for traumas, falls and fractures, life style related diseases and all-cause mortality. Recognizing the poor physical condition of SUD patients, effective physical training, targeting muscle strength and aerobic capacity should be implemented in clinical treatment to improve physical and mental health.

Abbreviations

1RM: one repetition maximum; CG: control group; HAD: hospital anxiety & depression scale; ISI: insomnia severity index; M_{max}: maximal M-wave amplitude; MVC: maximal voluntary contraction; RFD: rate of force development; SUD: substance use disorder; TG: training group; V_{max}: maximal V-wave amplitude; V/M- ratio: maximal V-wave amplitude / maximal M-wave amplitude.

Competing interests

The authors declare that they have no competing interests.

Authors' contributions

RU has contributed as main author of the paper as well as physical testing. GF has contributed with subject recruitment, training and physical testing. JH has contributed with study design and writing of the paper. EW has contributed with study design and writing of the paper. All authors have read and approved the final version of the manuscript.

Acknowledgements

The authors would like to thank the subjects who volunteered to participate in this study for their time and efforts. The study was funded by the Norwegian University of Science and Technology.

Author details

[1]Department of Circulation and Medical imaging, Faculty of Medicine, the Norwegian University of Science and Technology, Prinsesse Kristinas gt. 3, 7006 Trondheim, Norway. [2]Department of Research and Development, Clinic of Substance Use and Addiction Medicine, St. Olav University Hospital, Trondheim, Norway. [3]Department of Physical Medicine and Rehabilitation, St. Olav University Hospital, Trondheim, Norway. [4]Division of Psychiatry, Department of Østmarka, St. Olav University Hospital, Trondheim, Norway. [5]Department of Internal Medicine, University of Utah, Salt Lake City, Utah, USA.

References

1. Nordentoft M, Wahlbeck K, Hallgren J, Westman J, Osby U, Alinaghizadeh H, et al. Excess mortality, causes of death and life expectancy in 270,770 patients with recent onset of mental disorders in Denmark, Finland and Sweden. PLoS One. 2013;8(1):e55176. doi:10.1371/journal.pone.0055176.
2. Stenbacka M, Leifman A, Romelsjo A. Mortality and cause of death among 1705 illicit drug users: a 37 year follow up. Drug Alcohol Rev. 2010;29(1):21–7. doi:10.1111/j.1465-3362.2009.00075.x.
3. Richards JR, Bretz SW, Johnson EB, Turnipseed SD, Brofeldt BT, Derlet RW. Methamphetamine abuse and emergency department utilization. West J Med. 1999;170(4):198–202.
4. Mosenthal AC, Livingston DH, Elcavage J, Merritt S, Stucker S. Falls: epidemiology and strategies for prevention. J Trauma. 1995;38(5):753–6.
5. Fang JF, Shih LY, Lin BC, Hsu YP. Pelvic fractures due to falls from a height in people with mental disorders. Injury. 2008;39(8):881–8. doi:10.1016/j.injury.2008.03.012.
6. Flemmen G, Wang E. Impaired aerobic endurance and muscular strength in substance use disorder patients: implications for health and premature death. Med (Baltimore). 2015;94(44):e1914. doi:10.1097/MD.0000000000001914.
7. Pijnappels M, van der Burg PJ, Reeves ND, van Dieen JH. Identification of elderly fallers by muscle strength measures. Eur J Appl Physiol. 2008;102(5):585–92. doi:10.1007/s00421-007-0613-6.
8. Jarvinen TL, Sievanen H, Khan KM, Heinonen A, Kannus P. Shifting the focus in fracture prevention from osteoporosis to falls. BMJ. 2008;336(7636):124–6. doi:10.1136/bmj.39428.470752.AD.
9. Hoff J, Tjonna AE, Steinshamn S, Hoydal M, Richardson RS, Helgerud J. Maximal strength training of the legs in COPD: a therapy for mechanical inefficiency. Med Sci Sports Exerc. 2007;39(2):220–6. doi:10.1249/01.mss.0000246989.48729.39.
10. Ruiz JR, Sui X, Lobelo F, Lee DC, Morrow Jr JR, Jackson AW, et al. Muscular strength and adiposity as predictors of adulthood cancer mortality in men. Cancer Epidemiol Biomarkers Prev. 2009;18(5):1468–76. doi:10.1158/1055-9965.EPI-08-1075.
11. Artero EG, Lee DC, Lavie CJ, Espana-Romero V, Sui X, Church TS, et al. Effects of muscular strength on cardiovascular risk factors and prognosis. J Cardiopulm Rehabil Prev. 2012;32(6):351–8. doi:10.1097/HCR.0b013e3182642688.

12. Ruiz JR, Sui X, Lobelo F, Morrow Jr JR, Jackson AW, Sjostrom M, et al. Association between muscular strength and mortality in men: prospective cohort study. BMJ. 2008;337:a439. doi:10.1136/bmj.a439.
13. Timpka S, Petersson IF, Zhou C, Englund M. Muscle strength in adolescent men and risk of cardiovascular disease events and mortality in middle age: a prospective cohort study. BMC Med. 2014;12(1):62. doi:10.1186/1741-7015-12-62.
14. Stenholm S, Mehta NK, Elo IT, Heliovaara M, Koskinen S, Aromaa A. Obesity and muscle strength as long-term determinants of all-cause mortality–a 33-year follow-up of the Mini-Finland Health Examination Survey. Int J Obes (Lond). 2014;38(8):1126–32. doi:10.1038/ijo.2013.214.
15. Mosti MP, Kaehler N, Stunes AK, Hoff J, Syversen U. Maximal strength training in postmenopausal women with osteoporosis or osteopenia. J Strength Cond Res. 2013;27(10):2879–86. doi:10.1519/JSC.0b013e318280d4e2.
16. Hill TR, Gjellesvik TI, Moen PM, Torhaug T, Fimland MS, Helgerud J, et al. Maximal strength training enhances strength and functional performance in chronic stroke survivors. Am J Phys Med Rehabil. 2012;91(5):393–400. doi:10.1097/PHM.0b013e31824ad5b8.
17. Fimland MS, Helgerud J, Gruber M, Leivseth G, Hoff J. Enhanced neural drive after maximal strength training in multiple sclerosis patients. Eur J Appl Physiol. 2010;110(2):435–43. doi:10.1007/s00421-010-1519-2.
18. Wang E, Helgerud J, Loe H, Indseth K, Kaehler N, Hoff J. Maximal strength training improves walking performance in peripheral arterial disease patients. Scand J Med Sci Sports. 2010;20(5):764–70. doi:10.1111/j.1600-0838.2009.01014.x.
19. Heggelund J, Morken G, Helgerud J, Nilsberg GE, Hoff J. Therapeutic effects of maximal strength training on walking efficiency in patients with schizophrenia - a pilot study. BMC Res Notes. 2012;5:344. doi:10.1186/1756-0500-5-344.
20. Storen O, Helgerud J, Stoa EM, Hoff J. Maximal strength training improves running economy in distance runners. Med Sci Sports Exerc. 2008;40(6):1087–92. doi:10.1249/MSS.0b013e318168da2f.
21. Hvid L, Aagaard P, Justesen L, Bayer ML, Andersen JL, Ortenblad N, et al. Effects of aging on muscle mechanical function and muscle fiber morphology during short-term immobilization and subsequent retraining. J Appl Physiol (1985). 2010;109(6):1628–34. doi:10.1152/japplphysiol.00637.2010.
22. Wyszomierski SA, Chambers AJ, Cham R. Knee strength capabilities and slip severity. J Appl Biomech. 2009;25(2):140–8.
23. Osteras H, Helgerud J, Hoff J. Maximal strength-training effects on force-velocity and force-power relationships explain increases in aerobic performance in humans. Eur J Appl Physiol. 2002;88(3):255–63. doi:10.1007/s00421-002-0717-y.
24. Aagaard P, Simonsen EB, Andersen JL, Magnusson P, Dyhre-Poulsen P. Increased rate of force development and neural drive of human skeletal muscle following resistance training. J Appl Physiol (1985). 2002;93(4):1318–26. doi:10.1152/japplphysiol.00283.2002.
25. Fimland MS, Helgerud J, Gruber M, Leivseth G, Hoff J. Functional maximal strength training induces neural transfer to single-joint tasks. Eur J Appl Physiol. 2009;107(1):21–9. doi:10.1007/s00421-009-1096-4.
26. Linke SE, Ussher M. Exercise-based treatments for substance use disorders: evidence, theory, and practicality. Am J Drug Alcohol Abuse. 2015;41(1):7–15. doi:10.3109/00952990.2014.976708.
27. Mamen A, Martinsen EW. Development of aerobic fitness of individuals with substance abuse/dependence following long-term individual physical activity. Eur J Sport Sci. 2010;10(4):255–62. doi:10.1080/17461390903377126.
28. Cassilhas RC, Antunes HK, Tufik S, de Mello MT. Mood, anxiety, and serum IGF-1 in elderly men given 24 weeks of high resistance exercise. Percept Mot Skills. 2010;110(1):265–76.
29. Martinsen EW, Hoffart A, Solberg O. Comparing aerobic with nonaerobic forms of exercise in the treatment of clinical depression: a randomized trial. Compr Psychiatry. 1989;30(4):324–31.
30. Doyne EJ, Ossip-Klein DJ, Bowman ED, Osborn KM, McDougall-Wilson IB, Neimeyer RA. Running versus weight lifting in the treatment of depression. J Consult Clin Psychol. 1987;55(5):748–54.
31. Ortega FB, Silventoinen K, Tynelius P, Rasmussen F. Muscular strength in male adolescents and premature death: cohort study of one million participants. BMJ. 2012;345, e7279. doi:10.1136/bmj.e7279.
32. Brown RA, Abrantes AM, Read JP, Marcus BH, Jakicic J, Strong DR, et al. Aerobic exercise for alcohol recovery: rationale, program description, and preliminary findings. Behav Modif. 2009;33(2):220–49. doi:10.1177/0145445508329112.
33. Flemmen G, Unhjem R, Wang E. High-intensity interval training in patients with substance use disorder. Biomed Res Int. 2014;2014:616935. doi:10.1155/2014/616935.
34. McLellan AT, Kushner H, Metzger D, Peters R, Smith I, Grissom G, et al. The fifth edition of the addiction severity index. J Subst Abuse Treat. 1992;9(3):199–213.
35. Hermens HJ, Freriks B, Disselhorst-Klug C, Rau G. Development of recommendations for SEMG sensors and sensor placement procedures. J Electromyogr Kinesiol. 2000;10(5):361–74.
36. Bastien CH, Vallieres A, Morin CM. Validation of the insomnia severity index as an outcome measure for insomnia research. Sleep Med. 2001;2(4):297–307. doi:10.1016/S1389-9457(00)00065-4.
37. Vaeroy H. Depression, anxiety, and history of substance abuse among Norwegian inmates in preventive detention: reasons to worry? BMC Psychiatry. 2011;11:40. doi:10.1186/1471-244X-11-40.
38. Helgerud J, Karlsen T, Kim WY, Hoydal KL, Stoylen A, Pedersen H, et al. Interval and strength training in CAD patients. Int J Sports Med. 2011;32(1):54–9. doi:10.1055/s-0030-1267180.
39. Karlsen T, Helgerud J, Stoylen A, Lauritsen N, Hoff J. Maximal strength training restores walking mechanical efficiency in heart patients. Int J Sports Med. 2009;30(5):337–42. doi:10.1055/s-0028-1105946.
40. Moreland JD, Richardson JA, Goldsmith CH, Clase CM. Muscle weakness and falls in older adults: a systematic review and meta-analysis. J Am Geriatr Soc. 2004;52(7):1121–9. doi:10.1111/j.1532-5415.2004.52310.x.
41. Skelton DA, Kennedy J, Rutherford OM. Explosive power and asymmetry in leg muscle function in frequent fallers and non-fallers aged over 65. Age Ageing. 2002;31(2):119–25.
42. Sale DG, Martin JE, Moroz DE. Hypertrophy without increased isometric strength after weight training. Eur J Appl Physiol Occup Physiol. 1992;64(1):51–5.
43. Behm DG, Sale DG. Intended rather than actual movement velocity determines velocity-specific training response. J Appl Physiol (1985). 1993;74(1):359–68.
44. Aagaard P, Simonsen EB, Andersen JL, Magnusson P, Dyhre-Poulsen P. Neural adaptation to resistance training: changes in evoked V-wave and H-reflex responses. J Appl Physiol (1985). 2002;92(6):2309–18. doi:10.1152/japplphysiol.01185.2001.
45. Del Balso C, Cafarelli E. Adaptations in the activation of human skeletal muscle induced by short-term isometric resistance training. J Appl Physiol (1985). 2007;103(1):402–11. doi:10.1152/japplphysiol.00477.2006.
46. Vila-Cha C, Falla D, Correia MV, Farina D. Changes in H reflex and V wave following short-term endurance and strength training. J Appl Physiol (1985). 2012;112(1):54–63. doi:10.1152/japplphysiol.00802.2011.
47. Sparr LF, Moffitt MC, Ward MF. Missed psychiatric appointments - who returns and who stays away. Am J Psychiat. 1993;150(5):801–5.
48. Ball SA, Carroll KM, Canning-Ball M, Rounsaville BJ. Reasons for dropout from drug abuse treatment: symptoms, personality, and motivation. Addict Behav. 2006;31(2):320–30. doi:10.1016/j.addbeh.2005.05.013.
49. Mamen A, Pallesen S, Martinsen EW. Changes in mental distress following individualized physical training in patients suffering from chemical dependence. Eur J Sport Sci. 2011;11(4):269–76. doi:10.1080/17461391.2010.509889.
50. Martinsen EW, Medhus A, Sandvik L. Effects of aerobic exercise on depression - a controlled-study. Brit Med J. 1985;291(6488):109.
51. Galper DI, Trivedi MH, Barlow CE, Dunn AL, Kampert JB. Inverse association between physical inactivity and mental health in men and women. Med Sci Sport Exer. 2006;38(1):173–8. doi:10.1249/01.mss.0000180883.32116.28.
52. Mota-Pereira J, Silverio J, Carvalho S, Ribeiro JC, Fonte D, Ramos J. Moderate exercise improves depression parameters in treatment-resistant patients with major depressive disorder. J Psychiatr Res. 2011;45(8):1005–11. doi:10.1016/j.jpsychires.2011.02.005.
53. Myers J, Prakash M, Froelicher V, Do D, Partington S, Atwood JE. Exercise capacity and mortality among men referred for exercise testing. N Engl J Med. 2002;346(11):793–801. doi:10.1056/NEJMoa011858.

23

A systematic review of financial incentives given in the healthcare setting; do they effectively improve physical activity levels?

Claudia C. M. Molema[1,2*], G. C. Wanda Wendel-Vos[2], Lisanne Puijk[2], Jørgen Dejgaard Jensen[4], A. Jantine Schuit[2,3] and G. Ardine de Wit[2,5]

Abstract

Background: According to current physical activity guidelines, a substantial percentage of the population in high-income countries is inactive, and inactivity is an important risk factor for chronic conditions and mortality. Financial incentives may encourage people to become more active. The objective of this review was to provide insight in the effectiveness of financial incentives used for promoting physical activity in the healthcare setting.

Methods: A systematic literature search was performed in three databases: Medline, EMBASE and SciSearch. In total, 1395 papers published up until April 2015 were identified. Eleven of them were screened on in- and exclusion criteria based on the full-text publication.

Results: Three studies were included in the review. Two studies combined a financial incentive with nutrition classes or motivational interviewing. One of these provided a free membership to a sports facility and the other one provided vouchers for one episode of aerobic activities at a local leisure center or swimming pool. The third study provided a schedule for exercise sessions. None of the studies addressed the preferences of their target population with regard to financial incentives. Despite some short-term effects, neither of the studies showed significant long-term effects of the financial incentive.

Conclusions: Based on the limited number of studies and the diversity in findings, no solid conclusion can be drawn regarding the effectiveness of financial incentives on physical activity in the healthcare setting. Therefore, there is a need for more research on the effectiveness of financial incentives in changing physical activity behavior in this setting. There is possibly something to be gained by studying the preferred type and size of the financial incentive.

Keywords: Financial incentive, Physical activity, Healthcare setting, Systematic review

Background

In high-income countries, 41 % of men and 48 % of women have an inactive lifestyle, based on the World Health Organisation (WHO) Global physical activity guidelines [1, 2]. According to the WHO, physical inactivity is defined as not adhering to physical activity guidelines, thus spending less than 150 min of moderate-intensity aerobic physical activity throughout the week, or less than 75 min on vigorous-intensity aerobic physical activity throughout the week or less than an equivalent combination of moderate—and vigorous-intensity activity [2]. Physical inactivity has negative consequences for people's health, as it is the fourth leading risk factor for mortality worldwide and it increases the risk of cardiovascular diseases, obesity and diabetes [1–3]. Physical activity can reduce the risk of several

* Correspondence: Claudia.molema@rivm.nl
[1]Department of Tranzo, Scientific Center for Care and Welfare, Tilburg University, PO Box 901535000LE Tilburg, The Netherlands
[2]National Institute for Public Health and the Environment, Centre for Nutrition and Health Services, Bilthoven, The Netherlands
Full list of author information is available at the end of the article

chronic conditions, such as diabetes and cardiovascular diseases. Moreover, it is associated with more favorable outcomes in the course of disease. If people would achieve the recommended level of activity, an all-cause mortality risk reduction of almost 30 % would be possible [4]. Still, a substantial proportion of the high-income population is insufficiently active. It is therefore important to find ways to improve physical activity levels, particularly among those who are the least active. However, behavior such as physical activity is complex and therefore difficult to change, implying a serious challenge concerning program adherence and maintaining results after program completion [5, 6].

One setting from which physical activity programs are initiated is the healthcare setting. Many people with (a high risk of) a chronic disease are already within the healthcare setting for treatment of their condition. For these people being physically active to a sufficient extent may be important to prevent a deterioration of their condition. At the same time, healthcare providers can play an important role in motivating patients to participate in a physical activity program [7]. However, research shows that long-term adherence varies greatly between 10 % and 80 % in therapeutic exercise interventions for diabetes patients [8]. There are many reasons that people find it difficult to adhere to exercise schemes, one of which is motivation One of many ways to address motivation is to include financial incentives in the intervention.

Financial incentives provide economic encouragement for people to show desired behavior, such as increasing their physical activity level [9]. Incentives can be either positive or negative. Positive incentives reward individuals either for participation or for when they fulfill the desired outcome of certain health behavior. Negative incentives or disincentives penalize individuals if they do not participate, or if they do not meet the required outcomes established [10].

Financial incentives have the potential to affect both participation rates and program adherence [11, 12]. An important point to address however when studying and discussing effectiveness of financial incentives on behavioral change, is the general notion that a financial incentive constitutes an external motivation for changing behavior. According to the health promotion literature, people need skills and knowledge (intrinsic motivation) to change their lifestyle behavior and simply giving them a financial incentive is not expected to teach them these skills [10, 13, 14]. Building intrinsic motivation takes time and needs work, but financial incentives may help, for instance to increase program adherence to an intervention that teaches these skills and knowledge. Financial incentives can be provided on many levels in healthcare, for example incentives for insurers to promote the financing of exercise programs, for healthcare providers to incorporate physical activity in treatment and rehabilitation, for employers to establish training facilities at work places, or for patients to participate. The providers of the incentives also vary, depending on the healthcare system in a country. Incentives can be provided by the government, insurers, employers or non-profit organizations. The government may have an interest in this, if the benefits to society and/or the government budget (in terms of potential for saved healthcare spending in the long run) exceed the cost of providing the incentive. Similar rationales may apply for insurer—and employer-financed incentive schemes.

Hypotheses on the effectiveness of direct financial incentives to improve physical activity levels vary. One opinion is that offering rewards may be counterproductive in the sense that this extrinsic motivation may crowd out the intrinsic motivation already present. Therefore any increase in physical activity during the time of the intervention, as well as part of the activity level present before the intervention started, will disappear after the incentives are removed [15–17]. A competing hypothesis states that getting people interested in physical activity by giving financial incentives may very well contribute to habit formation. This theory assumes that if exercising is a form of habitual behavior, giving financial incentives to motivate people to exercise for a certain period, may increase future utility from exercising [15, 18]. Previous studies on the effect of financial incentives to change relatively simple health-related behaviors, such as attending appointments at clinics and take up of child immunization, indicate that financial incentives are effective [10, 15]. Systematic reviews on effectiveness of financial incentives to increase physical activity showed positive results in both community- and school setting, particularly in the short term [11, 12]. No such systematic review has been carried out for the healthcare setting. The objective of this study was to systematically review the literature with respect to the effectiveness of direct financial incentives used to promote physical activity in the healthcare setting.

Methods

Data sources

A systematic literature search was conducted, using three literature databases (Medline, EMBASE and SciSearch) to find eligible studies on the effect of financial incentives to promote physical activity within a healthcare setting. A combination of search terms covering the healthcare setting (e.g. primary care, delivery of healthcare), financial incentives (e.g. financial support, access and price) and physical activity (e.g.

leisure center, active transport) was used to identify all relevant articles (see Appendix 1 for the full search strategy). The search was restricted to publications in English and Dutch and included publications up until April 2015.

Inclusion and exclusion criteria

The primary inclusion criterion was that the paper under consideration had to address physical activity promotion initiated from or within the healthcare setting, including the use of one or more direct financial incentives given to patients. Included studies had to use a prospective design to be able to measure differences over time in individuals and at group level, and provide one or more study arms in which the financial incentive was the exclusive factor, while the goal was to increase people's physical activity. Effectiveness had to be studied quantitatively in terms of physical activity outcome measures or weight loss. Reviews, editorials and other papers not describing individual studies were excluded. Figure 1 shows the flowchart that contains all exclusion criteria. If one of the criteria was not met, we scored this item a '1'. The criteria were scored in a fixed order; if a criterion was scored a '1', assessment of further criteria became redundant.

Study selection

Publications were selected using a standardized process. Four reviewers (LP, WV, CM and AW) worked in pairs. The first reviewer (LP, CM or WV) selected eligible papers by checking the title against

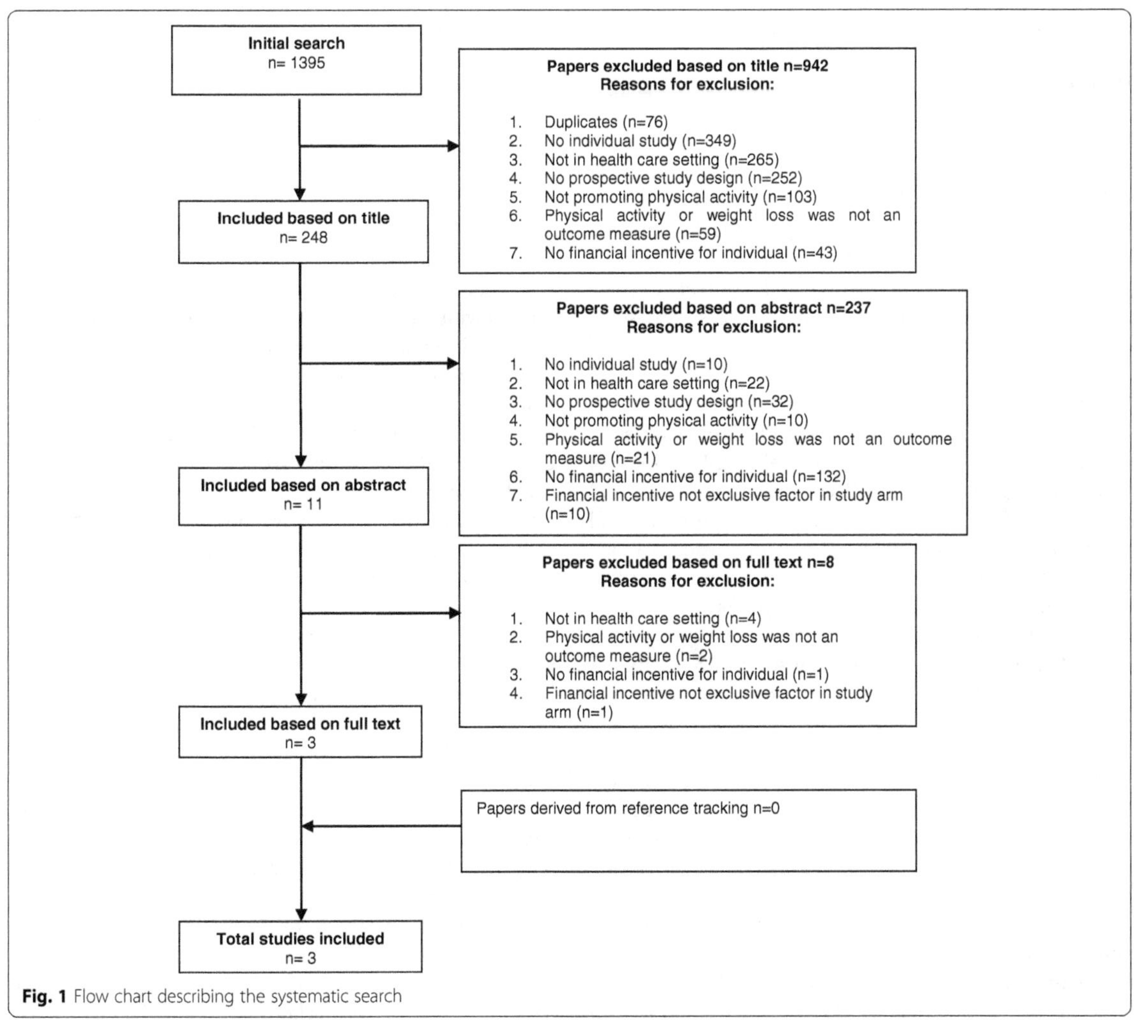

Fig. 1 Flow chart describing the systematic search

the in- and exclusion criteria and if necessary the process was repeated for the abstract. Another reviewer checked whether the exclusion of the paper by the first reviewer was correct. Any disagreement between reviewers was resolved by consensus. References from the selected full text publications based on their abstract ($n = 11$) were searched for more eligible publications, but did not result in the inclusion of additional publications to be included. Duplicate studies were removed. The process of study selection and reasons for excluding studies are shown in Fig. 1.

Data extraction

Information was extracted about the first author, year of publication, the setting in which the study was conducted, the study population, description of the intervention and the given incentive, and relevant outcome measures and quantitative results. Table 1 provides a structured overview of the characteristics of the studies included in this review.

Results

Search

In total 1395 papers were found of which 76 papers were duplicates. Based on title and abstract, 1308 publications were excluded. Eleven full-text papers were selected and scored according to the in- and exclusion criteria individually by two reviewers. Finally, three papers, describing randomized controlled trials (RCT) were included (Fig. 1). These studies are summarized in Table 1.

Study populations, designs and settings

All three included studies describe a RCT. Harland et al. evaluated the effectiveness of several combinations of methods to promote physical activity using brief (one) or extended (six) motivational interviews and a financial incentive for PA promotion (30 vouchers each for one episode of aerobic activities at a local leisure center or swimming pool). This study was performed in the United Kingdom in the primary care setting and involved the local leisure center. In total, 523 adults between 40 and 64 years old were recruited from one urban general practice in a socioeconomically disadvantaged region of Newcastle.

The study of Duggins et al. was designed to address the question, of whether eliminating financial barriers to physically activity leads to weight loss. This study was performed in the USA in the primary care setting in combination with the local Young Men's Cristian Association (YMCA). In total, 83 children between 5 and 17 years old were recruited in two family medicine clinics and a specialized pediatrics clinic. Patients were eligible if they had a BMI at or above the 85th percentile for age and sex, and the socioeconomic status of the participants varied widely. In the study, participating families were randomized in an intervention group and a control group. Both groups received nutrition advice through four nutrition classes, and to promote physical activity the intervention group received a financial incentive (family membership of the local YMCA). The materials were available in English and Spanish in order to also include Spanish-speaking families.

The study of Islam evaluates a financial incentive in a physical activity program for 22 women of at least 18 years old, who have used cocaine regularly in their lives. The study was performed at Rubcion, a non-profit organization for substance abuse in the USA. Women were eligible if they were approved for 60 days of residential treatment at Rubicon and received medical clearance from the physician to participate. Both groups had an exercise schedule of three weekly sessions for a period of six weeks. In addition, the intervention group had an incentive scheme. If they met their targets in their exercise schedule, participants were allowed to draw tokens from a prize gym bag.

Financial incentives

All three studies have combined a financial incentive with some other technique, such as motivational interviewing, education or exercise sessions. However, these additional techniques were provided to the individuals in both the intervention group and the control group. As studies were only included in this review when the financial incentive was the only difference between study groups, any effect observed can be assigned to the financial incentive. The incentives in the included studies diverge in their characteristics, such as the value they represent, the requirements to receive the incentive and the moment of handing out the incentive.

Both the studies of Harland et al. and Duggins et al. chose an incentive that is linked to physical activity. The study of Islam chose an incentive in the form of simply a compliment or presents of different values, such as toiletries, jewelry or a digital camera. The higher the value of the incentive, the lower the chance they could grab that prize from the prize gym bag. The study of Islam set requirements in such a way that the participants were only allowed to grab a prize from the prize gym bag if they met their target of 30 min of observed treadmill walking. Some additional prizes could be earned if their adherence to the program was high. In contrast with the study of Islam, the studies of Harland et al. and Duggins et al.

Table 1 Characteristics and outcomes of the reviewed studies

Author, year	Setting	Study design & study population	Intervention	Outcome measures	Results
Harland et al., 1999 [20]	GP practice in a socio-economically disadvantaged area.	RCT 523 adults aged 40–64 years: C: $n = 105$ I1: $n = 105$ I2: $n = 106$ I3: $n = 104$ I4: $n = 103$	C • Baseline body measurements and information about PA. I1 • Baseline body measurements and information about PA. • Brief motivational interviewing ($n = 1$) during 12 weeks intervention period. I2 • Baseline body measurements and information about PA. • Brief motivational interviewing (n = 1) during 12 weeks intervention period. • 30 vouchers, each for one episode of aerobic activities, at local leisure center or swimming-pool. I3 • Baseline body measurements and information about PA. • Extended motivational interviewing (n = 6) during 12 weeks intervention period. I4 • Baseline body measurements and information about PA. • Extended motivational interviewing (n = 6) during 12 weeks intervention period. • 30 vouchers, each for one episode of aerobic activities, at local leisure center or swimming pool.	• Self-reported physical activity (shortened version of the National Fitness Survey questionnaire).	12 weeks: • No significant effect on PA was found due to the introduction of vouchers or more than one interview. • Significant interaction between providing vouchers and more than one interview: the highest proportion of participants with increased physical activity scores was in the group offered both multiple interviews and vouchers. • Proportion of participants with an improvement on vigorous activity or moderate activity was significantly higher for all intervention groups combined compared to the control group. • No significant effect within the intervention groups due to interviews, vouchers or interactions between them for vigorous or moderate activity. 12 months: • Increases in PA reported at 12 weeks by participants in all intervention groups were not maintained at one year, regardless of the intensity of the intervention.
Duggins et al., 2010 [19]	Family Medicine Clinics and specialized Pediatrics clinics with patients that represented a wide variety of socioeconomic backgrounds.	RCT 83 children aged 5–17 years, with BMI at or above the 85th percentile for age and sex: C: $n = 39$ I: $n = 44$	C • 4 dietician-led nutrition classes (over a 9 months period), discussing diet, nutrition, eating habits and meal planning. In addition, written materials (handbook) were provided. I • 4 dietician-led nutrition classes (over a 9 months period), discussing diet, nutrition, eating habits and meal planning. In addition, written materials (handbook) were provided. • Free 1-year family membership to local YMCA, providing access to all activities, such	• Year change in BMI-for-age percentile and weight loss	12 months: • No significant differences between groups were found in BMI or change in weight. • The relationship between the number of visits to the YMCA and the loss of either BMI or weight was positive, but very small and not statistically significant.

Table 1 Characteristics and outcomes of the reviewed studies *(Continued)*

			as swimming, water aerobics, a track for walking or jogging and weights in a variety of sizes. Patients were asked to complete a diary of activities and were reinforced by study staff.		
Islam, 2013 [21]	Rubicon Centre, a facility that provides residential care facility that provides treatment for women with substance abuse disorder	RCT 22 women aged at least 18 years old, who have used cocaine regularly in her lifetime, be approved for 60 days of residential treatment at Rubicon and received medical clearance from the physician to participate: C: $n = 10$ I: $n = 12$	C • Three core exercise sessions scheduled weekly for six weeks, with the opportunity to engage in additional exercise. I • Three core exercise sessions scheduled weekly for six weeks, with the opportunity to engage in additional exercise. • Participants had the opportunity to draw tokens from a prize gym bag if they met the target of 30 min of observed treadmill walking at any intensity. Every time a participant completed the 30 min at a level, she received an escalating number of prize draws. Escalation resumed from baseline (two draws) until the participant completed three consecutive sessions that met the completion of 30 min of exercise criteria. At that time, the number of draws returned to the level achieved prior to reset. Participants received bonus draws if they completed moderate exercise up to 3 times a week.	• Compliance • Anthropometric measurements (BMI and WHR) • Attitudes about exercise (ECS,EBBS and IPAQ-S) • Physical activity levels	6 weeks: • No significant differences were found in minutes spent in exercise sessions, number of completed scheduled 30-min exercise sessions, number of consecutive exercise sessions. • No differences over time were found for both intervention- and control group in BMI and WHR. • No differences over time were found for both intervention- and control group on patients' attitudes about exercise and in the perception of individuals concerning the benefits of and participating in exercise. • No differences over time were found between intervention- and control group in physical activity levels

Abbreviations used: *BMI* Body Mass Index; *C* control group; *EBBS* Exercise Benefits/Barriers Scale; *ECS* Exercise Confidence Scale; *GP* general practitioner; *I* intervention group; *IPAQ-S* International Physical Activity Questionnaire – Short; *PA* physical activity; *RCT* Randomized Controlled Trial; *YMCA* Young Men's Christian Association; *WHR* Waist-to-hip ratio

did not have requirements that the participants had to meet before they received the incentive.

The studies of Harland et al. and Duggins et al. did not report that the content of the financial incentive was matched with the preferences of the target group. The study of Islam surveyed the participants beforehand and during the intervention to identify which prizes were preferred and whether they were still incentivizing during the intervention. They did not report that they surveyed the preferences for other characteristics, such as the moment of handing out and the requirements for receiving the incentive.

Study outcomes

Harland et al. evaluated the effectiveness of several combinations of methods to promote physical activity. Data were collected at baseline, at 12 weeks, and after one year. After 12 weeks of intervention, significantly more participants in the intervention group had improved physical activity scores compared to the control group (38 % vs. 16 %, $p = 0.001$). A significant interaction was found between the two intervention conditions (interviews and vouchers) with the greatest effect in the group offered both vouchers and extended interviewing. In general, this pattern was also found when focusing on only vigorous and moderate physical activity. Comparing the matching groups with regard to the number of motivational interviews, no statistically significant effects were found for providing vouchers as a financial incentive as opposed to not providing this incentive. Moreover, effects found at 12 weeks were not maintained one year after the intervention, regardless of the intensity of the intervention. However, the use of vouchers was higher (44 % versus 27 %) among the group that received the intensive intervention (vouchers + six interviews) than in the group that received the brief intervention (vouchers + one interview).

In the study of Duggins no differences in Body Mass Index (BMI) or weight change were seen between the intervention and control group after the one-year intervention period. In the intervention group, the relationship between the number of visits to the YMCA and the loss of either BMI or weight was positive, but very small and not statistically significant.

After the six week intervention period, the study of Islam reported no significant changes over time in both groups for attitude and perception on benefits of participating in exercise, physical activity levels, compliance, BMI, and Waist Hip Ratio (WHR).

Discussion

The objective of this systematic review was to provide an insight in the effectiveness of financial incentives used for physical activity promotion in the healthcare setting. The search revealed only three eligible studies (two RCTs among adults and one among children) that specifically studied the effect of a financial incentive on improving physical activity measured by physical activity outcomes or weight loss [19–21]. Two of the three studies combined a financial incentive with other methods, such as motivational interviewing or nutrition classes [19, 20]. Despite short-term differences between intervention groups in one study, no differences were found between the control and intervention group over a longer period of time (12 months) in these studies [19, 20]. The study of Islam measured only short term effects and found almost no significant improvements in the intervention group [21]. The included studies do not indicate that financial incentives stimulate physical activity in the healthcare setting.

Two studies included in this review found no long-term effects of the financial incentive. The third study did not measure long-term effects, but did not find important effects in the short term [21]. Harland et al. found some short-term effects. Possibly, the duration and/or intensity of intervention activities in these studies were not enough to alter behavior, since effects regardless of the incentive were small or absent. A well-known physical activity intervention strategy in the healthcare setting is exercise on prescription, which is usually integrated into multidisciplinary combined lifestyle interventions. Such programs tend to include physical activity promotion, improvement of diet, and reduction of psychological barriers using motivational interviewing [22]. Two studies included in this review did not consist of a strong and structured physical activity component, which might have caused participants to focus on other aspects of the intervention than actually becoming physically active [19, 20]. The study of Islam had a structured physical activity component, but the duration was just six weeks [21].

Although the effectiveness of financial incentives on increasing physical activity levels and accomplishing weight loss was generally absent in our review, in other settings, such as the community setting, at least short term effects of financial incentives on physical activity behavior were found [11, 12]. The review of Mantzari et al. has evaluated the effect of financial incentives on health-related behavior, which includes for example healthier eating, physical activity, and smoking cessation. In this review it is also acknowledged that effects are not sustained when the incentive is removed [23].

In all three studies included in our systematic review, a motivation was lacking as to why this particular incentive was chosen for the particular population. It is likely that preferences for a certain type of financial incentive differ between target groups. For example, women may be more risk adverse than men so a financial incentive in the form of a lottery might not be as effective for men as for women [24]. If the specific type of incentive does not fit the preferences of the target population, this may partially explain the lack of its effect on behavior. There is research available that elucidates the importance of some attributes of financial incentives. A broader scoped review on the effectiveness of financial incentives on physical activity showed that for an incentive to be effective it should at least be conditional to the targets set in the intervention [25]. Promberger et al. [26] have performed a discrete choice experiment on the acceptability of financial incentives to change health related behavior. They have found that a preference for the type of incentive for smoking cessation is different than the preferred incentive for weight loss [26]. Moreover, the size of the incentive matters [10] and includes an optimum [27]. Therefore, one important recommendation would be to study preferences of the target group to determine a suitable financial incentive before designing and implementing a study.

In a recently published review of reviews the effectiveness of physical activity promotion interventions in the primary care are shown. These interventions seem to have small positive effects [28]. Combining a lifestyle intervention with a financial incentive that is preferred by the target population, might increase the effects on physical activity levels of the individuals. Future research should focus on the most effective combination of the lifestyle intervention and the preferred financial incentive of the target population.

Theoretically, the benefits of the investment in a financial incentive returns to the provider of the incentive, for example in the form of decreased use of healthcare. In national health systems such as in the UK, the provider of the incentive in the healthcare setting is automatically the collector of the benefits. In managed competition systems, insurers might be the provider of incentives with the underlying principle of return on investment, but also gain a competitive advantage in a market with many healthcare insurance providers. It should be acknowledged that financial incentives in the healthcare systems of developing countries might be a bridge too far. The theory of return on investment is a concept that might function as well in healthcare as in the work setting. A review shows that giving incentives in the work setting to employees by providing free wellness programs, and sometimes incentives to increase participation, returns in less healthcare expenditures and less costs for absenteeism [29]. As mentioned before, the present systematic review includes only three studies. We believe however that this is a true reflection of the level of knowledge, despite the fact that the use of financial incentives is fairly common. For example, during many physical activity interventions, participants can freely access sports and/or leisure accommodations or they receive a small reward for participating in the intervention [30, 31]. However only a few studies explicitly address the effectiveness of the incentive given in a separate arm of the study, as was one of the inclusion criteria in our study. There were some studies excluded from the review that stated as their aim to evaluate the effect of changing physical activity behavior by giving financial incentives. A closer look at the study methods revealed that this statement could not be justified because of different reasons. These suboptimal study designs prevented drawing definite conclusions on the effectiveness of financial incentives on physical activity behavior, because for example the effect of the financial incentive could not be distinguished from the other components of the study or the study did not have a control group [24, 30–32].

We decided not to perform a quality check for the included studies. With a yield of only three very diverse interventions addressing the effect of financial incentives on physical activity our review, although systematic in nature, may be characterized as explorative rather than thoroughly addressing the effectiveness of financial incentives in promoting physical activity from the healthcare setting.

One could argue that extending our search with other databases such as EconLit, Psychlit and Sportsdiscus might have increased the yield of the review. However, if we would have missed a key publication, we would have expected it to be found through reference tracking of the studies already included. The limited set of appropriate study designs is confirmed in other systematic reviews. Two other systematic reviews evaluating the effect of financial incentives on physical activity irrespective of the setting included as few as 10 and 11 studies [11, 12]. Moreover, most of the studies included in these reviews defined 'attendance' as the incentivized behavior instead of behavioral change. This could also partly explain why few studies are found to be effective in actually changing physical activity behavior. Perhaps incentives may only offer the particular behavior that has been incentivized.

Conclusion

Few studies have evaluated the effect of a financial incentive on changing physical activity behavior in the healthcare setting. The three studies included in this systematic review did not show effects that could be attributed to the incentive used. However, study designs were not particularly strong and there seems to have been little thought given to whether or not particular incentives suit particular study populations. Nevertheless, based on results in other settings, financial incentives seem promising instruments to increase people's physical activity.

It is recommended that in future research on the effectiveness of financial incentives on physical activity some basic requirements are met. First, the study protocol should include intervention arms in such a way that effectiveness of incentives can be studied. Second, it is recommended to first study the preferences of the target population with regard to financial incentives to maximize the chance that the incentive will indeed help to increase the intended behavior. Assuming that the control condition will include a program aiming to increase physical activity, it is recommended to consider multidisciplinary combined lifestyle interventions in order to maximize the chance of habit formation and long-term maintenance of behavioral change.

Appendix 1

Table 2 Full search strategy

1	(incentive* or reward* or voucher or free access or lottery or lotteries or voucher*1 or prize* or monetary support or financial support or financial assist* or cost sharing or medical fees or subsidy or subsidies or cash payment* or contingent payment* or bonus* or loan* or credit* or member* or financing or disincentive* or penalty or penalties).tw.
2	financial support/or financing, organized/or financing, government/ or cost sharing/or fees, medical/or "fees and charges"/or public assistance/
3	(access or participation rate* or "frequency of participation" or sustained participation or increased participation or repeated participation or attendance or (complet* adj3 program) or referral uptake or "used the prescription" or "uptake rate*" or (received adj3 pedometer*) or offered or half price).tw.
4	exercise therapy/ut or "referral and consultation"/ut or counseling/ ut or health promotion/ut or health services/ut
5	1 or 2 or 3 or 4
6	(intervention* or program*1 or project*1 or pilot*1 or policy or policies or trial* or increas* or campaign or sustain* or encourag* or motivat* or promot* or improv* or counsel?ing or participation or health facilit*).ti.
7	intervention studies/or health promotion/or health plan implementation/or healthy people programs/or national health programs/or government programs/or program development/or program evaluation/or pilot projects/or exp clincial trials/or counseling/or health facilities/or exercise therapy/or motivation/
8	(excercise referral* or referral program* or exercise program* or excercise promotion or exercise advice*).tw.
9	6 or 7 or 8
10	(physical activit* or exercise or aerobics or aerobic capacit* or aerobic class* or aerobic activ* or physical exert* or moderate activ* or vigorous activ* or sport* or fitness or "keep fit" or gymnas* or gym or walking or walk or running or run or jogging or jog or cycle or cycling or bicycl* or bike*1 or biking or swimming or swim or swims or dancing or gardening or stair*1).ti.
11	(aqua* or yoga* or pilates* or rollerblad* or rollerskat* or skate or skates or skating).ti. or (leisure centre* or leisure center*).tw.
12	(active travel* or active transport* or active commut* or multimodal transportation or alternative transport* or alternative travel* or pedestrianis* or pedestrianiz).ti.
13	motor activity/or exp exercise/or exercise therapy/or exp sports/ or fitness centers/or walking/or running/or jogging/or bicycling/ or swimming/or dancing/or gardening/or "physical education and training"/or gymnastics/or physical fitness/
14	10 or 11 or 12 or 13
15	9 and 14
16	(health care or health care or primary care or primary health care or preventive care or preventive medicine or health promotion or integrated care or behavi?r therap* or referral scheme* or hospital* or physician* or nurse* or nursing or general practi* or gp or family practi* or doctors or public health).tw.
17	delivery of health care/or delivery of health care, integrated/or primary health care/or preventive medicine/or preventive health services/or primary prevention/or behavior therapy/or hospitals/or physicians/or physicians, family/or physicians, primary care/or family practice/or general practice/or general practitioners/or nursing/or nurses/or "referral and consultation"/or public health/
18	16 or 17
19	5 and 15 and 18
20	(employee* or worker* or work or job or jobs or occupational or school* or pupils or student* or athletes or athletic* or sports medicine or wounds or injuries or injury or incontinence or pregnancy or pregnant or pain or cancer).tw. or injuries.fs.
21	work/or occupational health/or occupational health services/or occupational health physicians/or employee incentive plans/or schools health services/or schools/or students/or student health services/or athletes/or athletic performance/or sports medicine/or exp "wounds and injuries"/or urinary inconticence/or exp pregnancy/or rehabilitation/or exp pain/or pain management/or exp neoplasms/or sports/px
22	19 not (20 or 21)
23	22 and (english or dutch).lg.
24	remove duplicates from 23

Abbreviations

BMI, body mass index; C, control group; EBBS, exercise benefits/barriers scale; ECS, exercise confidence scale; GP, general practitioner; I, intervention group; IPAQ-S, international physical activity questionnaire – short; PA, physical activity; RCT, randomized controlled Trial; YMCA, young men's christian association; WHO, World Health Organisation; WHR, waist-to-hip ratio

Funding

This research was supported by ZonMw. ZonMw is the Dutch national organisation for health research and healthcare innovation.

Authors' contributions

JS, AW, WV and JJ made substantial contributions to the design of the review. CM, WV, AW, and LP have performed the selection of the studies eligible for the review. CM has written the main part of the manuscript. All authors critically reviewed the manuscript and read and approved the final manuscript.

Competing interests

The authors declare that they have no competing interests.

Consent for publication

Not applicable.

Ethics approval and consent to participate

Not applicable.

Author details

[1]Department of Tranzo, Scientific Center for Care and Welfare, Tilburg University, PO Box 901535000LE Tilburg, The Netherlands. [2]National Institute for Public Health and the Environment, Centre for Nutrition and Health Services, Bilthoven, The Netherlands. [3]Institute of Resource Economics and Food Policy, University of Copenhagen, Copenhagen, Denmark. [4]Department of Health Science, VU University, Amsterdam, The Netherlands. [5]Julius Center for Health Sciences and Primary Care, University Medical Center Utrecht, Utrecht, The Netherlands.

References

1. World Health Organisation. Noncommunicable Diseases - Country profiles. 2011.
2. World Health Organisation. Global Recommendations on Physical Activity for Health. 2010.

3. World Health Organisation. Physical activity. Factsheet N°385. World Health Organisation; 2014. http://www.who.int/mediacentre/factsheets/fs385/en/.
4. Physical Activity Guidelines Advisory Committee. Physical activity guidelines advisory committee report, 2008. Washington: U.S. Department of Health and Human Services; 2008.
5. Pettee Gabriel KK, Morrow Jr JR, Woolsey AL. Framework for physical activity as a complex and multidimensional behavior. J Phys Act Health. 2012;9 Suppl 1:S11–8.
6. Trost SG, Owen N, Bauman AE, Sallis JF, Brown W. Correlates of adults' participation in physical activity: review and update. Med Sci Sports Exerc. 2002;34(12):1996–2001. doi:10.1249/01.MSS.0000038974.76900.92.
7. Estabrooks PA, Glasgow RE, Dzewaltowski DA. Physical activity promotion through primary care. JAMA. 2003;289(22):2913–6. doi:10.1001/jama.289.22.2913.
8. Praet SF, van Loon LJ. Exercise therapy in type 2 diabetes. Acta Diabetol. 2009;46(4):263–78. doi:10.1007/s00592-009-0129-0.
9. Flodgren G, Eccles M, Shepperd S, Scott A, Parmelli E, Beyer F. An overview of reviews evaluating the effectiveness of financial incentives in changing healthcare professional behaviours and patient outcomes (Review). The Cochrane Library. 2011;7:CD009255.
10. Jochelson K. Paying the Patient; improving health using financial incentives: King's fund. 2007.
11. Mitchell MS, Goodman JM, Alter DA, John LK, Oh PI, Pakosh MT, et al. Financial incentives for exercise adherence in adults: systematic review and meta-analysis. Am J Prev Med. 2013;45(5):658–67. doi:10.1016/j.amepre.2013.06.017.
12. Strohacker K, Galarraga O, Williams DM. The impact of incentives on exercise behavior: a systematic review of randomized controlled trials. Annals BehavMed. 2014;48(1):92–9. doi:10.1007/s12160-013-9577-4.
13. Alm-Roijer C, Stagmo M, Uden G, Erhardt L. Better knowledge improves adherence to lifestyle changes and medication in patients with coronary heart disease. Eur J Cardiovascular Nursing. 2004;3(4):321–30. doi:10.1016/j.ejcnurse.2004.05.002.
14. Whittemore R. Strategies to facilitate lifestyle change associated with diabetes mellitus. J Nursing Scholarship. 2000;32(3):225–32.
15. Charness G, Gneezy U. Incentives to exercise. Econometrica. 2009;77(3):909–31.
16. Gneezy U, Rustichini A. Pay Enough or Don't Pay at All. Quarterly J Economics. 2000;115(3):791–810. doi:10.1162/003355300554917.
17. Gneezy U, Rustichini A. A fine is a price. J Leg Stud. 2000;29(1 PART I):1.
18. Becker GS, Murphy KM. A theory of rational addiction. J Political Economy. 1988;96(4):675–700.
19. Duggins M, Cherven P, Carrithers J, Messamore J, Harvey A. Impact of family YMCA membership on childhood obesity: a randomized controlled effectiveness trial. J Am Board Fam Med. 2010;23(3):323–33. doi:10.3122/jabfm.2010.03.080266.
20. Harland J, White M, Drinkwater C, Chinn D, Farr L, Howel D. The Newcastle exercise project: a randomised controlled trial of methods to promote physical activity in primary care. BMJ. 1999;319:828–32.
21. Islam L. Using Behavioral Incentives to Promote Exercise Compliance in Women with Cocaine Dependence. 2013. p. 3231. VCU Theses and DIssertations.
22. Berendsen BA, Hendriks MR, Verhagen EA, Schaper NC, Kremers SP, Savelberg HH. Effectiveness and cost-effectiveness of 'BeweegKuur', a combined lifestyle intervention in the Netherlands: rationale, design and methods of a randomized controlled trial. BMC Public Health. 2011;11:815. doi:10.1186/1471-2458-11-815.
23. Mantzari E, Vogt F, Shemilt I, Wei Y, Higgins JP, Marteau TM. Personal financial incentives for changing habitual health-related behaviors: A systematic review and meta-analysis. Prev Med. 2015;75:75–85. doi:10.1016/j.ypmed.2015.03.001.
24. Croson R, Gneezy U. Gender differences in preferences. J Econ Lit. 2009; 47(2):448–74. doi:10.1257/jel.47.2.448.
25. Barte JC, Wendel-Vos GC. A Systematic Review of Financial Incentives for Physical Activity: The Effects on Physical Activity and Related Outcomes. Behav Med. 2015. doi:10.1080/08964289.2015.1074880.
26. Promberger M, Brown RC, Ashcroft RE, Marteau TM. Acceptability of financial incentives to improve health outcomes in UK and US samples. J Med Ethics. 2011;37(11):682–7. doi:10.1136/jme.2010.039347.
27. Wanders JO, Veldwijk J, de Wit GA, Hart HE, van Gils PF, Lambooij MS. The effect of out-of-pocket costs and financial rewards in a discrete choice experiment: an application to lifestyle programs. BMC Public Health. 2014; 14:870. doi:10.1186/1471-2458-14-870.
28. Sanchez A, Bully P, Martinez C, Grandes G. Effectiveness of physical activity promotion interventions in primary care: A review of reviews. Prev Med. 2015;76(Suppl):S56–67. doi:10.1016/j.ypmed.2014.09.012.
29. Baicker K, Cutler D, Song Z. Workplace wellness programs can generate savings. Health Aff (Millwood). 2010;29(2):304–11. doi:10.1377/hlthaff.2009.0626.
30. Finkelstein EA, Brown DS, Brown DR, Buchner DM. A randomized study of financial incentives to increase physical activity among sedentary older adults. Prev Med. 2008;47(2):182–7. doi:10.1016/j.ypmed.2008.05.002.
31. Jeffery RW, Wing RR, Thorson C, Burton LR. Use of Personal Trainers and Financial Incentives to Increase Exercise in a Behavioral Weight-Loss Program. J Consult Clin Psychol. 1998;66(5):777–83.
32. Jeffery RW, French SA. Preventing weight gain in adults: the pound of prevention study. Am J Public Health. 1999;89(5):747–51.

Permissions

All chapters in this book were first published in BSSMR, by BioMed Central; hereby published with permission under the Creative Commons Attribution License or equivalent. Every chapter published in this book has been scrutinized by our experts. Their significance has been extensively debated. The topics covered herein carry significant findings which will fuel the growth of the discipline. They may even be implemented as practical applications or may be referred to as a beginning point for another development.

The contributors of this book come from diverse backgrounds, making this book a truly international effort. This book will bring forth new frontiers with its revolutionizing research information and detailed analysis of the nascent developments around the world.

We would like to thank all the contributing authors for lending their expertise to make the book truly unique. They have played a crucial role in the development of this book. Without their invaluable contributions this book wouldn't have been possible. They have made vital efforts to compile up to date information on the varied aspects of this subject to make this book a valuable addition to the collection of many professionals and students.

This book was conceptualized with the vision of imparting up-to-date information and advanced data in this field. To ensure the same, a matchless editorial board was set up. Every individual on the board went through rigorous rounds of assessment to prove their worth. After which they invested a large part of their time researching and compiling the most relevant data for our readers.

The editorial board has been involved in producing this book since its inception. They have spent rigorous hours researching and exploring the diverse topics which have resulted in the successful publishing of this book. They have passed on their knowledge of decades through this book. To expedite this challenging task, the publisher supported the team at every step. A small team of assistant editors was also appointed to further simplify the editing procedure and attain best results for the readers.

Apart from the editorial board, the designing team has also invested a significant amount of their time in understanding the subject and creating the most relevant covers. They scrutinized every image to scout for the most suitable representation of the subject and create an appropriate cover for the book.

The publishing team has been an ardent support to the editorial, designing and production team. Their endless efforts to recruit the best for this project, has resulted in the accomplishment of this book. They are a veteran in the field of academics and their pool of knowledge is as vast as their experience in printing. Their expertise and guidance has proved useful at every step. Their uncompromising quality standards have made this book an exceptional effort. Their encouragement from time to time has been an inspiration for everyone.

The publisher and the editorial board hope that this book will prove to be a valuable piece of knowledge for researchers, students, practitioners and scholars across the globe.

List of Contributors

Mathias Wolfrum
Institute of General Practice and for Health Services Research, University of Zurich, Zurich, Switzerland
Cardiovascular Center Cardiology, University Hospital Zürich, Zürich, Switzerland

Christoph Alexander Rüst and Thomas Rosemann
Institute of General Practice and for Health Services Research, University of Zurich, Zurich, Switzerland

Romuald Lepers
INSERM U1093, Faculty of Sport Sciences, University of Burgundy, Dijon, France

Beat Knechtle
Institute of General Practice and for Health Services Research, University of Zurich, Zurich, Switzerland
Gesundheitszentrum St. Gallen, Vadianstrasse 26, 9001 St. Gallen, Switzerland

Jeffrey A. Brown
School of Kinesiology and Health Science, York University, 357 Bethune College, 4700 Keele Street, Toronto M3J 1P3ON, Canada

Marc Dalecki
School of Kinesiology and Health Science, York University, 357 Bethune College, 4700 Keele Street, Toronto M3J 1P3ON, Canada
Centre for Vision Research, York University, Toronto, Canada

Cindy Hughes and Alison K. Macpherson
School of Kinesiology and Health Science, York University, 357 Bethune College, 4700 Keele Street, Toronto M3J 1P3ON, Canada
York University Sport Medicine Team, York University, Toronto, Canada

Lauren E. Sergio
School of Kinesiology and Health Science, York University, 357 Bethune College, 4700 Keele Street, Toronto M3J 1P3ON, Canada
Centre for Vision Research, York University, Toronto, Canada
York University Sport Medicine Team, York University, Toronto, Canada
Southlake Regional Health Centre, Newmarket, ON, Canada

David C Nieman and Mary Pat Meaney
Appalachian State University, Human Performance Lab, North Carolina Research Campus, 600 Laureate Way, Kannapolis, NC 28081, USA

R Andrew Shanely and Kevin A Zwetsloot
Department of Health and Exercise Science, Appalachian State University, Boone, NC, USA

Gerald E Farris
Department of Emergency Medicine, Carolinas Medical Center NorthEast, Concord, NC, USA

Ellen L de Hollander
National Institute for Public Health and the Environment, Centre for Nutrition, Prevention and Health Services, PO Box 1, 3720 BA Bilthoven, Netherlands

Eline Scheepers and Albertine J Schuit
National Institute for Public Health and the Environment, Centre for Nutrition, Prevention and Health Services, PO Box 1, 3720 BA Bilthoven, Netherlands
Department of Health Sciences and EMGO institute for Health and Care Research, VU University Amsterdam, De Boelelaan 1085, 1081 HV Amsterdam, Netherlands

Harm J van Wijnen and Elise EMM van Kempen
National Institute for Public Health and the Environment, Centre for Sustainability, Environment and Health, PO Box 1, 3720 BA Bilthoven, Netherlands

Pieter JV van Wesemael
Department of the Built Environment, Technical University Eindhoven, PO Box 513, 5600 MB Eindhoven, Netherlands

Wanda Wendel-Vos
Department of Health Sciences and EMGO institute for Health and Care Research, VU University Amsterdam, De Boelelaan 1085, 1081 HV Amsterdam, Netherlands

Patricia Olaya-Contreras
Department of Orthopedics, Institute of Clinical Sciences at the Sahlgrenska Academy, University of Gothenburg, Gothenburg, Sweden
Department of Postgraduate Studies, Faculty of Nursing, University of Antioquia, Calle 70 No 52-21, Apartado Aereo, 1226 Medellín, Antioquia, Colombia
Unit for Health Promotion Research, University of Southern Denmark, Esbjerg, Denmark

Jorma Styf, Karin Frennered and Tommy Hansson
Department of Orthopedics, Institute of Clinical Sciences at the Sahlgrenska Academy, University of Gothenburg, Gothenburg, Sweden

Daniel Arvidsson
Unit of Clinical Physiology and Nuclear Medicine, Department of Translational Medicine, Lund University, Malmö, Sweden
RICH/EXE, Institute of Sports Science and Clinical Biomechanics, University of Southern Denmark, Odense, Denmark

Gøran Paulsen
Department of Physical Performance, Norwegian School of Sport Sciences, Oslo, Norway
Norwegian Olympic Sport Center, Oslo, Norway

Kristoffer T Cumming, Håvard Hamarsland and Truls Raastad
Department of Physical Performance, Norwegian School of Sport Sciences, Oslo, Norway

Elisabet Børsheim
University of Arkansas for Medical Sciences, Arkansas Children's Nutrition Center, Arkansas Children's Hospital Research Institute, Little Rock, Arkansas, USA

Sveinung Berntsen
Department of Public Health, Sport and Nutrition, Faculty of Health and Sport Sciences, University of Agder, Kristiansand, Norway

James E. Gaida
University of Canberra Research Institute for Sport and Exercise (UCRISE), Canberra, Australia
Discipline of Physiotherapy, University of Canberra, ACT 2601 Canberra, Australia
Department of Surgical and Perioperative Sciences, Sports Medicine, Umeå University, Umeå, Sweden
Department of Integrative Medical Biology, Anatomy Section, Umeå University, Umeå, Sweden

Håkan Alfredson
Department of Community Medicine and Rehabilitation, Umeå University, S-901 87 Umeå, Sweden
Institute of Sport Exercise and Health, University College Hospital London, London, UK

Sture Forsgren
Department of Integrative Medical Biology, Anatomy Section, Umeå University, Umeå, Sweden

Jill L. Cook
La Trobe University Sport and Exercise Medicine Research Centre, Melbourne, Australia

Ali E. Wolpern, Dara J. Burgos, Jeffrey M. and Lance C. Dalleck
Recreation, Exercise, and Sport Science Department, Western State Colorado University, 600 N. Adams St., Gunnison, CO 81230, USA

Janot
Department of Kinesiology, University of Wisconsin - Eau Claire, 105 Garfield Ave, PO Box 4004, Eau Claire, WI 54702, USA

Jarle Stålesen, Frøydis Nordgård Vik and Sveinung Berntsen
Department of Public Health, Sport and Nutrition, Faculty of Health and Sport Sciences, University of Agder, P.O. Box 422, NO-4604 Kristiansand, Norway

Bjørge Herman Hansen
Department of Sports Medicine, Norwegian School of Sport Sciences, Oslo, Norway

Henny Solleveld and Arnold Goedhart
SportsInjuryLab, Box 3141, 3760 DC Soest, The Netherlands

Luc Vanden Bossche
Physical Rehabilitation and Sports Medicine, Ghent University Hospital, De Pintelaan 185, 9000 Ghent, Belgium

Dennis Caine
Department of Kinesiology and Public Health Education, University of North Dakota, Grand Forks, ND, USA

Laura Purcell
Department of Pediatrics, David Braley Sport Medicine and Rehabilitation Centre, McMaster University, Hamilton, ON, Canada

Nicola Maffulli
Sports and Exercise Medicine, Queen Mary University of London, Barts and The London School of Medicine and Dentistry, William Harvey Research Institute, Centre for Sports and Exercise Medicine, Mile End Hospital, 275 Bancroft Road, London E1 4DG, UK

K. W. Douma, C. P. van der Schans
Research and Innovation Group in Healthy Aging, Allied Health Care and Nursing, Hanze University of Applied Sciences Groningen, Groningen, The Netherlands
Department of Rehabilitation Medicine, University of Groningen, University Medical Center Groningen, Groningen, The Netherlands

G. R. H. Regterschot
University of Groningen, University Medical Center Groningen Center for Human Movement Sciences Groningen, Groningen, The Netherlands

W.P. Krijnen
Research and Innovation Group in Healthy Aging, Allied Health Care and Nursing, Hanze University of Applied Sciences Groningen, Groningen, The Netherlands

G. E. C. Slager
School of Health Care Studies Hanze University of Applied Science Groningen, Groningen, The Netherlands

W. Zijlstra
Institute of Movement and Sport Gerontology, German Sport University, Cologne, Germany

Brendan Marshall, Chris Richter and Shane Gore
Sports Medicine Department, Sports Surgery Clinic, Santry Demesne, Dublin, Ireland
School of Health and Human Performance, Dublin City University, Dublin, Ireland
Insight Centre for Data Analytics, Dublin City University, Dublin, Ireland

Andrew Franklyn-Miller
Sports Medicine Department, Sports Surgery Clinic, Santry Demesne, Dublin, Ireland
Centre for Health, Exercise and Sports Medicine, University of Melbourne, Melbourne, Australia

Kieran Moran
School of Health and Human Performance, Dublin City University, Dublin, Ireland
Insight Centre for Data Analytics, Dublin City University, Dublin, Ireland

Enda King
Sports Medicine Department, Sports Surgery Clinic, Santry Demesne, Dublin, Ireland

Siobhán Strike
Department of Life Sciences, Roehampton University, London, UK

Éanna Falvey
Sports Medicine Department, Sports Surgery Clinic, Santry Demesne, Dublin, Ireland
Department of Medicine, University College Cork, Cork, Ireland
Centre for Health, Exercise and Sports Medicine, University of Melbourne, Melbourne, Australia

Armin Kibele and Claudia Classen
Institute for Sports and Sport Science, University of Kassel, Damaschkestr. 25, Kassel 34121, Germany

Thomas Muehlbauer and Urs Granacher
Division of Training and Movement Science, University of Potsdam, Potsdam, Germany

David G Behm
School of Human Kinetics and Recreation, Memorial University of Newfoundland, St. John's, Newfoundland, Canada

Thea J. M. Kooiman, Wim P. Krijnen and Cees P. van der Schans
Research group Healthy ageing, Allied health care and Nursing, Hanze University of Applied Sciences, Groningen, The Netherlands

Manon L. Dontje
CBO Groningen: Center for Physical Activity and Research, Groningen, The Netherlands
Quantified Self Institute, Hanze University of Applied Sciences, Groningen, The Netherlands

Siska R. Sprenger
CBO Groningen: Center for Physical Activity and Research, Groningen, The Netherlands

Martijn de Groot
Research group Healthy ageing, Allied health care and Nursing, Hanze University of Applied Sciences, Groningen, The Netherlands
Quantified Self Institute, Hanze University of Applied Sciences, Groningen, The Netherlands

Andrew John Greene
Postgraduate Medical Institute, Faculty of Medical Science, Anglia Ruskin University, Chelmsford, UK
Discipline of Exercise and Sport Science, Faculty of Health Science, The University of Sydney, Sydney, Australia

Max Christian Stuelcken
School of Health and Sport Sciences, Faculty of Science, Health, Education and Engineering, University of the Sunshine Coast, Queensland, Australia

Richard Murray Smith
Discipline of Exercise and Sport Science, Faculty of Health Science, The University of Sydney, Sydney, Australia

Benedicte Vanwanseele
Department of Kinesiology, KU Leuven, Leuven, Belgium
Chair of Health Innovation and Technology, Fontys University of Applied Sciences, Eindhoven, Netherlands

Rochelle M. Eime, Jack T. Harvey and Melanie J. Charity
Institute of Sport, Exercise and Active Living, Victoria University, PO Box 14428, Melbourne, Victoria 8001, Australia
School of Health Sciences and Psychology, Federation University, Ballarat, Australia

Meghan M. Casey
School of Health Sciences and Psychology, Federation University, Ballarat, Australia

Hans Westerbeek and Warren R. Payne
Institute of Sport, Exercise and Active Living, Victoria University, PO Box 14428, Melbourne, Victoria 8001, Australia

Mohamed Chedly Jlid and Mohamed Souheil Chelly
Research Unit of Sport Performance and Health, Higher Institute of Sport and Physical Education of Ksar Said, Tunis, Tunisia

Nicola Maffulli
Department of Musculoskeletal Disorders, Faculty of Medicine and Surgery, University of Salerno, 84081 Baronissi, Salerno, Italy
Centre for Sports and Exercise Medicine, Mile End Hospital, Barts and The London School of Medicine and Dentistry, London, UK

Nisar Souissi
Unité de Recherche Evaluation, Sport, Santé, Centre National de Médecine et Science en Sport, Tunis, Tunisie

Thierry Paillard
Laboratoire Activité Physique, Performance et Santé (EA 4445), Université de Pau et des Pays de l'Adour, Département STAPS, ZA Bastillac Sud, 65000 Tarbes, France

Laurent Ballaz and Martin Lemay
Department of kinanthropology, Université du Québec à Montréal, Montreal, Qc, Canada
Research & Engineering Chair Applied to Pediatrics (RECAP), Marie Enfant Rehabilitation Centre (CRME) - Research Center - Sainte-Justine UHC, and École Polytechnique de Montréal, Montreal, Qc, Canada

Maxime Raison
Department of mechanical engineering, École Polytechnique de Montréal, Montreal, Qc, Canada
Research & Engineering Chair Applied to Pediatrics (RECAP), Marie Enfant Rehabilitation Centre
(CRME) - Research Center - Sainte-Justine UHC, and École Polytechnique de Montréal, Montreal, Qc, Canada
CRME - Research Center, Office GR-123, 5200, East Bélanger Street, H1T 1C9 Montréal, QC, Canada

Christine Detrembleur
Institute of NeuroSciences (IoNS), Université catholique de Louvain, Bruxelles, Belgium

Guillaume Gaudet
Department of mechanical engineering, École Polytechnique de Montréal, Montreal, Qc, Canada
Research & Engineering Chair Applied to Pediatrics (RECAP), Marie Enfant Rehabilitation Centre (CRME) - Research Center - Sainte-Justine UHC, and École Polytechnique de Montréal, Montreal, Qc, Canada

Karianne Vassbakk-Brovold
Oncologic Department, Southern Hospital Trust, Postbox 416, 4604 Kristiansand, Norway
Department of Health and Sport Science, University of Agder, Postbox 422, 4604 Kristiansand, Norway

Christian Kersten and Svein Mjåland
Oncologic Department, Southern Hospital Trust, Postbox 416, 4604 Kristiansand, Norway

Liv Fegran
Oncologic Department, Southern Hospital Trust, Postbox 416, 4604 Kristiansand, Norway
Department of Health and Nursing Science, University of Agder, Postbox 4224604 Kristiansand, Norway

Odd Mjåland
Surgical Department, Southern Hospital Trust, Postbox 4164604 Kristiansand, Norway

Stephen Seiler and Sveinung Berntsen
Department of Health and Sport Science, University of Agder, Postbox 422, 4604 Kristiansand, Norway

Marília Santos Andrade, Fabiana de Carvalho Koffes and Antonio Carlos da Silva
Departamento de Fisiologia, Universidade Federal de São Paulo (UNIFESP), Rua Botucatu, 862, 5° andar, Vila Clementino, São Paulo, SP CEP: 04023-062, Brazil

Ana Amélia Benedito-Silva
Escola de Artes, Ciências e Humanidades, Universidade de São Paulo (USP), Av. Arlindo Béttio, 1000, Ermelino Matarazzo, São Paulo, SP CEP: 03828-000, Brazil

Claudio Andre Barbosa de Lira
Setor de Fisiologia Humana e do Exercício, Faculdade de Educação Física e Dança, Universidade Federal de Goiás (UFG), Avenida Esperança s/n, Campus Samambaia, Goiânia, GO CEP: 74690-900, Brazil

Runar Unhjem
Department of Circulation and Medical imaging, Faculty of Medicine, the Norwegian University of Science and Technology, Prinsesse Kristinas gt. 3, 7006 Trondheim, Norway

Grete Flemmen
Department of Circulation and Medical imaging, Faculty of Medicine, the Norwegian University of Science and Technology, Prinsesse Kristinas gt. 3, 7006 Trondheim, Norway
Department of Research and Development, Clinic of Substance Use and Addiction Medicine, St. Olav University Hospital, Trondheim, Norway

Jan Hoff
Department of Circulation and Medical imaging, Faculty of Medicine, the Norwegian University of Science and Technology, Prinsesse Kristinas gt. 3, 7006 Trondheim, Norway
Department of Physical Medicine and Rehabilitation, St. Olav University Hospital, Trondheim, Norway

Eivind Wang
Department of Circulation and Medical imaging, Faculty of Medicine, the Norwegian University of Science and Technology, Prinsesse Kristinas gt. 3, 7006 Trondheim, Norway
Division of Psychiatry, Department of Østmarka, St. Olav University Hospital, Trondheim, Norway
Department of Internal Medicine, University of Utah, Salt Lake City, Utah, USA

Claudia C. M. Molema
Department of Tranzo, Scientific Center for Care and Welfare, Tilburg University, PO Box 901535000LE Tilburg, The Netherlands
National Institute for Public Health and the Environment, Centre for Nutrition and Health Services, Bilthoven, The Netherlands

G. C. Wanda Wendel-Vos and Lisanne Puijk
National Institute for Public Health and the Environment, Centre for Nutrition and Health Services, Bilthoven, The Netherlands

Jørgen Dejgaard Jensen
Department of Health Science, VU University, Amsterdam, The Netherlands

A. Jantine Schuit
National Institute for Public Health and the Environment, Centre for Nutrition and Health Services, Bilthoven, The Netherlands
Institute of Resource Economics and Food Policy, University of Copenhagen, Copenhagen, Denmark

G. Ardine de Wit
National Institute for Public Health and the Environment, Centre for Nutrition and Health Services, Bilthoven, The Netherlands
Julius Center for Health Sciences and Primary Care, University Medical Center Utrecht, Utrecht, The Netherlands

Index

A

Accelerometer, 68, 85-86, 90, 147, 153, 155, 191, 193, 197, 199

Achilles Tendinopathy, 66-68, 71-75

Active Advice, 45-47, 49-53

Active Transportation, 34

Activity Trackers, 145-155

Acute Low Back Pain (albp), 45

Adolescent Athlete, 101, 103, 105, 107

Age Profiles, 166-171, 173, 175

Anterior Cruciate Ligament (acl) Tear, 99

Antioxidants, 54-55, 58, 61-62, 64-65

B

Balance Training, 134-135, 142, 144, 182

Ball Throwing Velocity, 200-201, 203-205

Biomarkers, 66-67, 69-71, 73-75, 215

Biomechanical Symmetry, 121-123, 125, 127, 129, 131, 133

Biomechanics, 13, 52, 120, 123, 133, 156-157, 165, 181-182, 190, 206

Bland-altman Plots, 145, 147, 149-153, 193, 195

Breaststroke Swimming, 2-3, 5, 7, 9, 11, 13

C

Cancer Patients, 191-193, 195-199

Cardiorespiratory Fitness, 76-77, 82-84

Cardiovascular Disease, 53, 76-77, 84, 207, 213, 216

Chemotherapy, 191-193, 195-199

Cognitive-motor Integration, 15-17, 19, 21, 23-25

Concussion, 15-17, 19-25, 99-100, 102-108

Cyclic Flexion-extension, 183, 185, 187, 189

Cytokines, 61, 66-67, 69, 71-73, 75, 92, 95, 98

D

Data Analysis Techniques, 121, 132

Dental Plaque, 91-92, 98

Dominant Versus Non-dominant, 121, 131

Dynamic Tasks, 121-123, 125-127, 129, 131, 133

E

Exercise Intensity, 76-77, 79-81, 83-84, 199, 202

Exercise Prescription, 76-77, 79-80

External Ankle Support, 156-157, 159, 161, 163-165

F

Financial Incentive, 217-220, 222-224

Free-living, 53, 145-155, 198

Freestyle Swimming, 1-3, 5-6, 8-9, 11, 13-14

G

Gender Difference, 1, 13

Gingival Diseases, 91

H

Healthcare Setting, 217-219, 221, 223-225

I

Inclinometer, 85-86, 88

Indirect Calorimetry, 85-86, 89, 154

Instability Resistance Training, 134-135, 143

Inter-limb Symmetry, 122, 126, 132

Internal Valgus Moment, 156

Intraclass Correlation Coefficient (icc), 109, 145, 202

Inverse Dynamics, 183-185, 190

Isokinetic Dynamometer, 200-201

Isometric Quadriceps, 109, 111, 113, 115, 117, 119

J

Joint Torque Variability, 183-185, 187, 189

K

Kinematic Solidification, 183

Knee Joint Loading, 156, 163

L

Limits of Agreement (loa), 109, 113

Lower Limb, 13, 67, 101, 133, 154, 156-157, 159, 161-165, 177, 180-181, 206

M

Metastability, 134-135, 137, 139, 141-143
Mild Traumatic Brain Injury, 15, 25, 107
Movement Control, 15-16, 23, 122, 130, 179
Muscle Biopsy, 27-29, 31, 33
Muscle Glycogen, 27-33
Muscle Mass, 54, 57, 59-61, 180
Muscle Strength, 54, 109-111, 113-115, 117-120, 177, 180, 183, 189, 199-201, 204-208, 211, 213-216
Musculoskeletal Pain, 66, 98

N

Neuromuscular Performance, 144, 176-177, 179-181

O

Oncology, 191-192, 198
Oral Health, 91-98

P

Pedometer Step Count, 45
Physeal Injury, 99-100, 105, 107
Physical Activity (pa), 34-35, 166, 191-192
Postural Control, 176-181
Pre-pubertal Males, 176-177, 179, 181
Prediction Model, 15
Primary Prevention, 76, 83, 225
Protocol Paper, 54
Psychosocial Factors, 47, 91-92

R

Rate of Force Development, 135, 207-208, 212, 215-216
Repeatability, 183-189
Route Features, 34-41, 43

S

Sedentary Time, 85-90
Sex-related Difference, 1, 6, 9, 11-13
Shoulder Strength, 200, 204-206
Side Step Cutting, 156-157, 160, 162-164
Skeletal Muscle, 27, 29, 31-33, 64-65, 70, 75, 119
Sport Participants, 166-167, 169-173, 175
Sport Performing Nation, 166
Sports Injuries, 91-92, 97, 99-100, 105
Sprint Running, 176-177, 181-182
Strength Training, 55, 57, 59, 61-65, 70, 75, 120, 135, 143-144, 206-209, 211-216
Stretch-shortening Cycle, 134-135, 137, 139
Substance Use Disorder (sud), 207
Supplementation, 33, 54-55, 57, 59, 61-65
Swimming Speed, 1-3, 5-8, 12-13

T

Taekwondo, 176-177, 179, 181-182
Test-retest Reliability, 109-110, 114, 120, 123-124, 145-148, 155, 190, 202
Three Activity Monitors, 85-89
Threshold-based Model, 76-77, 79, 81, 83
Traffic Safety, 34, 36, 40, 42-43
Transport Choice, 34-44
Tumor Necrosis Factor Alpha, 66

U

Ultrasonic Assessment, 29, 31, 33
Unstable Surfaces, 134-135, 137, 139, 141-143

V

Validation Study, 27, 145, 191-193, 196-197
Vastus Lateralis, 27-28, 30-32, 60-61
Vertical Jump, 106, 135, 144, 176-178, 180-182

www.ingramcontent.com/pod-product-compliance
Lightning Source LLC
Chambersburg PA
CBHW061939190326
41458CB00009B/2784

* 9 7 8 1 6 3 2 3 9 8 7 9 6 *